ENDOVASCULAR AND OPEN VASCULAR RECONSTRUCTION

A Practical Approach

ENDOVASCULAR AND OPEN VASCULAR RECONSTRUCTION

A Practical Approach

Edited by

Sachinder Singh Hans, MD, FACS

Medical Director Vascular and Endovascular Services, Henry Ford Macomb Hospital, Clinton TWP, MI, USA
Chief of Vascular Surgery, St. John Macomb Hospital, Warren, MI, USA
Clinical Assistant Professor of Surgery, Wayne State University School of Medicine, Detroit, MI, USA

Alexander D Shepard, MD, FACS

Senior Staff Surgeon, Division of Vascular Surgery
Betty Jane and Alfred J. Fisher Chair in Vascular Surgery, Henry Ford Hospital, Detroit, MI, USA
Professor of Surgery, Wayne State University School of Medicine, Detroit, MI, USA

and

Mitchell R Weaver, MD, FACS

Senior Staff Surgeon, Henry Ford Hospital, Detroit, MI
Clinical Assistant Professor of Surgery
Wayne State University School of Medicine, Detroit, MI

Paul G Bove, MD, FACS

Vascular Surgeon, William Beaumont Hospital, Royal Oak, MI, USA
Associate Professor of Surgery
Oakland University William Beaumont School of Medicine, Royal Oak, MI, USA

Graham W Long, MD, FACS

Vascular Surgeon, Medical Director, Surgical Clinical Trials Office
William Beaumont Hospital, Royal Oak, MI, USA
Associate Professor of Surgery
Oakland University William Beaumont School of Medicine, Royal Oak, MI, USA

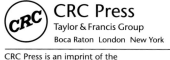

CRC Press
Taylor & Francis Group
Boca Raton London New York

CRC Press is an imprint of the
Taylor & Francis Group, an **informa** business

CRC Press
Taylor & Francis Group
6000 Broken Sound Parkway NW, Suite 300
Boca Raton, FL 33487-2742

© 2018 by Taylor & Francis Group, LLC
CRC Press is an imprint of Taylor & Francis Group, an Informa business

No claim to original U.S. Government works

Printed and bound in India by Replika Press Pvt. Ltd.

Printed on acid-free paper

International Standard Book Number-13: 978-1-4987-6055-3 (Pack – Book and eBook)

Library of Congress Cataloging-in-Publication Data

Names: Hans, S. S. (Sachinder Singh), editor. | Weaver, Mitchell R., editor. | Bove, Paul G., editor. | Long, Graham W., editor.
Title: Endovascular and open vascular reconstruction : a practical approach / [edited by] Sachinder Singh Hans,
    Mitchell R. Weaver, Paul G. Bove, Graham W. Long.
Description: Boca Raton : CRC Press, 2017. | Includes bibliographical references. |
    Description based on print version record and CIP data provided by publisher; resource not viewed.
Identifiers: LCCN 2017005996 (print) | LCCN 2017005021 (ebook) | ISBN 9781498760652 (eBook VitalSource) |
    ISBN 9781498760560 (eBook PDF) | ISBN 9781498760553 (hardback bundle : alk. paper).
Subjects: | MESH: Endovascular Procedures | Vascular Surgical Procedures | Reconstructive Surgical Procedures.
Classification: LCC RD598.5 (print) | LCC RD598.5 (ebook) | NLM WG 170 | DDC 617.4/13--dc23
LC record available at https://lccn.loc.gov/2017005996

Visit the Taylor & Francis Web site at
http://www.taylorandfrancis.com

and the CRC Press Web site at
http://www.crcpress.com

Contents

SECTION II: OPEN VASCULAR RECONSTRUCTIONS

SECTION III: ENDOVASCULAR AND OPEN VENOUS RECONSTRUCTIONS

Foreword

Dr. Hans and colleagues are to be congratulated on this excellent text. The editors and contributors are thoughtful, scholarly, and highly experienced vascular surgeons. I have an abiding respect for them as physicians. They have a wealth of clinical experience in treating vascular disorders. Their emphasis is to describe state-of-the-art vascular surgical practice. The text respects the basic sciences that underlie contemporary practice and acknowledges the well-documented epidemiology and natural history of common vascular clinical presentations.

This text is focused on optimal clinical practice. It is concise, has tightly written chapters, uses appropriate illustrative case examples, and is intelligently illustrated.

Detailed and nuanced descriptions of the technical steps in both routine and complex, nonroutine cases are provided. The description of how to deal with a high carotid bifurcation with skull-base carotid plaque extension, the use of hybrid open and endovascular techniques, and the advice to routinely use ultrasound guidance for vessel localization and vascular access demonstrate an experienced, knowledgeable, and safe surgical approach.

I believe this text will prove valuable to surgical trainees and established surgeons. It will become a standard addition to the library of all interested in the optimal care of the vascular patient.

Gerald B. Zelenock, MD

Preface

This book is the brainchild of the senior-most editor, who felt that vascular surgeons could benefit from a quick "how-to" reference before heading to the operating room or endovascular suite to perform a vascular procedure. Despite strongly worded admonitions that similar volumes had already been published, he persisted in his perspective that a new book focusing primarily on technique would be a valuable addition to the literature. It was also his opinion that there was enough vascular surgical expertise within the immediate geographic area that we did not need to reach beyond contributors with a southeast Michigan connection. Designed as a quick guide to the techniques of contemporary vascular surgery, this book is the result and early reviewers have strongly confirmed that the senior-most editor was correct in both of his opinions!

We focused specifically on the technical steps involved in standard vascular procedures and avoided discussions of disease presentation, diagnosis, and alternative surgical therapy. Each chapter is written by a surgeon expert in the performance of the prescribed procedure, whether an acknowledged academic leader or a well-respected community surgeon. The technical tips outlined in these chapters have been gained from a lifetime of case experiences and lessons sometimes learned the hard way. Illustrations and figures have been carefully chosen to highlight these tips and maximize teaching points. Case vignettes accompany many chapters to contextualize the described procedures.

It was felt that this book should focus on both endovascular and open reconstructions, as both types of procedures are still very much a part of routine vascular practice. While open surgery is being increasingly supplanted by endovascular approaches, the former will never completely disappear. Even the most ardent of endovascular adherents must understand and occasionally use open surgery techniques. In addition, newer practitioners of vascular surgery may find their exposure to some open surgery methods so limited that a few tips from an accomplished senior practitioner would be most welcome before undertaking such an operation.

We are grateful to the many contributors to this book who gave unselfishly of their time and energies to bring it to life. From the outset, we endeavored to tap into the vascular surgery strength of the Midwest and especially the State of Michigan, home to several premier vascular programs. Many of the authors were drawn from the Henry Ford Hospital Program, established in 1976 by the late Dr. D. Emerick Szilagyi, and we are particularly indebted to his legacy. We also need to thank Miranda Bromage and Cherry Allen of CRC Press for seeing the value of this project and providing the time, support, and energy to see it through from concept to publication. The Editors wish to acknowledge the remarkable work of editing by Kate Nardoni and Sonia ST Cutler. They kept the editing process at a fast pace in order to meet the time deadlines.

Finally, we want to thank our wives Mona, Karen, Jeanne, Kristen, and Randi for allowing us the time away from family to complete this project. We need to specifically acknowledge the special contributions of Dr. Mona Hans to this book. In providing sage advice to both the senior editor and the other members of the editorial board, she has had a hand in this book since day 1. By opening up her house (and kitchen) to us for our regular editorial meetings, she offered us a home away from home where colleagues became friends, and friends became family. None of this would have been as much fun without her steadfast help and support and it is only fitting that this book be dedicated to her.

For the editors,
Alexander D. Shepard, MD

Contributors

Emily Abbott DO
Surgery Resident
William Beaumont Hospital
Royal Oak, MI, USA

Jason Q. Alexander MD
Department of Vascular and Endovascular Surgery
Minneapolis Heart Institute, Abbott Northwestern Hospital
Adjunct Assistant Professor of Surgery
University of Minnesota
Minneapolis, MN, USA

Wesley R. Barnes MD
Surgery Resident
William Beaumont Hospital
Royal Oak, MI, USA

Hisham Bassiouny MD
Chief, Vascular Surgery and Endovascular Therapy
Dar Al Fouad Hospital
Giza, Egypt

Jamil Borgi MD
Division of Cardiac Surgery
Henry Ford Hospital
Detroit, MI, USA

Paul G. Bove MD
Section of Vascular Surgery
William Beaumont Hospital
Associate Professor of Surgery
Oakland University William Beaumont School of Medicine
Royal Oak, MI, USA

P.C. Balraj MD
Division of Vascular Surgery
Henry Ford Hospital
Clinical Assistant Professor of Surgery
Wayne State University
Detroit, MI, USA

Jae S. Cho MD
Salinas Valley Medical Clinic
Salinas, CA, USA

Dawn M. Coleman MD
Section of Vascular Surgery
Frankel Cardiovascular Center
Assistant Professor of Surgery
University of Michigan
Ann Arbor, MI, USA

Anthony J. Comerota MD
Director of Research, Jobst Vascular Institute
The Toledo Hospital
Toledo, OH, USA
Adjunct Professor of Surgery
University of Michigan
Ann Arbor, MI, USA

Mark F. Conrad MD
Division of Vascular and Endovascular Surgery
Massachusetts General Hospital
Associate Professor of Surgery, Harvard Medical School
Boston, MA, USA

Robert Crawford MD
Division of Vascular Surgery
Associate Professor of Surgery
University of Maryland
Baltimore, MD, USA

Robert F. Cuff MD
Assistant Professor of Surgery
Michigan State University
Department of Vascular Surgery
Spectrum Health Hospital
Grand Rapids, MI, USA

Frank M. Davis MD
Vascular Surgery Resident
Section of Vascular Surgery
University of Michigan
Ann Arbor, MI, USA

Trevor Downing MD
Interventional Radiology Fellow
University of Michigan
Ann Arbor, MI, USA

Matthew J. Eagleton MD
Department of Vascular Surgery
Associate Professor of Surgery
Cleveland Clinic Lerner School of Medicine
Cleveland Clinic
Cleveland, OH, USA

Jonathan L Eliason MD
Section of Vascular Surgery
Frankel Cardiovascular Center
Lindenauer Professor of Surgery
Associate Professor
University of Michigan
Ann Arbor, MI, USA

Danon Garrido MD
Vascular Surgery Fellow
University of Maryland
Baltimore, MD, USA

Marika Gassner DO
Surgery Resident
Henry Ford Macomb Hospital
Clinton Township, MI, USA

Lindsay Gates MD
Vascular Surgery Resident
Yale University - New Haven Hospital
New Haven, CT, USA

Todd M. Getzen MD
Department of Radiology, Henry Ford Hospital
Detroit, MI, USA

Bruce L. Gewertz MD
Surgeon-in-Chief
H & S Nichols Distinguished Chair in Surgery
Chair, Department of Surgery
Vice President, Interventional Services
Vice Dean, Academic Affairs
Cedars-Sinai Medical Center
Los Angeles, CA, USA

Derrick Green MD MBA
University of Minnesota Vascular Surgery Fellow
Minneapolis, MN, USA

Arielle Hodari-Gupta MD
Fellow Surgical Critical Care
Henry Ford Hospital
Department of Surgery
Detroit, MI, USA

G. Haddad MD
Division of Vascular Surgery
Henry Ford Hospital
Clinical Associate Professor of Surgery
Wayne State University
Detroit, MI, USA

Sachinder Singh Hans MD
Medical Director Vascular and Endovascular Services
Henry Ford Macomb Hospital
Clinton TWP, MI, USA
Chief of Vascular Surgery
St. John Macomb Hospital
Warren, MI, USA
Clinical Assistant Professor of Surgery
Wayne State University School of Medicine
Detroit, MI, USA

Rob Harriz MD
Research Assistant
Vascular Surgery
Henry Ford Hospital
Detroit, MI, USA

Karem Harth MD MHS
Assistant Professor of Surgery
Department of General Surgery
Division of Vascular Surgery and Endovascular Therapy
UH Harrington Heart & Vascular Institute
Cleveland, OH, USA

Homayoun Hashemi MD
Chief of Surgery
INOVA Fair Oaks Hospital
Fairfax, VA, USA

Mounir J. Haurani MD
Assistant Professor of Surgery
Division of Vascular Diseases and Surgery
The Ohio State University
Columbus, OH, USA

Peter K. Henke MD
Leland Ira Doan Professor of Surgery
Professor of Surgery
Section of Vascular Surgery
University of Michigan
Ann Arbor, MI, USA

Hernan Hernandez MD
University of Nebraska School of Medicine
Omaha, NE, USA

Joseph Herrmann DO
Vascular Surgery Fellow
Detroit Medical Center
Wayne State University
Detroit, MI, USA

Maen Aboul Hosn MD
Surgery Resident
Department of Vascular Surgery
University of Iowa Hospitals and Clinics
Iowa City, IA, USA

Zachary Hothem DO
Surgery Resident
William Beaumont Hospital
Royal Oak, MI, USA

Iyad N. Isseh MD
Medical Resident
Henry Ford Hospital
Detroit, MI, USA

Arjun Jayaraj MD
The RANE Center for Venous and Lymphatic Diseases,
    St. Dominic Hospital
Jackson, MS, USA

Jacob Johnson DO
Vascular Surgery Fellow
Detroit Medical Center
Wayne State University School of Medicine
Detroit, MI, USA

Loay Kabbani MD
Division of Vascular Surgery
Henry Ford Hospital
Clinical Assistant Professor of Surgery
Wayne State University of Medicine
Detroit, MI, USA

Arnoud V. Kamman MD
Department of Cardiac Surgery
Frankel Cardiovascular Center, University of Michigan
Ann Arbor, MI, USA

Joseph Karam MD
Department of Vascular and Endovascular Surgery
Minneapolis Heart Institute
Abbott Northwestern Hospital
Adjunct Assistant Professor of Surgery
University of Minnesota
Minneapolis, MN, USA

Vikram S. Kashyap MD
Chief, Division of Vascular Surgery and Endovascular
    Therapy
Professor of Surgery, Case Western Reserve University
University Hospitals Cleveland Medical Center
Cleveland, OH, USA

Neelima Katragunta MD
Department of Vascular Surgery
Clinical Assistant Professor
University of Iowa Hospitals and Clinics
Iowa City, IA, USA

Yasaman Kavousi MD
Resident, Department of Surgery
Henry Ford Hospital
Detroit, MI, USA

Elias Kfoury MD
Vascular Surgery Fellow
Baylor College of Medicine
Houston, TX, USA

Hannah Kim DO
Valley Health Vascular Surgeons
Department of Vascular Surgery
Winchester Medical Center
Winchester, VA, USA

Adriana Laser MD MPH
The Vascular Group
Albany Medical College
Albany, NY, USA

Judith C. Lin MD PhD MPH
Division of Vascular Surgery
Henry Ford Hospital
Associate Professor of Surgery
Wayne State University School of Medicine
Detroit, MI, USA

Graham W. Long MD
Vascular Surgeon, Medical Director, Surgical Clinical Trials Office
William Beaumont Hospital, Royal Oak, MI, USA
Associate Professor of Surgery
Oakland University, William Beaumont School of Medicine,
    Royal Oak, MI, USA

Rashad Majeed MD
Surgery Resident
Howard University
Washington DC, USA

M. Ashraf Mansour MD
Chair, Department of Surgery
Spectrum Health Medical Group
Professor of Surgery Michigan State University
Grand Rapids, MI, USA

Farah Mohammad MD
Surgery Resident
Henry Ford Hospital
Detroit, MI, USA

Robert G. Molnar MD
Michigan Vascular Center
Clinical Professor of Surgery
Michigan State University
Flint, MI, USA

Mark D. Morasch MD
Director and Head, Division of Vascular and Endovascular
    Surgery
Department of Cardiac, Thoracic, and Vascular Surgery
Billings Clinic
Billings, MT, USA

Dipankar Mukherjee MD
Chief of Vascular Surgery
INOVA Fairfax Hospital
Falls Church, VA, USA

Semeret T. Munie MD
Surgery Resident
Henry Ford Hospital
Detroit, MI, USA

Timothy J. Nypaver MD
Head, Division of Vascular Surgery
Szilagyi Chair in Vascular Surgery
Henry Ford Hospital
Assistant Professor of Surgery
Wayne State University
Detroit, MI, USA

William Oppat MD
Program Director Vascular Surgery
Detroit Medical Center
Wayne State University
Detroit, MI, USA

Himanshu J. Patel MD
Chief, Department of Cardiac Surgery
Frankel Cardiovascular Center
Professor of Surgery
University of Michigan
Ann Arbor, MI, USA

Iraklis I. Pipinos MD
Chief, Vascular Surgery
Nebraska and Western Iowa VA Medical Center
Professor of Surgery
University of Nebraska
Omaha, NE, USA

Sherazuddin Qureshi MD
Vascular Surgeon
Centegra Physician Care – Surgical Associates
McHenry, IL, USA

Joseph Rabin MD
Assistant Professor of Surgery
University of Maryland
Baltimore, MD, USA

Seshadri Raju MD
The RANE Center for Venous and Lymphatic Diseases,
    St. Dominic Hospital
Jackson, MS, USA

Daniel J. Reddy MD
Professor of Surgery
Wayne State University
Detroit, MI, USA

Rehan Riaz MD
Radiology Resident
Henry Ford Hospital
Detroit, MI, USA

Scott T. Robinson MD PhD
Vascular Surgery Resident
Section of Vascular Surgery
University of Michigan
Ann Arbor, MI, USA

Jeffrey R. Rubin MD
Chief, Vascular Surgery
Detroit Medical Center
Professor of Surgery
Wayne State University
Detroit, MI, USA

Rodrigo Ruiz-Gamboa MD
Vascular Fellow
Jobst Vascular Institute
The Toledo Hospital
Toledo, OH, USA

Jason Ryan MD
Vascular Surgery Fellow
Henry Ford Hospital
Detroit, MI, USA

Constantine G. Saites MD
Surgery Resident
Henry Ford Hospital
Detroit, MI, USA

Timur P. Sarac MD
Chief, Vascular Surgery
Yale-New Haven Hospital
Professor of Surgery
Yale University
New Haven, CT, USA

Rajabrata Sarkar MD PhD
Chief, Vascular Surgery
Barbara Bauer Dunlap Professor of Surgery
University of Maryland
Baltimore, MD, USA

Shahab Tour Savadkohi MD
Assistant Professor of Surgery
University of Maryland School of Medicine
College Park, MD, USA

Shruti Sevak MD
Surgery Resident
William Beaumont Hospital
Royal Oak, MI, USA

Aamir Shah MD
Cardiothoracic and Vascular Surgery
Cedars-Sinai Medical Center
Associate Professor of Surgery
Los Angeles, CA, USA

Mel J. Sharafuddin MD
Department of Vascular Surgery
Clinical Associate Professor
University of Iowa Hospitals and Clinics
Iowa City, IA, USA

Alexander D. Shepard MD
Betty Jane and Alfred J. Fisher Chair in Vascular Surgery
Henry Ford Hospital
Detroit, MI, USA
Professor of Surgery, Wayne State University
Detroit, MI, USA

Scott M. Silver MD
Section of Vascular Surgery
William Beaumont Hospital
Assistant Professor of Surgery
Oakland University William Beaumont School of Medicine
Royal Oak, MI, USA

Sunita D Srivastava MD
Department of Vascular Surgery
Cleveland Clinic
Assistant Professor of Surgery
Cleveland Clinic Lerner School of Medicine
Cleveland, OH, USA

James C. Stanley MD
Section of Vascular Surgery
Frankel Cardiovascular Center
Professor Emeritus of Surgery
University of Michigan
Ann Arbor, MI, USA

Sarah E.B. Strot DO
Vascular Surgery Resident
Spectrum Health
Michigan State University
Grand Rapids, MI, USA

Timothy M. Sullivan MD
Chair Vascular and Endovascular Surgery
Minneapolis Heart Institute
Abbott Northwestern Hospital
Adjunct Professor of Surgery
University of Minnesota
Minneapolis, MN, USA

Robert W. Thompson MD
Section of Vascular Surgery
Professor of Surgery
Radiology and Cell Biology and Physiology
Washington University
St. Louis, MO, USA

Jessica M. Titus MD
Department of Vascular and Endovascular Surgery
Minneapolis Heart Institute, Abbott Northwestern Hospital
Adjunct Assistant Professor of Surgery
University of Minnesota
Minneapolis, MN, USA

Shahab Toursavadkohi MD
Division of Vascular Surgery
University of Maryland
Baltimore, MD, USA

Maciej Uzieblo MD
Section of Vascular Surgery
William Beaumont Hospital
Assistant Professor of Surgery
Oakland University
William Beaumont School of Medicine
Royal Oak, MI, USA

Jason VonDerHaar MD
Surgery Resident
Cedars-Sinai Medical Center
Los Angeles, CA, USA

Thomas W. Wakefield MD
Chief, Section of Vascular Surgery
Stanley Professor of Vascular Surgery
Professor of Surgery
University of Michigan
Ann Arbor, MI, USA

Mitchell R. Weaver MD
Senior Staff Surgeon
Henry Ford Hospital
Detroit, MI
Clinical Assistant Professor of Surgery
Wayne State University School of Medicine
Detroit, MI

Charles A. West Jr. MD
Director of Vascular and Endovascular Surgery
Texas Health Vascular Surgical Care
Fort Worth, TX, USA

David M. Williams MD
Department of Radiology, Division of Vascular and
   Interventional Radiology
Professor of Radiology and Internal Medicine
University of Michigan
Ann Arbor, MI, USA

Bo Yang MD PhD
Department of Cardiac Surgery, Frankel Cardiovascular
   Center
Assistant Professor of Surgery
University of Michigan
Ann Arbor, MI, USA

Taehwan Yoo MD
Clinical Instructor
Department of Surgery
The Ohio State University
Columbus, OH, USA

Baraa Zuhaili MD
Vascular Surgery Fellow, Michigan Vascular Center
McLaren Regional Medical Center
Flint, MI, USA

Hannah Zwibelman MD
Vascular Surgery Resident
Spectrum Health
Grand Rapids, MI, USA

SECTION I

Endovascular Procedures

Carotid angioplasty and stenting

ROBERT G. MOLNAR AND BARAA ZUHAILI

CONTENTS

INTRODUCTION

Open carotid surgery with carotid endarterectomy (CEA) was first introduced in 1954 by Eastcott, Pickering & Rob.[1] More than two decades later, a percutaneous balloon angioplasty of a carotid artery stenosis was performed in 1977.[2] However, it was not until 1989 that a balloon-expandable stent was deployed in the carotid artery.[3,4] Balloon-expandable stents were subsequently substituted with self-expanding stents;[5] the latter has become the standard stent type used for endovascular carotid intervention. While there are several stent manufacturers with U.S. Food & Drug Administration (FDA)-approved stent systems that include both open/closed cell design and straight/tapered configurations, this chapter concentrates on the techniques required to perform the procedure safely and effectively.

Several clinical trials have assessed the safety and efficacy of carotid artery stenting (CAS).[6–11] The CREST trial (Carotid Revascularization Endarterectomy versus Stenting Trial)[12] is arguably the trial that has shaped current practice regarding CEA and carotid stenting. CREST enrolled both symptomatic and asymptomatic standard-risk patients. There was no statistical significance between the two groups in the primary composite end point of stroke, myocardial infarction (MI), or death from any cause during the periprocedural period, or ipsilateral stroke within 4 years after randomization. However, the periprocedural stroke rate was statistically more significant in the carotid stent group, and periprocedural MI was higher in the open carotid surgery group.

While it is anticipated that the ongoing CREST-2 (Carotid Revascularization and Medical Management for Asymptomatic Carotid Stenosis Trial) trial will provide additional useful data on determining for whom CAS or CEA should be considered, the current guidelines for using carotid stent have been mainly driven by the Center for Medicare and Medicaid Services (CMS) reimbursement criteria. According to the most recent reconsideration memorandum published in 2009,[13] Medicare covers percutaneous transluminal angioplasty of the carotid artery concurrent with the placement of an FDA-approved carotid stent with distal protection for the following situations:

- patients who are at high risk for CEA and who also have symptomatic carotid artery stenosis ≥70%;
- patients who are at high risk for CEA and have symptomatic carotid artery stenosis between 50 and 70%, in accordance with the Category B investigational device exemption (IDE) clinical trials regulation or in accordance with the national coverage determination (NCD) on CAS postapproval studies;
- patients who are at high risk for CEA and have asymptomatic carotid artery stenosis ≥80%, in accordance with the Category B IDE clinical trials regulation or in accordance with the NCD on CAS postapproval studies.

Currently, asymptomatic patients outside of FDA-approved clinical trials are not approved for reimbursement by the CMS. Until sufficient data is available to provide more clarity on the safety and efficacy of CAS, the role of carotid stenting is limited based on reimbursement decisions.

PROCEDURE PLANNING

When initially beginning a carotid stent program, it may be helpful to obtain a preprocedure aortic arch evaluation either with a computed tomography angiography, magnetic resonance angiography, or a diagnostic aortic arch and carotid angiogram. This is performed to assess arch anatomy (type I, II, or III) and to determine whether carotid cannulation can be performed safely and effectively. Excessive calcification, tortuosity, a severe type II or a type III aortic arch should be avoided and surgical endarterectomy performed. It is very important to note that a meticulous approach to any carotid intervention is mandatory, because the consequences of embolization or thrombosis are much more devastating than in other vascular beds treated via endovascular means. Patients can also be approached with an aortic arch and carotid arteriogram with the intent to treat, recognizing that unfavorable arch anatomy, excessive calcification, or unfavorable carotid anatomy might lead to a diagnostic study based only on the procedural findings.

Periprocedural recommendations

All patients should be counseled on expectations during the procedure and a detailed neurologic examination completed to document their baseline status. If not already on dual antiplatelet therapy, they should receive 300 mg clopidogrel if not contraindicated and should also be on aspirin therapy. The conduct of the procedure should be reviewed with the patient so they are comfortable with instructions on breathing and head positioning. The importance of not moving during image acquisition should be stressed. It is often helpful to review the instructions to be used during the procedure. Patients should be counseled in the preprocedure area. They should be informed that, for the acquisition of a few images, they are required to take a breath and hold it while keeping still. It may be helpful to have a standard verbal direction that is routinely used, such as: "Take a small breath in, blow it out, take in another small breath in and hold it—don't breathe, don't move, don't swallow, and keep very still." If they anticipate these instructions and know that their breath hold will only be approximately 10 seconds, image quality will be greatly enhanced.

Procedures

Patients are placed in a standard supine position and blood pressure (BP), electrocardiogram tracing, and pulse oximetry are monitored. Supplemental oxygen should be available and used routinely with conscious sedation. Prepare both groins to allow access to the best femoral artery for safe access. Standard angiographic equipment is used and strict attention to avoiding air embolization is critical.

Once safe femoral access is obtained, the patient is anticoagulated with either weight-based heparin, argatroban,

or an anticoagulant of choice. Activated clotting time (ACT) levels should be between 250 and 300 seconds. A pigtail catheter is inserted into the ascending aortic arch and the image intensifier is then rotated until the catheter is visualized in its widest plane. Most textbooks report using a standard 30-degree left anterior oblique view; however, occasionally the best angle may be up to 50 degrees. This becomes very important because some patients with an aortic arch that appears to be a steep type II at 30 degrees may be a type I or mild type II at a steeper angle (e.g., >30 degrees).

After the aortic arch arteriogram has been assessed and it appears the carotid intervention is going to proceed, the anticoagulation level is confirmed by ACT. The contralateral carotid is cannulated with your catheter of choice. For a standard type I aortic arch and many mild type II aortic arches, a JB-1 or Berenstein catheter is usually an excellent selection. For a type II or severely angulated origin to the aortic arch, use a Simmons 1 or Vitek catheter. It is best to have a few catheters that are used routinely, as this familiarity with the catheters allows you to develop a significant "feel" for the catheter and how it reacts with tortuosity and resistance, and how it reacts to your manipulations. In summary, the routine catheters used are the pigtail for a flush arch aortogram, a JB-1 for cannulation of most type I aortic arches, and a Simmons 1 for type II or bovine arch configurations (**Figure 1.1**). While there are many brands and shapes available for selective catheterization of the great vessels, it is most important that you identify a few as your catheters of choice to allow for a reliable response during manipulation and avoid excessive "attempts" that increase the risk of embolization.

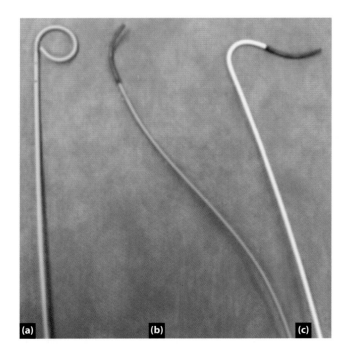

Figure 1.1 Basic diagnostic catheters. (**a**) Pigtail. (**b**) JB-1 or Berenstein. (**c**) Simmons 1.

Assuming the disease is distal to this segment, the selective catheter should be advanced to the mid-common carotid artery (CCA); anterior–posterior (AP), lateral, and oblique images should be obtained, including intracerebral runs. Pay specific attention to the AP intracranial runs to assess for cross-filling from one hemisphere to the other. Once the contralateral artery is assessed, the ipsilateral or treatment side is selected. Again, baseline AP, lateral, and oblique images are obtained to quantify and measure the degree of stenosis. Visualizing bony landmarks as to the distal extent of the lesion assists with stent positioning and deployment.

Vessel reference measurements are made and include the diameter of the mid-to-distal internal carotid artery (ICA) where filter placement would be anticipated. The CCA just proximal to the bifurcation determines the size of the stent used. Most have tended towards using 40-mm long stents in most cases to fully cover the index lesion. The stent size is chosen to be a minimum of 1-mm wider than the CCA measurement. Tapered stents have become widely used, most commonly a 6–8-mm taper by 40-mm length, but many interventionists also use straight stent configurations successfully. The distal filter size is slightly larger than the diameter of the distal ICA. If post-dilation is anticipated, a size equal to the distal ICA reference is chosen. Once all the equipment is prepared/flushed and ready for use, a short, floppy-tip Amplatz wire (1-cm floppy tip) is slowly advanced through the selective catheter and the wire tip is placed to the distal CCA. The authors routinely do not cross the bifurcation nor select the external carotid artery (ECA) to avoid crossing any diseased segment without distal protection. However, for extreme tortuosity or type II arches, selection of the ECA helps with safe sheath positioning. Maintaining fluoroscopic monitoring of the wire tip, the short femoral sheath is removed and a 90-cm sheath is slowly advanced over the Amplatz wire. As the sheath is slowly advanced while the wire tip is monitored, the sheath is placed into the CCA and the dilator is held in place as the sheath is advanced to the distal CCA. It is very important to note that the dilator for the sheath can extend beyond the sheath tip by 4–6 cm. For this reason, the authors secure the dilator and slowly advance the sheath to the distal CCA or 2 cm proximal to a lesion in the CCA.

With the sheath in place, the wire and dilator are slowly removed and the sheath is thoroughly debubbled. A Tuohy Borst valve is recommended, but a self-sealing hemostatic valve can be used. The sheath is connected to a power-assisted injector and the line is prepped and debubbled using the three-way stopcock. A manifold system can also be used, but strict adherence must be maintained to avoid air embolization. An additional magnified angiogram is obtained with attention to centering the lesion on the viewing monitor. This allows for the proximal CCA to the distal ICA to be imaged. A pre-assessment neurologic check is made by having the patient squeeze a squeaky toy or follow motor commands with assessment by cath lab staff. Under fluoroscopic guidance, the distal protection device is advanced past the lesion and positioned in the distal ICA, preferably in a straight segment. Should there be significant tortuosity in the ICA, it may be safer to approach the lesion with retrograde flow protection using the Mo.Ma® Ultra (Medtronic, Minneapolis, MN, USA) device or with the ENROUTE® transcarotid artery revascularization (TCAR) system (Silk Road Medical, Inc., Sunnyvale, CA, USA). TCAR uses a supraclavicular incision to gain access to the proximal CCA. The reverse flow system uses a femoral venous catheter that is the outflow from a CCA-placed sheath. Between the two vascular accesses is a filter system and manifold that allows for confirming brisk retrograde flow as well as halting flow for brief arteriograms. TCAR is especially advantageous in unfavorable arch anatomies and tortuous distal ICAs that make filter positioning distal to the lesion difficult or impossible. With standard transfemoral approaches, after the filter is deployed, a small amount of contrast is delivered to ensure antegrade flow through the filter and to make sure that the location of the lesion has not moved from the bony landmarks established with the placement of the filter wire. If the stenosis is severe, pre-dilation should be considered to facilitate safe stent placement and stent delivery system removal. The stent is advanced over the wire and past the lesion, then slowly brought back to the target lesion based on the bony landmarks to remove any redundancy in the system and to help prevent the stent from jumping during deployment. A small puff of contrast is administered to ensure positioning before the stent is deployed. If the stent delivery system occludes the antegrade flow, the stent can still be deployed using the bony landmarks established before the antegrade flow was lost.

After the stent has been deployed, another small puff of contrast is administered to check for antegrade flow and a neurologic test is performed. If the stent has a ≤30% residual stenosis, it is left as is. If the residual stenosis is >30%, angioplasty is performed based on the reference vessel diameter of the ICA. If angioplasty is performed, the patient can be given atropine for possible bradycardia at the interventionist's discretion. After two orthogonal views are obtained to ensure no additional intervention is required, the filter is recaptured and another neurologic test is completed. AP and lateral views, including intracranial views, are obtained to document postprocedure flow. The shuttle sheath is then withdrawn over a J-tipped wire and exchanged for a short sheath. There is no need to reselect the contralateral carotid artery for the completion arteriogram. A closure device is used as needed.

Postprocedural care

Patients are admitted for a 23-hour observation, which includes monitoring BP, evaluating the access site, and undertaking neurologic assessments. Any hypotension or hypertension should be appropriately treated and any change in the neurologic examination immediately assessed. Periprocedural strokes can occur because of late embolization through the stent struts or because of thrombus formation. Patients should be continued on dual antiplatelet medication as well as a cholesterol-lowering/stabilizing agent. Carotid duplex exams should be performed at 1, 6, and 12 months followed by yearly examinations to assess for restenosis.

CONTRAINDICATIONS AND PITFALLS TO AVOID

Aortic arch anatomy is one detail that cannot be overlooked nor its importance disregarded. Steep aortic arches in which the origins of the great vessels have shifted to a right inferior orientation to the apex of the aortic arch make cannulation and safe delivery of the stent delivery catheter difficult; it can also lead to inadvertent embolization from the aortic arch itself. The standard classification of aortic arch anatomy as it pertains to safe cannulation of the great vessel rates the complexity of the arch as type I, II, and III. In general, because the great vessels come off more proximally on the ascending aorta, the ability to traverse up the descending aorta, over the peaked aortic arch, inferiorly into the ascending aorta followed by acute angulations to the origins of the great vessels becomes more difficult. This results in additional manipulation of catheters in a potentially diseased aortic arch. While some cannulations are nearly impossible, others can be performed with excellent endovascular skills; yet, this entails accepting a significant additional embolization risk. **Figure 1.2** provides angiographic depictions of three examples of aortic arch anatomy.

Concentric calcification or severe complexity of the lesion itself (**Figure 1.3**), thrombus/near-occlusion (**Figure 1.4**), and excessive tortuosity of the distal ICA if distal filter protection is to be used (**Figure 1.5**) are all relative and, depending on severity, can be definitive contraindications to CAS.

CONCLUSIONS

In certain patient populations, CAS has been established as a safe and effective alternative to CEA. While there are patients who are at high risk for endarterectomy because of medical comorbidities or surgical exposure limitations, it is now becoming clear that there are patients who are also at high risk for CAS. Despite the exemplar credentials of the initial CREST interventionalists, nearly 12% of octogenarians enrolled in the lead-in phase of CREST suffered a stroke.[14] This early recognition that octogenarians

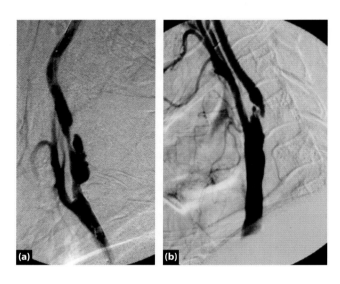

Figure 1.3 Complex lesions (**a,b**) prone to embolization with intervention.

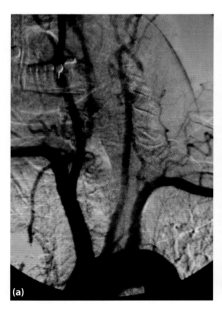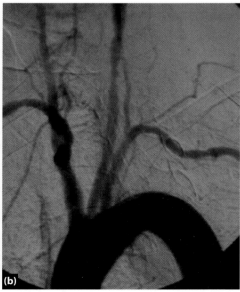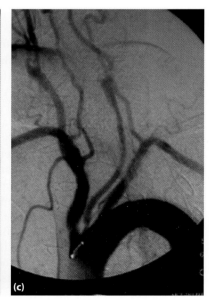

Figure 1.2 Proximal progression of the origins of the great vessels for a type I (**a**), II (**b**), and III (**c**) aortic arch.

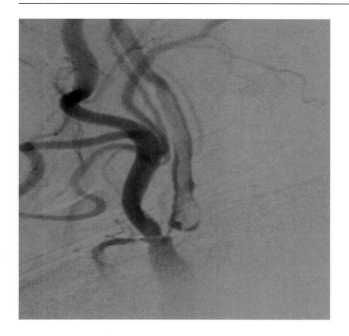

Figure 1.4 Thrombus present at severe carotid stenosis.

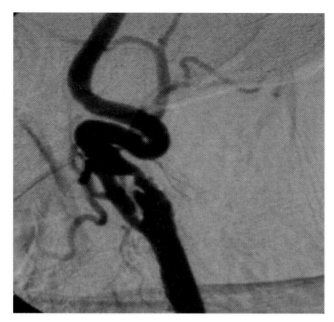

Figure 1.5 Excessive internal carotid artery tortuosity making filter placement contraindicated.

may have a higher risk of stroke with CAS has helped to define risk profiles associated with carotid interventions. The authors' recent analysis of carotid stent fractures also addressed concerns of long-term durability of stents used to treat carotid occlusive disease and points to a need for continued scrutiny of both outcomes and durability. The recent publication of 10-year follow-up data from the original CREST trial demonstrates that both CEA and CAS outcomes remain statistically equivalent.[12] It is important to continue a critical assessment of carotid stent technology to finely focus on those characteristics that create a higher risk for patients undergoing CAS and to better define who is best suited for CAS versus CEA. While this clarity is being defined, it is of critical importance that interventionists who either perform or wish to perform carotid interventions pay close attention to a meticulous approach to patient selection and procedural technique.

REFERENCES

1. Eastcott HH, Pickering GW, Rob CG. Reconstruction of internal carotid artery in a patient with intermittent attacks of hemiplegia. *Lancet.* 1954;**267**:994–996.
2. Mathias K. [A new catheter system for percutaneous transluminal angioplasty (PTA) of carotid artery stenosis]. [Article in German]. *Fortschr Med.* 1977;**95**:1007–1011.
3. Diethrich EB, Ndiaye M, Reid DB. Stenting in the carotid artery: initial experience in 110 patients. *J Endovasc Surg.* 1996;**3**:42–62.
4. Marks MP, Dake MD, Steinberg GK, et al. Stent placement for arterial and venous cerebrovascular disease: preliminary experience. *Radiology.* 1994;**191**:441–446.
5. Roubin GS, New G, Iyer SS, et al. Immediate and late clinical outcomes of carotid artery stenting in patients with symptomatic and asymptomatic carotid artery stenosis: a 5-year prospective analysis. *Circulation.* 2001;**103**:532–537.
6. Naylor AR, Bolia A, Abbott RJ, et al. Randomized study of carotid angioplasty and stenting versus carotid endarterectomy: a stopped trial. *J Vasc Surg.* 1998;**28**:326–334.
7. Yadav JS, Wholey MH, Kuntz RE, et al. Protected carotid-artery stenting versus endarterectomy in high-risk patients. *N Engl J Med.* 2004;**351**:1493–1501.
8. CAVATAS Investigators. Endovascular versus surgical treatment in patients with carotid stenosis in the Carotid and Vertebral Artery Transluminal Angioplasty Study (CAVATAS): a randomised trial. *Lancet.* 2001;**357**:1729–1737.
9. Ringleb PA, Allenberg J, Brückmann H, et al. 30 day results from the SPACE trial of stent-protected angioplasty versus carotid endarterectomy in symptomatic patients: a randomised non-inferiority trial. *Lancet.* 2006;**368**:1239–1247.
10. Ederle J, Dobson J, Featherstone RL, et al. Carotid artery stenting compared with endarterectomy in patients with symptomatic carotid stenosis (International Carotid Stenting Study): an interim analysis of a randomised controlled trial. *Lancet.* 2010;**375**:985–997.
11. Mas JL, Chatellier G, Beyssen B, et al. Endarterectomy versus stenting in patients with symptomatic severe carotid stenosis. *N Engl J Med.* 2006;**355**:1660–1671.
12. Brott TG, Hobson RW 2nd, Howard G, et al. Stenting versus endarterectomy for treatment of carotid-artery stenosis. *N Engl J Med.* 2010;**363**:11–23.

13. Centers for Medicare & Medicaid Services. *Decision Memo for Percutaneous Transluminal Angioplasty (PTA) of the Carotid Artery Concurrent with Stenting (CAG-00085R7).* Available from: https://tinyurl.com/k6xdfct (accessed May 11, 2017).

14. Hobson RW 2nd, Howard VJ, Roubin GS, et al. Carotid artery stenting is associated with increased complications in octogenarians: 30-day stroke and death rates in the CREST lead-in phase. *J Vasc Surg.* 2004;**40**:1106–1111.

2

Stenting for occlusive disease of the aortic arch branches

TIMOTHY M. SULLIVAN AND JESSICA M. TITUS

CONTENTS

INTRODUCTION

The branches of the aortic arch include the Brachiocephalic (Innominate) (BCA), arising from the arch and dividing into the right subclavian and right common arteries, the left common carotid artery (CCA), and the left subclavian artery (LSA). Multiple disease processes can affect these vessels including atherosclerosis, vasculitis, radiation-induced injury, dissection, and aortic aneurysmal disease. Occlusive disease due to atherosclerosis is the most common cause of symptoms requiring treatment in this region. Flow disturbance from occlusive disease may result in both ischemic and embolic sequelae presenting as arm claudication, cerebrovascular accident, vertebrobasilar insufficiency, or even myocardial ischemia in situations where the patient has had a previous internal mammary coronary artery bypass graft (CABG).

Consensus dictates that symptomatic disease warrants intervention. Criteria for intervention are not as clear for asymptomatic disease. Some recommend intervention for asymptomatic severe disease, defined as >75% stenosis in the involved vessels, if the patient has good surgical risk. However, observation for even severe lesions is reasonable while the patient remains asymptomatic, as there is a robust collateral network between the head and neck vessels. The exception to this is a patient with an existing or planned ipsilateral internal mammary CABG and severe subclavian stenosis. In this situation, the patient should be treated to avoid the potential complication of coronary subclavian steal syndrome.

PATIENT SELECTION

Options for treatment of occlusive disease of the brachiocephalic arteries include direct revascularization by endarterectomy or bypass, extra-anatomic bypass, or endovascular intervention including angioplasty or stenting. Direct revascularization has long been established as the gold standard; however, it carries a significant risk of morbidity and mortality. Extra-anatomic bypass avoids the risks associated with sternotomy but is limited as an approach to multivessel disease. Endovascular treatment has become an increasingly used approach for its low operative risk and minimal recovery time for the patient along with evidence of good patency rates.

Although peripheral vessels were being treated with balloon angioplasty as soon as 1970, treatment of the supra-aortic trunks was not performed until 1980. This is largely because of concern for cerebral embolization during intervention. However, with advances in protection devices, endovascular equipment, and physician experience, endovascular intervention in this distribution has become a viable and even attractive alternative to open surgery.

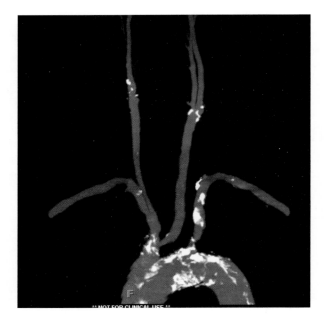

Figure 2.1 Computed tomography angiogram maximum intensity projection reconstruction demonstrating severe multivessel disease that would be best considered for open surgical treatment.

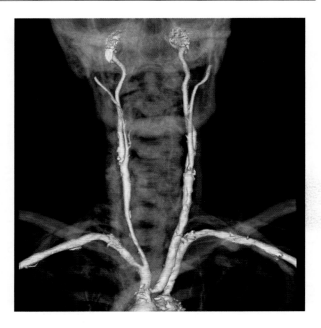

Figure 2.2 Computed tomography angiogram showing diffuse disease with a bovine arch configuration.

Selecting the best approach for the individual patient is based on a combination of lesion characteristics along with assessment of the patient's overall operative risk and medical comorbidities. Multivessel disease is best treated with direct revascularization unless patient factors preclude this method (**Figure 2.1**). Lesion characteristics that are most amenable to endovascular intervention include stenoses not involving the vessel origin. Anatomic factors that make intervention more difficult include severe vessel tortuosity in the treatment area, heavy calcification, or plaque ulceration. In these cases, consideration should be given to other approaches. During treatment of subclavian lesions, proximity to the vertebral artery makes an endovascular approach riskier in terms of posterior circulation embolization or possible coverage of the vertebral artery origin during stenting.

PREOPERATIVE PLANNING

When considering an endovascular intervention of the aortic arch branches, preoperative planning is often the most important step. A thorough evaluation of imaging, thoughtful plan for access, and embolic protection maneuvers, along with stent selection and sizing, are a necessity for successful intervention with avoidance of complications.

Imaging should be obtained both for disease diagnosis and planning of operative approach. High-quality computerized tomography angiography or magnetic resonance imaging angiography are the most used methods to evaluate aortic arch disease because they avoid the potential complications associated with manipulation of catheters within the arch and access-related complications in angiography. Three-dimensional reconstructions of these images can be extremely helpful to measure vessel size and evaluate disease severity. Both modalities also have the advantage of providing information about access vessel disease to allow planning for specific approaches. Transesophageal echocardiography can also provide information about complex aortic arch disease; however, it should not be used as the sole imaging modality for surgery planning. Important factors to consider when evaluating imaging along with the access sites are the presence of atheromatous disease in the aortic arch, lesion characteristics, and aortic arch configuration because up to 20% of people will have aberrant aortic arch anatomy, which can affect the intervention (**Figure 2.2**).

Special consideration should be given to the planning of access sites for intervention. Multiple access sites may be advantageous in different situations including total occlusions, brachiocephalic lesions, and cases where neuroprotection is planned. Access site possibilities include CCA through cutdown and femoral or brachial access by either percutaneous or open means. Additional discussion about specific access can be found later in the chapter, in the sections on specific vessel interventions.

As stated earlier, balloon angioplasty was the initial method used for Brachiocephalic (Innominate) interventions. In the 1990s, the use of stents began and it has now become the primary mode of therapy. Technical success rates have improved with this modality to as high as 96% even in cases of total occlusions. Patency rates have been shown to be excellent, with primary patency rates of 96% at 2 years and secondary patency >98% in recent studies. The use of covered stents has been described for traumatic injuries in the brachiocephalic arteries with good outcomes; however, there remains a paucity of literature regarding their use in occlusive disease. Balloon-expandable stents offer more radial force and should be used for ostial lesions; they also offer the advantage of more precise deployment. Tortuous lesions, especially when not involving the vessel origin, are better treated with self-expanding stents to prevent kinking and occlusion of the stent.

SURGICAL TECHNIQUE

General considerations

Regardless of the vessel being treated, femoral access, unless contraindicated, is usually warranted. Percutaneous femoral access is obtained with a micropuncture system; the authors recommend the use of ultrasound (US)-guided access especially when the use of larger sheaths is planned. Initially, a 5-Fr sheath can be placed and a hydrophilic wire passed into the aortic arch followed by a diagnostic, multiple sidehole flush catheter for arch aortography. The use of a straight flush catheter in the aortic arch is not recommended because it can lead to dissection with the high-pressure injections used in the aortic arch. In general, a formal arch aortogram is performed regardless of the vessel to be treated for intervention planning. This is best performed in a left anterior oblique (LAO) projection. If a marker pigtail catheter is used as the flush catheter, a good guide to assist with projection is to use the steepness of obliquity that shows even spacing between the markers. Otherwise, a 45-degree LAO will generally be enough to "open up" the aortic arch. Once the arch angiogram has been performed, if the decision is made to proceed with the intervention, ancillary access may be obtained if needed by either percutaneous brachial artery, CCA, or brachial artery cutdown. Once completed, the patient should be given heparin to obtain an activated clotting time of 250–300 seconds for intervention.

At this point, the femoral access sheath should be exchanged for a longer sheath to build a more stable system for crossing the lesion and to deploy the stent. However, if one of the ancillary access sites is planned to be the "working" access for intervention and the femoral access will be solely used for imaging, then the longer sheath is unnecessary.

Aortic arch vessel selection can usually be achieved with a simple forward-facing, minimum angle catheter, such as the angled Glide (Terumo Medical Corporation, Somerset, NJ, USA) or the vertebral (Cook Medical Inc., Bloomington, IN, USA). If cannulation can be achieved with these catheters, the simple angles will facilitate easier advancement into the vessel and exchanges. More complex aortic arch anatomy with severe degrees of angulation may require the use of increased angle catheters, such as the C2 (Cook Medical Inc.) or the JR 4 (Cordis de Mexico, S.A. de C.V., Juarez, Mexico). In even more complex cases, the use of a reverse curve catheter, such as a Simmons, may

be necessary. If it is necessary to use one of these catheters, great care should be taken with the formation of the catheter in the aortic arch and movement because catheter manipulation can cause disruption of debris in the aortic arch and lead to embolic stroke.

Once the vessel is accessed, an angiogram is performed and one can proceed with the planned intervention. Details for specific vessels are outlined later in the chapter. One other consideration regardless of the vessel involved is the relative location of other vessel origins. Aortic arches with vessel origins located very close to one another expose the other vessels to risk during the intervention of another, especially in a heavily calcified lesion. In these situations, disruption of the calcium during the intervention can cause a shift leading to compromise of the adjacent vessel origin. This should be anticipated on evaluation of the preoperative imaging or at least the arch angiogram. To protect the adjacent vessel origin, a balloon can be inflated during the intervention. This requires cannulation through an ancillary access or placement of a buddy wire through the femoral access (**Figure 2.3**). The protective balloon should not be oversized and perhaps even slightly undersized to the vessel diameter to avoid vessel dissection or injury during inflation.

LSA INTERVENTIONS

The LSA is the most frequently intervened-on vessel in the brachiocephalic distribution. Open surgery bypass has excellent outcomes but carries a higher risk of complications and even mortality. Therefore, endovascular therapy has really become the first-line consideration for treatment of subclavian artery lesions especially as patency rates have continued to improve and are now reported as >90% secondary patency at 1 and 5 years.

Once the subclavian artery has been cannulated, a hydrophilic wire such as a 0.035-inch Glidewire® (Terumo Medical Corporation), either stiff or floppy, is used to

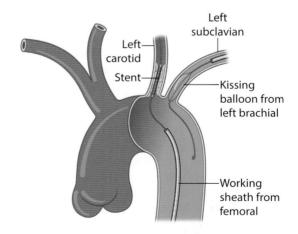

Figure 2.3 Kissing balloon technique during intervention on a left subclavian artery whose origin is very near that of the left common carotid artery. The balloon in the carotid helps to protect that origin during stenting of the subclavian lesion.

cross the lesion. If a stiff guidewire is used, it can be left in place to advance the catheter or sheath across the lesion. If a floppy guidewire was chosen, this must be exchanged for a stiffer wire, such as the stiff Glidewire® or Rosen wire (Cook Medical Inc.) for sheath advancement and intervention. The catheter must be advanced across the lesion for this exchange. In circumstances where a reverse curve catheter was used to cannulate the subclavian origin, it may be safer to exchange this catheter for a simple curve catheter (e.g., Quick-Cross Support Catheter; Spectranetics, Colorado Springs, CO, USA) because attempting to advance the reverse curve catheter over a floppy guidewire may result in loss of wire access or embolization during advancement.

Once a stiff wire and catheter have been advanced across the lesion, repeat imaging can be performed to confirm placement within the true lumen and confirm sizing for intervention. This also helps confirm the location of the vertebral artery origin before intervention. Pre-dilation should be performed at this time with a 4–6-mm balloon to ensure there is no impediment to stent advancement. The balloon should be slightly undersized to avoid injury to the artery or vertebral origin during pre-dilation; the goal is not to treat yet to gain enough lumen to advance the stent. Some interventionists want to deliver a stent in "protected" fashion, especially across occlusions or tight stenoses. In this case, the sheath would be advanced across the lesion after pre-dilation also and then pulled back after the stent has been positioned.

The stent should be sized to the vessel diameter or just slightly oversized by 1 mm, keeping in mind that balloon-expandable stents can be overdilated if needed, but realizing this will cause some foreshortening of the stent. The length of the stent should be selected to project into the aorta 1–2 mm and extend beyond the lesion by at least 2 mm to ensure treatment of the entire lesion and avoid compromise of the subclavian origin. After deployment, post-dilation is performed in cases either where a self-expanding stent was used or where more aggressive dilation of a balloon-expandable stent is needed. A larger balloon can also be used to "flare" the portion of the stent extending into the aorta, thereby further opening the origin and facilitating access for future interventions. Once completed, completion angiography is performed (**Figure 2.4**).

The vertebral artery origin is often located close to the subclavian disease. In situations where treatment of the lesion could result in inadvertent coverage of the vertebral origin, protection of the vessel should be considered. The risk of emboli to the vertebral distribution is low so, although placement of protection devices has been described, they are not widely used. In situations of subclavian steal syndrome, where reversal of flow has been confirmed by US, the patient is already protected from an embolic standpoint and protection devices would expose the artery to unnecessary risk of vessel injury. Vertebral artery origin protection during subclavian intervention can be achieved in a variety of ways. If brachial access

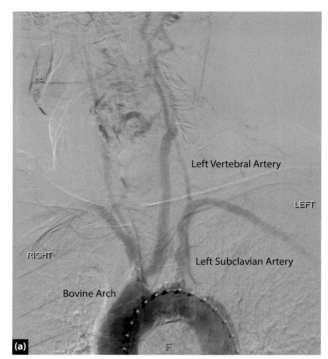

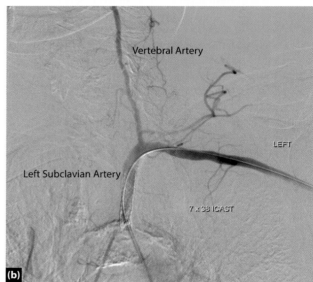

Figure 2.4 Left subclavian intervention before (**a**) and after (**b**) stent placement. This patient was only symptomatic from a left upper extremity standpoint so the disease in the brachiocephalic artery was not treated at this setting. Note the more robust filling of the vertebral artery postintervention.

has been obtained, a wire and catheter can be positioned in the vertebral origin to ensure against coverage during intervention. If only femoral access is used, a buddy wire may be used. This requires slight oversizing of the sheath to allow for the passage of two wires. One wire is extended into the axillary artery while the other is advanced into the vertebral artery. Both wires can be exchanged for 0.014-inch wires; a balloon-expandable stent can be advanced over these wires for deployment. If the stent cannot be advanced over both wires, it should be passed over the axillary wire to avoid injury to the vertebral origin during intervention.

Brachial access is an important adjunct to subclavian intervention. Surgeons may only be able to cross occlusions involving the origin from a retrograde approach because introduction of a catheter into the origin from the aortic arch in these cases may not be possible. Access-related complications for the brachial artery have been reported to be higher, causing some to avoid its use; however, providing the sheath size is kept to <6 Fr and pressure is held by an experienced provider, those complications can be kept to a minimum. An alternative, especially when using larger sheaths, is to perform a cutdown at the end with direct brachial repair. This can be easily done under local sedation with a small incision. In the authors' experience, cutdown at completion is preferred over at the start because percutaneous access allows increased stability from the surrounding tissues during recanalization and intervention. Once the lesion is crossed from the brachial approach, the wire can be snared by the femoral access and intervention proceeds as described earlier.

LEFT CCA INTERVENTIONS

Interventions of the left CCA proceed in very similar fashion to the LSA. A fair number of patients, up to 20%, may have "bovine" arch anatomy wherein the left CCA arises from the Brachiocephalic (Innominate). In these situations, special consideration must be given to alternative therapy, given the risk to both cerebral hemispheres in the treatment of this location. Treatment can be safely performed in this situation; further discussion is detailed in the section on treatment of Brachiocephalic (Innominate) lesions.

Internal carotid artery (ICA) protection should be considered for interventions on the CCA. This can be achieved with placement of the protection device of choice over the working wire placed into the ICA. In angled or tortuous lesions, this can expose the ICA to significant torque and possible dissection. To avoid this, a buddy wire can be placed into the external carotid artery (ECA) to gain support and stability (**Figure 2.5**). The stent should still be advanced over the protection device wire to be able to recapture and remove it with the least risk.

It is not unusual for patients to have both CCA and ipsilateral ICA disease. For purposes of intervention, both should be considered as separate entities with respect to their own indications to intervene. For example, there would be no reason to perform an endarterectomy on a patient with an asymptomatic 50% ICA stenosis just because a CCA intervention is planned and vice versa. Preoperative imaging will generally indicate if an inflow lesion is significant enough to treat.

There are two described ways to proceed with the technical conduct of the operation. The first method involves exposure of the ICA, ECA, and CCA in the usual manner for carotid endarterectomy (CEA). Once exposed, a clamp is placed on the ICA above the level of the disease. The CCA below the level of the disease is then accessed

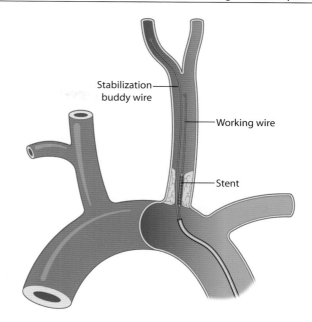

Figure 2.5 Depiction of buddy wire technique for stabilization during left common carotid artery intervention.

percutaneously and intervention is performed on the common or brachiocephalic lesion. Once this is completed, the CCA is clamped above the stent, the artery is opened, and endarterectomy is performed. The debris from stent placement is flushed out by opening the CCA clamp. A second method is to perform the CEA initially and then percutaneously access the patch for intervention. A clamp can be placed during the stent portion of the procedure for embolic protection and the debris is flushed out through the patch at the removal of the sheath.

Because of significant recurrence with angioplasty alone, stent placement is performed as primary intervention.

BRACHIOCEPHALIC (INNOMINATE) INTERVENTIONS

The Brachiocephalic (Innominate) can be the most difficult to access from the aortic arch because it usually has the most angulation. In a difficult aortic arch, consideration should be given to brachial access using a through-and-through technique as described for subclavian artery intervention. Also, unique to the Brachiocephalic (Innominate) is the need to clearly see the branch point of the right carotid and subclavian arteries. The origin may be best viewed in an LAO projection, but the bifurcation is usually best "opened up" using a right anterior oblique projection. It is imperative to see the bifurcation clearly during the intervention to avoid "jailing" the origin of the right CCA.

Both the right CCA and right vertebral distributions are at risk during a Brachiocephalic (Innominate) intervention. However, as stated earlier, risk of embolization seems to be low overall. Right CCA protection can be performed in similar fashion to the procedure outlined in the section on left CCA interventions.

Disease at the origin may be treated with stent placement like the one outlined in the section on LSA interventions.

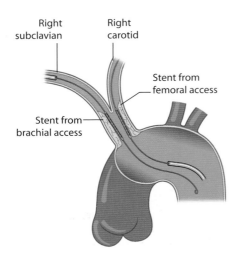

Figure 2.6 Placement of "kissing" stents for brachioce-phalic artery disease that encroaches on the bifurcation into the carotid and subclavian arteries.

However, if the left CCA arises from the Brachiocephalic (Innominate) one must make sure there is enough room for stent placement without encroaching on the origin of the left CCA. Alternative considerations for a bovine arch in this situation would be extra-anatomic bypass of the left CCA with subsequent coverage of the origin, or open revascularization of the Brachiocephalic (Innominate) or its branches.

In circumstances where the disease involves or encroaches on the bifurcation of the Brachiocephalic (Innominate) treatment by endovascular means can still be performed by placement of "kissing" stents (**Figure 2.6**). This requires two access sites, usually femoral and brachial, although carotid is possible if necessary and even preferred if done in conjunction with an endarterectomy.

The carotid stent is placed over the femoral access while the subclavian stent is performed through the brachial route. Carotid artery protection can still be performed through the femoral access.

POSTOPERATIVE CONSIDERATIONS

Patients are usually discharged after a short observation period. Some prefer to monitor patients overnight, especially if brachial or carotid cutdown were performed. Patients with renal insufficiency should be hydrated both before and after the procedure.

Patients should be maintained on aspirin. The addition of clopidogrel has been shown to be beneficial in the carotid stent literature; based on this, its use is also recommended in aortic arch interventions. Clopidogrel can generally be discontinued after a period of 6 weeks, continuing aspirin alone thereafter.

SUGGESTED READING

Aiello F, Morrissey NJ. Open and endovascular management of subclavian and innominate arterial pathology. *Semin Vasc Surg.* 2011;**24**:31–35.

Bicknell CD, Subramanian A, Wolfe JH. Coronary subclavian steal syndrome. *Eur J Vasc Endovasc Surg.* 2004;**27**:220–221.

Brountzos EN, Petersen B, Binkert C, et al. Primary stenting of subclavian and innominate artery occlusive disease: a single center's experience. *Cardiovasc Intervent Radiol.* 2004;**27**:616–623.

Rhodes JM, Cherry KJ Jr., Clark RC, et al. Aortic-origin reconstruction of the great vessels: risk factors of early and late complications. *J Vasc Surg.* 2000;**31**:260–269.

3

Endovascular intervention for mesenteric ischemia

MAEN ABOUL HOSN, NEELIMA KATRAGUNTA, AND MEL J. SHARAFUDDIN

CONTENTS

INTRODUCTION

Mesenteric ischemia can be classified as either acute or chronic. Acute mesenteric ischemia presents with symptom onset over hours to days and demands prompt diagnosis and revascularization, as well as open or laparoscopic abdominal exploration to assess gut viability and to resect nonviable intestinal segments. The role of endovascular management of acute mesenteric ischemia remains limited to hybrid retrograde stenting of an underlying superior mesenteric artery (SMA) stenosis.

Chronic mesenteric ischemia, on the other hand, is caused by long-standing atherosclerotic disease involving two or more mesenteric vessels, and occasionally an isolated, high-grade SMA lesion. Its classic presentation is postprandial abdominal pain (abdominal angina), "food fear," and weight loss. Endovascular revascularization has been the mainstay of therapy in recent years, offering lower morbidity compared with open revascularization, albeit with higher restenosis and reintervention rates.

PRINCIPLES OF TREATMENT

- Diagnosis with duplex ultrasound (US), computed tomography angiography (CTA), or magnetic resonance angiography
- In multivessel disease, the SMA should be the focus of treatment with revascularization of the remaining vessels, if feasible.
- Either a transfemoral or transbrachial approach can be used; the latter offers superior stability and support in cases of chronic occlusion or steep caudal angle of the mesenteric vessel. The authors prefer an open approach to the brachial artery, because of the high rate of thrombosis or brachial sheath hematoma in percutaneous brachial access, although percutaneous access is also an accepted method.
- Dual antiplatelet therapy is recommended for at least 6 weeks postoperatively, including a loading dose of clopidogrel, preferably before the intervention. Aspirin is continued indefinitely, along with a statin medication, if tolerated.

TECHNIQUES FOR INTERVENTION

The femoral or brachial artery is percutaneously accessed using a micropuncture technique under US guidance. A pigtail/flush catheter is used to perform an aortogram in two projections, demonstrating blood flow patterns and anatomy of the celiac axis and SMA. Lateral aortography is used to delineate and assess for ostial lesions. Once the decision to intervene is made, the patient is administered intravenous heparin to achieve an activated clotting time of at least 250 seconds. The standard-length sheath is exchanged for a 45–55-cm, 6- or 7-Fr flexible sheath. Selection of the diseased vessel is accomplished using a curved catheter/0.035-inch guidewire combination (multipurpose guide catheter or JB catheter for brachial access; Cobra I and II, Simmons 1–3, or SOS Omni catheter for femoral access). The guidewire is maneuvered into the artery and the lesion is crossed. Sometimes, a straight-tipped 0.018-inch or 0.14-inch guidewire may cross the lesion more easily. The lesion is carefully crossed with the catheter. If there is a chronic occlusion, support catheters can be helpful in crossing the lesion (CXI®; Cook Medical Inc., Bloomington, IN, USA; Quick-Cross™; Spectranectics, Colorado Springs, CO, USA).

Once accessed, it is imperative to perform selective mesenteric angiography to confirm the presence of the catheter tip within the true lumen, because wire manipulation can cause dissection. Pre-dilation is mandatory with a 3–4-mm, low-profile angioplasty balloon catheter, which can also be valuable in stent sizing. Next, the pre-dilated lesion is traversed with the sheath and a balloon-expandable stent or stent graft is delivered, positioned, and deployed to cover the entire lesion, with 2–3 mm of the stent flaring into the aorta. Care should be taken to avoid covering any branch vessels, especially the middle colic artery, when using a stent graft. A selective completion angiogram is performed through the sheath, confirming patency of the stent without embolization. Any residual stenosis should be <30% in diameter. A flush aortogram is performed to ascertain position and patency of the stent. Hemostasis is achieved at the puncture site.

RETROGRADE MESENTERIC STENTING DURING LAPAROTOMY (HYBRID APPROACH)

The hybrid approach is valuable in patients presenting with acute or acute-on-chronic nonembolic mesenteric ischemia undergoing laparotomy for evaluation of bowel viability. The advantages of this technique include its minimal access requirement (inframesocolic exposure) and the use of mesenteric thrombectomy and arteriotomy for retrograde sheath access. This technique can restore flow to the gut faster and less invasively than a mesenteric bypass in a critically ill patient.

After the abdominal cavity is entered, the SMA is exposed at the root of the mesentery and a sufficient segment is controlled inferior to the transverse colon mesentery. In cases of confirmed secondary thrombosis of the SMA, access is established via a transverse arteriotomy. If the vessel is diseased, a longitudinal arteriotomy is performed and later closed with a vein patch. Balloon thrombectomy is performed. A 7-Fr sheath with a tip marker is introduced retrograde several centimeters into the SMA. The ostial stenosis is carefully traversed with a directional catheter/guidewire combination. Once true lumen re-entry into the aorta is confirmed angiographically, access is exchanged for a stiff wire and balloon angioplasty/stenting is performed, flaring the stent 2–3 mm into the aortic lumen. Position and patency of the stent are confirmed with lateral aortography. The arteriotomy is closed primarily or using a vein patch.

COMPLICATIONS

Complications associated with any endovascular procedure include access site hematoma or vessel thrombosis. A brachial sheath hematoma with resulting median nerve damage is a dreaded complication. Wire and catheter manipulation in a "shaggy" atherosclerotic aorta can lead to distal atheroembolization. Unrefined cannulation and wire manipulation can lead to mesenteric arterial dissection or occlusion. A risk of false lumen entry is present during recanalization of a chronic total occlusion (CTO) and must be avoided. It is crucial to confirm true lumen position of the guidewire angiographically before angioplasty and stent deployment. Finally, contrast-induced nephropathy can also occur. With the exception of false lumen entry during recanalization of a CTO, these complications can be kept to <2% each.

CASE EXAMPLES

Case example 1

An 80-year-old man presented with postprandial pain and weight loss. He was found to have a 7-cm juxtarenal abdominal aortic aneurysm and occlusion of both celiac axis and SMA (**Figure 3.1a**). Recanalization of the SMA was deemed necessary before fenestrated endovascular repair (**Figure 3.1b,c**).

Case example 2

A 47-year-old woman with a history of chronic mesenteric ischemia who had undergone SMA stent placement 1 year earlier, presented with recurrent symptoms of postprandial pain, diarrhea, and failure to thrive. A computed tomography angiography showed in-stent restenosis, as well as extensive disease involving the mid-SMA at about the level of the middle colic branch (**Figure 3.2a**).

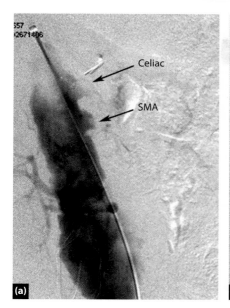
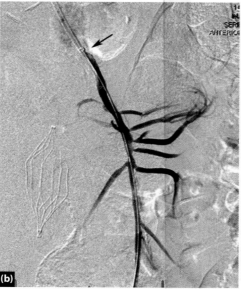
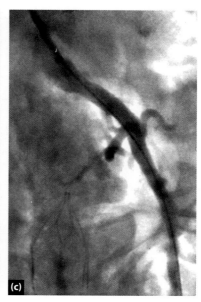

Figure 3.1 Juxtarenal abdominal aortic aneurysm and occlusion of both celiac axis and superior mesenteric artery (SMA). (a) Aortogram with lateral projection showing occlusion of both celiac axis and SMA (arrows) with visible stumps. (b) After recanalization and pre-dilation, a 6-Fr Flexor® sheath (Cook Medical Inc.) was advanced past the stenosis (arrow). (c) Completion angiogram after the SMA stent was deployed and flared into the aorta.

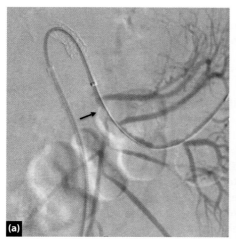
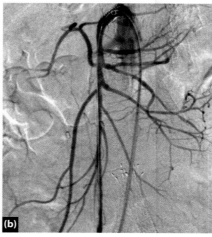

Figure 3.2 Digital subtraction angiogram showing in-stent restenosis and extensive SMA disease. (a) Angiogram demonstrating passage of the sheath through the in-stent restenosis and high-grade stenosis proximal to the middle colic artery origin (arrow). (b) Completion angiogram following deployment and proximal flaring of a 7 × 22-mm iCast™ stent graft and drug-coated balloon angioplasty of the mid-segment disease. There was restoration of brisk antegrade flow with no residual stenosis in the stent or mid-superior mesenteric artery.

She had a patent celiac artery and an occluded inferior mesenteric artery.

Using a femoral access, the restenosed stent was recanalized and pre-dilation balloon angioplasty was performed. The sheath was passed through the stent beyond the stenosis. Angiography confirmed a long segment of diffuse critical atherosclerotic stenosis of the mid-SMA segment with a high-grade stenosis just proximal to the middle colic artery origin. These were dilated using a 5 × 60-mm Lutonix® drug-coated balloon (Bard Peripheral Vascular, Inc., Tempe, AZ, USA), followed by relining of the in-stent stenosis using a 7 × 22-mm iCast™ stent graft (Atrium Medical Corporation, Hudson, NH, USA) (**Figure 3.2b**).

Case example 3

A 45-year-old woman with a history of postprandial abdominal pain and weight loss presented acutely with severe, unrelenting abdominal pain. She had a known ostial SMA stenosis from a previous abdominal CTA. CTA on presentation showed new segmental total thrombosis of the SMA down to the jejunal branch origin. She underwent exploratory laparotomy with open retrograde thrombectomy of the SMA from an inframesocolic approach using a transverse arteriotomy (**Figure 3.3a**). This was followed by retrograde recanalization of the occluded SMA (**Figure 3.3b**) and deployment of a 6 × 16-mm iCast™ stent graft (**Figure 3.3c**).

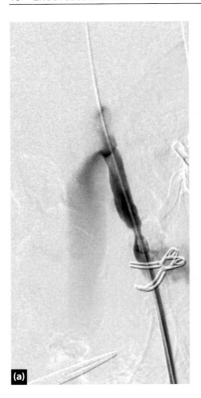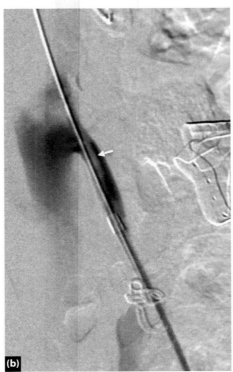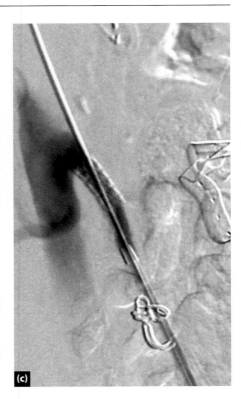

Figure 3.3 Open retrograde SMA revascularization. (**a**) Retrograde access of the superior mesenteric artery (SMA) with a 7-Fr sheath through a transverse arteriotomy, following open thromboembolectomy. Note the bulldog clamps used for distal arterial control. (**b**) Following recanalization of the tight ostial stenosis, a nearly occlusive stenosis was seen in the proximal SMA, due to the disrupted plaque/dissection flap (arrow). (**c**) Final appearance after deployment of a 6 × 16-mm iCast™ stent graft (Atrium Medical Corporation) with restoration of flow and no residual stenosis.

SUGGESTED READING

Asciutto G, Sonesson B, Björses K, et al. Retrograde totally endovascular recanalization of occluded mesenteric arteries through the pancreaticoduodenal arcade. *EJVES Short Reports.* 2015;**29**:28–31.

Atkins MD, Kwolek CJ, LaMuraglia GM, et al. Surgical revascularization versus endovascular therapy for chronic mesenteric ischemia: a comparative experience. *J Vasc Surg.* 2007;**45**:1162–1171.

Blauw JT, Meerwaldt R, Brusse-Keizer M, et al. Retrograde open mesenteric stenting for acute mesenteric ischemia. *J Vasc Surg.* 2014;**60**:726–734.

Oderich GS, Erdoes LS, Lesar C, et al. Comparison of covered stents versus bare metal stents for treatment of chronic atherosclerotic mesenteric arterial disease. *J Vasc Surg.* 2013;**58**:1316–1323.

Sharafuddin MJ, Nicholson RM, Kresowik TF, et al. Endovascular recanalization of total occlusions of the mesenteric and celiac arteries. *J Vasc Surg.* 2012;**55**:1674–1681.

Zacharias N, Eghbalieh SD, Chang BB, et al. Chronic mesenteric ischemia outcome analysis and predictors of endovascular failure. *J Vasc Surg.* 2016;**63**:1582–1587.

4

Endovascular intervention for renal artery occlusive disease

JASON Q. ALEXANDER, DERRICK GREEN, AND TIMOTHY M. SULLIVAN

CONTENTS

INTRODUCTION

Historically, renal artery (RA) stenosis has been regarded as the most common curable cause of secondary hypertension. The rationale for intervention was based on stabilization of the renin–angiotensin pathway that is artificially elevated or theoretically accelerated when a kidney is exposed to decreased blood volume secondary to RA stenosis. Recent trials have cast doubt on both this pathway and its influence on patients with hypertension. The high incidence of essential hypertension in the atherosclerotic patient population further confuses the question of the impact of RA stenosis on this pathology. Considering 15% of patients undergoing coronary angiography are found to have a >50% stenosis of the RAs, blanket statements connecting RA stenosis and hypertension seems unwarranted. Putative benefits of renal parenchymal preservation in the face of RA stenosis are even more controversial. Thus, current evidence suggests that the medical field is at a point of change regarding both open and endovascular RA intervention for stenosis.

INDICATIONS FOR INTERVENTION ON THE RAs FOR STENOSIS

The completion of the CORAL (Cardiovascular Outcomes in Renal Atherosclerotic Lesions) trial has significantly decreased the indications for percutaneous intervention of the RAs for stenosis secondary to atherosclerotic disease.[1] The CORAL trial did not show a statistically significant reduction in blood pressure (BP) following percutaneous treatment of RA stenosis when compared with best medical management. Studies evaluating the use of percutaneous RA interventions for preservation of renal function have been even less promising. Thus, until new trials demonstrate significant benefit, indications for either open or endovascular revascularization of RAs due to atherosclerotic disease are limited. However, this does not mean that there are not indications for treatment. While traditional indications for RA intervention due to atherosclerotic disease may be less clear, the rapid expansion of new endovascular interventions including complex branched and fenestrated endograft placement or "chimney" endovascular aneurysm repair (chEVAR) procedures for abdominal aortic aneurysm (AAA) means that practitioners must still know how to obtain access and treat RA stenosis. Further, in the face of BP that cannot be controlled despite maximal management with four or more antihypertensive medications, treatment of RA stenosis may still be warranted if for no other reason than a lack of other options. Similar statements can likely be made for patients with poor BP control and episodes of flash pulmonary edema. Controversy will probably continue to present itself when practitioners are faced with the question of worsening RA stenosis in patients with single-functioning kidneys and progressive renal dysfunction.

RA stenosis secondary to nonatherosclerotic causes presents different issues with respect to intervention. Current evidence continues to support the use of percutaneous RA transluminal balloon angioplasty in cases of fibromuscular dysplasia (FMD) and associated hypertension. Placement of stents or open revascularization have fared less well in this presentation. Neurofibromatosis, though extremely rare, may be another nonatherosclerotic etiology of RA stenosis that benefits from a percutaneous approach. Once again, angioplasty may well be preferred over stenting, although the fibrotic nature of these lesions often requires a high-pressure balloon to counteract the potential for recoil. Takayasu arteritis-associated RA stenosis appears to respond better to open RA revascularization and it is likely the better option when available to the patient.

Finally, although rare, there is a role for percutaneous RA revascularization in the setting of trauma. Opportunities for revascularization in trauma are limited primarily by the short window of ischemia time to the kidney before function cannot be recovered. While several studies have argued for an even shorter window, there certainly does not appear to be any rationale to attempt revascularization in the face of RA occlusion due to thrombosis beyond 6 hours from the initial event. If, however, a patient presents within the appropriate timeframe and does not have any contraindications, an argument can be made to pursue percutaneous revascularization with pharmacologic or mechanical thrombolysis followed by stenting (preferably covered).

PREOPERATIVE EVALUATION

While an array of diagnostic functional studies have assessed renal function, many of these have likely become obsolete because of their relative inaccuracies or utility, particularly in the face of outcome studies such as CORAL. In those patients who have indications for intervention, imaging studies can be particularly helpful in preprocedural planning. Magnetic resonance angiography (MRA) and computed tomography angiography (CTA) can also identify stenosis or clarify etiology, and may help with decisions regarding an endovascular or open approach.

Preoperative imaging is extremely helpful in making decisions regarding choice of access site. Acute angles between RAs and the aorta may make arm access a better option. However, caution should be taken to ensure adequate evaluation of the route to the RA from the arm before this is pursued. The continued evolution of catheter-based technology has led to smaller sheath sizes with greater support, tracking, and maneuverability. Therefore, the brachial or radial arteries are viable options. Those patients with acute angles due to atherosclerotic disease are more likely to have occlusive subclavian artery disease and are also more likely to have highly torturous thoracic aortas that might make this choice of access less

straightforward than one would intuitively expect. Finally, access in the arms is almost always associated with manipulation across, at a minimum, the left vertebral artery. Wires, catheters, and sheaths also intrude on the aortic arch, all of which have the potential for the rare but potentially catastrophic consequence of stroke.

In the nonatherosclerotic patient undergoing percutaneous RA intervention, the femoral artery is usually the route of choice. However, because these patients tend to be a much younger cohort, the previously noted detriments of an arm approach are less pronounced.

Presented here are two cases of percutaneous intervention for RA stenosis. First, is a case of treatment for atherosclerotic RA stenosis leading to uncontrolled hypertension despite maximal medical management. The second case demonstrates percutaneous management of a young woman with FMD and persistent hypertension. While the goal of altering the renin–angiotensin cycle is the same in both cases, important differences between the approaches to these two different etiologies are highlighted.

PERCUTANEOUS INTERVENTION FOR RA STENOSIS

Case 1: Atherosclerotic RA stenosis

An older woman with a single functional kidney (right) presented with uncontrolled hypertension despite treatment with four antihypertensive medications. In addition, she was noted to have worsening renal function based on serial glomerular filtration rate evaluation. Preoperative imaging included an RA duplex scan and time-of-flight MRA. Both studies suggested high-grade stenosis of a single right RA at the origin of the vessel. Imaging also indicated a femoral approach would be feasible.

Ultrasound (US) guidance was used to identify and cannulate the common femoral artery with a 21-G needle (micropuncture).

For the case presented here, a carbon dioxide (CO_2)-based aortogram was completed to confirm the stenosis (**Figure 4.1**). CO_2 can be particularly helpful in patients with renal insufficiency or contrast allergies. A few important notes regarding the use of CO_2 as a contrast agent. Because of the buoyancy of the gas, patients may need to be tilted to allow best visualization of the arteries. While CO_2 can be used to perform all imaging for an RA case, some liquid-based contrast agent is usually helpful before deploying the stent. Further, obese patients can severely hamper imaging with CO_2. Finally, it may be helpful to provide an antiemetic to awake patients before using CO_2 because the injection incites nausea in some patients.

In patients with atherosclerosis as the underlying etiology of RA stenosis, the anatomic distribution of disease is typically an aortic plaque intruding into the lumen of the RA. Thus, imaging the origin of the artery is critical to confirm stenosis. This usually necessitates multiple right

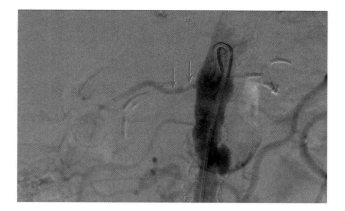

Figure 4.1 Carbon dioxide (CO_2) aortogram with angulation to display origin. Right anterior oblique projection with patient tilted to the left to allow visualization of the origin of the renal artery (arrows) and take advantage of the buoyancy associated with CO_2.

and left anterior oblique views to best visualize the origin of the RA (**Figure 4.1**).

Once imaging has confirmed stenosis, selection of the artery is performed. Multiple different catheter and wire combinations can be employed for this task. Usually, identifying a catheter that matches the angle of RA take-off is a best first option. Multiple different wire options may also be successful, although selection with a directional wire is the choice of most practitioners. Difficult selection may take place in patients with severe stenosis, severe angulation, excessive aortic plaque, or concomitant pathology (e.g., aortic aneurysm). In cases where selective catheterization is not possible, a different access route may be beneficial. This certainly includes arm access, although it may be prudent to first move to the opposite femoral artery. Access from the contralateral femoral artery sometimes changes the angle thereby allowing for easier selective catheterization. Finally, movement of the RA during respiration can dramatically change the access angle, particularly for the left RA. Having the patient hold their breath at either the end of inspiration or expiration may be an easy solution that provides the angle necessary for selection. In these situations, maintaining access to the vessel can be tenuous and care must be taken to avoid dislodgement. In extreme situations, a general anesthetic may be used to help with these issues (often when previous attempts or accesses have failed).

Many practitioners use a hydrophilic wire in combination with a directional catheter to select the vessel. While these wires are extremely maneuverable, caution must be taken to avoid creation of a dissection plane. There is also the potential for advancing the wire too far and even injuring the renal parenchyma. Once a catheter can be advanced into the artery and confirmed to be within the true lumen, trading out for a stiffer and less traumatic wire is advantageous. A 0.035-inch diameter system often provides the greatest stability for advancing a sheath or guide catheter. However, with appropriate anatomy, either 0.018

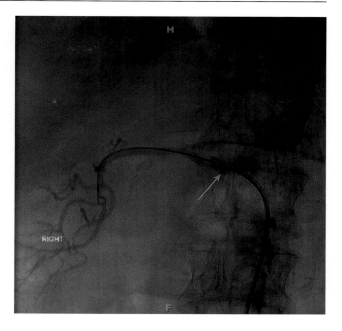

Figure 4.2 Nonsubtracted renal arteriogram with sheath engaged at the origin demonstrates renal artery stenosis and encroachment of aortic atherosclerosis into the renal artery as the etiology of stenosis (arrow).

or even 0.014-inch systems can certainly be employed. At this point, either a sheath or guide catheter can be advanced. Imaging with the RA orifice engaged can be helpful to provide sizing information with respect to stent selection (**Figure 4.2**). Ideally, the lesion itself can be crossed with the sheath or guide catheter, which eases the placement of a balloon-expandable stent. In those cases where crossing the lesion is not possible, pre-dilation with a small balloon catheter may facilitate these maneuvers with the sheath or guide catheter engaged at the RA origin. Routine pre-dilation of the artery is probably best avoided because of concerns about the potential for atheroembolization.

Use of distal embolic protection devices during RA intervention has been described and provides an intuitive advantage. However, further studies and technological advances will determine whether the potential benefit in preventing distal embolization outweighs the complexity and potential complications of employing these devices.

Once the sheath or guide catheter is in place and measurements are confirmed, a balloon-expandable stent is advanced and the guide catheter or sheath are withdrawn. A balloon-expandable stent provides the greatest precision for deployment. Self-expanding stents should be avoided because of the potential for movement during deployment. Arguments can be made for both covered and uncovered stents presently, but current data probably does not favor one choice over the other.

A common mistake with stent deployment is the failure to extend the stent significantly into the aorta (**Figure 4.3**). As the underlying etiology of stenosis is most often atherosclerosis from the aorta encroaching on the RA, stents that are deployed just within the RA are prone to restenosis.

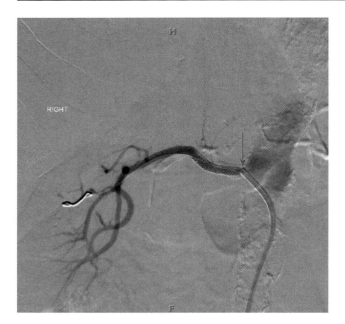

Figure 4.3 Recurrent proximal renal artery stenosis due to failure to extend the stent into the aorta (arrow).

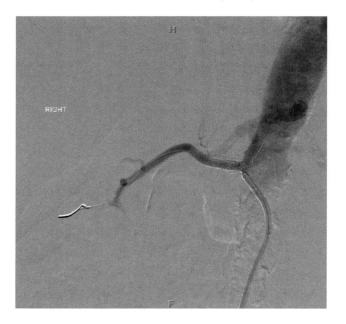

Figure 4.4 Renal artery stenting extended into the aorta (arrow) and flared to account for aortic atherosclerosis.

Extending the stent into the aorta and then flaring the intra-aortic portion with an oversize balloon is a useful technique (**Figure 4.4**). A completion angiogram is performed to confirm treatment and no residual stenosis/dissection or distal embolization.

Postoperative complications are most commonly access-related. However, some patients may have a dramatic response to the treatment and care should be taken to closely observe post-stent BP with treatment in the form of intravenous fluid resuscitation and vasopressors available in the case of hypotension.

Practitioners should place patients on a minimum of aspirin postprocedure; most prefer dual therapy to include clopidogrel.

Case 2: Nonatherosclerotic RA stenosis (FMD)

The technical approach to RA stenosis secondary to FMD differs from that due to atherosclerotic disease in several important ways. The population of patients presenting with FMD tend to be considerably younger and healthier. Rarely is there much tortuosity in the anatomy of this cohort of patients, making a femoral approach the feasible option in almost all cases. Preoperative imaging may once again be useful in helping predict best catheter and wire combinations for selection of the RA. The beaded or so-called "string of beads" appearance is classic for FMD. Preoperative imaging in the form of CTA or MRA can often confirm the diagnosis before a formal catheter-based angiogram. Importantly, however, evidence of disease in one RA should mandate close examination of the contralateral RA during a formal catheter-based angiogram, even if it appears disease-free on preoperative imaging. Preoperative imaging may also identify disease extending into one or more secondary branches of the RA. When this is identified, the practitioner may need to be prepared to place buddy wires into the RA to preserve access into the secondary branches. Finally, a reminder that patients diagnosed with FMD should undergo evaluation of other vascular beds, most importantly the cerebrovascular system.

The standard approach begins with femoral access gained under US visualization. An aortogram is then performed (**Figure 4.5**). Attention should be paid to the extent of disease within the RAs. FMD rarely is evident at the RA origin; however, RA origin images should be obtained to make sure that occult stenosis is not missed during treatment. Determination of the extent of the disease distally, as well as involvement of secondary branches, is critical in planning at this point. Selection of the RA is once again obtained with a matching selective catheter. Careful surveillance needs to be maintained if a hydrophilic wire is used. This is particularly true when the disease is rather extensive because movement of the distal end of the wire can quickly lead to intimal flaps or even damage to the renal parenchyma that will not be noted by the haptic feedback of the proceduralist. Typically, multiple hemodynamically significant lesions are present because of the multiple webs that develop in FMD.

Once wire access is obtained, a supporting sheath or guide catheter should be advanced to the origin of the RA. Unlike in atherosclerotic disease, crossing of the lesions with the sheath or guide catheter is usually not critical. However, engaging the origin of the RA is helpful to maintain support and obtain selective digital subtraction angiography runs (**Figure 4.6**). With the lesion (lesions) crossed by a wire and a sheath or guide catheter in place, selective runs should be obtained to determine the length

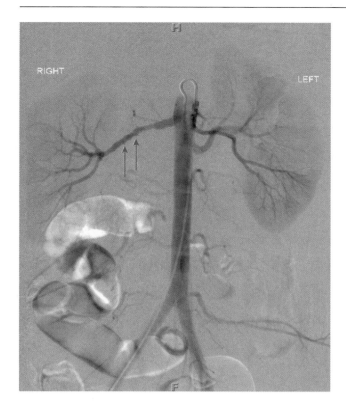

Figure 4.5 Fibromuscular dysplasia aortogram showing the "string of beads" (arrows) appearance in the right renal artery.

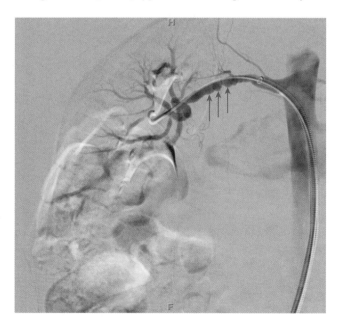

Figure 4.6 Fibromuscular dysplasia renal artery sheath injection showing "string of beads" appearance (arrows).

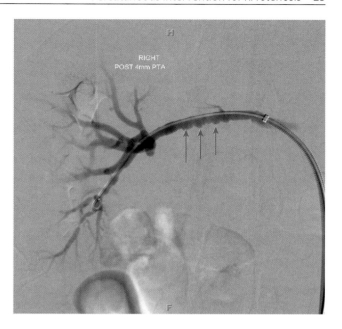

Figure 4.7 Sheath injection renal angiogram showing residual disease (arrows) after inadequate angioplasty.

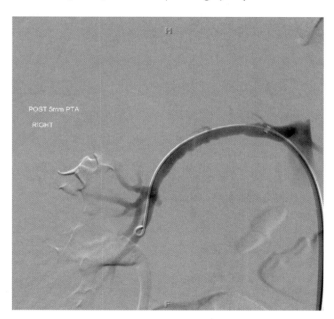

Figure 4.8 Sheath injection renal angiogram showing resolution of stenosis.

and width of subsequent balloon dilation. Balloon angioplasty is the treatment modality of choice for FMD and stents should be avoided except in the most unusual or bailout situations. Balloon diameter sizing is best based on a normal segment of the artery. If no normal artery exists, the contralateral RA can sometimes be used for guidance.

Multiple-view completion angiography is often useful following angioplasty because of the tendency for occult webs to be present that are uncovered with further views (**Figure 4.7**). The authors' practice is to perform pull-back pressure measurements across the artery to assure that all the lesions have been treated (**Figure 4.8**). Unfortunately, in some cases (small RAs being an example), pull-back pressures are unobtainable. Intravascular US is an option in these situations, although practitioners need to feel very comfortable with the set-up and interpretation of this technology, if used. However, even with all precautions taken, the incidence of missed lesions or recurrence of disease in these patients is not trivial and patients should be warned that the possibility of multiple treatments exists.

Following completion of the case, patients should be maintained on antiplatelet therapy. Like those treated for atherosclerotic lesions, patients should be carefully observed for hypotension after treatment has been completed. Surveillance studies may be helpful in identifying untreated occult lesions or restenosis, although this is also often guided by the patient's clinic response with respect to hypertension or antihypertensive medication requirements.

ACCIDENTAL RA COVERAGE

A final comment on percutaneous RA intervention should be reserved for inadvertent coverage of the RA during EVAR (**Figure 4.8**). Current endovascular devices allow for more precise positioning or even repositioning, which make this potentially devastating complication a less frequent event. Multiple different solutions exist for this problem. Sadly, no solution is perfect and ultimately an open intervention may be necessary to preserve kidney function. In the early setting, when an endograft has been deployed across the RA or arteries, pulling the graft down can be attempted. Use of a balloon is usually ineffective in this situation because it tends to seat the graft into position. Alternatively, using a snare to cross the flow divider with a wire and pulling down from both groins simultaneously with a "body floss" technique sometimes allow for enough movement of the graft to uncover the RAs. Obviously, extreme care needs to be taken in this situation because of the potential damage from this technique. When coverage is because of a cuff, this technique is even less likely to be successful.

More often, the best chance of percutaneous revascularization is via cannulation of the covered artery from a brachial approach. The lay of the graft makes a femoral approach of limited utility. Even when the RA can be accessed from the brachial artery, considerable effort may be exhausted maintaining position. Early placement of a long sheath before RA selection can be helpful, because maintaining access can be tenuous and easily lost when a sheath is being advanced after RA selection. Constant vigilance is necessary to prevent loss of access to the RA. Intuitively, increased radial strength in the stent makes sense. Thus, a first choice would be a balloon-expandable covered stent. However, data from early reviews of the chE-VAR literature suggests that it may be best to match a covered stent with the type/material of the endograft placed. Fewer subsequent endoleaks appear to be present when self-expanding nitinol stents are matched with similar grafts (e.g., GORE-TEX®/polytetrafluoroethylene grafts) while balloon-expandable stents may work more favorably with other endograft options (e.g., woven/polyethylene terephthalate grafts). Future studies may help to clarify the juxtaposition of these stents. Regardless, overlap of the

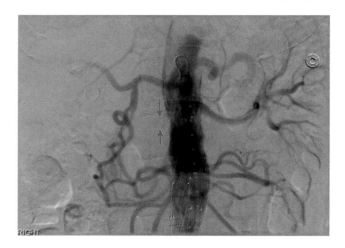

Figure 4.9 Angiogram showing a nonenhancing right renal artery (RRA) that was covered after the endovascular stent graft was placed. The previously placed RRA stent is still visible (arrows).

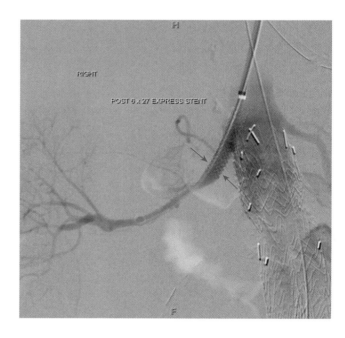

Figure 4.10 Angiogram showing a patent right renal artery (arrows) that was stented after being covered by an endovascular stent graft. The stent extended well above the endograft.

stent into the aorta and ideally well above the top of the endograft is likely beneficial to prevent recurrence or stent thrombosis (**Figures 4.9** and **4.10**).

CONCLUSION

Recent trials have made the rationale for treatment of atherosclerotic RA stenosis by a percutaneous approach less clear. Regardless, indications for percutaneous management of RA disease, particularly for some nonatherosclerotic etiologies, remain the standard of care. With the expansion in endovascular technologies, notably complex juxta, para, and suprarenal AAA repair, practitioner familiarity with endovascular approaches and treatment of the RAs remains critical.

REFERENCE

1. Cooper CJ, Murphy TP, Cutlip DE, et al. Stenting and medical therapy for atherosclerotic renal-artery stenosis. *N Engl J Med.* 2014;**370**:13–22.

5

Endovascular management of aortoiliac occlusive disease

HANNAH KIM, KAREM HARTH, AND VIKRAM S. KASHYAP

CONTENTS

INTRODUCTION

Aortoiliac occlusive disease (AIOD) typically involves the aortic bifurcation and proximal common iliac arteries (CIAs), and slowly progresses both proximally and distally. Clinical presentation can vary depending on the extent of the involved segment, from intermittent claudication of the hip, buttock, thigh, or calf, to severe claudication, rest pain, and limb-threatening tissue loss with concurrent, multilevel occlusive disease. Vascular interventions are indicated typically for those patients with severe claudication, rest pain, tissue loss (Rutherford stages 3–6), or distal embolization, such as blue toe syndrome. With rapidly advancing technology in vascular imaging, and balloon and stent angioplasty, over the last decades, endovascular treatment of AIOD has demonstrated high success rates of revascularization and limb salvage, with low morbidity. Endoluminal therapies have been used for focal stenosis or occlusions (TransAtlantic Inter-Society Consensus (TASC) II A and B lesions). Recently, the endovascular approach has been extended even in advanced AIOD, which includes TASC II C and D lesions.

When a patient's symptoms warrant an intervention, primary evaluation of the location and extent of the occlusive disease begins with physical examination, including a complete pulse examination, and noninvasive arterial study, including arterial duplex imaging and ankle–brachial pressure index (ABPI). Diminished femoral pulses and decreased thigh segmental pressure suggest AIOD; however, a normal pulse exam and ABPI can be obtained in patients in the presence of mild AIOD with iliac stenosis. In these patients, obtaining an ABPI before and after exercise may help determine the presence of hemodynamically significant AIOD. Vascular imaging studies include duplex ultrasound (US), computed tomography angiography (CTA), and magnetic resonance angiography (MRA). CTA is particularly useful in procedural planning because of its ability to provide the anatomy and severity of disease in three-dimensional views. However, the risks of employing this modality must be carefully weighed, especially the use of iodinated contrast that can lead to contrast-induced nephropathy. Gadolinium-based MRA is contraindicated in patients with renal insufficiency because of the risk of nephrogenic systemic fibrosis.

Diagnosis of concomitant aortic or common femoral artery (CFA) disease is important to determine the type of approach to be used. Specifically, the location and extent of the lesion and the anatomy of the aortoiliac system would determine: (1) the feasibility of endovascular versus open revascularization; (2) percutaneous versus hybrid approach; and (3) the ipsilateral, contralateral, or brachial approach for endovascular recanalization. Lesions in the aorta and iliac segments tend to be eccentric with heavy calcifications; therefore, care should be taken to closely monitor hemodynamic changes to avoid complications of aortic or iliac artery rupture. Hemodynamically significant lesions can be determined by measuring the intra-arterial pressure. This can be obtained typically by "pullback" method; an end-hole catheter connected to the arterial pressure monitoring system is "pulled" from proximal to distal across the lesion over a guidewire. If the systolic pressure gradient is >10 mmHg or the mean gradient >5 mmHg, it is considered to be hemodynamically significant and should be considered for treatment. Hemodynamically significant, concomitant CFA stenosis often warrants a hybrid approach; a groin cutdown to expose the femoral arteries, femoral endarterectomy with or without patch angioplasty, retrograde canalization of the ipsilateral iliac arteries, and balloon or stent angioplasty are performed.

TECHNIQUES FOR INTERVENTION

Determination of approach

Arterial access can be obtained via an ipsilateral retrograde versus a contralateral transfemoral or transbrachial approach, depending on the extent of the disease and the tortuosity of the vessel. For aortoiliac artery stenosis, ipsilateral retrograde transfemoral access is typically obtained using a hydrophilic catheter. A contralateral up-and-over technique can be used; however, this technique may be disadvantaged over ipsilateral access, since there is minimal support from the catheter, especially because tortuous vessel anatomy and steeply angled aortic bifurcation hinder the advancement of the supporting sheath. Transbrachial arterial access, usually via the left side, is a useful alternative to recanalize the aortoiliac segment; however, care should be taken especially in female patients whose vessels tend to be smaller. Because of the brachial artery's smaller diameter compared to the femoral arteries, there can be limitations in selecting larger-sized sheaths for interventions. Brachial artery cutdown may have to be performed to safely access the artery and reduce access-related complications; however, it does not prevent the possibility of embolic complications from catheter manipulation within the aortic arch.

Stent selection

Selecting the appropriate size of balloons and stents is paramount to successful angioplasty. Preoperative assessment of the diameter of a stenotic or occlusive vessel segment becomes important and can often be obtained from vascular imaging studies, such as computed tomography (CT) or magnetic resonance,

performed before the procedure. If such imaging studies are not available, intraoperative, pretreatment measurement of the vessel diameter can be performed with a marker catheter or with the operative imaging computer system. For heavily calcified, severely stenotic, and occlusive lesions, balloon angioplasty before the stent is deployed may be indicated. The length of the balloon or stent should cover the diseased segment only without damaging the normal vessel. Slow insufflation of undersized balloons, with small increments in size, can be used if the initial result is not satisfactory. Slightly oversized stents, typically 5–10%, are used unless the vessel is heavily calcified and there is concern that oversizing may rupture the vessel. Different types of stents are available: covered versus uncovered; balloon-expandable versus self-expanding. Covered stents are usually employed in proximal CIAs with heavy, eccentric plaques that are at high risk of rupture. However, meticulous calculation of stent length should be taken into consideration to avoid inadvertent coverage of the internal iliac artery. Balloon-expandable stents allow for precision of stent placement, and provide hoop strength and excellent radiolucency on fluoroscopy. However, they can permanently deform if enough external force is applied by a heavily diseased vessel wall, because of its reduced flexibility. Self-expanding stents can be used for tortuous vessels; because of their flexibility, they can also be deployed more easily via contralateral access.

Aortic bifurcation lesions

"Kissing" balloons and stents, that is, simultaneous balloon insufflation or stent deployment of bilateral CIAs, are typically used for lesions at the aortic bifurcation even with a unilateral lesion, and concerns for contralateral CIA compression, plaque dislodgement with subsequent distal embolization, or dissection. When there are any concerns of distal aortic disease just proximal to the bifurcation, the stents can be deployed from this level down to the CIAs in a kissing stent fashion.

Chronic total occlusion lesions

Recanalization of chronic total occlusions of the aortoiliac segment can be done via the true lumen or via a subintimal path followed by reentry into the true lumen. Support from a good outer sheath is usually necessary. A combination of a stiff hydrophilic wire and a low-profile, angled, hydrophilic-coated catheter is often used. These are most successfully achieved by ipsilateral retrograde transfemoral or transbrachial access, since support and pushability can be provided. Once the lesion is crossed using this technique, the hydrophilic wire is exchanged for stiffer, nonhydrophilic guidewires to provide greater support for balloon or stent angioplasty and catheter exchanges. If reentry into the true lumen is unsuccessful with these maneuvers, reentry devices are commercially available. Various types from different manufacturers that use differently sized guidewires or intravascular US (IVUS) are available. Understanding the nuances and limitations of each device and the operator's comfort level using each device determines the success rate.

MAJOR COMPLICATIONS SPECIFIC TO THE PROCEDURE

Arterial access-related complications include: pseudoaneurysm; arterial dissection; arteriovenous fistula below the CFA bifurcation; and retroperitoneal hematoma from above the inguinal ligament. US-guided arterial access has been shown to reduce these access-related complications. Stent-related complications include: stent dislodgement in the delivery system; misplacement; migration; and embolization from undersizing, infection, and stent fracture. Rupture of an artery caused by an oversized balloon in a calcified vessel may result in significant morbidity and mortality. In-stent stenosis from intimal hyperplasia, and progression of atherosclerotic disease and thrombosis in the stented vessel, as well as distal embolization following endovascular repair may occur. Therefore, gentle handling of wires and catheters, and accurate sizing of the vessel diameter should be routinely obtained with preoperative CTA, calibrated catheters, IVUS, or angiography systems in angiography suites.

CASE EXAMPLES

Case example 1

A 76-year-old woman presented with rest pain in her bilateral lower extremities and no palpable femoral pulses on examination, with an ABPI of 0.31 on the right and unobtainable left ABPI or Doppler signal (**Figure 5.1a,b**). Noncontrast CT and MRA of the abdomen and pelvis demonstrated significant stenosis of the infrarenal abdominal aorta with bilateral AIOD. With these findings, an aortogram was obtained (**Figure 5.2a–d**) via US-guided right transfemoral arterial access using a micropuncture set; this demonstrated a calcified aorta that was very small in diameter. The aorta was recanalized with a guidewire (Glidewire®; Terumo Medical Corporation, Somerset, NJ, USA) and glide catheter; pre-stent deployment balloon angioplasty was performed using a 6-mm balloon. The authors then upsized to a 6-Fr long sheath and brought a self-expanding 10-mm stent (Absolute Pro®; Abbott Vascular, Santa Clara, CA, USA) into the aorta. Of note, preoperative imaging with noncontrast CT indicated a calcified wall-to-wall diameter of approximately 11 mm. The authors deployed the stent and then carried out post-stent deployment angioplasty with a percutaneous transluminal angioplasty 10-mm balloon dilatation catheter (Dorado®; BARD Peripheral Vascular, Inc., Tempe, AZ, USA) to remedy the significant waist of the stent. Final imaging demonstrated rapid blood flow through the stented segment. There was still a 10–15% waist; however, given the calcified artery and the fact that further intervention may have

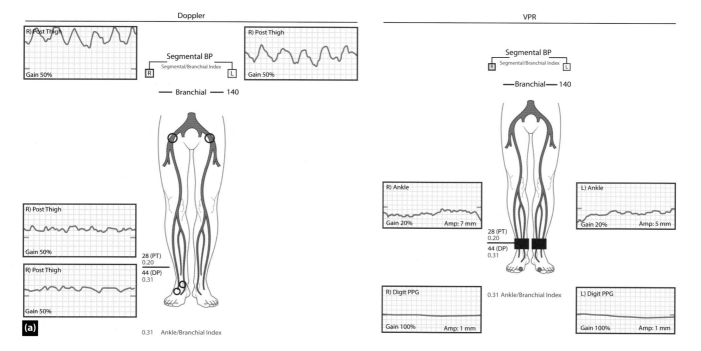

Figure 5.1 76-year-old woman presenting with rest pain in her bilateral lower extremities and no palpable femoral pulses on examination. (**a**) Preoperative ankle–brachial pressure index (ABPI)/pulse volume recording (PVR) of bilateral lower extremities.

(Continued)

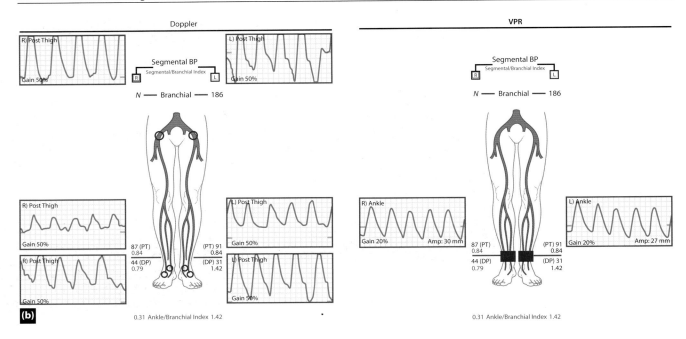

Figure 5.1 (Continued) 76-year-old woman presenting with rest pain in her bilateral lower extremities and no palpable femoral pulses on examination. (**b**) Postoperative ABPI/PVR of bilateral lower extremities.

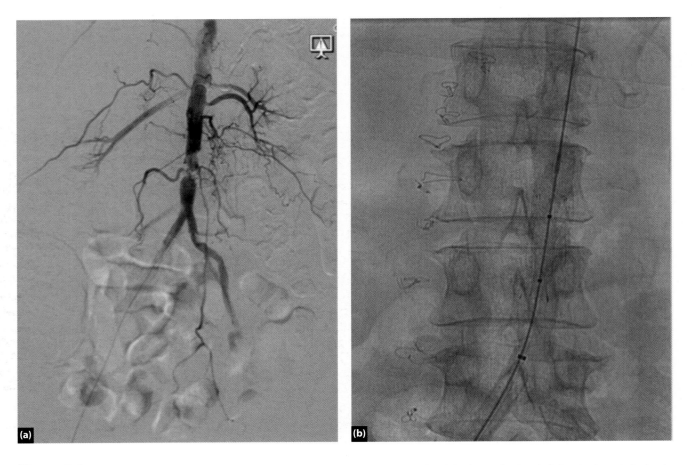

Figure 5.2 Aortogram of 76-year-old woman. (**a**) Aortogram demonstrating a focal, high-grade, distal abdominal aortic lesion in a small aorta. (**b**) Positioning of the 10 mm × 30-mm self-expanding stent (Absolute Pro®; Abbott Vascular, Santa Clara, CA, USA) via right transfemoral approach.

(Continued)

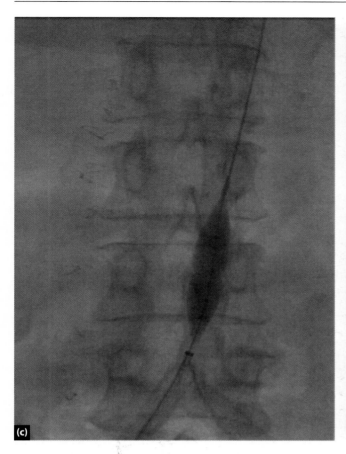
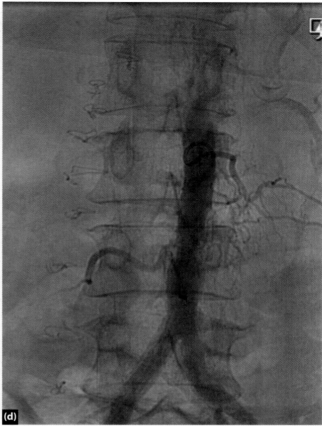

Figure 5.2 (Continued) Aortogram of 76-year-old woman. (**c**) Post-stent deployment balloon angioplasty (10 mm × 30-mm Dorado® catheter; BARD Peripheral Vascular, Inc., Tempe, AZ, USA). (**d**) Completion aortogram demonstrating rapid blood flow through the stented segment with a residual 10–15% waist.

caused plaque rupture, the authors stopped at this point. Postprocedure ABPI/pulse volume recording (PVR) was repeated and demonstrated a significant improvement to 0.81 on the right and 0.84 on the left side.

Case example 2

A 66-year-old woman presented with a 6-month history of rest pain in the left lower extremity. On physical examination, no femoral pulses were palpable, with monophasic dorsalis pedis/posterior tibial pulses obtained bilaterally. Preoperative ABPI/PVR of the bilateral lower extremities was obtained and was 0.31 on the right and 0.28 on the left (**Figure 5.3a**). A preoperative CTA of the abdomen and pelvis was obtained. It demonstrated near-occlusion of the distal aorta just proximal to the bifurcation, with occlusion of the bilateral iliac arteries and reconstitution of CFAs, and severe atherosclerotic disease and superficial femoral artery occlusion. With concomitant bilateral femoral artery disease, bilateral groin cutdown for exposure of femoral arteries was performed. Retrograde recanalization of the iliac arteries was attempted bilaterally via an open surgical field using a hydrophilic guidewire and catheter; however, because of chronic total occlusive lesions, these

attempts were not successful. At this point, the authors proceeded with left brachial artery access and successfully recanalized the distal aorta. A 6-Fr sheath was then advanced over the guidewire to the distal aorta just proximal to the bifurcation, and successfully recanalized via the subintimal plane out into the true lumen under direct vision in the groin cutdown surgical field for both sides (**Figure 5.4a–d**). Next, bilateral external iliac artery (EIA), CIA, and profunda femoris endarterectomy with bovine pericardial patch angioplasty was performed: 2–3 mm of the patch was left open along the middle, medial side; an 8-Fr sheath was introduced; and kissing stent angioplasty of the bilateral CIAs was performed with covered balloon-expandable stents (**Figure 5.4c**) after pre-stent deployment balloon angioplasty with smaller-diameter balloons. The authors ensured that the large lumbar arteries just proximal to the aortic occlusion were not covered by these stents. The bilateral EIAs also successfully underwent angioplasty with uncovered, self-expanding stents. A completion aortogram was then performed and demonstrated excellent rapid blood flow via the stented aorta, and the bilateral CIAs and EIAs; readily palpable common femoral pulses were noted. Postoperatively, much improved Doppler signals at the foot as well as ABPI/PVR (**Figure 5.3b**) were obtained, with resolution of rest pain.

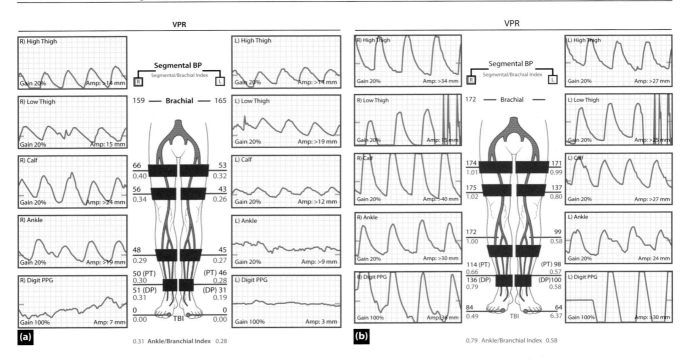

Figure 5.3 66-year-old woman presenting with a 6-month history of rest pain in the lower left extremity. (**a**) Preoperative ankle–brachial pressure index (ABPI)/pulse volume recording (PVR). (**b**) Postoperative ABPI/PVR.

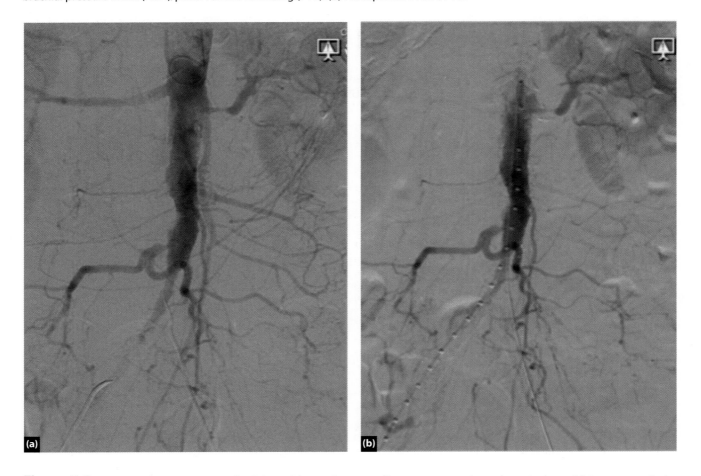

Figure 5.4 Intraoperative aortogram after bilateral femoral artery endarterectomy with patch angioplasty. (**a**) Aortogram via the left transbrachial approach with distal aortic and left proximal common iliac artery (CIA) occlusion, occluded bilateral external iliac arteries (EIAs), with large lumbar arteries. (**b**) Transbrachial recanalization of bilateral iliac arteries with hydrophilic guidewires and retrograde introduction of pigtail marker catheter via the right femoral artery. *(Continued)*

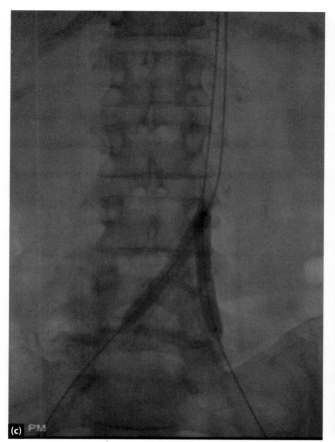
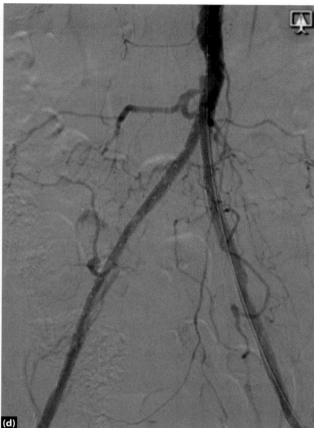

Figure 5.4 (Continued) Intraoperative aortogram after bilateral femoral artery endarterectomy with patch angioplasty. (**c**) Kissing stent angioplasty of bilateral CIAs using covered stents. (**d**) Completion aortogram demonstrating successful recanalization of the aorta, CIAs, and EIAs bilaterally.

SUGGESTED READING

Arko F, Mattauer M, McCollough R, et al. Use of intravascular ultrasound improves long-term clinical outcome in the endovascular management of atherosclerotic aortoiliac occlusive disease. *J Vasc Surg.* 1998;4:614–623.

Bosch JL, Hunink MG. Meta-analysis of the results of percutaneous transluminal angioplasty and stent placement for aortoiliac occlusive disease. *Radiology.* 1997;**204**:87–96.

Gardiner GA Jr., Meyerovitz MF, Stokes KR, et al. Complications of transluminal angioplasty. *Radiology.* 1986;**159**:201–208.

Greiner A, Dessl A, Klein-Weigel P, et al. Kissing stents for treatment of complex aortoiliac disease. *Eur J Vasc Endovasc Surg.* 2003;**26**:161–165.

Henry M, Amor M, Ethevenot G, et al. Percutaneous endoluminal treatment of iliac occlusions: long-term follow-up in 105 patients. *J Endovasc Surg.* 1998;5:228–235.

Henry M, Klonaris C, Amor M, et al. State of the art: which stent for which lesion in peripheral interventions? *Tex Heart Inst J.* 2000;**27**:119–126.

Kashyap VS, Pavkov ML, Bena JF, et al. The management of severe aortoiliac occlusive disease: endovascular therapy rivals open reconstruction. *J Vasc Surg.* 2008;**48**:1451–1457.

Krishnamurthy VN, Eliason JL, Herve PK, et al. Intravascular ultrasound-guided true lumen reentry device for recanalization of unilateral chronic total occlusions of iliac arteries: technique and follow-up. *Ann Vasc Surg.* 2010;**24**:487–497.

Leville CD, Kashyap VS, Clair DG, et al. Endovascular management of iliac artery occlusions: extending treatment to TransAtlantic Inter-Society Consensus class C and D patients. *J Vasc Surg.* 2006;**43**:32–39.

Moise MA, Kashyap VS. Treatment of aortoiliac occlusive disease: medical versus endovascular versus surgical therapy. *Curr Treat Options Cardiovasc Med.* 2011;**13**:114–128.

Murphy TP, Ariaratnam NS, Carney WI Jr., et al. Aortoiliac insufficiency: long-term experience with stent placement for treatment. *Radiology.* 2004;**231**:243–249.

Norgren L, Hiatt WR, Dormandy JA, et al. Inter-Society Consensus for the Management of Peripheral Arterial Disease (TASC II). *J Vasc Surg.* 2007;**45(Suppl S)**:S5–67.

Timaran CH, Ohki T, Gargiulo NJ 3rd, et al. Iliac artery stenting in patients with poor distal runoff: influence of concomitant infrainguinal arterial reconstruction. *J Vasc Surg.* 2003;**38**:479–484.

Upchurch GR, Dimick JB, Wainess RM, et al. Diffusion of new technology in health care: the case of aorto-iliac occlusive disease. *Surgery.* 2004;**136**:812–818.

Whiteley MS, Ray-Chaudhuri SB, Galland RB. Changing patterns in aortoiliac reconstruction: a 7-year audit. *Br J Surg.* 1996;**83**:1367–1369.

6

Percutaneous intervention for femoropopliteal artery occlusive disease

FARAH MOHAMMAD AND TIMOTHY J. NYPAVER

CONTENTS

INTRODUCTION

The femoropopliteal segment is the most common location of lower extremity peripheral arterial occlusive disease. Atherosclerotic lesions within the superficial femoral artery (SFA) tend to be long and diffuse, rending interventions more challenging, both in their approach and durability. Furthermore, the SFA and popliteal arteries are high-resistance and low-flow in character and subject to mechanical stresses from joint flexion, all variables that adversely affect long-term patency of any endovascular intervention. The decision to intervene is based on three factors: (1) symptoms; (2) the natural history of the disease process; and (3) whether the patient will experience a meaningful benefit from a technically successful procedure. Most important is the distinction between claudication, which is non-limb-threatening, from critical limb ischemia (CLI), which is associated with major limb loss. Multiple anatomic classification systems can guide the decision-making process for intervention, the most common of which is the TransAtlantic Inter-Society Consensus (TASC) II classification.[1,2] General recommendations from the TASC Working Group include endovascular treatment for type A and B lesions and open surgical treatment for type D lesions (**Table 6.1**). While there is debate over the treatment methods for types B, C, and even D lesions, conventional bypass achieves outstanding results and should always be considered. In practice, the vascular surgeon must consider a variety of factors, which include the patient's surgical risk, symptom severity, wound depth and extent, ambulatory ability, functional status, and the durability of the planned intervention, to make the most appropriate treatment recommendation.

INDICATION FOR INTERVENTION: CLAUDICATION

Claudication is defined as major muscle group pain with ambulation that occurs at a level below that of atherosclerotic disease. For lesions within the SFA and popliteal artery, this typically occurs in the calf. The natural history of claudication secondary to SFA and popliteal artery occlusive disease is relatively benign with <5% of patients progressing to CLI.[1-4] Confirmation of the disease (measurement of an ankle–brachial pressure index (ABPI) and toe pressures) and risk factor modification are the mandatory initial steps in patient management. Intervention is recommended if the claudication symptoms are severe, progressive, and not well managed with a 45–90-day trial

Table 6.1 TransAtlantic Inter-Society Consensus (TASC) for the management of peripheral arterial disease: classification of femoropopliteal lesions (TASC II)

Lesion type	Description	Recommendation
A	Single stenosis ≤10 cm in length	Endovascular
	Single occlusion ≤5 cm in length	
B	Multiple lesions, each ≤5 cm in length	Endovascular
	Single stenosis or occlusion ≤15 cm (not involving the infrageniculate popliteal artery)	
	Heavily calcified occlusion ≤5 cm in length	
	Single popliteal stenosis	
C	Multiple stenoses or occlusions >15 cm (with or without heavy calcification)	Endovascular or bypass
	Recurrent stenoses or occlusions	
D	Chronic occlusion of CFA or SFA >20 cm (involving the popliteal artery)	Bypass
	Chronic occlusion involving the popliteal artery and proximal trifurcation vessels	

Note: CFA: common femoral artery; SFA: superficial femoral artery.

of medical therapy. Many patients improve their ambulation distance with cessation of tobacco use, a supervised exercise program, lipid-lowering agents, antiplatelet agents, and selective use of cilostazol, and never require intervention.[5] For those with persistent lifestyle-limiting or disabling claudication, evaluation with computed tomography angiography (CTA) is indicated to define the anatomic disease pattern and suitability for endovascular intervention. As lesion length is the major factor affecting long-term patency, it is accurate to imply that the shorter the lesion (i.e., the lower the TASC classification), the more likely the patient is to experience a beneficial and durable intervention.

INDICATION FOR INTERVENTION: CRITICAL LIMB ISCHEMIA

CLI is defined as chronic peripheral arterial disease with either ischemic rest pain or tissue loss with nonhealing ulcers or gangrene.[1,2] This is often associated with an ankle pressure of <40 mmHg or toe pressure of <30 mmHg for rest pain or an ankle pressure of <60 mmHg in patients with tissue loss. A recently introduced classification system, the WIfI (Wound, Ischemia, and foot Infection) classification scheme, adopted by the Society for Vascular Surgery, provides more granular data to allow meaningful analysis of outcomes. This validated scoring system correlates with the overall risk of major amputation and time to wound healing.[6,7] The natural history of CLI, compared with claudication, is considerably worse with >25% of patients progressing to major limb amputation within 1 year. Of those patients initially presenting with CLI, 10–40% will require primary amputation because of major tissue loss, infection, nonreconstructible occlusive disease, nonambulatory status, or high risk of revascularization failure.[1,7,8] Revascularization is recommended in functional patients whenever possible.

An endovascular-first approach has been adopted by many centers specializing in limb salvage, although limited numbers of studies exist directly comparing open

and endovascular options. The BASIL (Bypass versus Angioplasty in Severe Ischemia of the Leg) study, conducted in the United Kingdom, concluded that there was no significant difference at 2 years in amputation-free survival or quality of life measures between those undergoing endovascular treatment compared to bypass surgery for CLI. The surgery group resulted in one-third greater costs than the angioplasty group at 1 year. By 3 years, this difference was no longer significant because of a higher need for reintervention in the angioplasty group. Importantly, endovascular treatment was limited to angioplasty alone.[9] As new endovascular treatment modalities develop, it is anticipated that results for endovascular intervention will improve. The BEST-CLI (Best Endovascular vs. Best Surgical Therapy in Patients with CLI) study is an ongoing multicenter, prospective, randomized study comparing the best endovascular intervention versus the best surgical therapy in the initial treatment of CLI patients. Hopefully this study will yield some guidelines as to what the best initial form of intervention is in these anatomically and medically complex patients.

TECHNIQUES FOR INTERVENTION

Endovascular approach

Once an endovascular approach has been deemed warranted, the set-up in terms of access, imaging, wire crossing, and intervention is critically important to achieve the optimal patient outcome. A hybrid operating endovascular suite provides the optimal resolution and field of view to accomplish these percutaneous interventions, but a mobile C-arm is satisfactory. Anesthesia generally consists of intravenous (IV) sedation with local anesthesia. Groin access is used in most cases; however, the following arteries have also been used: brachial; radial; popliteal; posterior tibial; and anterior tibial. Alternate sites are chosen depending on disease location, any previous aortic operation, and the success of previous attempts. Except in rare cases, the patient is positioned supine; the left arm is tucked, padded, and supported (unless brachial access is used), and the right arm is left out for IV access and monitoring. Common femoral access options include a retrograde puncture contralateral to the diseased section of the SFA versus antegrade ipsilateral to the side of the disease. The authors prefer a retrograde approach, unless there is a contraindication, such as a previous aortobifemoral bypass graft or endovascular aneurysm repair in which the graft bifurcation angle is too steep to successfully pass a sheath to the contralateral side. Also, the presence of significant common

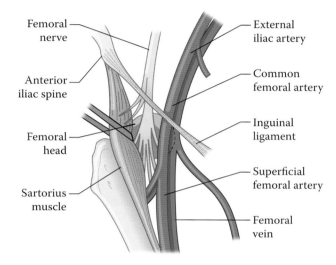

Figure 6.1 Anatomy of the femoral artery and its relationship with the femoral vein and nerve and the underlying femoral head. Anterior iliac spine should read "anterior superior iliac spine." The line indicating the common femoral artery needs to point to the artery distal to the inguinal ligament, so probably need to exchange the positions of "common femoral artery" and "inguinal ligament."

femoral artery (CFA) occlusive disease on the side being punctured (contralateral to the disease being intervened on) represents a relative contraindication to the retrograde approach. Preprocedural maneuvers to limit access site complications include control of hypertension (HTN) and the review of any previous diagnostic angiograms or CTAs. Details about the access artery including its length, concomitant atherosclerotic disease, and the presence of any previously inserted stents are noted.

Vascular access/diagnostic angiography

While topographic and fluoroscopic anatomy can assist femoral artery access, the anatomic relation of the groin crease to the CFA is unreliable. Thus, the authors use adjunctive ultrasound (US) guidance in all cases. US not only guides identification of the CFA and its bifurcation, but also demonstrates arterial calcification and the external iliac-CFA junction. The adjacent common femoral vein is evident by its compressibility. A review of the anatomic relationship of the CFA to the vein, nerve, and adjacent structures is warranted (**Figures 6.1** and **6.2**). If US is not available, fluoroscopic imaging identifies the probable location of the CFA. In >80% of patients, the CFA overlies the medial one-third of the femoral head.

From a procedural standpoint, the US probe and gel are placed in a sterile sleeve. A micropuncture access needle is inserted at 45 degrees directly over the CFA; in most cases, it can be visualized in the CFA lumen (**Figure 6.3**). With blood return, the wire is inserted and the microaccess sheath is placed. Arterial flow is confirmed, a J-tip wire is advanced, and the microaccess sheath exchanged for a 5-Fr sheath. If no prior imaging is available, a full diagnostic aortogram with runoff is performed. With recent imaging available, the plan is for immediate access

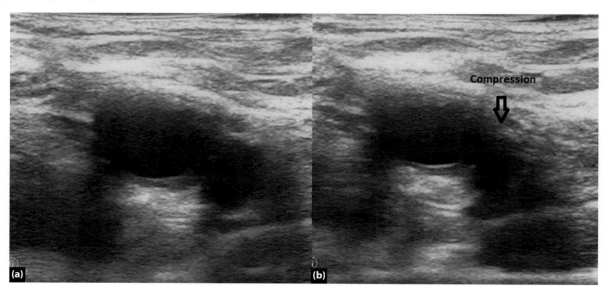

Figure 6.2 Access ultrasound demonstrating the compression of the femoral vein. (**a**) Noncompressed image. (**b**) Image showing femoral vein compression.

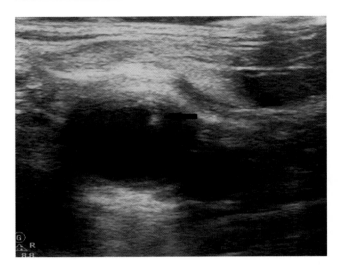

Figure 6.3 Access ultrasound demonstrating the tip of the needle in the lumen of the femoral artery (arrow).

to the symptomatic limb through a retrograde approach and an "up-and-over" technique. The authors favor the Omni™ Flush catheter (AngioDynamics, Latham, NY, USA) for wire passage to the contralateral extremity; however, many catheters can serve this purpose (e.g., Rösch inferior mesenteric (RIM); Cobra 1, 2, 3; pigtail) (**Figure 6.4**). The authors prefer to use a stiff 260-cm, 0.035-inch hydrophilic Glidewire® (Terumo Medical Corporation, Somerset, NJ, USA) for passage to the contralateral extremity. If there is known proximal SFA disease, the Glidewire® is passed into the profunda femoris

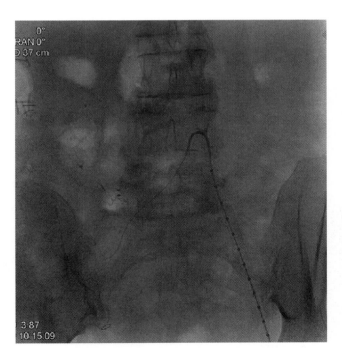

Figure 6.4 Fluoroscopy image of a patient where a flush catheter and advancing guidewire up and over the aortic bifurcation were used.

artery. If the SFA is free of disease, the Glidewire® is positioned into the proximal or mid-SFA. The 5-Fr sheath is removed while maintaining wire position and a 45-cm, 6-Fr Destination® guiding sheath (Terumo Medical Corporation) is advanced over the bifurcation into the CFA. Occasionally, and especially in patients with iliac artery calcification, it may be difficult to obtain contralateral access, and the authors have used other guidewires of increasing stiffness (e.g., Amplatz Super Stiff™; Boston Scientific Corporation, Marlborough, MA, USA) to facilitate placement. An additional technique for crossing a difficult aortic bifurcation is with an angioplasty balloon in the contralateral iliac artery. The balloon is inflated to maintain the position of the stiff guidewire and enhances the ability to track the sheath over the aortic bifurcation. The balloon is slowly deflated while simultaneously advancing the sheath over the balloon catheter. Once access to the contralateral side is achieved, IV heparin is administered (70 IU/kg) and a confirmatory lower extremity angiogram is obtained. To reduce contrast volume and the incidence of contrast-induced nephropathy, the authors liberally employ carbon dioxide (CO_2) angiography in almost all cases, irrespective of baseline creatinine. This is performed via a closed circuit with slow injection of 30 cc of CO_2; it is prudent to wait 2 minutes between injections so that the extra CO_2 equilibrates.

Crossing the lesion

The success of the procedure is directly tied to the ability of the interventionalist to cross the lesion. The authors use a stiff Glidewire® with an angled tip supported by a 135-cm support catheter (Quick-Cross®; Spectranetics Corporation, Colorado Springs, CO, USA) for the initial attempt. If the SFA or popliteal disease has been determined to be a stenosis, the success of crossing these lesions approaches 100%. The Glidewire® and catheter are advanced together with the Glidewire® out 2–3 cm. One looks for deflection of the tip of the Glidewire® and feels for any resistance in advancing the guidewire/catheter combination. The Glidewire® is advanced outward in areas of the disease to "test" or feel the stenosis with the intention of maintaining the wire intraluminally. Once the lesion is crossed, wire resistance dissipates and one advances the support catheter over the Glidewire® and a distal angiogram is performed to confirm the intraluminal position. The authors then pass a stiff 0.014-inch wire through the support catheter, allowing for subsequent passage of any balloons, devices, and stents for the intervention being performed. When the artery is occluded, the authors initially attempt to remain "intraluminal" with a similar approach. If this is unsuccessful, after a relatively short period of time, the authors proceed with crossing the lesion in the subintimal plane—this is accomplished by allowing a loop to form and then advancing the loop past the disease to a predetermined area where the artery reconstitutes and is relatively disease-free (**Figure 6.5**).

With passage of the catheter, the guidewire is straightened out and one attempts to regain access intraluminally. This often occurs spontaneously or with the assistance of an angled catheter. It is important not to allow the subintimal dissection to continue beyond the designated arterial reentry point so as not to destroy a potential target artery for bypass. When unsuccessful, the authors have used reentry devices, such as the OUTBACK® LTD® Re-Entry Catheter (Cordis Corporation, Baar, Switzerland) with very good success in regaining entry back into the lumen (**Figure 6.6**). This is performed by passing the device to the area of reentry, orienting it toward the lumen and advancing the needle forward with the goal of positioning the needle tip intraluminally (**Figure 6.7**). Retrograde access from a distal reconstituted vessel beyond the lesion with bidirectional crossing of the lesion is also an option.

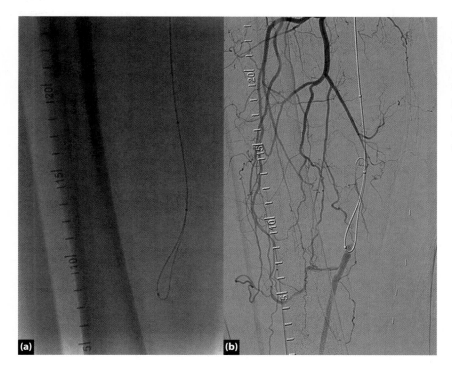

Figure 6.5 The success of the procedure is directly linked to crossing the lesion. (**a**) Fluoroscopy image showing loop created with the stiff Glidewire® (Terumo Medical Corporation, Somerset, NJ, USA) to allow subintimal passage and advancement. (**b**) Subtraction image showing the location of the loop in relationship to the reconstituted popliteal artery.

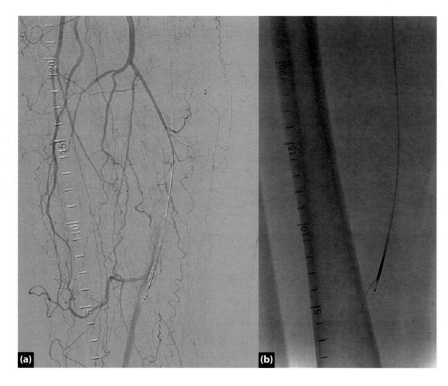

Figure 6.6 Using reentry devices to regain entry back into the lumen. (**a**) Subtraction image showing the appropriate orientation of the reentry catheter in relationship to the artery in preparation for reentry. (**b**) Fluoroscopy image showing successful advancement of the tip of the 0.014-inch wire into the lumen.

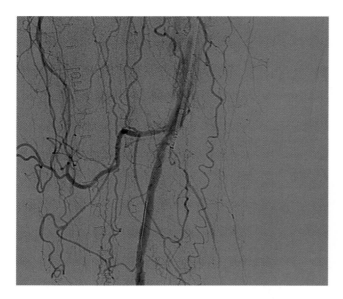

Figure 6.7 Subtraction image showing the 0.014-inch guidewire passed further down into the lumen with confirmation of intraluminal position.

Endovascular management of femoropopliteal stenosis

When the lesion is relatively short (<10 cm in length), the authors presently favor drug-coated balloons (DCBs) (Lutonix®, BARD Peripheral Vascular, Inc., Tempe, AZ, USA; IN.PACT Admiral, Medtronic, Minneapolis, MN, USA) for intervention. Pre-dilation of the lesion is performed with a similarly sized balloon to that of the DCB. The DCB is then used to treat the lesion. If a good technical result is obtained, no further intervention is required. If the lesion intervention results in a significant dissection or residual stenosis (>30%), a self-expanding stent is placed, sizing the stent 1–2 mm over the artery diameter. Longer lesions are treated similarly; however, the authors would be less likely to use DCBs because the likelihood of requiring placement of a self-expanding nitinol stent increases. The authors avoid stents in the popliteal artery if possible, preferring to use a percutaneous transluminal angioplasty balloon catheter (AngioSculpt® PTA Scoring Balloon Catheter, Spectranetics Corporation).

Endovascular management of femoropopliteal occlusion

The management of occlusion, once the lesion is crossed, does not vary significantly from what has been discussed previously. The lesion is dilated with an appropriately sized balloon and re-evaluated angiographically. Once the postangioplasty angiogram is obtained, the authors selectively stent the areas of significant residual disease or dissection. DCBs are reserved for patients with relatively short occlusions or for those lesions through which

they thought the wire passed intraluminally. Alternately, debulking devices, such as the orbital atherectomy device (DiamondBack 360® Peripheral Orbital Atherectomy System, Cardiovascular Systems, Inc., St. Paul, MN, USA) can be used. The theoretical advantage would be to debulk the lesion, following which a DCB is used to try to reduce stent insertion and potentially improve patency. The authors have reserved the use of these debulking devices for lesions that show a high degree of eccentric calcification. Deposition of calcium into the arterial wall has a negative impact on the technical and procedural success of femoropopliteal interventions. This is especially true in those lesions characterized by focal irregular and eccentric calcified atherosclerotic plaque. Calcified lesions decrease the ability to manipulate and advance devices because the inherent drag builds up, preventing and limiting advancement and successful positioning. Sequential balloon dilation to allow the passage of larger devices may be necessary.

COMPLICATIONS

Complications can be divided into access site complications (ASCs) and procedural complications (involving the artery being treated). Risk factors for ASCs include: older age; female sex; smaller body mass index; use of antiplatelets and anticoagulants; uncontrolled HTN; arterial calcification; larger sheath size; therapeutic procedures; and a history of previous catheterization. Common ASCs include hematoma and acute bleeding with an incidence rate of 1.2–8.9%.[10] Multiple unsuccessful access attempts, puncturing of the back wall, and inadequate manual pressure can result in a hematoma and a pseudoaneurysm. Other rare complications include: dissection (0.4%); arteriovenous fistula (0.6%); and thrombosis (0.1%) Nerve injury is rare in femoral access (0.2%) but well documented in transbrachial access with an incidence of 0.4–12.7%. Overall, with the selective use of appropriate closure devices, reversal of anticoagulation (IV protamine sulfate is routinely administered), and enactment of a postprocedural sheath removal policy, including the timing and technique of manual compression, the authors have reduced the risk of ASCs to <2%. Procedural complications include: stent maldeployment; embolization of friable plaque or thrombus; and arterial wall dissection or perforation. Perforation is relatively rare and typically does not lead to significant bleeding. It can be managed with inflation of a balloon matching the size of the artery, providing internal compression. Rarely, a stent graft will have to be deployed.

POSTOPERATIVE RESULTS AND SURVEILLANCE

In general, for stenotic lesions, technical success is at or near 100%. For occlusions, the authors have found that with the approach described previously, technical success is nearly 95%. Endovascular procedures have decreased patency rates compared to open surgery bypass; however, the benefits of a less invasive and morbid procedure often outweigh this reduction in patency. For SFA interventions, patency results have been as poor as 50% at 1–2 years and as high as 75% at 3 years.[11] Of course, endovascular interventions, especially for those lesions in the femoro-popliteal segment, are continually evolving with newer devices and approaches influencing long-term durability. Postprocedurally, the authors have followed any endovascular intervention as they would do with a bypass patient: performance of an ABPI and arterial imaging every 4 months for the first year; every 6 months for the second year; and annually thereafter. While the technical success of femoropopliteal interventions is expected to be high, one must employ sound judgement in the decision and justification to intervene, thereby optimizing patient outcomes both in terms of symptom relief and limb salvage.

REFERENCES

1. Norgren L, Hiatt WR, Dormandy JA, et al. Inter-Society Consensus for the Management of Peripheral Arterial Disease (TASC II). *J Vasc Surg.* 2007;**45(Suppl S)**:S5–67.

2. Dormandy JA, Rutherford RB. Management of peripheral arterial disease (PAD). TASC Working Group. TransAtlantic Inter-Society Consensus (TASC). *J Vasc Surg.* 2000;**31(1 Pt 2)**:S1–296.

3. Kannel WB, Skinner JJ Jr., Schwartz MJ, et al. Intermittent claudication. Incidence in the Framingham Study. *Circulation.* 1970;**41**:875–883.

4. Conte MS, Pomposelli FB, Clair DG, et al. Society for Vascular Surgery practice guidelines for atherosclerotic occlusive disease of the lower extremities: management of asymptomatic disease and claudication. *J Vasc Surg.* 2015;**61(3 Suppl)**:2S–41S.

5. Greenhalgh RM, Belch JJ, Brown LC, et al. The adjuvant benefit of angioplasty in patients with mild to moderate intermittent claudication (MIMIC) managed by supervised exercise, smoking cessation advice and best medical therapy: results from two randomised trials for stenotic femoropopliteal and aortoiliac arterial disease. *Eur J Vasc Endovasc Surg.* 2008;**36**:680–688.

6. Stoner MC, Calligaro KD, Chaer RA, et al. Reporting standards of the Society for Vascular Surgery for endovascular treatment of chronic lower extremity peripheral artery disease. *J Vasc Surg.* 2016;**64**:e1–21.

7. Mills JL Sr., Conte MS, Armstrong DG, et al. The Society for Vascular Surgery Lower Extremity Threatened Limb Classification System: risk stratification based on wound, ischemia, and foot infection (WIfI). *J Vasc Surg.* 2014;**59**:220–234.e1–2.

8. Abou-Zamzam AM Jr., Gomez NR, Molkara A, et al. A prospective analysis of critical limb ischemia: factors leading to major primary amputation versus revascularization. *Ann Vasc Surg.* 2007;**21**:458–463.

9. Bradbury AW, Adam DJ, Bell J, et al. Bypass versus Angioplasty in Severe Ischaemia of the Leg (BASIL) trial: analysis of amputation free and overall survival by treatment received. *J Vasc Surg.* 2010;**51(5 Suppl)**:18S–31S.

10. AbuRahma AF, Robinson PA, Boland JP, et al. Complications of arteriography in a recent series of 707 cases: factors affecting outcome. *Ann Vasc Surg.* 1993;**7**:122–129.

11. Antoniou GA, Chalmers N, Georgiadis GS, et al. A meta-analysis of endovascular versus surgical reconstruction of femoropopliteal arterial disease. *J Vasc Surg.* 2013:**57**:242–253.

7

Percutaneous intervention for infrapopliteal occlusive disease

SARAH E.B. STROT AND ROBERT F. CUFF

CONTENTS

INTRODUCTION

Atherosclerotic peripheral arterial disease (PAD) has a prevalence of 15–20% in those older than 70 years and 3–10% in younger individuals. It affects more than 10 million people in the USA and is more common in those who smoke or have diabetes.[1] The gold standard in limb salvage for infrapopliteal disease resulting in critical limb ischemia (CLI) has long been open surgical revascularization with autologous saphenous vein. Endovascular treatment offers a lower-risk alternative and may be more beneficial for those with medical comorbidities. With the increased availability of endovascular devices and improved skill of interventionalists, there has been a move toward an "endovascular-first" approach for revascularization within the infrapopliteal region.

TREATMENT

Treatment of infrapopliteal disease includes the anterior tibial artery, tibioperoneal trunk, posterior tibial artery, peroneal (fibular) artery, and pedal arteries. This region is plagued with vessels that are often heavily calcified, have diffuse, high-grade stenosis, or even total occlusions. Diffuse involvement of tibial vessels is common within the diabetic population presenting with ischemic foot lesions. Poor distal runoff increases the risk of restenosis which adds to difficult decision-making processes regarding best treatment options.

PATIENT SELECTION

In those with lifestyle-limiting, intermittent claudication due to infrapopliteal PAD, standard of care involves optimizing medical therapy and improving aortoiliac or femoropopliteal inflow disease. If, however, symptoms worsen or are not alleviated with this initial intervention, then it is reasonable to progress toward revascularization of infrapopliteal disease via endovascular means.

ACCESS

There are several ways to access the infrapopliteal arteries, including a retrograde or antegrade femoral and a more recently described retrograde pedal approach. The approach should be decided before the procedure takes place, based on patient and vessel characteristics to anticipate the supplies needed and situate the angiographic suite appropriately, but both groins are typically prepared for access.

It is advisable to access the common femoral artery (CFA) over the femoral head, which can be accomplished with fluoroscopic and ultrasound (US) guidance. Once access is obtained, a hemostatic sheath (typically 5 Fr) is used with a 5-Fr diagnostic catheter for aortography. The sheath will likely need to be exchanged for a longer sheath (55, 70, or 90-cm length) to provide adequate support to cross infrapopliteal occlusions and allow for angiographic imaging with minimal contrast. Intervention of the infrapopliteal region is accomplished with 0.018-inch or 0.014-inch guidewire platforms; therefore, a 5-Fr sheath is usually adequate.

Retrograde femoral approach via the contralateral limb

Infrainguinal disease has traditionally been accessed in a retrograde femoral manner via the contralateral limb and this remains appropriate for intervention within the proximal tibial vessels. This approach allows for an aortogram with runoff to be easily obtained, assessing the need for intervention of inflow disease. The main limits of this approach are the length of guidewires, catheters, and devices required to access and treat the distal tibial lesions and potential difficulty crossing over the aortic bifurcation in some patients.

An up-and-over maneuver crossing the aortic bifurcation with the assistance of a hook-shaped catheter, such as the Omni™ flush (AngioDynamics, Latham, NY, USA), Rösch inferior mesenteric (Cook Medical Inc., Bloomington, IN, USA), or SOS Omni® (AngioDynamics), minimizes the contrast used in patients with normal inflow vessels. Typically, the authors use a stiff, hydrophilic guidewire (Glidewire®; Terumo Medical Corporation, Somerset, NJ, USA) for crossing the aortic bifurcation and tibial occlusions. Access to the target lesion can be attained through retrograde access on the contralateral side with a long sheath up and over the bifurcation. Once the sheath is in place, the patient is systemically heparinized with 50–100 IU/kg for an activated clotting time >250 seconds to avoid thrombosis within the vessel. A long, steerable Glidewire® (Terumo Corporation) or other steerable 0.014- or 0.018-inch guidewire is then used, depending on the characteristics of the lesion, to cross the lesion with the assistance of a hydrophilic catheter. After crossing the lesion with the guidewire, the catheter can be advanced through the lesion and the guidewire removed to obtain angiography confirming runoff and true lumen access before intervention. Supplies that may be encountered during this approach can be found in **Table 7.1**.

Antegrade femoral approach via the ipsilateral limb

An antegrade femoral approach via the ipsilateral limb allows for more distal lesions to be intervened on. This approach also enables better control of the guidewires and catheters and does not require the additional length needed when accessing the contralateral limb. It is beneficial to use an ipsilateral approach if the iliac vessels are known to be tortuous or if the aortic bifurcation is

Table 7.1 Retrograde femoral access via the contralateral limb

Category	Type	Use	Diameter	Length	Notes
Guidewires	Bentson[a]	Starting	0.035 inch	145 cm	Long, soft tip
	Glidewire[b]	Selective, therapy	0.035, 0.018 inch	150, 260 cm	Steerable
	Rosen[a]	Exchange	0.035 inch	180 cm	Sheath placement
	Amplatz[a]	Exchange, therapy	0.035 inch	180 cm	Sheath placement
	Iron Man[c]	Therapy	0.014 inch	190, 300 cm	
Catheters	Omni™ Flush[d]	Flush, selective	4 Fr	65 cm	Multiside hole
	Straight[d]	Flush, exchange	5 Fr	90 cm	
Crossing catheters	DAV[a]	Selective, exchange	4 Fr, 5 Fr	100 cm	Angled tip
	Quick-Cross[e]		0.018, 0.014 inch	90, 135, 150 cm	Straight tip, low profile
Sheaths	Destination®[b]	Guide sheath	5 Fr, 6 Fr	45 cm	Straight
	Flexor® Raabe[a]	Guide sheath	6 Fr	55, 70, 90 cm	Straight

[a] Cook Medical Inc. Bloomington, IN, USA
[b] Terumo Medical Corporation, Somerset, NJ, USA
[c] Abbott Vascular, Santa Clara, CA, USA
[d] AngioDynamics, Latham, NY, USA
[e] Spectranetics Corporation, Colorado Springs, USA.

Table 7.2 Antegrade femoral access via the ipsilateral limb

Category	Type	Use	Diameter	Length	Notes
Guidewires	Wholey™[a]	Starting, selective	0.035 inch	145 cm	Steerable
	Glidewire[b]	Selective, therapy	0.035, 0.018 inch	150, 180 cm	Steerable
	Rosen[c]	Exchange	0.035 inch	180 cm	Sheath placement
	Iron Man[d]	Therapy	0.014 inch	190 cm	
Catheters	Kumpe[c]	Selective, exchange	5 Fr	40 cm	Short, angled tip
Crossing catheters	DAV[c]	Selective, exchange	4 Fr, 5 Fr	65, 70 cm	Angled tip
	Quick-Cross[e]		0.018, 0.014 inch	90, 135, 150 cm	Straight tip, low profile
Sheaths	Standard	Access, guide	5 Fr, 6 Fr	12–55cm	Straight

[a] Medtronic, Minneapolis, MN, USA
[b] Terumo Medical Corporation
[c] Cook Medical Inc.
[d] Abbott Vascular
[e] Spectranetics Corporation

known to be heavily diseased because the up-and-over maneuver is not required. Workspace, however, is somewhat limited and this approach can be more difficult in obese patients.

For this approach, it is best to ensure that the proximal CFA is accessed over the femoral head to more easily enter the superficial femoral artery (SFA). After diagnostic angiography, a steerable guidewire should be advanced anteromedially into the SFA and up to the area of intended treatment. The sheath is upsized if necessary to an appropriately sized French sheath that allows for intervention via the interventionalist's preferred modality; the patient is then systemically heparinized as previously described. Again, low-profile hydrophilic guidewires and catheters could prove beneficial to cross the intended lesion. Supplies that may be useful for this approach can be found in **Table 7.2.**

Retrograde tibial/pedal access

This is an additional option for access if a femoral approach (via the ipsilateral or contralateral side) is ineffective at crossing the diseased segment. Antegrade recanalization of infrapopliteal occlusions can fail in up to 20% of those with CLI.[2,3] Though this technique has mostly been used after failure of antegrade recanalization resulting in an antegrade-retrograde approach (see the case example), a totally retrograde approach has been described.[4] Access to an artery distal to the lesion (tibial or pedal) can be obtained with a micropuncture access kit under US guidance. The foot should be placed in plantar flexion when accessing the dorsalis pedis or anterior tibial artery and with added inversion if accessing the distal peroneal artery. Patients are heparinized following sheath insertion. Commonly, the lesion is crossed with a 0.018-inch wire. Once the lesion is crossed, the guidewire is snared with a microsnare from an antegrade approach and brought through the sheath in the groin. Intervention can then be

performed in an antegrade fashion.[3] A pedal access kit, including an access micropuncture needle, guidewire, and tapered sheath is available from Cook Medical Inc. to help facilitate retrograde pedal access.

TREATMENT MODALITIES

Once access is obtained, the sheath is placed, the lesion is crossed, and angiography confirms that the guidewire is intraluminal, there are several treatment modalities that may be considered. Options available to the interventionalist include angioplasty with standard, drug-coated or cutting balloons, stenting with bare-metal stents (BMS) or drug-eluting stents (DES), or using an atherectomy device.

Percutaneous balloon angioplasty

Balloon angioplasty has long been the predominant endovascular treatment offered and studied. Intervention via percutaneous transluminal angioplasty (PTA) occurs with a radial force exerted causing plaque fracture and intimal injury, which subsequently creates a larger channel. PTA can cause a dissection plane requiring stent placement if the dissection is determined to be flow-limiting. There are several balloons to choose from depending on the lesion characteristics encountered. If multiple lesions are to be treated, the authors recommend PTA to the more distal lesion first and progressing proximally. A cutting balloon may be used if unsuccessful with traditional PTA. The cutting balloon contains microrazors on its surface that cut through regions of intimal hyperplasia during insufflation.

When preparing for balloon insufflation, a mixture of contrast and saline is used so that the balloon can be visualized under fluoroscopy. Sizing of the balloon depends on the diameter of the vessel and the size of the target lesion, keeping in mind that the average diameter of popliteal arteries is 3–6 mm and tibial arteries is 1–4 mm. Balloon length should be chosen based on lesion length so that the balloon does not extend beyond the lesion by a significant amount. Once the balloon is advanced over the guidewire and placed across the lesion, insufflation is initiated and a "waist" is identified, signifying that the lesion has been engaged. The "waist" resolves with increasing balloon pressure and this pressure should be held for 30–60 seconds. The lesion can be ballooned again with a higher pressure or a larger balloon if there is residual stenosis. It is important to be mindful of the nominal and rated burst pressures associated with each type of balloon.

Stent placement

Early elastic recoil in tibial vessels has been shown to occur as early as 15 minutes post angioplasty and may play a significant role in restenosis. To escape early recoil, stent placement has been advocated. Stents have also been used in bailout procedures within the popliteal vessels after PTA if flow-limiting dissection is detected. Both BMS and DES have been used in infrapopliteal disease.

As with PTA, it is important to keep in mind the vessel and lesion characteristics when choosing an appropriate stent. Typically, in the authors' center, lesions are pre-dilated with a balloon before stent placement; this also allows the determination of the luminal diameter. Among the types of stents to choose from are balloon-expandable and self-expanding. Balloon-expandable stents are deployed more precisely and may be dilated past the reported diameter (with some shrinkage in length), but are more rigid and not as suitable for use in mobile or tortuous vessels. Self-expandable stents require better operator stabilization and must be upsized 1–2 mm because they cannot be post-dilated. A post-stent angiogram should reveal adequate diameter of the vessel with brisk flow within the stent and into the distal arteries.

Atherectomy

Atherectomy is performed to remove plaque endoluminally and has been used effectively in PAD. Several devices serve this purpose, but generally they work to cut, shave, sand, or vaporize plaque. As with most endovascular treatment of infrapopliteal disease, more research is necessary before solid recommendations can be made.

CONCLUSION

Endovascular interventions for infrapopliteal PAD continue to evolve and provide additional options for patients with limited surgical targets or conduits, or those who are poor surgical candidates. Improvements in the devices, balloon and stent platforms, and access techniques have improved patency rates and increased the number of patients that are amenable to endovascular treatment. There remain both substantial health care and overall costs to society associated with the management of PAD and CLI. Although new devices may allow for increasingly complex infrapopliteal lesions to be treated, one must weigh treatment with device cost. Each patient with infrapopliteal disease deserves an individualized approach and it is important to adopt a multidisciplinary treatment regimen that comprises the best medical therapy, optimized pre- and postprocedural wound care, revascularization, and postprocedural surveillance with the possible need for future reintervention to achieve the best outcomes.

CASE EXAMPLE

A 63-year-old woman with a history of peripheral vascular disease, ongoing tobacco use, hypertension, coronary artery disease, and a sedentary lifestyle presented with left foot pain and discoloration of her left great toe. She also had a history of a right above-knee amputation after multiple revascularization attempts. The ankle-brachial pressure index was 0.44 on the left and demonstrated a flat photoplethysmographic tracing of the left great toe.

A left lower extremity angiogram revealed diffuse atherosclerotic disease with the tibial vessels completely occluded. There was reconstitution of the anterior tibial artery via collaterals. Atherectomy and balloon angioplasty were completed successfully to more proximal vessels. Occlusion of the anterior tibial artery would not accommodate cannulation from an antegrade approach, so retrograde access of the anterior tibial artery was obtained with a micropuncture kit (Cook Medical Inc.). A V-18™ ControlWire guidewire (Boston Scientific Corporation, Marlborough, MA, USA) was used to cross the occlusion via a retrograde approach. This opened the origin of the anterior tibial artery and access was gained with a guidewire (Glidewire Advantage®; Terumo Medical Corporation) in an antegrade fashion. Angioplasty of the occluded segment was performed resulting in in-line flow to the foot via the anterior tibial artery (**Figure 7.1**).

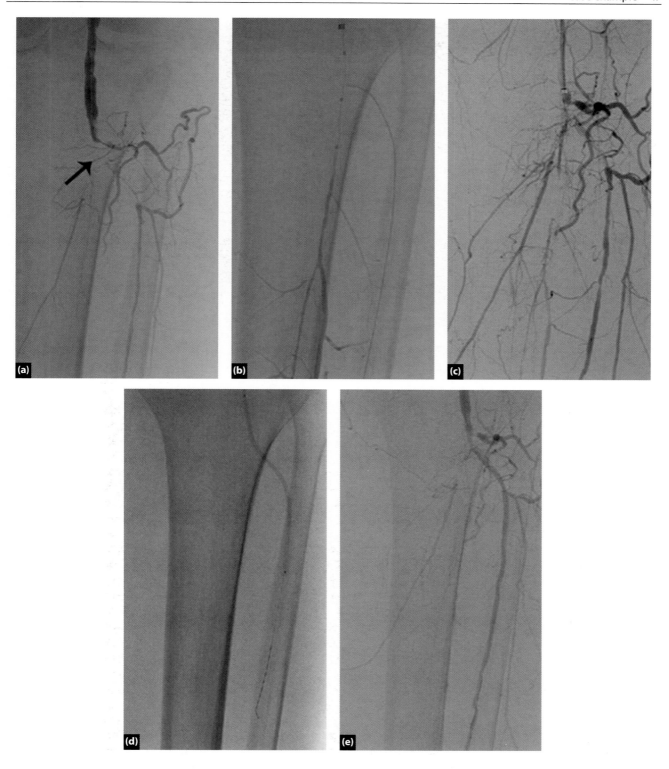

Figure 7.1 Angioplasty of occluded segment in a 63-year-old woman. (**a**) Antegrade approach with occlusion of the anterior tibial origin. (**b**) Retrograde access via the distal anterior tibial artery using a micropuncture kit. A retrograde V-18™ ControlWire guidewire (Boston Scientific Corporation) is shown traversing the anterior tibial artery occlusion and meeting the retrograde access. (**c**) Antegrade guidewire can now enter the anterior tibial artery. (**d**) V-18 wire™ ControlWire with 2.5 × 120-mm balloon for angioplasty of the distal popliteal and anterior tibial arteries. (**e**) Completion angiogram with restored in-line flow to the anterior tibial artery.

REFERENCES

1. Norgren L, Hiatt WR, Dormandy JA, et al. Inter-Society Consensus for the Management of Peripheral Arterial Disease (TASC II). *J Vasc Surg.* 2007;**45(Suppl)**:S5–67.

2. Adam DJ, Beard JD, Cleveland T, et al. Bypass versus angioplasty in severe ischaemia of the leg (BASIL): multicentre, randomised controlled trial. *Lancet.* 2005;**366**:1925–1934.

3. El-Sayed H, Bennett ME, Loh TM, et al. Retrograde pedal access and endovascular revascularization: a safe and effective technique for high-risk patients with complex tibial vessel disease. *Ann Vasc Surg.* 2016;**31**:91–98.

4. Huang ZS, Schneider DB. Endovascular intervention for tibial artery occlusive disease in patients with critical limb ischemia. *Semin Vasc Surg.* 2014;**27**:38–58.

8

Endovascular repair of infrarenal abdominal aortic aneurysms

PAUL G. BOVE

CONTENTS

INTRODUCTION

The endovascular treatment of infrarenal abdominal aortic aneurysms (AAAs) with stent grafts has become the most common mode of treating these aneurysms. Achieving a successful outcome with this intervention requires precise preoperative planning based on high-quality imaging. The surgeon also requires access to high-quality imaging capabilities and comprehensive endovascular tools in the operating room to obtain the best results.

CLINICAL DECISION-MAKING

Generally accepted indications for AAA repair include any patient with a symptomatic AAA, or an aneurysm with a diameter of ≥5.5 cm in a patient with acceptable surgical risk. Repair may also be considered for AAAs with a diameter of 5.0 cm for women or in certain circumstances of progressive growth.

PATIENT SELECTION: ANATOMIC CHARACTERISTICS

To perform a successful repair, the anatomic characteristics of the abdominal aorta, iliac arteries, and common femoral arteries (CFAs) must provide satisfactory proximal and distal seal zones, and adequate access size for delivery of the stent graft (**Figures 8.1–8.3**). The proximal seal zone is the infrarenal aortic neck, which is generally defined as the linear distance between the lowest renal artery (RA) and the aneurysm sac. Most manufacturer's instructions for the use of commercially available stent grafts require an aortic neck length of at least 10–15 mm, with an absolute neck diameter between 18 and 32 mm and no variation in diameter >20% within that distance. Angulation of the aortic neck, from the visceral segment of the aorta to the RAs, and the angle between the aortic neck and the aortic sac also require consideration. An optimal aortic neck angle is <45 degrees, although some devices allow for treatment of more severe angulation. The presence of neck angulation may also have an impact on the decision to use a device with suprarenal fixation. The presence of a densely calcified plaque or significant thrombus within the aortic neck may prevent successful stent graft fixation and sealing. These findings on computed tomography (CT) are usually best accessed with the preset bone windows on the arterial phase or the noncontrast phases. If a significant thrombus or calcified plaque are present, and one proceeds with the endograft, both findings should optimally be <30% of the aortic neck circumference. For most devices, the diameter of the graft is based on the

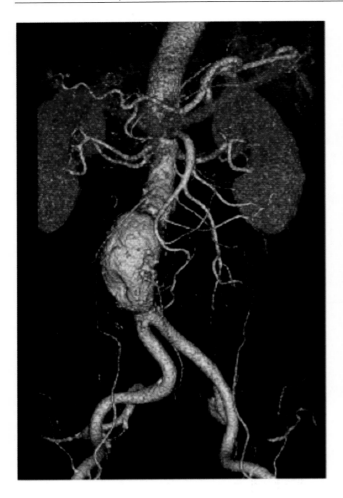

Figure 8.1 Reformatted computed tomography angiography demonstrating a clear anatomic candidate for endovascular aneurysm repair.

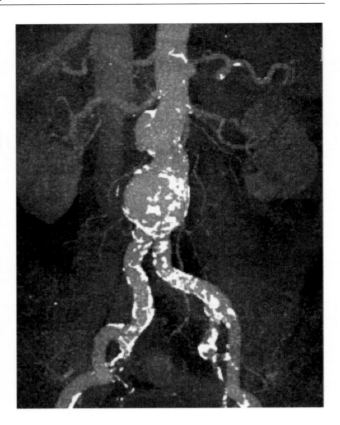

Figure 8.2 Reformatted computed tomography angiography demonstrating anatomy not amenable to endovascular infrarenal abdominal aortic aneurysm repair because of aneurysm proximity to the renal arteries.

diameter of the aortic neck with oversizing of 10–20%. Therefore, each aortic stent graft system will have a variety of sizes and limits of aortic diameters that can be treated.

Next, the iliac arteries are evaluated for an adequate seal zone and, along with the CFAs, for an adequate access size. Seal zones for commercially available devices typically can accommodate arterial diameters of 8–25 mm and require landing zone lengths of typically 20 mm. The optimal scenario would allow adequate lengths of the common iliac artery (CIA) extending to the iliac bifurcations to allow for adequate seal zones for the distal aspect of the grafts. If an inadequate seal zone is present in the CIA, in cases such as aneurysmal dilatation of the CIA, consideration can be made to extend the graft into the external iliac artery (EIA) with coil embolization of the hypogastric (internal iliac) artery (HGA), or preserve the HGA, if possible, with newer branched devices.

Delivery of most main body devices requires the CIAs/EIAs to have a diameter close to 7 mm; delivery of the contralateral limbs requires a diameter close to 5 mm. Along with size, the degree of calcification and tortuosity also need to be evaluated, to determine whether the endograft components

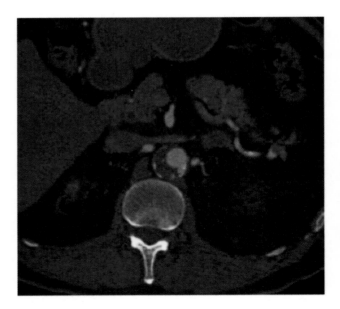

Figure 8.3 Computed tomography angiography demonstrating significant aortic thrombus mandating open aortic reconstruction with a suprarenal clamp.

can be successfully delivered to their intended target sites. If the access vessels are not satisfactory, alternative access measures should be considered. These may include serial dilatation with progressively larger dilators, the performance of balloon angioplasty, or stenting the iliac arteries before advancing the stent graft. In the case of extensive EIA occlusive disease, an access conduit based on the CIA using an 8-mm expanded polytetrafluoroethylene graft from the CIA to the CFA should be created via a small retroperitoneal incision. Endoluminal "paving" can be considered, using covered vascular stents as the iliac system is dilated to an appropriate size to allow passage of the stent graft. Because of advanced atherosclerotic disease in the femoral artery, a femoral endarterectomy may need to be performed.

Once the patient has met the anatomic criteria acceptable for the placement of an aortic stent graft, then the choices of device are numerous. A thorough understanding of the nuances of each type of device being used is mandatory. Having a close working relationship with the industry clinical specialist is always beneficial.

PREPARATION OF PATIENT

As AAAs have a significant association with cardiovascular disease, appropriate assessment and optimization of the comorbidities of surgical candidates is appropriate, with special emphasis on cardiac, pulmonary, and renal disease. For those patients with chronic kidney disease, preprocedural hydration, minimizing the use of iodinated contrast, and using carbon dioxide angiography should be employed to reduce the risk of contrast-induced nephropathy. A thorough assessment should include the identification of any medication allergies; specifically, allergies to iodinated contrast need to be identified and pretreated with diphenhydramine and prednisone.

PROCEDURAL SET-UP

Aortic stent grafting is performed in a sterile operating room with high-quality imaging, preferably a fixed fluoroscopic imaging unit or, if not available, a mobile C-arm. The imaging table should allow for fluoroscopic visualization of the entire length of the body. Appropriate radiation safety measures should be employed. The patient is positioned and, after inserting a Foley catheter, is prepped and draped from the level of the nipples to the knees. Generally, a radial arterial line is inserted as well as adequate large-bore venous access. With supportive anesthesia staff, these procedures can be performed with general anesthesia, regional anesthesia, or in select cases local anesthesia and sedation. Preoperative antibiotics are administered intravenously within an hour of initiation of the procedure, with redosing up to every 4 hours as needed based on the antimicrobial agent chosen.

A comprehensive inventory of endovascular tools is necessary, including access sheaths, multiple guidewire varieties, including soft-tip access guidewires, angled hydrophilic guidewires and stiff support wires for the delivery of the endograft, as well as simple directional catheters to aid in advancing the guidewires, and multihole pigtail catheters. A variety of balloons and stents to perform angioplasty or stenting if necessary should also be available, and an aorta-sized balloon to aid in fixation of the graft at the end of the procedure as well as serving as an aortic occlusion balloon if necessary. The availability of covered stents may be necessary to treat iliac arterial trauma due to delivery systems or angioplasty ruptures. Having long instrument tables that can accommodate the length of the devices and guidewires is helpful; positioning these near the foot of the operating room table in an "L" configuration can be advantageous.

ACHIEVEMENT TO ACCESS VESSELS

Traditionally, access is obtained by direct exposure of the femoral arteries. This can be performed with vertical or oblique incisions. Data suggests that fewer surgical site complications may occur with the oblique technique. The dissection should extend from the inguinal ligament to the femoral bifurcation; vascular control can be performed with vessel loops on the CFA and its branches. Adequate access is needed to insert the access needle, delivery sheaths, and ultimately the device. The presence of atherosclerotic disease in this location does not usually mandate femoral endarterectomy, but this can be considered. When adequately sized, disease-free femoral arteries are present, percutaneous access can be achieved with the assistance of the Perclose ProGlide® Suture-Mediated Closure System (Abbott Vascular, Santa Clara, CA, USA).

PERFORMANCE OF THE PROCEDURE

Each device has its unique deployment methods and each graft is engineered differently; therefore, it is beyond the scope of this chapter to discuss the nuances of each available device. Most commercially available aortic stent grafts are based on modular components that include a bifurcated main body and component overlapping iliac limbs. The following discussion is meant to be a description of such a stent grafting technique.

INITIAL IMAGING, ACCESS, MAIN BODY POSITIONING, AND DEPLOYMENT

Having obtained femoral access, a marked pigtail catheter is inserted into the abdominal aorta through the side predetermined to be contralateral to the main body, and an abdominal aortogram is performed. This allows confirmation of the arterial anatomy with regard to the lengths, diameters, and side of delivery for the devices that have been preselected. Therapeutic heparin is given and monitored with activated clotting times after the initial bolus and at 30-minute intervals. Via the side chosen for delivery of the main body

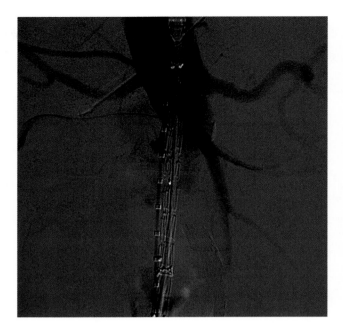

Figure 8.4 Magnified fluoroscopic imaging of an aortic stent graft with radiopaque markers demonstrating the limits of the covered portion of the stent graft to the renal artery level. Note that the image includes the contralateral gate.

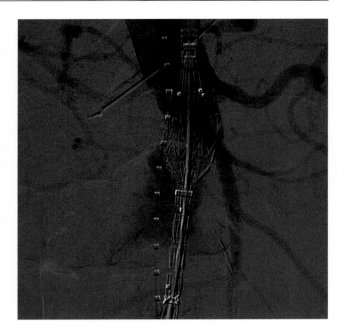

Figure 8.5 Partial deployment of the aortic body now positioned immediately below the lowest renal artery.

graft (ipsilateral side), a stiff support wire (Lunderquist® Extra-Stiff Wire Guide; Cook Medical Inc., Bloomington, IN, USA) is advanced through the femoral artery up into the descending thoracic aorta. The exact location of this stiff delivery wire should be confirmed with fluoroscopy to ensure that it is not within the aortic arch; the location of the end of the wire on the table is noted with a surgical marker for a reference point. Placement of this stiff wire also offers an opportunity to evaluate how the guidewire will react to tortuous anatomy involving either the aorta or the iliac arteries. The main body of the bifurcated device is oriented with respect to the contralateral limb and its intended position within the patient and is loaded onto a stiffened wire and advanced into the abdominal aorta. If significant resistance is encountered, passing serial tapered dilators, performing balloon angioplasty, or attempting contralateral main body access may be considered. The main body delivery system is positioned so that the most proximal portion that is covered with fabric is at the level of the RAs. Because the proximal aortic neck often has some degree of anterior angulation, and often some lateral angulation, appropriate cranial-caudal adjustment and lateral adjustment of the C-arm is performed to optimize imaging of the aortic neck and location of the RAs. The magnification of the fluoroscopy unit should be increased to allow focused visualization of the aortic landing zone, to clearly identify the lowest RA and include the gate of the docking limb within the field of view to avoid the need to move the fluoroscopy unit during deployment. Angiography is then performed and the lowest RA is identified (**Figure 8.4**). Once the graft position is optimized with respect to the RAs and the intended deployment

position of the contralateral docking gate, the main body may be deployed. Initially, it is deployed partially and repeated imaging is performed to ensure stable position in relation to the RAs (**Figure 8.5**); once this is accomplished, it is deployed to allow the docking section to emerge. For grafts with suprarenal fixation, this is deployed at this point. Frequently, positioning the docking gate somewhat anteriorly or even in a manner that will result in crossed iliac limbs can facilitate cannulation of the docking gate.

ILIAC DEPLOYMENT AND COMPLETION OF THE PROCEDURE

Next, the pigtail catheter is straightened and brought back to within the aortic sac. On occasion, the pigtail catheter itself may be used as a directional catheter to access the contralateral docking gate. More commonly, directional catheters, such as an angled catheter or a "shepherd's hook" design, will be used to assist in this maneuver with the aid of a hydrophilic guidewire. Once the docking gate has been accessed, it is crucial to confirm that it has been successfully accessed either by verifying that a pigtail catheter can rotate freely or by using contrast angiography. Another confirming maneuver is to rotate the fluoroscopy unit through the oblique positions to ensure that the guidewire remains within the confines of the framework of the docking section.

Once cannulation of the contralateral gate is confirmed, a stiffened support wire is advanced through the contralateral iliac system and into the docking limb through a catheter and it is positioned in the descending thoracic aorta. A marker pigtail catheter is placed on the wire with the markings aligned with the docking gate of the graft and into the iliac system. A retrograde iliac angiogram is performed through the contralateral sheath to verify the length of the iliac limb, and define and mark the iliac landing zone (**Figure 8.6**). Imaging of the iliac system and docking section should be optimized; often, oblique imaging is needed to visualize the origin of the internal iliac artery (IIA).

The pigtail catheter is removed and the appropriate iliac limb is advanced over the supportive guidewire and into the docking section and deployed according to the roadmap image. Once the contralateral limb is deployed and the delivery system is removed, then the iliac portion of the main body is deployed fully and the delivery system removed from the body according to the manufacturer's instructions. Additional iliac components are placed at this time as needed, as in the case of a bimodular device or if additional distal iliac coverage is needed.

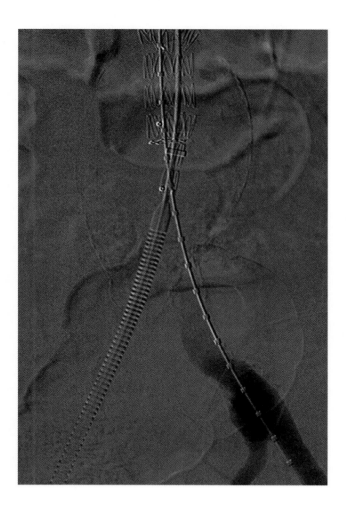

Figure 8.6 Retrograde iliac angiography performed with the marked pigtail catheter left in place. Note is made of the distance from the intended landing zone within the docking section to the intended iliac landing zone. The docking section is positioned so that the iliac limbs are crossed to facilitate cannulation of the docking section. Optimization of docking section location can be performed with any of the modular type devices.

The presence of iliac aneurysmal disease can alter the treatment algorithm. If a patient's CIAs are dilated to 28 mm, there is an option to treat the CIA with a large iliac limb or aortic cuff to achieve a seal. Alternatively, or for CIAs >28 mm, it is common to occlude the IIA (this can be performed in a staged manner with an earlier procedure) with a variety of devices including intravascular plugs, embolization coils, and embolization balloons. Once this is performed, the iliac limb is extended to the EIA. This transition point from CIA to EIA can be a point of kinking of the device that can contribute to early or late thrombosis; therefore, any significant stricture should be studied and treated, if necessary, to prevent limb occlusion. There are devices available now that can potentially save IIAs; snorkel techniques can be used to maintain internal iliac flow, particularly if both IIAs are at risk.

Having deployed all components of the stent graft, a low-pressure aortic balloon is advanced through each iliac system, up into the abdominal aorta, to press the aortic graft throughout the aortic seal zone, fully expand any overlapping components, and press the iliac portions of the grafts throughout both iliac seal zones. Care should be taken not to be too zealous because even a low-pressure balloon that is aggressively overinflated can cause vessel rupture of the treated segment or device failure due to rupturing the graft material itself.

A completion aortogram is performed with the pigtail catheter at the level of the RAs to confirm position, proximal seal, and RA patency (**Figure 8.7**). Fluoroscopic imaging

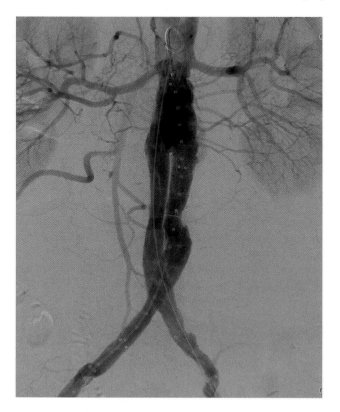

Figure 8.7 Completion angiogram demonstrating patency of the graft and native anatomy without obvious endoleak.

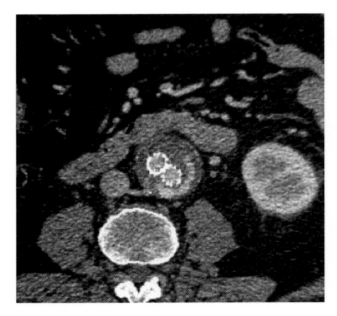

Figure 8.8 Computed tomography image of a type II endoleak from both lumbar and inferior mesenteric arteries with aneurysm growth requiring treatment.

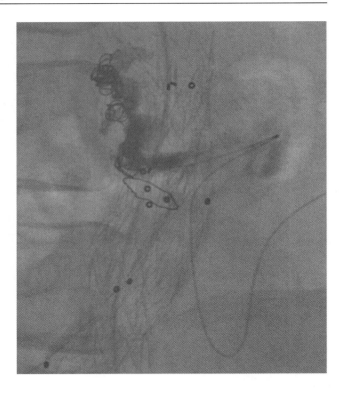

Figure 8.9 Coil embolization of the inferior mesenteric artery through the superior mesenteric and meandering arteries.

is prolonged to visualize any endoleaks. Commonly, the pigtail catheter is then drawn into the aortic graft for an additional injection to evaluate the iliac seal zones and IIA patency, and any evidence of type IB endoleaks. If there are concerns for a type I endoleak, additional angioplasty or aortic or iliac cuff placement may be necessary. Significant impingement on a RA can be addressed. If there is concern of kinking of iliac components as they transition into the iliac arteries, additional supportive stents, either covered or uncovered, may be necessary to treat any significant dissections in the iliac arteries. Once satisfactory insertion of the stent graft has been confirmed, the sheaths and catheters are removed. If an open surgical exposure was performed, the artery access sites are typically closed primarily with polypropylene suture in a transverse manner. More severely diseased atherosclerotic arteries may require endarterectomy and patch angioplasty. Percutaneous access is closed using the pre-close technique. For the percutaneous method of access, it is the author's preference to address the main body delivery site first, and once successful the contralateral side. After ensuring satisfactory distal lower extremity arterial perfusion, protamine sulfate may be administered.

POSTOPERATIVE CARE AND FOLLOW-UP

It is not uncommon for a patient to be able to be discharged within 48 hours, provided they have an uneventful course. Routine postoperative care for the aortic stent graft patient includes adequate volume hydration, with attention to

significant comorbidities, such as renal dysfunction and cardiopulmonary comorbidities. Adequate postoperative pain control is necessary and often requires the use of intravenous narcotics immediately perioperatively with a quick transition to oral analgesics. Monitoring of the patient's postoperative vascular status needs to be documented, as well as a period of hemodynamic monitoring to assess for any serious perioperative complications.

Lifelong follow-up is mandatory, because delayed complications, such as limb thrombosis, further aneurysmal degeneration of the aorta or iliac arteries, or aneurysm growth due to an endoleak may occur (**Figures 8.8 and 8.9**). Typically, postoperative imaging consisting of CT angiography (CTA) of the abdomen and pelvis (including delayed imaging) is carried out, with follow-up at 1 month, every 6 months during the first year, and annually thereafter with either CTA or possibly aortic duplex imaging as determined by what is most appropriate for that specific patient.

SUGGESTED READING

Chaikof EL, Brewster DC, Dalman RL, et al. The care of patients with an abdominal aortic aneurysm: the Society for Vascular Surgery practice guidelines. *J Vasc Surg.* 2009;**50**:S2–49.

9

Endovascular repair of iliac artery aneurysms

SHRUTI SEVAK AND GRAHAM W. LONG

CONTENTS

INTRODUCTION

Iliac artery aneurysms (IAAs) occur in 40% of patients with abdominal aortic aneurysms (AAAs) or as isolated entities. Approximately 80% affect the common iliac artery (CIA), with 20% involving the internal iliac artery (IIA). External iliac artery (EIA) aneurysms are rare. Patients with both AAA and CIA aneurysms have a greater likelihood of bilateral disease, while only 25% with isolated CIA aneurysms are bilateral.

Arterial degeneration remains the most common etiology with infection, anastomotic disorders, dissection, trauma, and collagen vascular disorders comprising the remainder. Risk of rupture remains the primary indication for repair. Up to 30% of patients with isolated IAAs present with rupture, which carries a 30–50% mortality. Given their deep location within the pelvis, IAAs are difficult to palpate on physical examination and are usually found incidentally on imaging performed for other indications or at the time of rupture. Others arise when the aneurysm enlarges to compress surrounding pelvic structures, such as the ureter or iliac veins, causing hydronephrosis, limb swelling, or venous thrombosis.

There is no consensus on either the annual risk of rupture for an IAA of a given size or the threshold for elective repair. In asymptomatic patients with isolated IAAs and acceptable risk factors, it is reasonable to proceed if the aneurysm diameter is 3–4 cm in size. Likewise, the threshold for elective repair based on aneurysm growth rate has not been defined.

ENDOVASCULAR APPROACH

Open surgical repair of IAAs is technically challenging because of their location deep within the pelvis. Blood loss from iliac vein injury and intestinal or ureteral injury are significant risks of this operation. Damage to sympathetic and parasympathetic nerves, resulting in erectile dysfunction or retrograde ejaculation, are additional risks. An endovascular approach mitigates these difficulties. It can be used for both primary degenerative iliac aneurysms and anastomotic pseudoaneurysms, but only as a bridge to definitive therapy in mycotic aneurysms. In addition, it provides an alternative in patients with prior abdominal or pelvic surgery or radiation, or in those at high risk because of medical comorbidities. Caution is advised in pursuing an endovascular approach for patients with venous or ureteral compressive symptoms, because the aneurysm is not sufficiently decompressed immediately after endograft placement resolve these symptoms.

Preoperative considerations

Preoperative computed tomography angiography (CTA) with three-dimensional reformatting is recommended for endograft sizing and planning. This study will demonstrate the size and extent of aneurysmal disease, length of proximal and distal landing zones, and degrees of vessel tortuosity and calcification. Digital subtraction angiography and intravascular ultrasound (US) may be used as adjuncts in obtaining length and diameter measurements. Potential proximal and distal landing zones are measured distal to the aortic bifurcation and proximal to the IIA ostium, respectively. In patients with an isolated CIA aneurysm with adequate proximal and distal landing zones, the diseased segment can be excluded with a covered stent or endograft limb. However, if there is a concomitant AAA, or if the proximal landing zone is <10–15 mm long, a bifurcated endograft is required.

If the IAA extends to its bifurcation, a decision is made as to which of a variety of options should be taken to obtain a distal seal. Optimally, antegrade flow is maintained in the IIA to prevent pelvic ischemic symptoms. These include buttock claudication, rectal ischemia, and erectile dysfunction. More serious complications include gluteal muscle necrosis and spinal cord infarction. These complications are more likely with bilateral IIA involvement or when a patent inferior mesenteric artery is covered by a bifurcated endograft. Ascertaining a widely patent superior mesenteric artery without the presence of an arc of Riolan or marginal artery of Drummond on CTA is an important aspect of planning when a bifurcated endograft is contemplated for IAA repair.

Listed here are the most common techniques used, each of which will be described in turn: (1) coil embolization/plug with endograft extension; (2) bell-bottom iliac limb; (3) iliac branch device; (4) snorkel technique; (5) EIA-IIA bypass with endograft extension; and (5) combined open and endovascular approach.

Coil embolization/plug with endograft extension

In cases where CIA dilation extends to or past the IIA orifice, an endograft can be extended unilaterally or bilaterally into the EIA, covering the IIA ostium. Periodically, coverage of the ostium by the endograft will prevent a type II endoleak. More frequently, it is necessary to actively exclude the IIA system. It should be preferentially occluded at its origin, proximal to the anterior and posterior divisions, to maximize pelvic collateral flow.

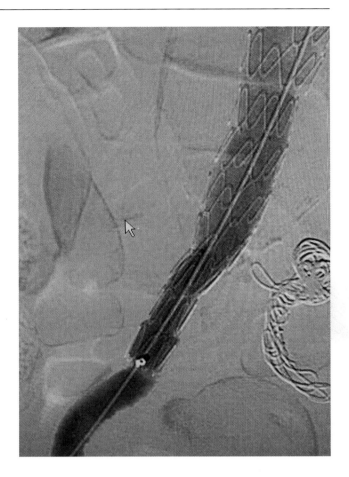

Figure 9.1 Completion digital subtraction angiogram after internal iliac artery coil embolization with iliac limb extension into the external iliac artery. Note the eggshell calcification of the aneurysm sac with no contrast opacification to suggest an endoleak.

This is achieved either by coil embolization (Cook Medical Inc., Bloomington, IN, and Penumbra, Inc., Alameda, CA, USA), placement of an Amplatzer™ vascular plug (St. Jude Medical, St. Paul, MN, USA), or surgical ligation of the IIA (**Figure 9.1**). Each of these can be performed simultaneously with endograft placement or in a staged fashion. In the case of bilateral CIA aneurysms, the IIAs are addressed in a staged fashion 4–6 weeks apart to allow pelvic collateral vessels to hypertrophy and lessen the risk of pelvic ischemia.

Procedurally, access to the IIA is achieved either from the ipsilateral or contralateral femoral artery, and less frequently with a left brachial artery approach. The patient is given systemic heparin (80 IU/kg) to decrease intraoperative thrombotic and embolic complications. Using the ipsilateral femoral approach, wire access is gained to the IIA using a recurved catheter (Rösch inferior mesenteric (RIM), Cobra; Cook Medical Inc.) and hydrophilic wire. Preferentially, a coaxial system consisting of a 30-cm, 5-Fr sheath, catheter, and 0.035-inch wire is used to achieve a stable platform and decrease the potential for inadvertent loss of access and coil placement into the femoropopliteal system. Alternatively, a coaxial system comprised of a 5-Fr catheter and a microcatheter and wire (PROGREAT® Microcatheter; Terumo Corporation, Somerset, NJ, USA) is placed into the IIA with 0.018-inch coils placed in sufficient numbers to markedly decrease contrast flow through the IIA outflow.

Periodically, the angle between the EIA and IIA is too acute to allow a catheter/guidewire combination to pass, and one of the other approaches is used. Using the contralateral common femoral approach, a RIM, Cobra, or SOS Omni catheter (Cook Medical Inc.) is used to cannulate the contralateral CIA and a hydrophilic wire is advanced into the iliofemoral artery system. A straight catheter is advanced over the aortic bifurcation into the superficial femoral artery. The hydrophilic wire is replaced with a stiff wire. The original groin sheath and straight catheter are exchanged for a 5-Fr or 6-Fr, 55-cm sheath that is advanced over the aortic bifurcation into the CIA. The IIA is addressed in the manner described earlier. The left brachial approach involves 5-Fr sheath placement under US guidance, with cannulation of the descending thoracic aorta with a RIM catheter and a 260–300-cm long stiff hydrophilic wire, which is used to cannulate the CIA aneurysm. A long 5-Fr or 6-Fr sheath or guide catheter of at least 90 cm is used to have sufficient length to advance it into the IIA. Once the IIA is addressed, the iliac endograft limb is extended from the proximal bifurcated endograft gate or the proximal CIA neck into the EIA to obtain a distal seal. Contrast arteriography is performed to rule out technical problems, assess correct endograft positioning, and visualize any endoleaks.

Bell-bottom iliac limb

This technique involves the use of a flared cuff, or "bell bottom," that anchors the stent graft device within a dilated distal CIA, preserving IIA patency and creating a seal. There are two approaches with this technique. The first involves a commercially available iliac limb in which the distal aspect is flared to varying sizes, the largest of which is 28 mm, and is oversized by 10–20% (**Figure 9.2**). The second approach is designated for CIA aneurysm diameters larger than the commercially available flared limbs. Planning for this strategy involves using a commercially available flared limb, keeping it short enough so that an aortic extension component can be telescoped into it distally without covering the IIA orifice. The aortic extension segment overlap is 50% within the proximal limb and 50% in the native CIA, which is sufficient to form a seal in each (**Figure 9.3**). The Zenith Flex® (Cook Medical Inc.), Endurant® II Stent Graft System (Medtronic, Minneapolis, MN, USA), and GORE® EXCLUDER® AAA Endoprosthesis (W. L. Gore & Associates, Inc., Flagstaff, AZ, USA) endografts have aortic extension components that can be used for this strategy. This approach is limited by the size of the CIA, since the largest-diameter aortic extension is 36 mm. It is helpful in patients with bilateral

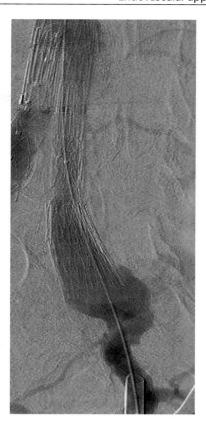

Figure 9.2 Completion digital subtraction angiogram of a flared iliac endograft limb to obtain a distal seal of a common iliac artery aneurysm, maintaining antegrade flow in the internal iliac artery.

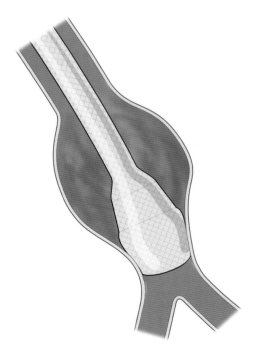

Figure 9.3 Diagram of a flared iliac endograft limb with an aortic endograft extension in place to obtain a seal of a larger iliac artery aneurysm.

CIA aneurysms, where one IIA is preserved and the other treated using the coil embolization/endograft extension strategy.

Iliac branch device

Each of the two techniques described in the previous sections has a potential issue regarding pelvic ischemia/buttock claudication versus distal type I endoleak. Iliac branched devices (IBDs) were designed to circumvent these risks by maintaining antegrade flow in the IIA. An IBD can be used with or without a conventional AAA stent graft and is composed of an iliac endograft limb with either a straight or helical side branch. A third iteration is a bifurcated-bifurcated endograft, which consists of a single-component bifurcated main body, attached iliac limb, and iliac limb side branch. It was designed for use in short-length CIA aneurysms (**Figure 9.4**). The GORE® EXCLUDER® Iliac Branch Endoprosthesis (W. L. Gore & Associates) is approved for use worldwide; the Zenith® Branch Iliac Endovascular Graft (Cook Medical Inc.) is in clinical trial in the USA, but it is available outside the USA. The helical and bifurcated-bifurcated devices from Cook Medical Inc. are available outside of the USA.

In terms of their placement, the straight and helical devices are delivered in a 20-Fr sheath with a preloaded wire and catheter passing external to its distal portion, entering the branch ostium and common iliac segment,

and exiting the sheath along a grooved pusher device. This wire is snared from the contralateral groin to establish through-and-through access. The proximal endograft and side branch are deployed and a 10–12-Fr sheath is inserted over the through-and-through wire directly into the branch from which wire access is gained into the IIA. The minimum requirements to accommodate the 12-Fr sheath passage over the aortic bifurcation and into the iliac branch are a 50-mm CIA aneurysm length and a 20-mm distal CIA diameter. A coaxial 7-Fr 45cm sheath is placed through the 12-Fr sheath into the IIA main body. A covered stent (iCAST™, Atrium Medical Corporation, Hudson, NH; GORE® VIABAHN®, W. L. Gore & Associates; Fluency® Plus, BARD Peripheral Vascular, Inc., Tempe, AZ, USA) is delivered through the 7-Fr sheath over a stiff wire, bridging the iliac branch and the IIA landing zone. The iliac branch device is proximally bridged with the aortic device using an iliac extension limb (**Figure 9.5**).

To deliver the bifurcated-bifurcated device, it is placed in the infrarenal position, and the helical branch is cannulated from the contralateral side by a fenestration opposite and superior to the branch ostium, which is later sealed by overlying endograft. A preloaded wire within the fenestration is snared from the contralateral groin and a 9–10-Fr

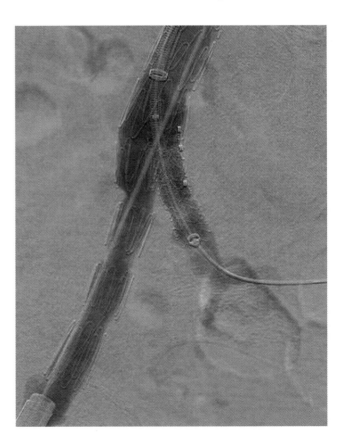

Figure 9.5 Completion digital subtraction angiogram of a patent iliac branch device with no kink or endoleak. The 12-Fr sheath is in place from the contralateral side with a coaxial 7-Fr sheath for deployment of the balloon-expandable bridging stent between the iliac branch and native internal iliac artery.

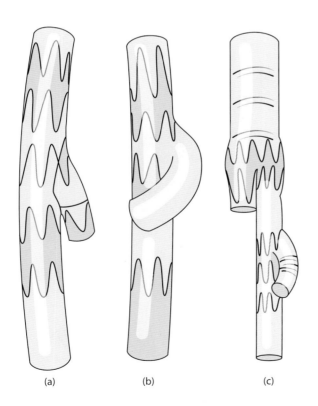

(a)　　　　(b)　　　　(c)

Figure 9.4 Images of iliac branch devices. (**a**) Straight iliac branch. (**b**) Helical iliac branch. (**c**) Bifurcated-bifurcated device.

Flexor sheath (Cook Medical Inc.) is placed to allow IIA access and stenting. The contralateral limb and proximal infrarenal aortic extension are placed in the standard fashion.

Snorkel technique

In this off-label approach, extensive preoperative planning is required to ascertain the appropriate iliac limb and covered stent lengths and diameters, and the IIA and EIA landing zones. A Powerlink® bifurcated stent graft (Endologix, Inc., Irvine, CA, USA) is deployed first. Because this endograft bifurcation sits on the native aortic bifurcation, the IIA adjacent to the CIA aneurysm can be cannulated with a 9-Fr Flexor sheath from the contralateral side. An 8–10 mm × 10-cm GORE® VIABAHN® (W. L. Gore & Associates) device is positioned from the distal IIA up to the proximal edge of the proximal iliac limb. An iliac limb extension of the same diameter as the proximal iliac limb is positioned from the ipsilateral side with sufficient length to line up with the proximal limb and extend into the ipsilateral EIA with a 2.5–3-cm overlap. The two devices are deployed and post-dilated simultaneously with appropriately sized balloons (**Figure 9.6**).

EIA-IIA bypass with endograft extension

In cases where preservation of the IIA system is necessary, such as with a contralateral IIA occlusion, a surgical bypass graft can be extended from the common femoral artery or distal EIA to the IIA main trunk to preserve pelvic flow. The IIA ostium is ligated and the iliac endograft limb extended into the proximal EIA to obtain a distal seal of the CIA aneurysm (**Figure 9.7**).

Combined open and endovascular approach

This alternative is helpful in patients with large bilateral CIA aneurysms, where it is not possible to obtain a distal seal with a flared limb in the distal CIA. An aorto-uni-iliac endograft that extends into the EIA, ipsilateral IIA embolization coils, and a femorofemoral artery bypass graft are placed. A covered stent is placed from the contralateral EIA to the IIA. This latter reconstruction is termed an endovascular EIA-to-IIA bypass. Procedurally, after cannulation of the IIA from the ipsilateral EIA, a stiff guidewire (Amplatz Super Stiff™ or Rosen; Boston Scientific, Marlborough, MA, USA) is placed. A 10–12-Fr, 30-cm Flexor sheath is softened in hot water and passed

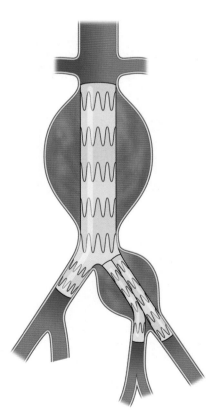

Figure 9.6 Diagram of completed Powerlink® bifurcated stent graft (Endologix, Inc., Irvine, CA, USA) with side-by-side stent grafts extending from the iliac limb into the internal and external iliac arteries, sealing off a large common iliac artery aneurysm.

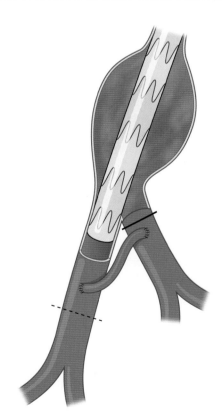

Figure 9.7 Diagram of a completed distal external iliac (EIA)-internal iliac (IIA) artery bypass graft with proximal IIA ligation (solid line) and iliac endograft limb extension into the proximal EIA to achieve distal seal of a large common iliac artery aneurysm. The dotted line represents the inguinal ligament.

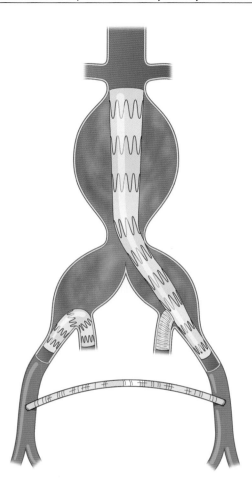

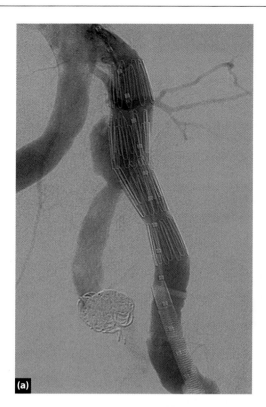

Figure 9.8 Diagram of an aorto-uni-iliac endograft with ipsilateral internal iliac artery (IIA) coil embolization, femoro-femoral artery bypass graft, and endovascular external iliac-IIA bypass for bilateral large common iliac artery aneurysms.

to the distal IIA. A covered stent (GORE® VIABAHN®; Fluency® Plus) is deployed just proximal to the IIA bifurcation. The covered stent is sized to seal the IIA and EIA, preventing retrograde flow into the CIA. Pelvic perfusion is retrograde from the aorto-uni-iliac endograft and femorofemoral bypass graft (**Figure 9.8**).

INTERNAL ILIAC ANEURYSMS

Preservation of the IIA is severely limited in patients with IIA aneurysms. Given their deep location within the pelvis, open repair is difficult; often, ligation and exclusion is are required. As such, an endovascular approach is preferred with coil embolization or plug placement in the anterior and posterior divisions and IIA aneurysm sac, with endograft coverage of the IIA origin (**Figure 9.9**). Rarely, if the proximal and distal landing zones permit, endograft placement may be feasible, but its durability is unknown.

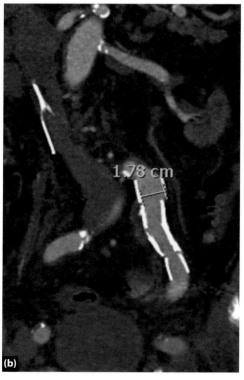

Figure 9.9 Endovascular repair of internal iliac artery (IIA) aneurysm. (**a**) Completion digital subtraction angiogram of completed coil embolization of the anterior and posterior divisions of an IIA aneurysm with endograft coverage of the IIA ostium. (**b**) Follow-up computed tomography angiography coronal image demonstrating a patent endograft and resolved endoleak.

SURVEILLANCE

Patients with endovascular IAA repair require lifelong surveillance with serial clinical examinations, color-flow duplex scan, and ankle–brachial pressure index measurements at 1, 6, and 12 months postoperatively and annually thereafter to assess endograft patency, migration, and endoleaks. Surveillance CTA for endografts placed for abdominal aortic and CIA aneurysms is limited to 1 and 12 months postoperatively if the reconstruction is intact without any endoleaks. However, in patients with an iliac branched graft, the utility of duplex US is often limited in the pelvis, especially when a detailed examination regarding IIA patency and sealing stent migration is required. As a result, CTA may be needed for a longer follow-up period despite the added expense, radiation, and contrast.

CLINICAL OUTCOMES

Endovascular IAA repair has excellent midterm results with >80% primary patency at 2 years, with shorter hospital stays and decreased morbidity and mortality rates compared to open repair. Postoperative complications are comparable to those of standard endovascular aneurysm repair and include aneurysm rupture, endoleak, iliac limb thrombosis, endograft infection or migration.

CONCLUSION

Currently, several techniques, whose utility and durability vary with the patient's anatomy, are available to address IAAs. With continued advances in technology and reports of long-term outcomes, there will be shifts in the applicability of each, with some becoming more useful and others becoming obsolete. For now, the techniques described in this chapter represent a list of commonly used strategies and are accompanied by the authors' thoughts on a hierarchy for their use.

SUGGESTED READING

Bacharach JM, Slovut DP. State of the art: management of iliac artery aneurysmal disease. *Catheter Cardiovasc Interv.* 2008;**71**:708–714.

Bergamini TM, Rachel ES, Kinney EV, et al. External iliac artery-to-internal iliac artery endograft: a novel approach to preserve pelvic inflow in aortoiliac stent grafting. *J Vasc Surg.* 2002;**35**:120–124.

Cronenwett JL, Johnston KW (eds.). *Rutherford's Vascular Surgery.* 8th ed. Philadelphia: Elsevier Saunders; 2014.

Dix FP, Titi M, Al-Khaffaf H. The isolated internal iliac artery aneurysm: a review. *Eur J Vasc Endovasc Surg.* 2005;**30**:119–129.

Kritpracha B, Pigott JP, Russell TE, et al. Bell-bottom aortoiliac endografts: an alternative that preserves pelvic blood flow. *J Vasc Surg.* 2002;**35**:874–881.

Lee WA, Nelson PR, Berceli SA, et al. Outcome after hypogastric artery bypass and embolization during endovascular aneurysm repair. *J Vasc Surg.* 2006;**44**: 1162–1168.

Lee WA, O'Dorisio J, Wolf YG, et al. Outcome after unilateral hypogastric artery occlusion during endovascular aneurysm repair. *J Vasc Surg.* 2001;**33**:921–926.

Murphy EH, Woo, EY. Endovascular management of common and internal iliac artery aneurysms. *Endovascular Today.* March 2012, pp. 76–81. Available from http://evtoday.com/2012/03/endovascular-management-of-common-and-internal-iliac-artery-aneurysms (accessed June 21 2017).

Wong S, Greenberg RK, Brown CR, et al. Endovascular repair of aortoiliac aneurysmal disease with the helical iliac bifurcation device and the bifurcated-bifurcated iliac bifurcation device. *J Vasc Surg.* 2013;**58**:861–869.

10

Endovascular repair of ruptured abdominal aortic aneurysms

M. ASHRAF MANSOUR AND HANNAH ZWIBELMAN

CONTENTS

INTRODUCTION

In the USA, an estimated 17 000 deaths are attributed annually to abdominal aortic aneurysms (AAAs). Screening programs, using abdominal ultrasound (US), in Europe and the USA have been useful in detecting patients with AAAs. The outcomes of elective repair, whether open or endovascular, are always more favorable than waiting for the AAA to rupture.

Several randomized trials comparing elective endovascular aneurysm repair (EVAR) to open surgical repair have shown improved outcomes, especially in frail patients. Recent data from the US Medicare population indicates that the rate of ruptured AAAs in the last few years has been cut in half.[1] The same database depicts a significant shift from open surgical repair to EVAR over time.

EVAR is now the preferred method of treatment in elective patients. Although randomized trials have been conducted to evaluate EVAR versus open surgical repair for ruptured AAAs, the results have been mixed. However, the authors, along with many investigators are firmly convinced that an endovascular-first approach for ruptured AAAs is best.[2] The purpose of this chapter is to describe the preoperative planning and intraoperative technique of EVAR for ruptured AAAs.

PREOPERATIVE PLANNING

To achieve good outcomes, a multidisciplinary and coordinated approach affords the best chance for the patient. As with many complex surgical cases, assigning roles and rehearsing the steps help with good preparation for the event. A true multidisciplinary approach should involve emergency and operating room personnel. The vascular surgeon and anesthesiologist should be informed as early as possible. Open lines of communication between team members are essential to execute plans and secure a good outcome.

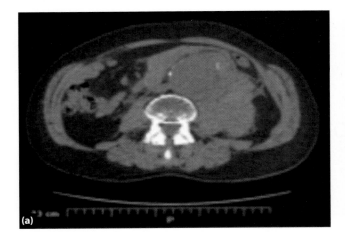

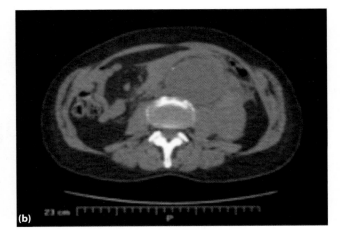

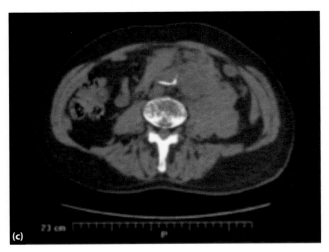

Figure 10.1 Abdominal computed tomography (**a–c**) without intravenous contrast, showing a 7-cm abdominal aortic aneurysm with retroperitoneal rupture.

CLINICAL PRESENTATION

Although the triad of abdominal or back pain, pulsatile mass, and shock is pathognomonic of a ruptured AAA, most stable patients undergo a computed tomography (CT) scan (**Figures 10.1a–c** and **10.2**). To obtain accurate measurements for graft selection, a thin-slice (2–3-mm) spiral CT angiogram is ideal. With compromised renal function, there may be a reluctance to administer intravenous contrast; in some hypotensive, unstable patients, it may be more prudent to proceed directly to the operating room without imaging (see the algorithm in **Figure 10.3**). It is still possible to get measurements of the aortic neck diameter from a non-contrast abdominal CT scan and confirm on initial aortogram (**Figure 10.4**).

GRAFT SELECTION

Many surgeons have a favorite aortic endograft they are comfortable using. It is important to select the endograft the surgeon is most familiar with and certainly not one they have never seen or used. In the authors' hospital, two endograft types are stocked on the shelf and the choice of

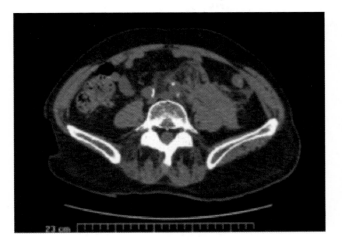

Figure 10.2 Pelvic computed tomography without intravenous contrast, showing the common iliac arteries with calcifications, but suitable for endovascular aneurysm repair.

endograft largely depends on the following features: proximal neck diameter and length; diameter of the external iliac arteries (EIAs); and general tortuosity of the aortic neck and iliac arteries.

A hybrid endovascular surgical suite is ideal to treat patients with ruptured AAAs. Even if the patient is not

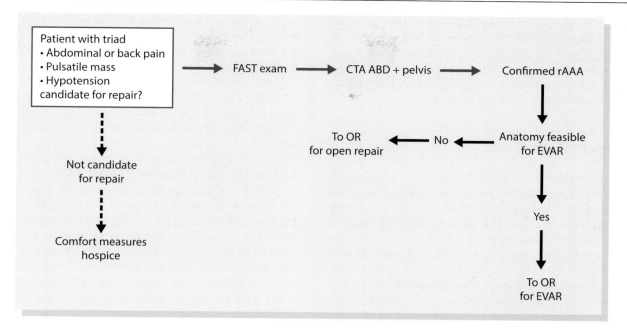

Figure 10.3 Treatment algorithm for endovascular aneurysm repair of ruptured abdominal aortic aneurysm. ABD: abdominal; CTA: computed tomography angiography; EVAR: endovascular aneurysm repair; FAST: focused assessment with sonography for trauma; OR: operating room; rAAA: ruptured abdominal aortic aneurysm.

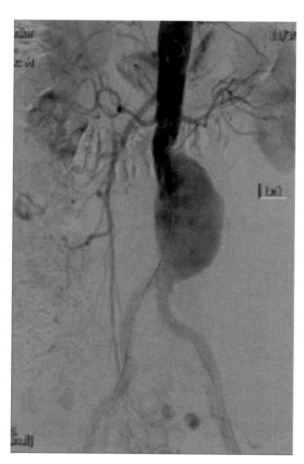

Figure 10.4 Initial intraoperative angiogram, showing a slightly angulated neck, but suitable for endovascular aneurysm repair.

suitable for EVAR, percutaneous placement of an intra-aortic occlusion balloon may be life-saving and certainly less morbid than an emergency thoracotomy or open supraceliac cross-clamp.

PROCEDURE

The primary objective of the surgical team is to get the patient to the endovascular suite as soon as possible. Everyone should be working in a purposeful and expeditious manner. Any undue delay is not in the patient's best interest. During the preoperative period, permissive hypotension is a good option to help maintain any temporary seal following AAA rupture. Keeping the room and patient warm is important to avoid worsening of a coagulopathy. The patient may be given mild sedation to relieve stress and anxiety, such as a small dose of midazolam and fentanyl.

Most importantly, avoiding anesthesia induction and muscle paralysis, until the patient is prepared and the surgeon is gowned and ready to access the groin, is crucial to avoid a sudden drop in blood pressure (BP). Many experienced surgeons prefer the patient awake to maintain sympathetic tone and avoid this potential problem.

Preparation

Skin preparation from the chest to the thighs (nipples to knees) as with any open AAA repair is essential. Hair clippers are used for hair removal in the groin area and a chlorhexidine-based solution is preferred to cleanse the skin. A Foley catheter and radial arterial line are ideal, but could be omitted in certain cases. Placing a central line is not necessary and should never be the cause of delaying the start of the procedure. Many experienced anesthesiologists use intraoperative transesophageal echocardiography monitoring to guide fluid resuscitation.

Emergent EVAR

The first step, after the patient is prepared and draped, is to perform a percutaneous US-guided puncture of the femoral artery. Unless the femoral arteries are severely diseased and calcified, the authors typically use the "pre-close" technique, deploying two ProGlide sutures (Abbott Vascular, Santa Clara, CA, USA) at 10 and 2 o'clock for later closure. If the surgeon is uncomfortable with this technique, an open femoral cutdown can be performed. Once the femoral artery is accessed with a micropuncture kit, an 8-Fr sheath is placed, and the first diagnostic angiogram can be performed using a pigtail catheter (**Figure 10.4**). If the patient is hypotensive or more unstable, a supraceliac aortic occlusion balloon can be placed. In cases where intra-aortic balloon occlusion is performed, it is important to keep track of how long the balloon is inflated to avoid sequelae of prolonged organ ischemia.

After the diagnostic angiogram, the surgeon now has a firm idea of what type of graft to use and if indeed EVAR is the best option (**Figure 10.4**). At this point, the authors typically give a heparin dose. In most cases, a full heparin dose is not necessary and the authors usually opt for a moderate dose of 40–50 U/kg heparin. If the patient is already coagulopathic, it is possible to proceed without additional anticoagulation.

Insertion of the main body of the graft is usually from the right side; however, in some cases, the surgeon may opt to use the left side to avoid calcification or narrowing of the right iliac artery, or to address an aortic neck angulation. Whether to keep the graft's short limb anatomic or cross the limbs depends on the angle of the iliac bifurcation (**Figure 10.5**). In general, angles of ≥90 degrees favor crossing the graft limbs. This simple maneuver can save a lot of time in trying to cannulate the short limb of the graft, especially when time is a factor. There are many techniques that have been described to help speed up the process of short gate cannulation. The authors typically use a Kumpe access catheter (Cook Medical Inc., Bloomington, IN, USA) and an angled guidewire; less frequently, the authors use other preformed catheters, such as a SOS Omni® (AngioDynamics, Latham, NY, USA) or Van Schie Beacon® Tip Seeking catheter (Cook Medical Inc.) for more difficult cannulations. Once the short gate is cannulated, the distance from the gate to the hypogastric artery (HGA) is measured, and an appropriate graft overlap is factored in; the proper length of limb is then selected and inserted (**Figure 10.6**). The ipsilateral side is then addressed. With the C3 GORE® EXCLUDER® stent graft (W. L. Gore & Associates, Flagstaff, AZ, USA), no additional pieces are necessary most of the time.

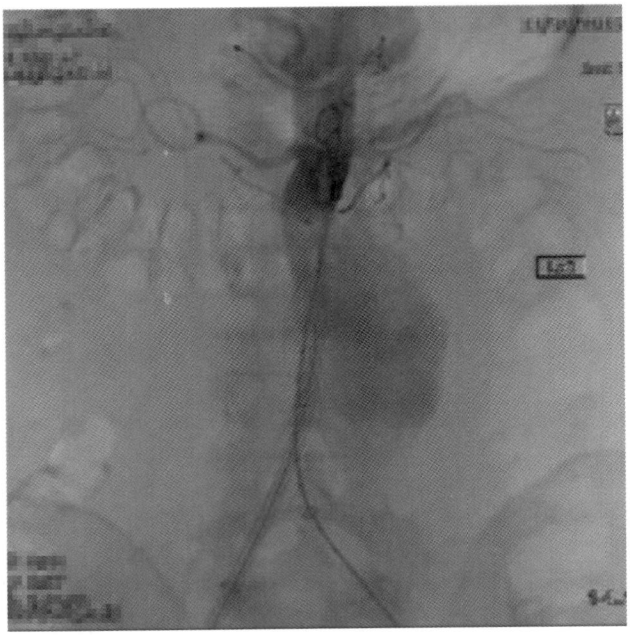

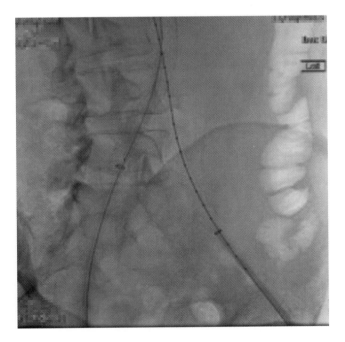

Figure 10.5 Angiogram with a device in place; accessory renal arteries are now seen. Note that the wires cross at the iliac bifurcation; this favors crossing the limbs of the graft (see **Figure 10.8**).

Figure 10.6 The device has been deployed and a pigtail catheter with centimeter markers has been used to measure the distance between the short leg of the graft and the left hypogastric artery, in an oblique view.

With the Zenith Flex® (Cook Medical Inc.), the ipsilateral limb is selected based on the length from the graft to the HGA and the diameter of the distal landing zone. It is generally a good policy to try to line the aorta and iliac arteries from the renal to hypogastric arteries, especially if the exact location of the rupture or leak is not known. This will save a lot of time after the graft is deployed and a persistent contrast blush is observed. If one iliac artery is aneurysmal, coverage of the HGA can be done by landing in the EIA. In an unstable patient, coiling is not advised.

Once the endograft is deployed, balloon inflation at the proximal end, graft-to-graft and distal junctions, a completion angiogram is performed (**Figure 10.7**). If no type I or type III endoleaks are observed, it is time to complete the procedure. If percutaneous access was used, and the pre-close technique was employed, these sutures are carefully tied and gentle manual compression is done for 5 minutes. It is reasonable to reverse the heparin effect with some protamine at this point, especially if there is evidence of unusual oozing.

If an open cutdown was done, the femoral artery is repaired with 5-0 or 6-0 polypropylene sutures and the wound is closed in layers. After closure, it is important to examine the legs and feet, and palpate the pedal pulses or check for Doppler signals. The abdomen is also examined. If the abdomen is tense, bladder pressure can be measured. If the anesthesiologist reports the need for high ventilator pressures, and the abdomen is tense, careful consideration should be given to releasing the abdominal compartment. In the authors' experience, this is necessary in only 10–15% of cases with ruptured AAAs.

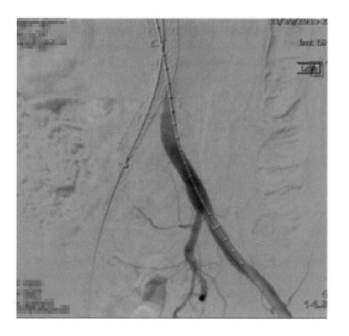

Figure 10.7 Angiogram showing the distance from gate to hypogastric artery to select the correct limb length.

COMPLICATIONS

Access site

With percutaneous access and the pre-close technique, careful selection of the puncture site to avoid anterior calcification is important. Despite proper technique, pre-close can fail in up to 5–8% of cases, and an open femoral cutdown must be performed. Other complications at the access site include inadvertently raising a flap thereby causing ischemia, or distal embolization. Occasionally, with the pre-close technique, the sutures break and open femoral artery repair is needed. If the femoral artery is badly diseased, it is sometimes necessary to perform an endarterectomy and patch closure.

Myocardial infarction

Patients with severe coronary artery disease do not tolerate hypotension and hemodynamic instability. Electrocardiogram changes or arrhythmias intraoperatively or postoperatively should prompt a cardiology consultation.

Contrast-induced nephropathy

Contrast-induced nephropathy is a known complication after EVAR. Using proper technique and avoiding excessive contrast volume are essential. Maintaining a normal BP postoperatively and crystalloid hydration can lessen the incidence of contrast-induced nephropathy.

Distal embolization

Atheroembolization occurs when the aortic graft snowplows through unstable aortic plaque or thrombus or there is excessive graft manipulation and torsion in the AAA. These maneuvers should be avoided if possible.

Abdominal compartment syndrome

If the ruptured AAA has caused excessive retroperitoneal bleeding, a large hematoma may lead to an abdominal compartment syndrome. Release of the abdominal compartment and placement of an abdominal vacuum dressing are the authors' preference. It is often feasible to close the abdomen in 36–48 hours when the hematoma is resorbed.

Graft limb occlusion

Acute graft limb occlusion can occur in cases of a severely diseased iliac artery or a tortuous one. If the endograft is not fully expanded in a narrow iliac artery,

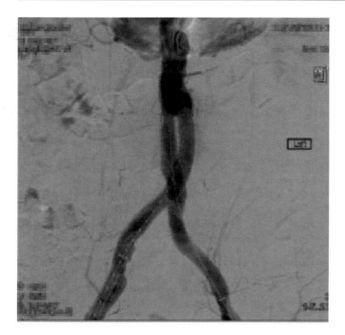

Figure 10.8 Completion angiogram in 83-year-old man. Note that the limbs are crossed.

this could lead to limb thrombosis. On the other hand, in very tortuous iliac arteries, the rigid graft may end up distorting the iliac artery and causing a functional occlusion. The latter problem can be averted sometimes by performing the completion angiogram without the stiff wire in place.

CASE EXAMPLE

An 83-year-old man was brought to the emergency department by ambulance. He had been complaining of severe flank and lower abdominal pain for about 6 hours before being admitted. He had no knowledge of an AAA, and denied any history of renal stones. He also denied hematuria. He had a history of lung transplant for severe chronic obstructive pulmonary disease.

On examination, he was awake and alert. He had a tender abdomen. He had palpable femoral and pedal pulses. He was not taking warfarin. He reported a good quality of life; he still lived at home with his wife. A noncontrast CT scan was available for review (**Figure 10.1**). The diagnosis was discussed with the patient and his wife. The options for treatment were outlined, including the choice of comfort measures only. The patient and his wife both were enthusiastic about proceeding. They gave informed consent for repair surgery.

The patient was taken to the operating room endovascular suite urgently where an emergency EVAR was performed. Bilateral percutaneous access was obtained as described. The graft was selected based on the preoperative CT scan. A pair of small accessory renal arteries (RAs), one on each side, were discovered on the intraoperative angiogram (**Figure 10.5**). These accessory RAs were intentionally covered to obtain an adequate proximal seal. The operation was otherwise uneventful. The completion angiogram showed no evidence of endoleak (**Figure 10.8**). After extubation, the patient was taken to the surgical intensive care unit and he had an uneventful early recovery.

CONCLUSION

To ensure the ideal outcomes for patients with ruptured AAAs, a multidisciplinary and coordinated approach needs to be adopted. While many randomized trials comparing EVAR for ruptured AAAs to traditional open surgical repair have failed to show a conclusive benefit for EVAR, most experts agree that an "EVAR-first" stance is best.[3,4] There will be patients with a difficult anatomy or hostile necks who are not good candidates for EVAR. However, if EVAR is feasible in a ruptured AAA, patients will be afforded the best chance of surviving this catastrophic event. Complication rates after emergent EVAR may be slightly higher, but overall survival is improved over open surgical repair.

REFERENCES

1. Schermerhorn ML, Bensley RP, Giles KA, et al. Changes in abdominal aortic aneurysm rupture and short-term mortality, 1995–2008: a retrospective observational study. *Ann Surg.* 2012;**256**:651–658.
2. McPhee J, Eslami MH, Arous EJ, et al. Endovascular treatment of ruptured abdominal aortic aneurysms in the United States (2001–2006): a significant survival benefit over open repair is independently associated with increased institutional volume. *J Vasc Surg.* 2009;**49**:817–826.
3. Holst J, Resch T, Ivancev K, et al. Early and intermediate outcome of emergency endovascular aneurysm repair of ruptured infrarenal aortic aneurysm: a single-centre experience of 90 consecutive patients. *Eur J Vasc Endovasc Surg.* 2009;**37**:413–419.
4. Kapma MR, Dijksman LM, Reimerink JJ, et al. Cost-effectiveness and cost-utility of endovascular versus open repair of ruptured abdominal aortic aneurysm in the Amsterdam Acute Aneurysm Trial. *Br J Surg.* 2014;**101**:208–215.

Endovascular repair of popliteal artery aneurysms

ZACHARY HOTHEM AND GRAHAM W. LONG

CONTENTS

INTRODUCTION

Popliteal artery aneurysms (PAAs) are the most common peripheral artery aneurysms, accounting for 70%, with a male-to-female ratio of 20:1. Fifty percent are bilateral and 40% have a concurrent abdominal aortic aneurysm.[1–4] Their natural history involves aneurysm thrombosis or embolization with ensuing acute or chronic ischemia and limb loss. Limb swelling and pain from venous or nerve compression and rupture are rare presentations. Most interventionalists use a 2-cm threshold for elective repair, with some proceeding when the aneurysm is twice the size of the adjacent normal artery, or if there is extensive mural thrombus within the aneurysm sac. Surveillance is usually performed with annual duplex ultrasound (US) imaging (**Figure 11.1a,b**).

The traditional approach to PAA repair has consisted of operative bypass graft placement, preferably with autogenous saphenous vein, and aneurysm exclusion. Advances in technology have created endografts that leverage the advantages of a minimally invasive approach, including shorter hospital stay and recovery times. Recent series that incorporated dual antiplatelet therapy into the postoperative medical regimen following endovascular popliteal aneurysm repair (EVPAR) reported improved patency rates of 80% with midterm follow-up.[5–8]

PLANNING

Preoperative evaluation consists of computed tomography angiography, magnetic resonance angiography, or conventional digital subtraction arteriography (DSA) with sizing catheter or ruler, extending from the aortoiliac to the pedal arterial systems. These examinations allow accurate assessment of the degree of aneurysmal and occlusive disease, tortuosity of the inflow and outflow vessels, and adequacy of the proximal and distal landing zones (**Figures 11.2** and **11.3a,b**). The most widely used stent graft for popliteal aneurysm repair is the GORE® VIABAHN® Endoprosthesis (W. L. Gore & Associates, Flagstaff, AZ, USA), which is available with or without a heparin bioactive surface. The GORE® VIABAHN® Endoprosthesis is constructed of polytetrafluoroethylene (PTFE) with a nitinol exoskeleton. Although not currently approved for repair of PAAs, it is approved by the U.S. Food & Drug Administration for treating symptomatic arterial occlusive disease of the iliac and superficial femoral arterial systems; it ranges in diameter from 5 to 13 mm with lengths from 25 to 250 mm.

Sizing and planning require the following to determine the patient's candidacy for endovascular repair: normal proximal and distal landing zones of at least 2 cm; diameter discrepancy between proximal and distal landing zones of ≤1 mm (**Figure 11.3a,b**); vessel tortuosity <45 degrees; and an aneurysm diameter <5 cm to prevent endograft kinking and displacement. Two-vessel runoff in the calf is preferred to maintain device patency. Young, active patients, or those with occupations or hobbies that require prolonged bending at the knee, such as gardening or carpentry, are more prone to thrombosis and may be better treated with surgical bypass.[6] Asymptomatic occluded PAAs are observed.

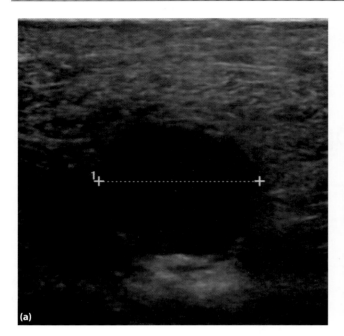

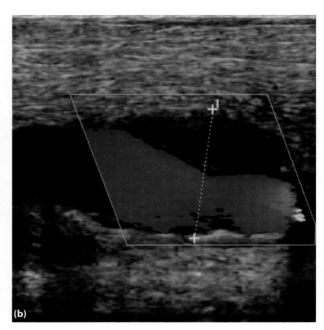

Figure 11.1 Duplex ultrasound images of a popliteal artery aneurysm. (**a**) Cross-sectional image. (**b**) Long-axis view showing mural thrombus and adjacent normal-caliber popliteal artery.

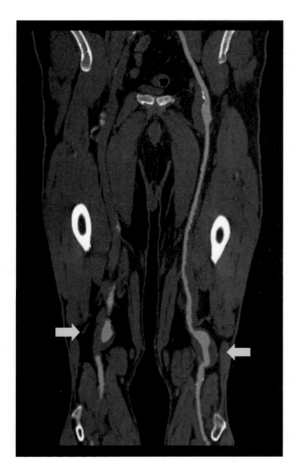

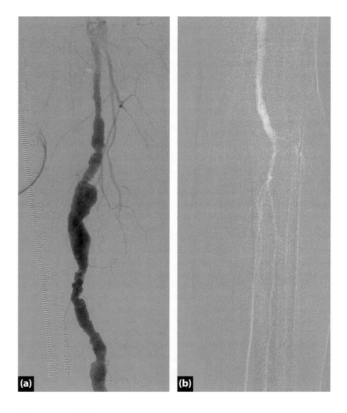

Figure 11.2 Computed tomography angiogram coronal view demonstrating bilateral popliteal artery aneurysms (arrows) with associated left common femoral artery aneurysm.

Figure 11.3 Digital subtraction angiograms demonstrating (**a**) long-segment femoropopliteal aneurysmal disease with significant concomitant calcified occlusive disease, and (**b**) two-vessel tibial runoff in the posterior tibial and peroneal arteries. Given the extent of occlusive disease and the inflow-to-outflow mismatch diameters, open surgical bypass was selected rather than endovascular repair.

The length of artery to be treated remains controversial. Covering all aneurysmal segments is important to minimize the development of a subsequent endoleak from migration or late aneurysmal degeneration. However, treating the entire length of the superficial femoral (SFA) and popliteal arteries increases the likelihood of acute limb ischemia with endograft thrombosis, due to collateral vessel coverage; also, the increased number of stent grafts used increases the number of overlap zones prone to fracture and thrombosis. A reasonable compromise involves coverage of all aneurysmal and ectatic segments with proximal and distal landing zones of 2 cm, preferably using only one covered stent.

Preoperative preparation involves medical optimization and placing the patient on dual antiplatelet therapy with aspirin and clopidogrel, prasugrel, or ticagrelor, which is continued for a minimum of 4–6 weeks postoperatively, if not indefinitely. Alternatively, if the patient takes an anticoagulant, dual therapy with aspirin is acceptable.

TECHNIQUE

Either ipsilateral/antegrade or contralateral/retrograde femoral artery access can be performed. New lower-profile devices permit up to an 8-mm diameter endograft to be delivered via a 7-Fr sheath using a 0.014 or 0.018-inch guidewire. This allows safe passage of a sheath or guide catheter over the aortic bifurcation from a contralateral/retrograde approach. Frequently, this cannot be performed safely with the higher profile sheaths required for delivery of larger-diameter devices. For these patients, an antegrade approach from either the ipsilateral common femoral artery (CFA) or SFA, percutaneously or via cutdown, is required. Specifically, 9–13-mm endografts require 9–12-Fr sheaths over a 0.035-inch guidewire for placement (**Table 11.1**).

After obtaining sheath access to the SFA, intravenous heparin is administered to maintain an activated clotting time (ACT) >250 seconds. Angiography of the target extremity is performed to confirm preoperative imaging

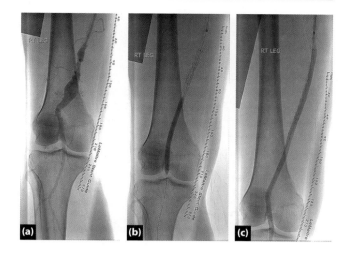

Figure 11.4 Angiographic demonstration of endovascular treatment of a popliteal artery aneurysm. (**a**) Diagnostic angiogram. (**b**) Angioplasty after endograft placement. (**c**) Completion angiogram with no evidence of endoleak.

findings (**Figure 11.4a–c**). If there is concern for mural thrombus along the landing zones, intravascular US (IVUS) can be used to complement DSA to ensure these sites are of good quality. Some interventionalists advocate obtaining additional lateral angiographic views with the knee flexed to determine the "hinge point" of the femoropopliteal arterial segment, usually a few centimeters above the actual knee joint. When multiple endografts are required for coverage, this hinge point is avoided as an area of overlap to reduce the risk of stent fracture. Likewise, avoiding placement of the end of the endograft at this point decreases the risk of thrombosis.

After angiographic anatomic confirmation, either a 0.035 or 0.018-inch stiff wire is advanced under fluoroscopic guidance through the femoropopliteal arterial system into the tibial arteries of the calf. The chosen covered stent should be oversized by 10–15% proximally and distally, which minimizes the potential for stent graft infolding. If there is significant occlusive disease within the femoral and popliteal arteries, advancing the delivery system "bareback" may not be possible. These lesions may tear the PTFE jacket enclosing the covered stent, deploying the device before it is correctly positioned. Advancing the access sheath with its dilator in place through these segments first facilitates placement of the delivery system to its intended position. Once the delivery system is advanced across the lesion, the sheath is retracted so the endograft is clear of its tip. Deployment is accomplished by pulling on a PTFE suture that opens the constraining PTFE jacket from around the device (**Figure 11.5a,b**). Deployment should be done under fluoroscopic visualization of the radiopaque markers using gentle, continuous traction on the PTFE suture to minimize device deflection and maintain the intended position. Deployment is in a "tip-to-hub" direction as the PTFE suture is removed. Aggressive tension on the PTFE suture can bow the tip of the delivery system,

Table 11.1 GORE® VIABAHN® Endoprosthesis[a] and access sheath sizing

Platform	Endograft size (mm)	Vessel diameter (mm)	Sheath size (Fr)
0.018- or 0.035-inch	5	4.0–4.7	6 or 7
	6	4.8–5.5	6 or 7
	7	5.6–6.5	7 or 8
	8	6.6–7.5	7 or 8
0.035-inch	9	7.6–8.5	9
	10	8.6–9.5	10
	11	9.6–10.5	11
	12	10.6–12.0	12

[a] W. L. Gore & Associates, Flagstaff, AZ, USA.

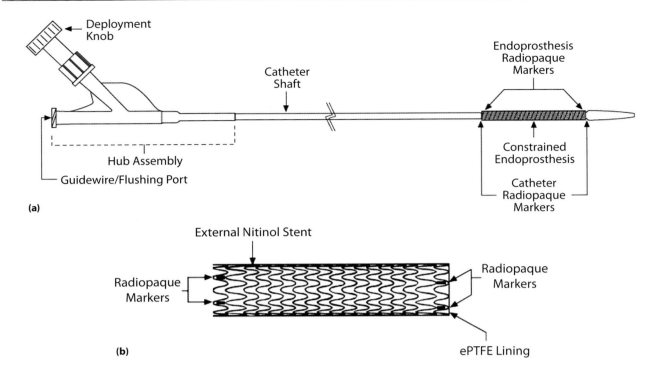

Figure 11.5 (**a**) GORE® VIABAHN® Endoprosthesis Delivery System. (**b**) GORE® VIABAHN® Endoprosthesis. (Reprinted with permission from W. L. Gore & Associates.)

resulting in deployment within the aneurysmal segment, and is known as the "bowstring phenomenon." If multiple endografts are used, there should be no more than a 1-mm size differential between overlapping devices. The smaller-diameter device is placed first and an overlap of 2–3 cm is maintained between them. Molding with an angioplasty balloon up to the native arterial diameter is performed on the first device before placing the second. Special attention is paid to molding of the overlapping endograft segments. The balloon is kept within the endograft to prevent dissection of the adjacent native artery.

Completion arteriography is performed via the introducer sheath to detect endoleaks, distal embolization, or significant kinking that impairs distal flow. If a type I endoleak is noted proximally, further inflation with an angioplasty balloon is performed, or an additional, appropriately sized endograft can be used for proximal extension. The same strategies are used for a distal endoleak with the caveat that the distal extension endograft should avoid covering a tibial outflow vessel. Some interventionalists advise imaging these reconstructions with the knee in both flexed and extended positions to ensure no significant graft kinking occurs.

ACUTE LIMB ISCHEMIA

Performing EVPAR in the acute ischemic setting is challenging because of the thrombosed PAA and frequent lack of runoff vessels. Catheter-directed, intra-arterial thrombolysis can improve distal runoff, making

subsequent surgical bypass or endograft placement feasible. Judgement is required to determine if the limb can tolerate the extended ischemic time for the lytic process to take place and if the patient is at reasonable risk for bleeding complications.

Typically, catheter-directed, intra-arterial thrombolysis is achieved via a 6-Fr sheath placed into the contralateral CFA and directed over the aortic bifurcation to the affected leg. A coaxial 5-Fr lytic catheter should be placed in the aneurysm sac with a lytic wire advanced through the catheter into one of the tibial outflow vessels. Tissue plasminogen activator (tPA) is infused with the patient monitored in the intensive care unit over 12–24 hours, with infusion rates 0.5–2 mg/hour. Heparin 500 IU/hour should be given via the 6-Fr access sheath to prevent thrombus formation around the catheter. Alternatively, a rheolytic percutaneous thrombectomy catheter may also be used to lace tPA (10 mg in 100 mL) directly into the thrombosed segments using the power-pulse spray technique, debulking the thrombus before thrombolytic infusion is initiated. This technique may hasten the lytic process and minimize the depth and length of the ischemic time. During infusion, partial thromboplastin time (PTT) and fibrinogen levels are monitored every 6 hours. Target PTT should be subtherapeutic (<50 seconds) to avoid bleeding complications. Lytic infusions can be continued for 24–48 hours, if fibrinogen levels remain >200 mg/dL. Infusion rates are cut in half if fibrinogen levels decrease to below 200 mg/dL and stopped if they drop below 150 mg/dL.

Angiography is repeated within 6–24 hours to reassess the popliteal-tibial artery outflow. Judgement is made as to whether there is adequate outflow present for bypass graft placement, or if the aneurysm sac is patent and there is the two-vessel runoff needed to maintain patency of an endograft. If there has been partial clearing of the thrombus, the infusion can be continued for another 24 hours. Otherwise, urgent thrombectomy and bypass graft placement is attempted.[7]

OUTCOMES

Postoperative surveillance is performed by duplex US imaging at 6 weeks and every 6 months for the first 2 years, along with a medical history and physical examination. Some interventionalists advocate for two-view plain radiographs with the knee extended and in full flexion to detect migration, strut fracture, and endograft kinking. The most common complications following EVPAR are stent thrombosis, migration, and endoleak. Thrombosis occurs most commonly and is usually secondary to kinking, fracture, or poor inflow or outflow. Early reported thrombosis rates were 10–15% at 12 months and 20–25% at 2 years. Recent experiences, which included clopidogrel in the postoperative medical regimen, demonstrated 5-year primary patency of 80%. Catheter-directed thrombolytic therapy is effective at recapturing these endografts with secondary patency rates ranging from 90 to 100% at 12 months and from 80 to 90% at 2 years.[5–8] Type I endoleaks require angioplasty or endograft extension, while type II endoleaks with concomitant sac expansion can be managed via percutaneous thrombin injection into the aneurysm sac under US guidance or with percutaneous coil embolization. If a minimally invasive approach is unsuccessful, an open surgical approach can be performed by opening the aneurysm sac and oversewing side branches to achieve proper exclusion.

SUMMARY

Currently, no endograft is approved for the treatment of PAAs. Nonetheless, there is an increasing use of this technique for this indication with significant variation in results. This chapter has outlined the principles for selection and the technique required to maximize endograft patency and aneurysm exclusion. Continued refinement in technique, technology, and postoperative medical regimen may improve primary patency of these reconstructions to achieve parity with that for surgical bypass.

REFERENCES

1. Jacobowitz G, Cayne NS. Lower extremity aneurysms. In: Cronenwett JL, Johnston KW, eds. *Rutherford's Vascular Surgery*. 8th ed. Philadelphia, PA: Saunders/Elsevier; 2014. pp. 2190–2205.
2. Gallala S, Verbist J, Van Den Eynde W, et al. Popliteal artery aneurysm: when open, when endo? *J Cardiovasc Surg (Torino)*. 2014;**55(Suppl)**:239–247.
3. Vallabhaneni R, Sanchez LA, Geraghty PJ. Endovascular treatment of popliteal aneurysm. In: Chaikof EL, Cambria RP, eds. *Atlas of Vascular Surgery and Endovascular Therapy: Anatomy and Technique*. Philadelphia, PA: Saunders/Elsevier; 2014. pp. 598–603.
4. Tielliu IF, Verhoeven ELG. Endovascular treatment of popliteal artery aneurysms. In: Stanley JC, Veith FJ, Wakefield TW, eds. *Current Therapy in Vascular and Endovascular Surgery*. Philadelphia, PA: Elsevier/Saunders; 2014. pp. 400–403.
5. Cina CS. Endovascular repair of popliteal aneurysms. *J Vasc Surg*. 2010;**51**:1056–1060.
6. Garg K, Rockman CB, Kim BJ, et al. Outcome of endovascular repair of popliteal artery aneurysm using the Viabahn endoprosthesis. *J Vasc Surg*. 2012;**55**:1647–1653.
7. Trinidad-Hernandez M, Ricotta JJ 2nd, Gloviczki P, et al. Results of elective and emergency endovascular repairs of popliteal artery aneurysms. *J Vasc Surg*. 2013;**57**:1299–1305.
8. Kumar HR, Rodriguez HE, Eskandari MK. Midterm outcomes of self-expanding covered stent grafts for repair of popliteal artery aneurysms. *Surgery*. 2015;**157**:874–880.

12

Endovascular repair of pararenal and thoracoabdominal aneurysms

MATTHEW J. EAGLETON

CONTENTS

INTRODUCTION

Endovascular aortic aneurysm repair, which was first described nearly two decades ago, allows for the treatment of aortic disease in a less invasive fashion. In direct comparison, infrarenal endovascular aneurysm repair (EVAR) demonstrates reduced perioperative mortality while providing long-term clinical equipoise with conventional surgery, but with the price of higher reintervention rates. Endovascular repair becomes more complicated when aneurysms involve or are near the renal and visceral segment of the aorta, such as in the treatment of pararenal abdominal aortic aneurysms (AAAs) and thoracoabdominal aortic aneurysms (TAAAs).

The development of fenestrated and branched endograft technology has allowed the application of this less invasive approach to aneurysm repair in these complex pathologies. For pararenal AAAs, fenestrated and branched EVAR (F/B-EVAR) has been limited to use in clinical trials. However, treatment of more advanced disease is possible with F/B-EVAR, but application of this technology has yet to reach the commercial arena and remains restricted to research programs within the USA.[1-5] In addition, given its still investigational nature, most fenestrated and branched endograft programs (at least in the USA) are limited to treating patients who are considered high risk for conventional surgery.[6]

PREOPERATIVE PLANNING

Planning is the key to success for all endografting. However, in complex endografting such as F/B-EVAR, preoperative planning becomes even more imperative. Appropriate case planning requires an expert knowledge of device construction and the properties of ancillary tools (such as covered bridging stent grafts), how the devices interact with one another, and what imaging protocols are necessary to obtain correct anatomic information so that device construction and implantation can be performed. It is during this stage that intraoperative problems can be anticipated with the development of alternate plans for critical points in the procedure.

Comprehensive aortic assessment is mandatory for procedural planning when using devices that incorporate branched vessels. This is accomplished with high-quality image acquisition, and the ability to manipulate the data in three-dimensional (3-D) workstations. Longitudinal or rotational misalignment can result in critical end organ loss, with potentially disastrous consequences. Currently available spiral computed tomography (CT) technology renders images of excellent quality. These can be used to design devices that incorporate the visceral, renal, iliac, internal, and even aortic arch vessels. The use of 0.75–1.0-mm slice image acquisitions is frequently employed. After acquisition, image reconstruction is

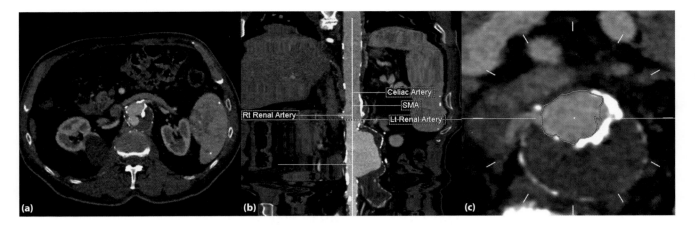

Figure 12.1 Preoperative image for sizing. (**a**) The use of thin-slice computed tomography imaging is necessary for the planning of fenestrated and branched aortic endografts. (**b**) Multiplanar reconstruction allows for the accurate assessment of the location of the appropriate proximal and distal seal/fixation zone and the location of the target vessels. (**c**) In addition, their rotational orientation is necessary, and is usually represented by either clock positions or arc length measurements.

performed with multiplanar techniques to allow for accurate measurements of a variety of arterial anatomic criteria, such as the proximal aortic neck, as well as location, distance, and rotational alignment of target branches. This is accomplished by analyzing renditions of aortic anatomy perpendicular to a centerline of flow that allows for accurate assessment of aortic anatomy (**Figure 12.1**). The use of 3-D workstations to plan for F/B-EVAR is essential.

Multiple different anatomic structures and their location must be considered when planning F/B-EVAR, including a thorough understanding of proximal and distal fixation/seal zones, and the corresponding location of the visceral and renal arteries in juxtaposition to these zones. For endovascular therapy to be effective and durable, a healthy proximal landing zone above the aneurysm is mandatory. Standard commercial EVAR requires a proximal landing zone between 10 and 15 mm in length according to most graft instructions for use. Commercial F/B-EVAR follows similar recommendations with the requirement of at least 15 mm of parallel, nondiseased aorta for a suitable neck. In branched aortic endograft placement, however, the author prefers to follow guidelines more akin to those for the placement of a thoracic endograft and extend the proximal landing zone to at least 25 mm of healthy-appearing aorta. The proximal and distal landing/seal zones should be free of significant atheroma and thrombus, and the aortic walls should be parallel. In addition to the proximal and distal seal zones, the linear and axial location of the visceral and renal vessels must be noted. This dictates where, on the graft, the location of the fenestrations or branches is to be constructed. The trajectory, whether caudal or cephalad, may also influence the decision whether to use a fenestration or directional branch.

When evaluating the patient's anatomy, the ability to deliver the graft system should also be considered. Most fenestrated and branched endografts are delivered through sheaths that are 20–22 Fr in diameter, and thus rely on the presence of adequate iliac artery diameters to accommodate placement of such a sheath. While methods that allow the endovascular placement of these larger sheaths have been described, the author has tended not to use these methods when placing branched endografts. It has been the author's experience that the presence of stents within the iliac system can reduce the ability to rotationally manipulate the graft delivery system, making it more difficult to accurately align the reinforced fenestrations or branches. In these situations, the author has preferred to place an iliofemoral conduit using a 10-mm graft. Typically, this has been done in a staged fashion (especially when the endograft procedure is quite complex).[7] With improvements in F/B-EVAR device design, lower-profile systems (18 Fr) are becoming available that will significantly reduce the need for iliac conduits and increase the rates of percutaneous access.

One of the significant risks of TAAA repair is the development of spinal cord ischemia.[8] To help mitigate this catastrophic complication, care must be exercised to maintain all collateral routes of spinal flow. When planning for surgery, the author routinely develops a treatment algorithm that preserves flow to both hypogastric and subclavian arteries whenever possible. This can be accomplished through the judicious use of iliofemoral conduits and placement of carotid-subclavian bypass grafts (or carotid-subclavian transpositions). Again, the author typically performs these procedures in a staged fashion before the endograft procedure.

GRAFT CONSTRUCTION

Most of the currently available devices are based on the Zenith system (Cook Medical Inc., Bloomington, IN, USA), although this is rapidly changing. Given that most reported experience is based on the Cook system, description of the devices is limited to that system, and much of the upcoming technology is based on similar principles.

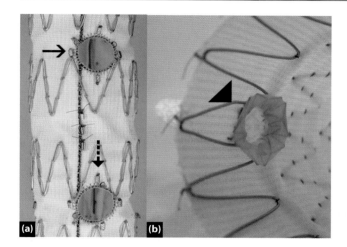

Figure 12.2 Example of a reinforced fenestration in an aortic stent graft. (**a**) The fenestration (arrow) is cut in the graft material so that it is not obstructed by one of the aortic supporting stent struts and in a location that allows it to align with the intended target vessels (renal or visceral). It is externally supported with a nitinol ring that allows it to mate and seal with a covered bridging stent. (**b**) The seal with the covered stent (arrow) allows continued flow to the target vessel and seals off the aneurysm.

To incorporate renal or visceral vessels into aortic repair, a "branch" must be constructed that allows for sealing of the aneurysm but preservation of flow to the target artery. This has been successfully accomplished with two structurally different types of approaches. The first type of design is termed a "reinforced fenestration" (**Figure 12.2**). This essentially involves holes, customized to the size and location of the target vessel, placed in the aortic graft and reinforced with a circumferential nitinol wire. These reinforced fenestrations are then mated with the target vessel with a balloon-expandable covered stent, which is flared within the fenestration to obtain a seal (**Figure 12.2**). Fenestrations that occur at the very proximal extent of the endograft are termed scallop fenestrations. Because these are located within the sealing stent of the aortic graft, they rarely require placement of a bridging stent except when it is necessary to preserve the scallop-target vessel alignment. The second type of branch is a directional branch; this is a sidearm attached directly to the main aortic component (**Figure 12.3**). These branches can take a variety of shapes; these have predominantly included a helical or a straight design. The directional branch allows for easier placement of the mating stent, more flexibility regarding orientation, and greater overlap with the mating stent. This greater overlap allows for the use of self-expanding covered stents, rather than balloon-expandable stents. Many graft designs incorporate a combination of reinforced fenestrations and directional branches. The decision to incorporate one over the other depends on the access vessels and aortic and target vessel morphology.

To assist with the placement of these devices, several attributes are designed within the delivery system to

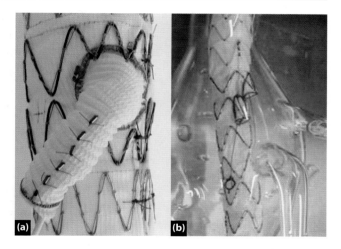

Figure 12.3 Directional branches are incorporated on the aortic stent graft to allow for mating (with balloon-expandable or self-expanding covered stents) with the target vessel. These branches can be of different shapes and lengths including (**a**) helical or (**b**) straight design.

facilitate accurate placement. The devices have several trigger wires that allow for the proximal and distal aspects of the stent graft to be attached to the delivery system (**Figure 12.4**). This is combined with a system that keeps the graft partially constrained even once it is deployed from the sheath. These attributes allow for limited cranial/caudal movement of the graft and some rotational maneuverability. This assists in aligning fenestrations and branches with the respective target vessels once the graft is unsheathed. Once the device is in the correct location and the target vessels have been successfully cannulated, these trigger wires can be released, thus fully deploying the graft. In addition, to aid access to the fenestrations and branches, catheters and wires can be incorporated into the delivery system; these allow for ipsilateral sheath placement directly to the fenestration or advancement of an additional sheath (through brachial/axillary artery access) into the directional branch.

INTRAOPERATIVE IMAGING

Endovascular device implantation requires skill in the orientation of 3-D devices based on two-dimensional angiographic imaging equipment. When performing branched endograft placement for pararenal AAAs and TAAAs, high-quality intraoperative imaging is needed. Imaging equipment is best housed in a hybrid operating room suite that allows for both open and endovascular procedures. When the complexity of the procedure increases, the ability to more accurately evaluate the 3-D architecture of the aortic tree before, during, and after surgery becomes increasingly important. Flat panel detectors have begun to replace the standard image intensifiers used with conventional fluoroscopy units. The application of this technology provides the ability to perform intraoperative

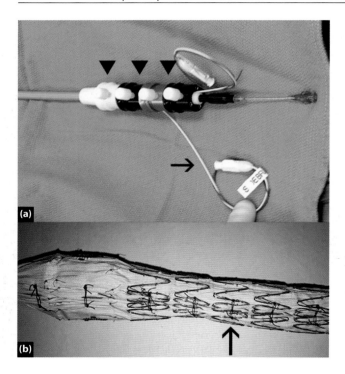

Figure 12.4 Example of a delivery system that (**a**) incorporates several trigger wires for controlled deployment of the graft (triangles). The "spools" are attached to wires that traverse the delivery system and help to keep the aortic endograft attached to the delivery system, allowing for rotational and cranial/caudal manipulation of the graft. In addition (**b**, arrow), the graft, once unsheathed, remains partially constrained, until the constraining wire is released fully and the graft is deployed. In some instances, additional catheters/wires in the delivery handle (**a**, arrow) are threaded into the fenestrations or directional branches facilitating ipsilateral access from below, or assisted access from above, via an axillary or brachial artery approach.

3-D imaging with rotational angiography, termed C-arm cone beam CT (CBCT). This technology can be used intraoperatively in the form of fusion imaging to guide device implantation. This is like the traditional roadmapping used with conventional angiography. Intraoperative CBCT images can be registered to the preoperative CT images, and these can be superimposed on the live fluoroscopic images (**Figure 12.5**). The superimposed image is updated in real time with movement of the C-arm gantry angle. The superimposed image can help to guide the placement of the fenestrated/branched endograft using the images to align the branches and fenestrations with their targets. Use of CBCT has been demonstrated to significantly decrease the volume of contrast used during these types of procedures.[9]

OPERATIVE PROCEDURE

Patients are positioned supine for the procedure, and the abdomen, pelvis, thighs, and left arm (when necessary)

are prepped and draped. The exact procedural steps vary based on the type of graft construction used. For the sake of completeness, the author describes the placement of a graft that used both reinforced fenestrated branches and directional branches for the treatment of a TAAA. Transverse incisions are performed in the inguinal region, and proximal and distal control of the femoral arteries is obtained. With device design enhancement and the development of lower-profile systems, grafts have increasingly been placed in a percutaneous fashion with a "pre-close" technique. If a directional branch is a part of graft construction, then an additional incision is made over the distal axillary artery in the upper arm. If this artery is not of adequate size to accommodate a 10–12-Fr sheath, then the incision is made more proximally in the infraclavicular location. If multiple sheaths are required from an antegrade approach, a conduit can be sewn to the axillary artery to facilitate placement of one larger sheath, or to allow for multiple smaller sheaths without having to puncture the native vessel in multiple locations.

After the patient is anticoagulated, intra-arterial access is obtained. Through the ipsilateral femoral artery, stiff wire access is obtained into the ascending aorta (for extensive aortic endografts). The wire can remain in the descending thoracic aorta for less extensive repairs such as would be performed with a standard fenestrated endograft for a juxtarenal AAA. Similar stiff wire access is obtained through the contralateral femoral artery. A large (20–24-Fr) sheath, depending on the number of reinforced fenestrations to be stented, is advanced to the aortic bifurcation under fluoroscopic imaging. Multiple smaller sheaths are then advanced into the larger sheath (**Figure 12.6**), and this allows for repeated access of multiple distal sites without having to reaccess the femoral artery.

Before the stent graft is placed, the target vessels must be localized to align the branches or fenestrations. This can be done with a variety of techniques, such as the fusion imaging described earlier. Alternatively, aortography can be performed. However, the author prefers to supplement the use of fusion imaging with the placement of catheters and wires in at least one of the target vessels to mark their location (**Figure 12.7**). While fusion imaging is helpful in assisting the placement of fenestrated/branched endografts, its accuracy is diminished in anatomies where there is significant vessel tortuosity. In these situations, with advancement of the stiff endograft systems, the location of the target vessel can shift making the location of the overlaid image inaccurate. When advancing the endograft, the additional placement of "marker" catheters can assist in positioning it along the length of the aortic axis and helping to align the branches/fenestrations with the target vessels without the use of contrast. Typically, if one target vessel is offset (usually in a cranial/caudal position), all the target vessels will be shifted similarly.

Before the endograft is inserted, it is oriented under fluoroscopy. There are several radiopaque markers on the graft that help with orientation. Typically, the reinforced fenestrations have four gold markers highlighting their

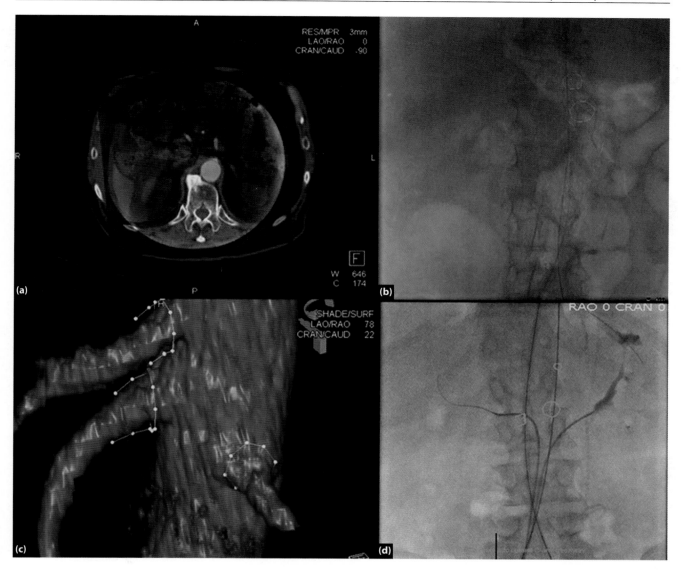

Figure 12.5 Example of an intraoperative imaging system that can facilitate fenestrated and branched aortic endografts. (**a**) Preoperative computed tomography (CT) imaging is "merged" or "registered" with the position of the patient on the fluoroscopy table. Historically, this was accomplished by performing an intraoperative cone beam CT, but with advancements in imaging technology it can be performed with multiple "single-shot" views. (**b**) Once registered, the preoperative CT image can be overlaid on the live fluoroscopy image. This can assist in placing the endograft and selecting the target vessels. (**c,d**) Alternately, the overlaid image can be replaced with graphic representation of areas of interest, such as highlighting only the origins of the renal and visceral vessels.

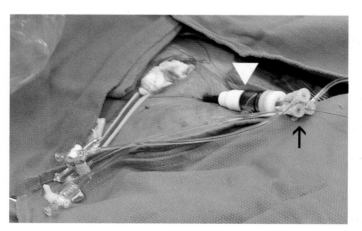

Figure 12.6 Example of right iliofemoral access with a 20-Fr, large-bore sheath. This allows for single puncture access of the femoral artery. Additional sheaths (arrow) can then be used to gain access into target vessels by puncturing the diaphragm of the larger sheath.

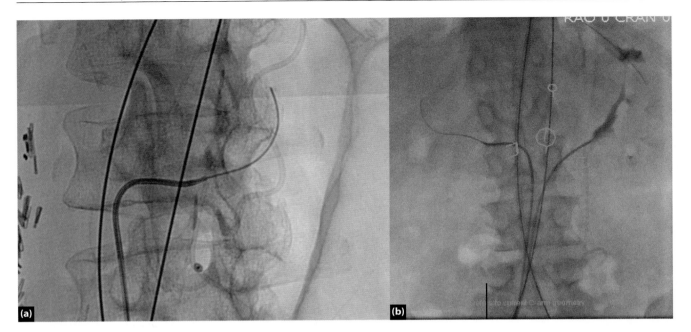

Figure 12.7 Example of the left renal artery being cannulated before the endograft is placed. (**a**) This marks the location of the vessel and decreases the need for additional contrast injection. (**b**) Overlay imaging can facilitate the placement of the fenestrated and branched endovascular aneurysm repair. The graphics outline the origin of the renal and visceral vessels. Again, catheter/wires have been placed in either renal artery (guided by overlay imaging). Note how overlay imaging is not perfectly accurate; this is because of the movement of the aorta and its branches with the advancement of stiff wire systems.

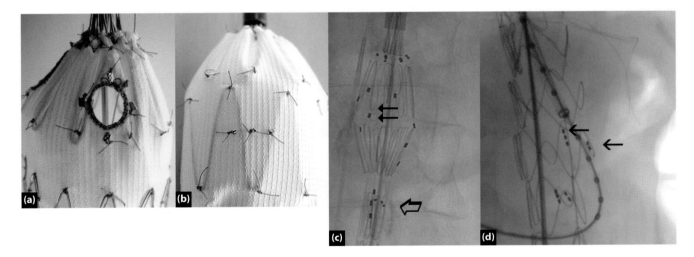

Figure 12.8 Images of endografts demonstrating some of the orientation markers. (**a**) Four gold markers outline the fenestrations. (**b**) In addition, gold markers are used to highlight the posterior and anterior aspect of the endograft. (**c**) When in vivo, these markers are easily visible under fluoroscopy and assist in the correct orientation and alignment of the stent graft. The double arrows show the four gold markers associated with a reinforced fenestration, while the open arrow shows a set of anterior and posterior orientation markers. (**d**) In addition, markers are placed on the directional branches to mark the opening and outlet of the branch (arrows).

peripheral circumference (**Figure 12.8**). Additional markers are placed to mark the location of the opening and exit of directional branches, and on the anterior and posterior aspects of the aortic component to help with rotational orientation. The exact configuration may vary depending on the profile of the graph and the incorporation of fenestrations and branches. Understanding the location

of these markers before the graft is inserted is necessary to assure proper graft placement during the procedure. Once oriented, the device is advanced through the femoral artery on the ipsilateral side. Care must be taken to assess for device rotation as it passes through tortuous iliac systems. When the graft is using directional branches, these frequently use preloaded catheter and wire systems, as described earlier, to facilitate sheath access into the branch. As the device is advanced into the aorta, a wire is advanced through the preloaded catheter system and snared through a sheath advanced through the axillary artery. The fenestrated/branched endograft is then advanced until the fenestrations and branches align with their target vessels, and the graft is unsheathed. Because the delivery system allows the graft to remain partially constrained until it is fully deployed, "fine tuning" can be performed with slight maneuvering of the graft in the cranial/caudal direction and rotationally.

Once in location and unsheathed, access from the femoral approach is obtained through the sheath in the contralateral femoral artery. Access is obtained into the body of the fenestrated/branched endograft, and the shorter, small-diameter sheath is exchanged for a larger (7–8-Fr) and longer (55-cm) sheath, which is advanced up to the reinforced fenestrations. Using a variety of different catheters and wires, depending on the orientation of the graft, target vessel access is obtained through the fenestration into the target vessel (**Figure 12.9**). The corresponding sheath is also advanced into the target vessel. This process is repeated for all the reinforced fenestrations. The marker catheters and wires are removed as each of the vessels is cannulated through the fenestration. For the directional branches, the process involves advancing the sheath (10 Fr) from the axillary artery, over the preloaded wire, into the corresponding branch. The sheath is counterpunctured and a catheter and wire are advanced through the sheath, into the branch and the target vessel. The wire is exchanged for a stiff wire, the through-and-through wire is removed, and the sheath is advanced into the target vessel. Once sheath access is obtained in the target vessels, the graft is completely deployed by releasing the constraining wire and the proximal and distal trigger wires, allowing removal of the delivery system.

Angiography is performed in the target vessels before stenting. The reinforced fenestrations are stented with balloon-expandable covered stents (**Figure 12.10**). These are dilated to a size appropriate for the diameter of the vessel, and then flared proximally in the fenestration to obtain a seal. If there is significant tortuosity in the target branch, the distal landing zone of the covered stent is transitioned with the placement of a self-expanding, bare-metal stent to avoid kinking and ultimate occlusion of that branch. Directional branches are stented with self-expanding covered stents (**Figure 12.11**). Aortography is performed

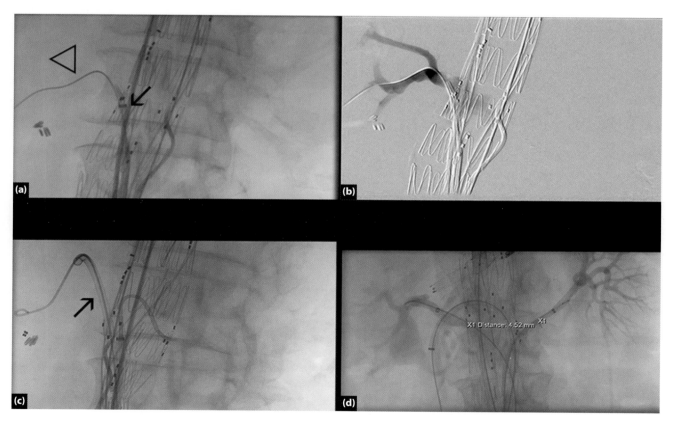

Figure 12.9 Images depicting access into a renal artery through a reinforced fenestration. (**a**) The graft is deployed after the fenestrations were aligned with the target vessel. A 6- or 7-Fr sheath is advanced from within the body of the fenestrated endograft up to the level of the reinforced fenestration (arrow). (**b**) Through this sheath, wire and catheter access is obtained in the target vessel. (**c**) The wire is exchanged for a stiffer wire and the sheath is advanced over its dilator into the target vessel through the fenestration (arrow). (**d**) These steps are repeated for each of the reinforced fenestrations until all the target vessels are cannulated. The graft can then be deployed fully.

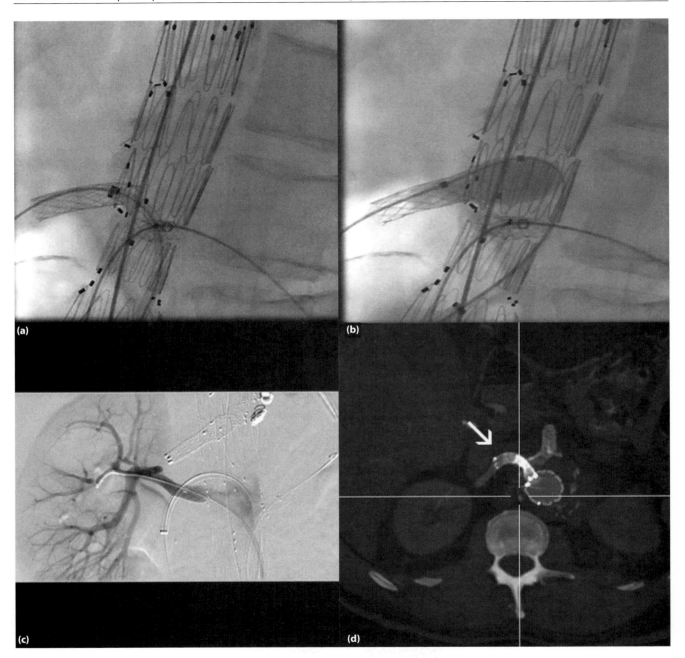

Figure 12.10 Placement of the bridging stent into a renal artery through a reinforced fenestration. This is performed with a balloon-expandable covered stent. (**a**) 4–5 mm of stent must extend into the aortic lumen; it is then flared (**b**) with an oversized balloon to achieve a seal. The size of the balloon depends on the diameter of the fenestration, but is typically at least 2 mm larger. (**c**) Completion arteriography is performed to verify patency and seal. (**d**) Care must be taken in the presence of tortuous target arteries. The placement of a stiff, balloon-expandable stent can cause the renal or visceral vessel to "kink" at the end of the stent. This can be overcome by prophylactic placement of a self-expanding stent (arrow). The need for this is best assessed preoperatively on cross-sectional imaging, which provides a better estimate of the anterior–posterior curvature of the vessel.

to assess for patency of the branches and to assess for the presence of a proximal endoleak.

Depending on the anatomy of the patient, a distal aortic extension may be necessary with either a straight endograft body piece or placement of a standard, modular, bifurcated component (**Figure 12.12**). Care must be taken when advancing any additional stent grafts so that the portions

of the bridging stents that extend into the aortic lumen are not crushed, with ultimate loss of vessel patency. To overcome this, if the delivery system appears to traverse adjacent to these stents (and it usually occurs in the vessel on the contralateral side of the aorta), sheath access is maintained in the bridging stent until after the bifurcated component is placed. In this case, if the stent becomes

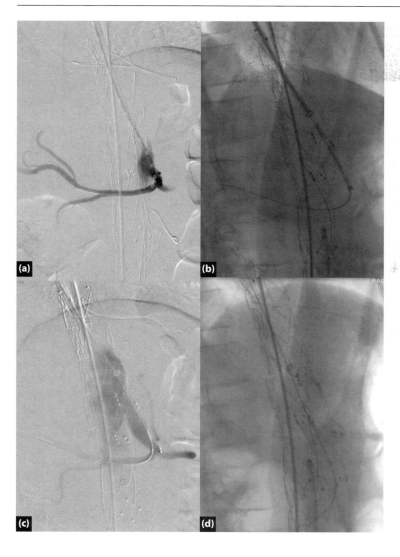

Figure 12.11 Placement of the bridging stent in a directional branch. Access into the branch is obtained via an antegrade approach through axillary or brachial artery access. Entrance into the branch can be facilitated by a preloaded guidewire and catheter system, which can be snared from above. (**a**) Once the sheath is into the branch, access into the target vessel is obtained and verified. In this case, the sheath is advanced into a straight directional branch and catheter access into the celiac artery is obtained. (**b**) Over a stiff wire, a covered self-expanding stent is placed and deployed. (**c**) Completion arteriography is performed to verify patency and the absence of an endoleak. If the overlap in the bridging stent is not sufficient, an additional covered stent can be placed, or the first stent graft can be anchored in place with a bare-metal, balloon-expandable stent. (**d**) This process is repeated for each of the directional branches.

malformed, access into it is maintained and it can be easily re-flared, maintaining patency and seal. The overlap zones undergo balloon angioplasty, as do the distal seal zone(s). Completion angiography is performed. Sheaths, catheters, and wires are removed, the arteriotomies are repaired with 5-0 or 6-0 polypropylene suture, and the wounds are closed in layers (provided the procedure was not performed in a percutaneous fashion).

POSTOPERATIVE MANAGEMENT

Patients undergoing repair of juxtarenal AAAs can be managed postoperatively on a standard nursing unit for vascular surgical patients. The author prefers to observe TAAA patients in the intensive care unit (ICU) following branched endograft repair. Time spent in the ICU is dependent on several factors, including the extent of the aneurysm that is repaired and the patient's underlying comorbidities. Depending on the length of aorta excluded, spinal drains are employed for up to 72 hours. As with any major surgery, urine output, blood pressure, and laboratory values are monitored closely. Most patients can eat on

the first postoperative day, and they are physically mobilized as soon as possible. Most patients remain hospitalized from 4 to 7 days.

Follow-up imaging is mandatory to assess for the adequate exclusion of the aneurysm and to assess for continued patency of the branch vessels. The protocol used by the author entails contrast, cross-sectional imaging (when renal function is not prohibitive), and duplex ultrasonography. These imaging tools are performed within 30 days of surgery, and then repeated annually. Reintervention may be necessary when an endoleak or branch vessel restenosis is present, but it has a very low incidence.[10] The ideal pharmacotherapy regimen to assist in branch vessel patency is not known. The author routinely has patients on lifelong aspirin therapy and a 3-month duration of clopidogrel therapy.

RADIATION SAFETY

With increasing complexity of aortic endograft procedures, there is a corresponding increase in fluoroscopy times and subsequent radiation exposure. Surgeons performing these procedures must be cognizant of the risks

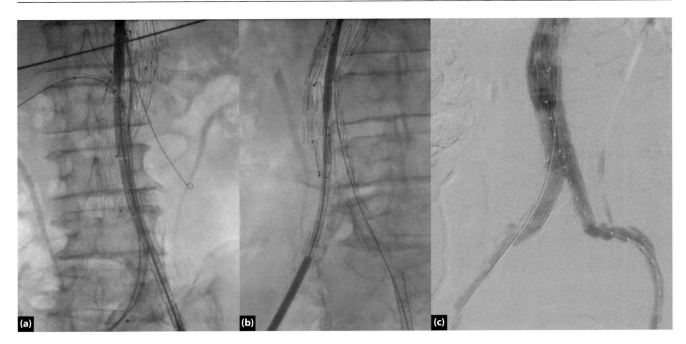

Figure 12.12 Depending on the distal seal zone, a bifurcated component may need to be placed. (**a**) Care must be taken in placing the bifurcated component because the delivery system can traverse near the stents extending into the aortic lumen and crush them. This can be prevented by maintaining sheath access in "at-risk" vessels during placement of additional aortic components. If the bridging stent becomes dislodged or malformed by the advancement of additional components, it can easily be re-flared. (**b**) Once the bifurcated component is placed, the iliac limbs are placed just as in standard endovascular aneurysm repair and (**c**) completion aortography performed.

of radiation exposure and be fluent in how exposure can be decreased. The deterministic effects are predictable, dose-related, and easier to manage. The stochastic effects, however, are cumulative in nature. Long-term exposure to radiation can cause untoward effects, with cancer potentially being the most feared. Surgeons must understand these mechanisms and the methods with which to reduce exposure risk to protect the patient and the treatment team. In an early evaluation of radiation exposure during F/B-EVAR, Panuccio and collaborators calculated that, at that time, the effective radiation dose of an endovascular TAAA repair was equivalent to two preoperative CT scans.[11] Certainly, intraoperative maneuvers can be performed to limit radiation exposure, including minimizing the use of digital subtraction acquisitions, avoiding lateral angulation, and being diligent about the use of shielding during fluoroscopy cases.[12] A number of adjuncts have more recently become available that can assist in limiting the amount of fluoroscopy time necessary to perform cases. One such adjunct is the use of image fusion to help guide the intervention.[9] The use of this technology has been associated with a reduction in procedure times and, therefore, a reduction in radiation exposure for patients and operators during both standard EVAR and complex aneurysm repair.[13,14] Any physician involved in the use of fluoroscopy, in particular with complex procedures, must become familiar with the mechanisms of fluoroscopy, the risk of radiation exposure, and the methods that can be used to reduce everyone's exposure.

REFERENCES

1. Greenberg RK, Sternbergh WC 3rd, Makaroun M, et al. Intermediate results of a United States multi-center trial of fenestrated endograft repair for juxtarenal abdominal aortic aneurysms. *J Vasc Surg.* 2009;**50**:730–737.e1.
2. Greenberg R, Eagleton M, Mastracci T. Branched endografts for thoracoabdominal aneurysms. *J Thorac Cardiovasc Surg.* 2010;**140(6 Suppl)**:S171–178.
3. Mastracci TM. Endovascular treatment of thoracoabdominal aneurysm. *Curr Treat Options Cardiovasc Med.* 2010;**12**:205–213.
4. Eagleton MJ, Follasbee M, Wolski K, et al. Fenestrated and branched endovascular aneurysm repair outcomes for type II and III thoracoabdominal aortic aneurysms. *J Vasc Surg.* 2016;**63**:930–942.
5. Mastracci TM, Eagleton MJ, Kuramochi Y, et al. Twelve-year results of fenestrated endografts for juxtarenal and group IV thoracoabdominal aneurysms. *J Vasc Surg.* 2015;**61**:355–364.

6. Bub GL, Greenberg RK, Mastracci TM, et al. Perioperative cardiac events in endovascular repair of complex aortic aneurysms and association with preoperative studies. *J Vasc Surg.* 2011;**53**:21–27.e1–2.

7. Abu-Ghaida AM, Clair DG, Greenberg RK, et al. Broadening the applicability of endovascular aneurysm repair: the use of iliac conduits. *J Vasc Surg.* 2002;**36**:111–117.

8. Greenberg RK, Lu Q, Roselli EE, et al. Contemporary analysis of descending thoracic and thoracoabdominal aneurysm repair: a comparison of endovascular and open techniques. *Circulation.* 2008;**118**:808–817.

9. Dijkstra ML, Eagleton MJ, Greenberg RK, et al. Intraoperative C-arm cone-beam computed tomography in fenestrated/branched aortic endografting. *J Vasc Surg.* 2011;**53**:583–590.

10. Mastracci TM, Greenberg RK, Eagleton MJ, et al. Durability of branches in branched and fenestrated endografts. *J Vasc Surg.* 2013;**57**:926–933.

11. Panuccio G, Greenberg RK, Wunderle K, et al. Comparison of indirect radiation dose estimates with directly measured radiation dose for patients and operators during complex endovascular procedures. *J Vasc Surg.* 2011;**53**:885–894.e1.

12. Mohapatra A, Greenberg RK, Mastracci TM, et al. Radiation exposure to operating room personnel and patients during endovascular procedures. *J Vasc Surg.* 2013;**58**:702–709.

13. Hertault A, Maurel B, Sobocinski J, et al. Impact of hybrid rooms with image fusion on radiation exposure during endovascular aortic repair. *Eur J Vasc Endovasc Surg.* 2014;**48**:382–390.

14. McNally MM, Scali ST, Feezor RJ, et al. Three-dimensional fusion computed tomography decreases radiation exposure, procedure time, and contrast use during fenestrated endovascular aortic repair. *J Vasc Surg.* 2015;**61**:309–316.

13

Endovascular repair of descending thoracic aortic aneurysms

FARAH MOHAMMAD, ROB HARRIZ, AND LOAY S. KABBANI

CONTENTS

INTRODUCTION

Descending thoracic aortic aneurysms (DTAA) are relatively rare, and comprise 2–5% of all degenerative aneurysms.[1] Dake and collaborators were the first to report endovascular aneurysm repair of a thoracic aneurysm using homemade "back-table" endografts.[2] The first commercially available thoracic endoprosthesis to treat DTAA was not approved by the U.S. Food & Drug Administration until 2005. Currently, thoracic endovascular aortic repair (TEVAR) for DTAAs has become the standard of care. Compared to open repair, TEVAR is associated with decreased length of stay, reduced blood transfusion, and earlier return to a baseline activity lifestyle. In addition, several studies have suggested that endoluminal grafting has an equal, or lower, incidence of neurologic complications.

INDICATIONS FOR TEVAR

Indications for repair of DTAAs include: a luminal diameter >5.5 cm; saccular aneurysm; and postoperative pseudoaneurysm. Currently, all patients with suitable anatomy and acceptable access should be considered for TEVAR.

CONTRAINDICATIONS FOR TEVAR

Absolute contraindications to TEVAR include inadequate landing zones (see the *Sealing (landing) zones* section of this chapter). Relative contraindications include unsuitable access anatomy, such as a severe tortuous aorta that may not allow the stent graft to track into position, or small access vessels. Other relative contraindications include mycotic or connective tissue disorder etiology, aortic severe angulation >60 degrees, or unreliable follow-up.

PATIENTS WITH SPECIAL CONSIDERATIONS

Severe intravenous dye allergy can usually be managed with premedication and steroid adjustment. In advanced renal insufficiency, contrast dose must be minimized. Intravascular ultrasound (IVUS) may be used to help address anatomic variations and decrease the amount of contrast needed. Octogenarians with major comorbidities need to have a lengthy, honest discussion with their surgeon about the survival benefits of treating the aneurysm weighed against the risks and patient's current quality of life.

OPERATIVE PLANNING

The single most important task that determines the success of these operations is preoperative planning. Remember the five Ps rule: Prior planning prevents poor performance! High quality cross-sectional imaging and its accurate interpretation is essential in preoperative planning. Look for poor access vessels, significant calcification, and tortuosity in the iliac arteries.

Imaging

Computed tomography angiography (CTA) with centerline reconstruction is ideal for preoperative planning. Centerline images can accurately estimate the diameter and length of the landing zones. Magnetic resonance angiography may be used if the patient has renal insufficiency or severe contrast allergy. For reporting purposes, the aorta has been divided into 11 zones (**Figure 13.1**). This landing zone classification has been supported by the Society for Vascular Surgery.[3]

Sealing (landing) zones

The patient should have appropriate landing zones, or "necks," proximal and distal to the aneurysm, to have a "seal" between the aortic wall and the endoprosthesis.

Ideally, the proximal landing zone should be sufficiently established beyond the origin of the subclavian artery (zones 3 or 4), and the distal landing zone should be proximal to the celiac artery (zone 5). Depending on device availability, the patient's landing zone diameter should be within the manufacturer's instruction for use. For example, the GORE® TAG® Thoracic Endoprosthesis (W. L. Gore & Associates, Flagstaff, AZ, USA) has a range of 16–42 mm (i.e., the proximal and distal landing zone diameters should not be <16 or >42 mm), and the landing zone length should be ≥20 mm. Typically, the endograft is oversized compared to the landing zone diameter by 10–20%. Excessive oversizing can lead to infolding with gutter formation and poor sealing, and excessive radial force that may accelerate degeneration of the neck. Placement of an undersized graft, on the other hand, increases the chance of endoleaks and graft migration.

Management of the arch and visceral arteries to extend the landing zones

Among patients undergoing TEVAR, 17–43% need coverage of the left subclavian artery (LSA) (zone 2), the left

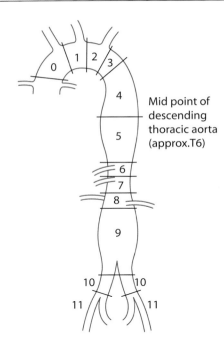

Figure 13.1 Zones of attachment in the aorta. (Adapted from Fillinger MF, Greenberg RK, McKinsey JF, et al. Reporting standards for thoracic endovascular aortic repair (TEVAR). *J Vasc Surg.* 2010;**52**:1022–1033.)

common carotid artery (CCA) (zone 1), or even the brachiocephalic artery (zone 0), to achieve an adequate proximal seal.[4] The left LSA is an important vessel for collateral perfusion the brain and spinal cord, through the left vertebral artery and internal mammary artery. Although generally well tolerated because of the rich collateral network, routine coverage of the LSA should be discouraged. Retrospective evidence suggests that not all patients can tolerate the occlusion safely. Complications with covering the LSA, such as arm and vertebrobasilar ischemia, have been reported in 6 and 2% of patients, respectively.[5] An increased risk for spinal cord ischemia (SCI) with LSA coverage was reported in the EUROSTAR (European Collaborators on Stent/Graft Techniques for Aortic Aneurysm Repair) registry data.[6] Revascularization of the LSA is prudent when extensive coverage of the thoracic aorta is planned, or TEVAR is being performed in patients with previous infrarenal aortic replacement, occluded internal iliac arteries, a dominant left vertebral artery with a hypoplastic or absent right vertebral artery, or termination of the left vertebral artery into the posterior inferior cerebellar artery. Other reasons to consider LSA bypass are a patent left internal mammary bypass to a coronary artery or the presence of left arm arteriovenous access for hemodialysis.

Standard options for revascularizing the LSA include left CCA-to-LSA bypass graft, or left CCA to LSA transposition. Less commonly used options include: open aortic arch debranching; endovascular debranching with a chimney technique; laser fenestration of the thoracic graft to revascularize the LSA with a short stent graft; or a pre-fabricated fenestrated endovascular graft.[7] The left CCA can be bypassed using an extra-anatomic carotid-carotid bypass, or, less commonly, endovascular debranching of the left CCA, which has been described with the chimney technique. The brachiocephalic artery can be debranched via a median sternotomy, with arch debranching originating from the ascending aorta or, less commonly, with an endovascular debranching technique (e.g. a chimney technique). The celiac artery can be covered if there are adequate collaterals between the superior mesenteric artery and the celiac artery, via the gastroduodenal artery. However, if revascularization is required, then options include open surgical revascularization, or endovascular techniques (e.g., with a periscope graft).[8]

ACCESS SELECTION

The femoral artery is the most common access site used to insert a thoracic endograft. The ideal size of the artery used for access is ≥7 mm, but this varies depending on the size of the endograft used (**Table 13.1**). Other than inadequate luminal size, limitations include severe occlusive disease, extensive calcification and tortuosity of the access vessel. Conduits may be used if the femoral, external, or common iliac arteries (CIAs) are unsuitable. Conduits are needed in approximately 15% of patients. Traditional conduits entail sewing an 8–10-mm graft to the distal aorta, or CIA. The conduit is tunneled out into the groin. The distal end is clamped and a separate puncture is made in the conduit to introduce the sheath and endograft (**Figure 13.2a**). Endoconduits require accessing the femoral artery, followed by placing a covered stent, and dilating the artery to the appropriate size. This is technically considered a controlled rupture of the artery, but the covered stent prevents blood extravasation (**Figure 13.2b**). Caution must be taken to prevent the rupture from reaching a patent internal iliac origin. Other options include a transcaval approach, or a transmediastinal approach. When dealing with a very tortuous aorta or an arch with a small radius, the "body floss" maneuver may be helpful in advancing the device through the arch. This is accomplished by passing a guidewire from the right brachial artery to the femoral artery; the device may then be advanced over this stabilized guidewire (**Figure 13.3**).

Table 13.1 Types of endografts available

Endograft	Diameter of endograft (mm)	Sheath size (Fr)
Zenith Alpha™[a]	15–46	16–20
GORE® TAG®[b]	16–46	20–24
Valiant® Thoracic[c]	28–42	20–22
RELAY®[d]	22–46	22–26

[a] Cook Medical Inc., Bloomington, IN, USA
[b] W. L. Gore & Associates, Flagstaff, AZ, USA;
[c] Medtronic, Minneapolis, MN, USA;
[d] Bolton Medical, Sunrise, FL, USA.

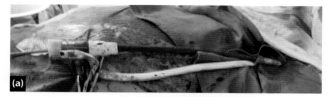
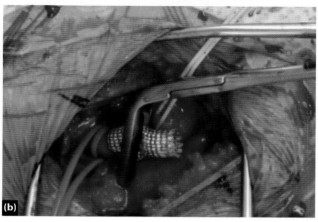

Figure 13.2 Conduits. (**a**) Open – 10 mm PTFE graft anastomosed to left common iliac and exited through a small groin incision; graft clamped distally and large sheath introduced proximally. (**b**) Endo – 8 mm covered stent exiting from right femoral artery, clamped distally.

NEUROPROTECTION

Patients at risk of SCI include those requiring long-segment descending thoracic aortic coverage and antecedent or concomitant abdominal aortic grafting. In addition to maintaining hemodynamic stability for adequate perfusion of the spinal cord, a spinal drain is recommended. The drain is usually inserted preoperatively, and maintained for 48–72 hours postoperatively. Cerebrospinal pressure is kept <10 cm H_2O. Postoperative has also been shown to reverse delayed-onset paraplegia after TEVAR. Complications, such as intracranial hemorrhage, have a reported incidence of 0–3% after spinal drain placement.[9]

OPERATIVE TECHNIQUE

A hybrid operating room is the safest set-up in which surgery can be performed. Surgery can be executed under local, regional, or general anesthesia. The authors prefer general anesthesia, to prevent patient movement during critical parts of the procedure, and to hold respirations when needed.

The patient is placed in the supine position. Bilateral groins are prepped. The left or right arm may be abducted and circumferentially prepped if the radial/brachial artery needs to be accessed. The contralateral groin is used to place a marker pigtail catheter. Percutaneous access is usually chosen if there is no extensive femoral artery disease. A femoral artery angiogram is performed to confirm the

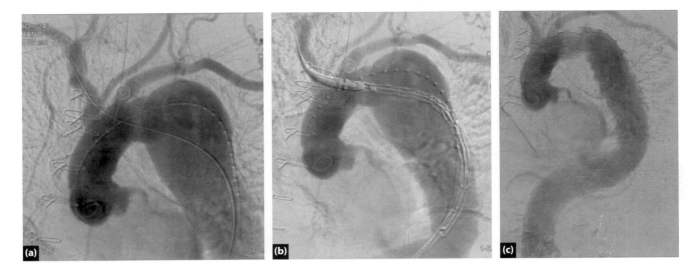

Figure 13.3 Endovascular deployment of a thoracic endograft. Note the placement of the stiff wire into the right subclavian artery to support advancement of the endograft ("body floss" maneuver). (**a**) Predeployment angiogram. (**b**) Endograft positioning. (**c**) Postdeployment (completion) angiogram.

access location (the common femoral artery) and rule out significant disease. Open exposure may be required if the artery is very calcified, or a femoral endarterectomy is required. An 0.35-cm flexible tipped wire is then passed in a retrograde fashion under direct fluoroscopic guidance to the ascending aorta, then exchanged for a stiff wire, such as a Lunderquist® Extra-Stiff Wire Guide (Cook Medical Inc., Bloomington, IN, USA). At this juncture, the patient is heparinized with approximately 100 IU/kg, to maintain an activated clotting time of >250 seconds. If the access artery(ies) are small serial dilators are used to dilate the artery to the size required to accommodate the introducer sheath for device delivery. The pigtail catheter is used to perform an aortogram of the area of interest. An aortic image is then taken in a left anterior oblique projection, with the proximal landing zone in a perpendicular plane to the image intensifier. IVUS can also be used to locate important branches and evaluate the landing zone for size, length, and presence of thrombus. The length and diameter of the proximal and distal landing zones may be measured using the preoperative CT scan, intraoperative IVUS, and angiogram. The chosen stent graft is delivered under fluoroscopic guidance. Before deployment, blood pressure may be reduced to below 100 mmHg systolic, to decrease the chance of caudal migration of the endograft. (This is less important with newer stent grafts that have tip capture devices in place.) The patient's breathing is held for stent graft deployment. Deployment is then carried out following the instructions for each device. Additional grafts may be required and should have an overlap of at least 5 cm to ensure adequate apposition and minimize the risk of type III endoleaks. Balloon molding may also be required and should be done in a proximal-to-distal sequence. Completion angiography is carried out to confirm placement and look for endoleaks. The arteriotomy is closed.

The distal pulses are checked; if they correspond to the preoperative baseline, heparin is reversed. The patient is then extubated in the operating room, and a neurologic assessment is made.

POSTOPERATIVE CARE

All patients with spinal drains are admitted to the intensive care unit postoperatively. Postoperative care includes: spinal drain care; maintaining hemodynamics; and neurologic assessment. A follow-up CTA is scheduled 6 weeks, 6 months (if problems on 6 week scan), and 12 months postoperatively and then yearly.

COMPLICATIONS

Mortality is between 2 and 10%.[10] Independent predictors of mortality include: severe coronary artery disease; congestive heart failure; chronic kidney disease; and emergency procedures. The incidence of complications ranges widely. For SCI, the incidence varies from 0 to 6%, and of stroke the incidence is between 2 and 5%.[11] The reported overall incidence of primary endoleaks ranges from 3 to 10%.[12] Most type II endoleaks appear to resolve without intervention. Type I endoleaks require treatment by extending the endograft or by performing additional procedures, such as coiling. Retrograde type A thoracic aortic dissection after transfemoral TEVAR has a reported incidence of around 2% and is associated with increased morbidity and mortality. Several stent graft-related late complications have been reported, including graft migration, endoleaks, and stent graft fractures.[12] It is important, therefore, to have periodic CT surveillance imaging to assess device integrity and positioning.

CASE EXAMPLE

A patient with an asymptomatic, rapidly enlarging, bilobed thoracic aneurysm had a poor landing zone distal to the LSA (zone 3) (**Figures 13.4** and **13.5a**). Therefore, a carotid subclavian bypass was performed and the landing zone was extended to zone 2 (**Figure 13.5a**). Preoperatively, a spinal drain was placed. At the time of the TEVAR operation, the LSA was embolized with an AMPLATZER™ Vascular Plug (St. Jude Medical, Inc., St. Paul, MN, USA) (**Figure 13.5b**). Since the iliac vessels were small, a right iliac endoconduit was placed using a 10-mm GORE® VIABAHN® Endoprosthesis (W. L. Gore & Associates, Flagstaff, AZ, USA). A postprocedure CTA revealed a covered DTAA, patent carotid subclavian bypass, occluded proximal LSA, and a patent right external iliac stent graft (**Figure 13.6**).

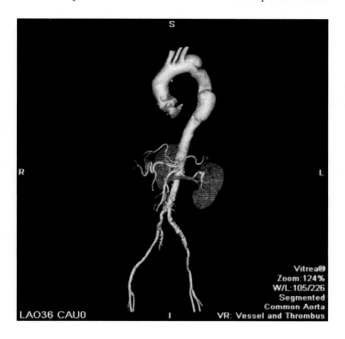

Figure 13.4 Preoperative computed tomography angiography of patient with an asymptomatic bilobed thoracic aneurysm.

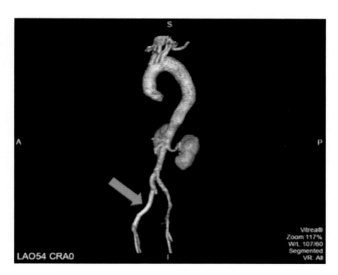

Figure 13.6 Post-thoracic endovascular repair computed tomography angiography. Note the endoconduit used to help deploy the iliac vessel (arrow).

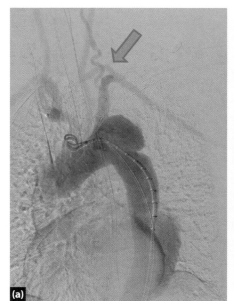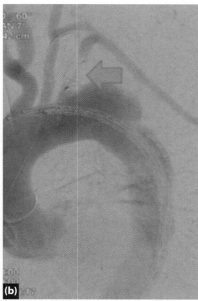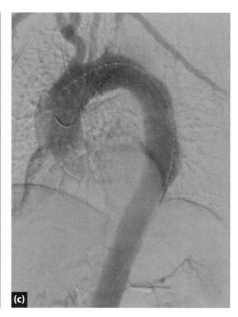

Figure 13.5 Same patient as in **Figure 13.4**. (**a**) Predeployment. Note the patent left carotid artery-to-subclavian bypass (arrow). (**b**) Positioning of endograft prior to deployment. Note the AMPLATZER™ Vascular Plug (St. Jude Medical, Inc., St. Paul, MN, USA) placed in the left subclavian artery (arrow). (**c**) Completion angiogram.

REFERENCES

1. Clouse WD, Hallett JW Jr., Schaff HV, et al. Improved prognosis of thoracic aortic aneurysms: a population-based study. *JAMA*. 1998;**280**:1926–1929.

2. Dake MD, Miller DC, Semba CP, et al. Transluminal placement of endovascular stent-grafts for the treatment of descending thoracic aortic aneurysms. *N Engl J Med*. 1994;**331**:1729–1734.

3. Fillinger MF, Greenberg RK, McKinsey JF, et al. Reporting standards for thoracic endovascular aortic repair (TEVAR). *J Vasc Surg*. 2010;**52**:1022–1033.

4. Matsumura JS, Rizvi AZ. Left subclavian artery revascularization: Society for Vascular Surgery Practice Guidelines. *J Vasc Surg*. 2010;**52(4 Suppl)**:65S–70S.

5. Rizvi AZ, Murad MH, Fairman RM, et al. The effect of left subclavian artery coverage on morbidity and mortality in patients undergoing endovascular thoracic aortic interventions: a systematic review and meta-analysis. *J Vasc Surg*. 2009;**50**:1159–1169.

6. Buth J, Harris PL, Hobo R, et al. Neurologic complications associated with endovascular repair of thoracic aortic pathology: incidence and risk factors. A study from the European Collaborators on Stent/Graft Techniques for Aortic Aneurysm Repair (EUROSTAR) registry. *J Vasc Surg*. 2007;**46**:1103–1110.

7. Redlinger RE Jr., Ahanchi SS, Panneton JM. In situ laser fenestration during emergent thoracic endovascular aortic repair is an effective method for left subclavian artery revascularization. *J Vasc Surg*. 2013;**58**:1171–1177.

8. Kabbani LS, Criado E, Upchurch GR Jr., et al. Hybrid repair of aortic aneurysms involving the visceral and renal vessels. *Ann Vasc Surg*. 2010;**24**:219–224.

9. Weaver KD, Wiseman DB, Farber M, et al. Complications of lumbar drainage after thoracoabdominal aortic aneurysm repair. *J Vasc Surg*. 2001;**34**:623–627.

10. Terzi F, Rocchi G, Fattori R. Current challenges in endovascular therapy for thoracic aneurysms. *Expert Rev Cardiovasc Ther*. 2016;**14**:599–607.

11. Yamaguchi D, Jordan WD Jr. Hybrid thoracoabdominal aortic aneurysm repair: current perspectives. *Semin Vasc Surg*. 2012;**25**:203–207.

12. Kamman AV, Jonker FH, Nauta FJ, et al. A review of follow-up outcomes after elective endovascular repair of degenerative thoracic aortic aneurysms. *Vascular*. 2016;**24**:208–216.

14

Endovascular repair of acute aortic dissection

LOAY S. KABBANI, JASON RYAN, AND IYAD N. ISSEH

CONTENTS

INTRODUCTION

The traditional classification for Stanford type B aortic dissection (TBAD) has been either acute (<2 weeks) or chronic (>2 weeks). Recently, a new classification has been proposed: hyperacute (symptom onset within 24 hours); acute (2–7 days); subacute (8–30 days); and chronic (>30 days).[1] In most cases, uncomplicated acute TBAD is treated medically, while complicated acute TBAD is offered surgery. Complicated acute TBAD is defined as: acute TBAD with rupture and hemodynamic instability (systolic blood pressure (BP) <90 mmHg); acute TBAD with impending rupture (defined as an increase in periaortic hematoma or hemorrhagic pleural effusion observed on two subsequent computed tomography examinations); or acute TBAD with malperfusion. Manifestations of malperfusion include: paresis or paraplegia in spinal cord malperfusion; abdominal pain, nausea, and bloody diarrhea in intestinal malperfusion; or decreased or absent lower extremity pulses with pain, paresthesia, and paralysis in lower extremity malperfusion. New-onset refractory hypertension despite three or more antihypertensive medications of different classes given at maximally recommended or tolerated doses may reflect renal malperfusion. Finally, refractory back or abdominal pain may be a clinical symptom indicative of complicated acute TBAD.[2,3]

MEDICAL MANAGEMENT OF ACUTE TBAD

The best medical therapy for acute TBAD aims to obtain pain control, lower systolic BP of 100–120 mmHg, and a heart rate of 60 bpm. This is attained with intravenous beta-blocking agents, with or without vasodilating drugs, such as sodium nitroprusside or nicardipine hydrochloride. Once stable BP and symptom relief are reached, the patient is transitioned to oral antihypertensive medication and discharged. Follow-up at 3 and 6 months and annually thereafter is essential to detect aneurysmal degeneration of the affected aortic segment, which affects 30–40% of patients within 5 years. For chronic TBAD, systolic resting BP should be kept at 130–150 mmHg, and BP during exercise should be kept below 180 mmHg.

Endovascular treatment for acute and subacute uncomplicated TBAD

Several studies have shown favorable aortic remodeling rates (increase in true lumen diameter and false lumen thrombosis) and improved long-term survival over medical therapy alone using thoracic endovascular aortic repair (TEVAR) for uncomplicated acute, subacute, and early chronic TBAD. Several clinical and radiographic variables have been identified as potential risk factors

Table 14.1 Risk factors for complicated type B aortic dissection

Category	Predictor of worse outcomes
History	Age <60 years
	White ethnicity
	Connective tissue disorder
	Persistent pain
Radiologic findings	Initial aortic diameter ≥40 mm
	Initial false lumen diameter ≥22 mm
	Large entry tear >10 mm
	Partially thrombosed false lumen
	Saccular aneurysm formation
	Entry tear on lesser curve

for subsequent complications (**Table 14.1**). Patients with one or more of these risk factors may benefit from early TEVAR.[4–10] However, early repair of uncomplicated acute TBAD remains controversial and more studies are needed to confirm this concept.

Endovascular treatment for acute complicated TBAD

TEVAR is an attractive alternative to open surgery in addressing complicated acute TBAD for both malperfusion and rupture. Hospital mortality is significantly lower than with open surgery (10 versus 34%).[11] Some surgeons advocate covering the thoracic aorta down to the celiac artery in all cases of malperfusion and rupture. The Provisional Extension to Induce Complete Attachment (PETTICOAT) concept takes the idea further by extending the stent graft scaffold distally with open-cell, bare-metal stents past the visceral vessels to correct distal malperfusion.[12]

TEVAR for chronic TBAD

Approximately 30–40% of patients develop aneurysmal degeneration along the dissected segments during follow-up. These are managed as descending thoracic aortic aneurysms or thoracoabdominal aortic aneurysms, and are discussed in Chapters 12, 13, and 35. When sizing and planning for TEVAR, the chronicity of the dissection flap should be considered, because the flap in chronic dissections may not allow dilation of the true lumen back to its original diameter.

Operative considerations in TEVAR for TBAD

All patients with TBAD should undergo dynamic CT angiography (CTA) with 1-mm cuts and phase delay imaging from the base of the skull to the femoral arteries. Phase delay imaging helps with delayed filling of branch vessels. CTA images give important information about: the type of dissection; proximal landing zones; true lumen compression; branch vessel obstruction; mechanism of obstruction (static versus dynamic); access vessel size; and associated aneurysmal disease. Reconstruction with centerline measurements, if available, is helpful in determining the suitability for TEVAR. Anatomic requirements for TEVAR include the presence of a 2-cm proximal landing zone that is relatively flat and not beaked or tapered (see Chapter 13 for further discussion on landing zones), and access vessels that are relatively straight and free of atherosclerotic disease and calcification with sufficient diameter to accommodate the endograft delivery system.

Intravascular ultrasound (IVUS) is essential to document that the wires and grafts remain in the true lumen throughout their trajectory from the common femoral arteries (CFAs) to the ascending aorta. A spinal drain is placed routinely and kept at a pressure of 10 cm H_2O. The left subclavian artery (LSA) can be covered without revascularization if there is an adequate right vertebral artery to compensate for the left. Covering the LSA without revascularization is discouraged in patients with a history of coronary artery bypass using the left internal mammary artery. The stent graft is deployed to cover the primary entry tear. The selected stent graft should have a diameter no more than 10% larger than the aortic diameter at the landing zone. As the true lumen expands, and flow through the false lumen is reduced or obliterated, any dynamic branch vessel compromise is usually ameliorated. After the stent graft has been deployed, graft molding with an angioplasty balloon is discouraged, as this increases the risk of retrograde type A thoracic aortic dissection.

Completion angiography and IVUS should be carried out routinely to ensure that the dynamic obstruction has resolved. If there is still a static or dynamic obstruction in one of the visceral or iliac arteries, pressure measurements can be obtained across the lesion to determine its significance. Significant stenosis is defined as a systolic gradient >20 mmHg. A self-expanding stent, sized to no more than 10% of the vessel diameter, is placed to correct this.

COMPLICATIONS

Early mortality for uncomplicated TBAD is reported to be 2–10% with a stroke rate of 1% and spinal cord ischemia (SCI) of 0.8%.[13,14] Complicated acute TBAD (rupture or malperfusion) occurs in 12–25% of patients who present with acute TBAD. TEVAR in complicated acute TBAD has a mortality rate of 7–16% with SCI and stroke occurring in 3 and 4%, respectively. Retrograde aortic dissection extension into the ascending aorta occurs in 0.4–7.5%.[11,12] Endoleaks, graft migration, renal failure, and device separation have also been reported.

CASE EXAMPLES

Case example 1

A 57-year-old man presented to the emergency department with sudden onset of severe, tearing chest and

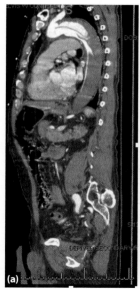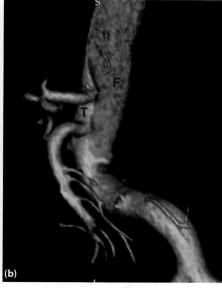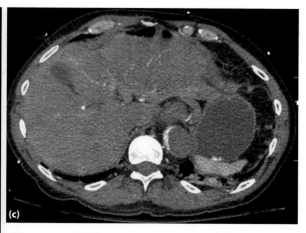

Figure 14.1 Computed tomography angiography of type B aortic dissection. (**a**) Sagittal view. (**b**) Three-dimensional reconstruction with true (T) and false (F) lumen. (**c**) Axial view.

back pain. He had a history significant for hypertension, and was 6 years status post-kidney transplant. He was a former smoker. On physical examination, his BP was 200/100 mmHg. He had strong distal pulses and no signs of malperfusion. A CT scan of his chest, abdomen, and pelvis demonstrated a TBAD, originating just distal to the LSA, and extending to the L2 vertebral body. The celiac axis, superior mesenteric artery, inferior mesenteric artery, and renal arteries were patent and arising from the true lumen (**Figure 14.1a,b**). The true lumen was severely narrowed from compression by the false lumen (**Figure 14.1c**). He was admitted to the cardiac intensive care unit (ICU) for anti-impulse therapy, and was placed on a labetalol drip. Despite becoming normotensive for 3 days, he continued to have debilitating chest pain that was refractory to medical treatment. The decision was made to repair the dissection with a thoracic stent graft in the acute setting.

The patient was taken to the operating room and a spinal drain was placed by the anesthesia staff. After arterial and central venous catheters were placed, US-guided percutaneous access was achieved in both CFAs. A hydrophilic wire was advanced bilaterally to the aortic arch. IVUS was used to confirm wire passage within the true lumen. After obtaining an aortogram, a GORE® TAG® Thoracic Endoprosthesis (W. L. Gore & Associates, Flagstaff, AZ, USA) was deployed just distal to the left common carotid artery, covering the LSA (**Figure 14.2**). A second component was deployed distally with 4 cm of overlap to an area just proximal to the celiac artery. Percutaneous closure devices were used to close the puncture sites.

The patient was transferred to the ICU for ongoing care. He was extubated and had no neurologic deficits. His chest pain was markedly improved postoperatively and he had no symptoms or signs of left upper extremity ischemia. The spinal drain was removed on postoperative day 2. He was discharged home on oral antihypertensives medication on postoperative day 3.

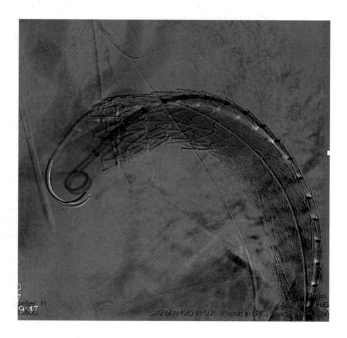

Figure 14.2 Completion digital subtraction angiography of the thoracic endograft. Note the complete coverage of the entry tear; the left subclavian artery was covered.

Case example 2

A 46-year-old woman presented to the emergency department at another institution with acute, sharp, and tearing chest pain radiating to her back. She had smoked 1 pack of cigarettes per day for the last 20 years, and had a history of untreated hypertension. Her BP on presentation was 220/120 mmHg. CTA revealed acute TBAD (**Figure 14.3a,b**). She was transferred to the authors' tertiary hospital. On arrival, she began reporting right foot pain with numbness and weakness that propagated up the right leg. On physical examination, the patient had

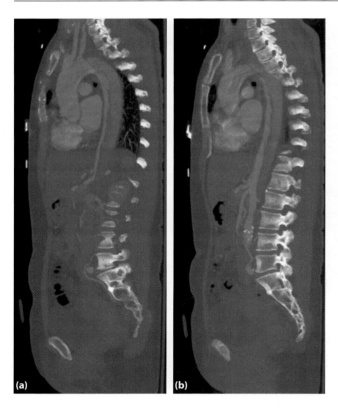

Figure 14.3 Computed tomography angiography demonstrating (**a**) type B aortic dissection and (**b**) sagittal cuts showing the celiac axis and superior mesenteric artery perfused by the true lumen.

palpable left femoral, posterior tibial, and dorsalis pedis pulses, but no palpable pulses in the right leg. Review of her CTA revealed that the visceral vessels and left iliac artery were patent and originated from the true lumen, but there was a severe narrowing involving her right common iliac artery (CIA) from the dissection flap (**Figure 14.4**). She was placed on anti-impulse therapy and, despite achieving good BP control, her right leg symptoms progressed. She was taken to the operating room.

Options to treat the right CIA narrowing included a left CFA-to-right CFA bypass, an iliac stent to open the

iliac artery, or a thoracic stent graft to close the proximal entry tear.

In the operating room, the anesthesia team placed an arterial line, a central venous catheter, and a spinal drain. The right CFA was surgically exposed and was pulseless. On opening the artery, no dissection flap or thrombus was seen. An 8-Fr sheath was placed into the artery. A wire was advanced up into the aorta, followed by a flush catheter. An aorto-bi-iliac angiogram was obtained. This demonstrated good flow through the infrarenal aorta and the left CIA and left external iliac artery. The dissection flap was visible in the infrarenal aorta and extended into the right iliac artery. There was poor flow in the right CIA. IVUS confirmed wire placement in the true lumen (**Figure 14.5**). Arterial pressure was obtained in the right CFA artery and was severely diminished at 30 mmHg, compared to the right arm systolic pressure of 120 mmHg. A 32 mm × 157 mm Valiant® Thoracic Stent Graft (Medtronic Inc., Minneapolis, MN, USA) was placed across the primary entry site, covering the LSA (**Figure 14.6a,b**). The stent graft was not molded into position with a compliant balloon. Following this, no significant pressure gradient remained between the right arm and the femoral arteries. IVUS confirmed proper placement of the graft with a patent true lumen, and no retrograde dissection (**Figure 14.7**). Because of the prolonged ischemia time, a right leg four-compartment fasciotomy was carried out in the standard fashion. The patient was extubated in the operating room and was found neurologically intact. She was transferred to the ICU for close monitoring. Six months after discharge, CTA revealed a healed dissection (**Figure 14.8a,b**).

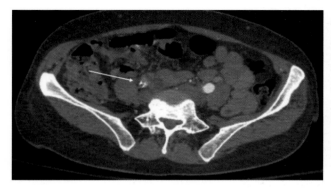

Figure 14.4 Computed tomography angiography axial image demonstrating extension of the dissection into the right common iliac artery with severe stenosis (arrow).

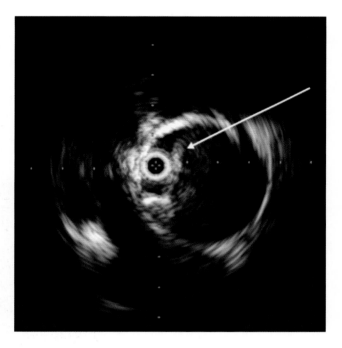

Figure 14.5 Intraoperative intravascular ultrasound image demonstrating that the probe and wire are within the severely compressed true lumen with the dissection flap (arrow) separating the true and false lumens.

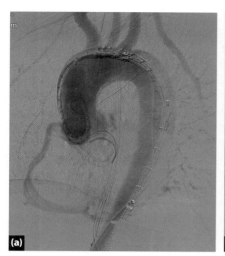
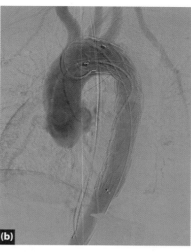

Figure 14.6 Intraoperative digital subtraction angiography images. (**a**) Predeployment of stent graft. (**b**) Postdeployment with complete coverage of entry tear.

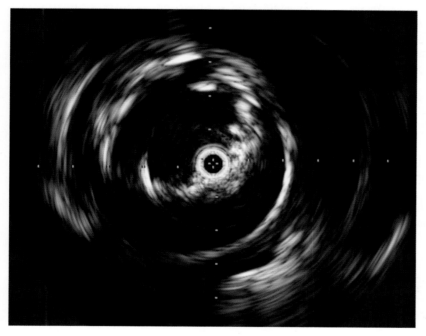

Figure 14.7 Intraoperative intravascular ultrasound image after placement of a thoracic endograft with expansion of the true lumen.

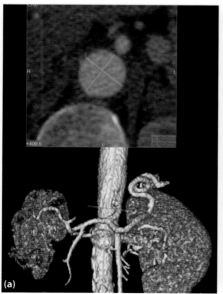
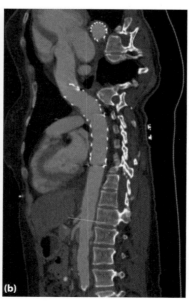

Figure 14.8 Six-month postoperative computed tomography angiography images. (**a**) Three-dimensional reconstruction with axial image (inset). (**b**) Sagittal image. Both images demonstrate a patent endograft with resolution of dissection.

REFERENCES

1. Booher AM, Isselbacher EM, Nienaber CA, et al. The IRAD classification system for characterizing survival after aortic dissection. *Am J Med.* 2013;**126**:730. e19–24.

2. Hiratzka LF, Bakris GL, Beckman JA, et al. 2010 ACCF/AHA/AATS/ACR/ASA/SCA/SCAI/SIR/STS/ SVM guidelines for the diagnosis and management of patients with Thoracic Aortic Disease: a report of the American College of Cardiology Foundation/American Heart Association Task Force on Practice Guidelines, American Association for Thoracic Surgery, American College of Radiology, American Stroke Association, Society of Cardiovascular Anesthesiologists, Society for Cardiovascular Angiography and Interventions, Society of Interventional Radiology, Society of Thoracic Surgeons, and Society for Vascular Medicine. *Circulation.* 2010;**121**:e266–369.

3. Nauta FJ, Trimarchi S, Kamman AV, et al. Update in the management of type B aortic dissection. *Vasc Med.* 2016;**21**:251–263.

4. Sueyoshi E, Sakamoto I, Hayashi K, et al. Growth rate of aortic diameter in patients with type B aortic dissection during the chronic phase. *Circulation.* 2004;**110(11 Suppl 1)**:II256–261.

5. Jonker FH, Patel HJ, Upchurch GR, et al. Acute type B aortic dissection complicated by visceral ischemia. *J Thorac Cardiovasc Surg.* 2015;**149**:1081–1086.e1.

6. Song JM, Kim SD, Kim JH, et al. Long-term predictors of descending aorta aneurysmal change in patients with aortic dissection. *J Am Coll Cardiol.* 2007;**50**:799–804.

7. Onitsuka S, Akashi H, Tayama K, et al. Long-term outcome and prognostic predictors of medically treated acute type B aortic dissections. *Ann Thorac Surg.* 2004;**78**:1268–1273.

8. Tolenaar JL, van Keulen JW, Jonker FH, et al. Morphologic predictors of aortic dilatation in type B aortic dissection. *J Vasc Surg.* 2013;**58**:1220–1225.

9. Marui A, Mochizuki T, Koyama T, et al. Degree of fusiform dilatation of the proximal descending aorta in type B acute aortic dissection can predict late aortic events. *J Thorac Cardiovasc Surg.* 2007;**134**:1163-1170.

10. Winnerkvist A, Lockowandt U, Rasmussen E, et al. A prospective study of medically treated acute type B aortic dissection. *Eur J Vasc Endovasc Surg.* 2006;**32**:349–355.

11. Fattori R, Tsai TT, Myrmel T, et al. Complicated acute type B dissection: is surgery still the best option? A report from the International Registry of Acute Aortic Dissection. *JACC Cardiovasc Interv.* 2008;**1**:395–402.

12. Lombardi JV, Cambria RP, Nienaber CA, et al. Aortic remodeling after endovascular treatment of complicated type B aortic dissection with the use of a composite device design. *J Vasc Surg.* 2014;**59**:1544–1554.

13. Fattori R, Cao P, De Rango P, et al. Interdisciplinary expert consensus document on management of type B aortic dissection. *J Am Coll Cardiol.* 2013; **61**:1661–1678.

14. Tsai TT, Fattori R, Trimarchi S, et al. Long-term survival in patients presenting with type B acute aortic dissection: insights from the International Registry of Acute Aortic Dissection. *Circulation.* 2006;**114**:2226–2231.

15

Endovascular management of splanchnic artery aneurysms

TIMUR P. SARAC AND LINDSAY GATES

CONTENTS

INTRODUCTION

Splanchnic artery aneurysms involve the celiac, superior mesenteric (SMA), inferior mesenteric (IMA), and renal arteries and their branches. The etiology is like other aneurysms, with atherosclerosis the primary etiology, followed by medial degeneration/dysplasia (24%), abdominal trauma (22%), infection and inflammatory disease (10%), connective tissue disorders, and hyper-flow conditions.[1] Because of low incidence, the natural history of visceral artery aneurysms is not completely elucidated.

Sixty percent of splanchnic artery aneurysms occur in the splenic artery, 20% in the hepatic artery, 8% in the SMA, 4% in the celiac artery, 4% in the gastric and gastroepiploic arteries, and 4% in the remaining splanchnic branches.[2] Splenic artery aneurysms (SAAs), the most common splanchnic artery aneurysms, have been estimated to occur in 0.8–4% of patients undergoing angiography.[3] In general, most splanchnic artery aneurysms are asymptomatic before rupture.[4] When pain is present, it often signifies acute aneurysmal growth. Rupture rates and subsequent mortality rates are reported to be 2–90% and 25–75%, respectively, depending on location and etiology.[3]

Traditionally, surgical therapy involves an open exposure for ligation or resection of the aneurysm with or without arterial reconstruction and possibly end organ resection (i.e., splenectomy, nephrectomy). However, percutaneous embolization with coils, glue, or plugs, placement of covered stents, and injection of endoluminal thrombin, polyvinyl alcohol particles or gel foam are also less invasive alternatives. In many situations, as with small atherosclerotic SAAs, these lesions may be safely observed.[5]

SPLENIC ARTERY ANEURYSMS

SAAs were first reported in 1770, when Beaussier[6] reported one in a 60-year-old woman at autopsy. Overall, 87% of patients with SAAs are women, the majority being multiparous women. Mortality from rupture is between 10 and 25% for those who are not pregnant and may be as high as 70% in pregnancy, with fetal mortality approaching 90%. Since the risk of mortality from prophylactic surgical treatment of noninflammatory SAAs is low, patients should undergo surgery if they are or may become pregnant, if the aneurysm is >2–2.5 cm, or if they have referred abdominal symptoms.[7]

Treatment for SAAs includes open surgical repair or endovascular repair. Open surgery for SAAs can carry a 1–3% mortality rate, together with a 9–25% perioperative complication rate from splenic or pancreatic injury.[5,8] Additionally, surgery for SAAs due to pancreatitis has an associated mortality rate of 30% because of the technical problems associated with persistent intra-abdominal sepsis, the presence of extensive inflammatory adhesions, pancreatic pseudocysts, multiple feeding vessels, and enteric erosions, as well as the possible need for splenectomy and

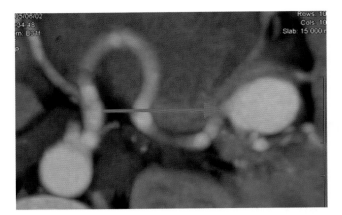

Figure 15.1 Splenic artery aneurysm embolized with coils (arrow).

partial pancreatectomy.[5] Therefore, percutaneous arterial embolism and thrombosis of the aneurysm is preferable and safer.

The outcomes reported from treating SAAs with minimally invasive endovascular techniques have been encouraging, and in most cases these therapies have become the preferred method of treatment. Treatment can include transcatheter embolization (coil or glue) and stent graft placement.[9] The more commonly used small embolic particles of polytetrafluoroethylene, polyvinyl acetal, or adhesive silicone are not used to cause thrombosis, because they are not retained in the aneurysm but embolize distally to the spleen. Instead, coils or glue are generally introduced into the arterial lumen. The coils expand after extrusion from the catheter, wedging within the lumen leading to thrombosis. Additionally, most coils are coated with Dacron strands, making them highly thrombogenic (**Figure 15.1**). For areas not amenable to coil or glue embolization, stent graft exclusion can be used. In these situations, sufficient vessel length and minimal tortuosity are needed to allow proper stent graft deployment. The overall success rates for all endovascular interventions have been reported to be between 72 and 98%.[10,11]

HEPATIC ARTERY ANEURYSMS (HAAs)

HAAs are the second most common location of splanchnic aneurysm formation (20%) and affect men 2–3 times as often as women. The majority (30%) of HAAs are degenerative (atherosclerotic).[12–14] Other important causes of HAAs are trauma and inflammation. Trauma accounts for 22% of HAAs. Blunt and penetrating trauma can cause both intrahepatic or extrahepatic aneurysms. Twenty percent of all HAAs are intrahepatic, and most these are caused by trauma and occasionally percutaneous transhepatic procedures.[15]

HAAs have the highest rupture rate of all SAAs and about 20% of patients present with right upper quadrant pain or rupture (**Figure 15.2**).[16] Asymptomatic patients are usually diagnosed incidentally from computed

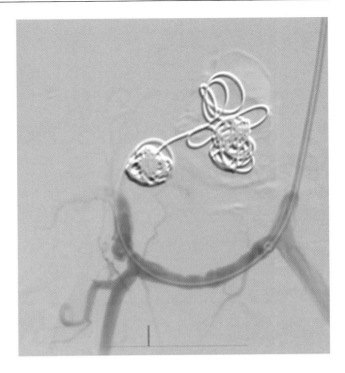

Figure 15.2 Ruptured hepatic artery aneurysm embolized with coils.

tomography (CT) scans. Occasionally, the diagnosis is based on vascular calcifications found incidentally on plain X-ray film imaging. In patients who have large aneurysms, displacement of neighboring structures, such as the biliary and gastrointestinal (GI) tracts, can provide a diagnostic clue. Rarely, these aneurysms will rupture into the portal vein, creating acute portal hypertension and bleeding varices. Rupture rates and subsequent mortality rates for HAAs are 20–44% and 35–82%, respectively.[15,16]

It is important to distinguish between true and pseudoaneurysms of the hepatic artery. Based on a study from the Cleveland Clinic, 92% of splanchnic pseudoaneurysms in their series presented with GI bleeding or hemobilia and required urgent intervention. They concluded that all pseudoaneurysms should be treated because of their higher risk for complications.[17]

The definitive diagnostic tool for planning treatment is selective celiac or hepatic artery angiography. Angiography can delineate the site and extent of the aneurysm, demonstrate an arteriovenous fistula, and can show arterial collaterals that have formed or enlarged portal venous collaterals if portal hypertension is present. It also outlines the anatomy of the liver's blood supply, which is via aberrant vessels in up to 40% of people. This is important information, as the arterial blood supply to the liver should be maintained following treatment, either through collaterals, normal aberrant arteries, or a prosthetic or autologous vein graft to replace the excised, diseased segment of artery.

While open surgery is still an option, endovascular outcomes have improved over time. Tulsyan and collaborators reported a 98% technical success rate with endovascular management, and complete aneurysm exclusion in 97% of patients on follow-up.[5] Invasive angiography can be used to thrombose HAAs and is the preferred method for the treatment of intrahepatic aneurysms that otherwise would be treated by ligation of the right or left hepatic artery or even by hepatic lobectomy. Percutaneous embolization and thrombosis is generally not recommended for the treatment of an extrahepatic aneurysm because of the importance of maintaining the arterial blood supply to the liver. There are reports of extrahepatic aneurysms being successfully treated by embolization and covered stent placement in patients with additional illnesses or where open repair in an inflammatory or hostile environment would be technically difficult and elevate the risk of major vascular reconstruction.[18]

SMA ANEURYSMS

Unlike SAAs and HAAs, SMA aneurysms (SMAAs) are rarely caused by trauma or medial degeneration, thus their overall incidence is proportionately lower. The most common etiology for SMAAs is infection (60%), with most patients presenting with subacute bacterial endocarditis.[19] *Streptococcus* species are commonly grown from the aneurysm, although in drug addicts *Staphylococcus aureus* is also likely. Mycotic aneurysms from septic emboli and dissections happen more often in the SMA than in the other splanchnic vessels (**Figure 15.3**). In a minority of patients, SMAAs are atherosclerotic in origin, and plain radiography may show ring-like calcification in the upper abdomen near the midline with a posterior defect in the circumference representing the origin of the SMA from the aorta.[20,21]

SMAAs are also unique in that the majority of symptomatic patients manifest symptoms from a vague colicky pain, intestinal angina, weight loss, or symptoms of intestinal ischemia before rupture.[21] At times, a pulsation can be appreciated and the patient may have positive blood cultures. Patients who have an SMAA from another cause can present with similar pain but no antecedent history. Asymptomatic aneurysms are most frequently discovered as an incidental finding from a CT scan.

The natural history of mycotic aneurysm wall is of painful enlargement and ultimately rupture. The history of atherosclerotic or other types of aneurysms is uncertain, though one could expect progressive enlargement and ultimate rupture like aneurysms in other locations. Rupture rates range from 38 to 50% with associated mortality rates of 30–90%.[22]

Excision of many SMAAs can be difficult, as they can adhere to important adjacent structures, including the superior mesenteric vein. Therefore, endovascular intervention with stent grafts or coil embolization are alternative treatments for SMAAs depending on the location, and in patients who are poor surgical candidates (**Figure 15.4**). In 2011, Jiang and collaborators reported treating five patients with endovascular stent graft repair. Postoperative follow-up showed no evidence of bowel ischemia in the stent graft group with 100% patency on follow-up.[23] They concluded that endovascular repair with stenting or embolization may be preferable in patients with severe cardiac or pulmonary disease or hostile abdomens because of shorter operative time and length of hospital stay and decreased operative mortality. However, many tributaries and collaterals originate proximal and distal to SMAAs and covering these vessels with a stent graft can cause bowel ischemia. Other reports have shown success with coil embolization. Occasionally, patients may have

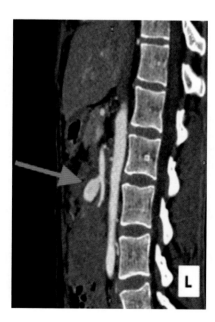

Figure 15.3 Saccular superior mesenteric artery aneurysm (arrow).

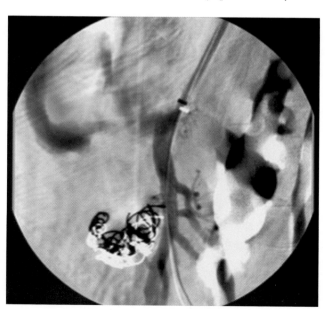

Figure 15.4 Stent graft and coils in the superior mesenteric artery and aneurysm sac.

saccular aneurysms, and these can be treated by combined coil embolization and stent grafts.

OTHER SPLANCHNIC ARTERY ANEURYSMS

Other locations are less common and include aneurysms of the celiac, gastric, gastroduodenal, pancreaticoduodenal, ileal and jejunal branches of the SMA, renal, and most rare of all, IMA. The majority are atherosclerotic degenerative aneurysms, or from increased flow through collateral branches in the case of a major trunk occlusion. However, some can arise following trauma to the arterial wall or from local inflammation, particularly in the case of the pancreaticoduodenal and gastroduodenal arteries in patients with pancreatitis.

Pancreaticoduodenal and gastroduodenal artery aneurysms caused by pancreatitis are usually identified serendipitously from a CT scan (**Figure 15.5**), but can present as bleeding from rupture into the pancreatic duct, biliary system, or adjacent bowel. These aneurysms should always be considered as possible points of origin of idiopathic intestinal bleeding. Most are from occlusion of the celiac artery and retrograde flow from small collaterals, which results in "flow" aneurysms.

Those in the celiac artery are usually fusiform aneurysms (**Figure 15.6**) and can be associated with celiac compression from the arcuate ligament or post-stenotic dilation. Stone and collaborators reported that 38% of patients with celiac artery aneurysms (CAAs) have other splanchnic artery aneurysms and 18% have abdominal aorta aneurysms.[24] Atherosclerosis is associated with 27% of CAAs.[24]

As in the case of SMAAs, 60% of patients with CAAs have abdominal discomfort before rupture and 30% have a pulsatile abdominal mass.[24,25] Rupture rates and subsequent mortality rates are 13% and 40%, respectively.[25]

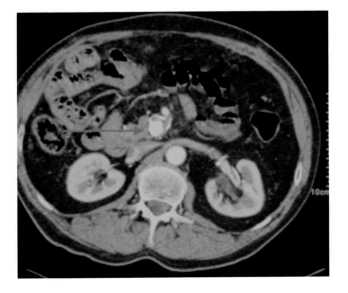

Figure 15.5 Pancreaticoduodenal artery aneurysm (arrow).

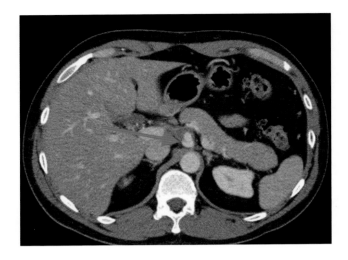

Figure 15.6 Celiac artery aneurysm (arrow).

Open surgery is successful in at least 90% of cases. Dissection in this area can be hazardous because the pancreas is in close juxtaposition; occasionally, a hybrid open and endovascular approach is an option.

Endovascular treatment by embolization has been described and may be appropriate in high-risk patients. Intact collateral circulation should allow for embolization of the inflow, outflow, and branches of the aneurysm without arterial reconstruction. Safe coverage/exclusion of the celiac artery has been described in the setting of thoracic artery aneurysm repair. However, to confirm adequate collateral circulation, selective arteriography through the SMA is appropriate.[26]

The close anatomic relationship of the gastroduodenal and pancreaticoduodenal arteries to the pancreas puts these arteries, like the splenic artery, at risk for development of inflammatory aneurysms. Sixty percent of gastroduodenal and 30% of pancreaticoduodenal aneurysms are caused by pancreatitis.[27] Another infrequent cause of aneurysm formation is concomitant celiac or SMA stenosis/occlusion. These patients have increased blood flow in the pancreaticoduodenal arcades predisposing them to aneurysm formation. Patients with pancreatitis-related aneurysms may have symptoms before rupture, but these may be difficult to differentiate from the symptoms of pancreatitis. Coil embolization and percutaneous transabdominal thrombin injection are other accepted forms of treatment in these patients, offering an excellent option in treating lesions that are challenging to access via an open surgical approach.[27]

GASTRIC AND GASTROEPIPLOIC ARTERY ANEURYSMS

Aneurysms of the gastric and gastroepiploic arteries occur through various mechanisms, the most common of which are atherosclerosis and medial degeneration. An unusual cause of gastric artery aneurysms (GAAs) is the so-called caliber-persistent artery of the stomach, also called cirsoid aneurysm, miliary aneurysm of the stomach, or Dieulafoy's vascular malformation. These lesions are probably congenital anatomic variants in which gastric vessels penetrate the submucosa without decreasing in size or joining in the normal submucosal anastomotic plexus of vessels.[1,5]

GAAs most commonly develop in the gastric, and not the gastroepiploic, vessels. Unlike other splanchnic aneurysms, most GAAs (70%) will rupture into the GI tract and not the peritoneal cavity.[28] Ninety percent of patients with these lesions present with aneurysm rupture as their initial symptom. The mortality rate for patients after rupture is 70%.[28] Because of the high rate of rupture leading to hemodynamic instability, emergency open surgery is the most common form of treatment. Ligation of the affected gastric vessel usually does not cause gastric ischemia because of the abundant collaterals. However, coil embolization is usually the first line of therapy.

RENAL ARTERY ANEURYSMS

Renal artery aneurysms are the rarest of all (**Figure 15.7**). They have the lowest rupture and growth rate, and observation is now recommended until they reach >3 cm in diameter.[29] Endovascular management can consist of stent graft placement, or coil embolization of saccular aneurysms or peripheral branches. However, open repair with bypass is still the gold standard.

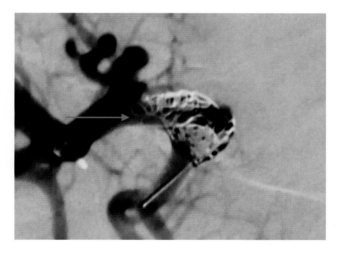

Figure 15.7 Renal artery aneurysm embolized with coils and pipeline stent (arrow).

REFERENCES

1. Gehlen JM, Heeren PA, Verhagen PF, et al. Visceral artery aneurysms. *Vasc Endovascular Surg.* 2011; **45**:681–687.
2. Deterling RA Jr. Aneurysm of the visceral arteries. *J Cardiovasc Surg (Torino).* 1971;**12**:309–322.
3. Stanley JC, Fry WJ. Pathogenesis and clinical significance of splenic artery aneurysms. *Surgery.* 1974;**76**:898–909.
4. Trastek VF, Pairolero PC, Joyce JW, et al. Splenic artery aneurysms. *Surgery.* 1982;**91**:694–699.
5. Tulsyan N, Kashyap VS, Greenberg RK, et al. The endovascular management of visceral artery aneurysms and pseudoaneurysms. *J Vasc Surg.* 2007;**45**:276–283.
6. Beaussier M. Sur un anévrisme de l'artère splénique dont les parois se sont ossifiés. [Article in French]. *J Med Toulouse.* 1770;**32**:157.
7. Al-Habbal Y, Christophi C, Muralidharan V. Aneurysms of the splenic artery: a review. *Surgeon.* 2010;**8**:223–231.
8. Pomerantz RA, Eckhauser FE, Strodel WE, et al. Splenic aneurysm rupture in cirrhotic patients. *Arch Surg.* 1986;**121**:1095–1096.
9. Cordova AC, Sumpio BE. Visceral artery aneurysms and pseudoaneurysms. Should they all be managed by endovascular techniques? *Ann Vasc Dis.* 2013;**6**:687–693.
10. Abbas MA, Stone WM, Fowl RJ. Splenic artery aneurysms: two decades experience at Mayo Clinic. *Ann Vasc Surg.* 2002;**16**:442–449.
11. Grotemeyer D, Duran M, Park EJ, et al. Visceral artery aneurysms: follow-up of 23 patients with 31 aneurysms after surgical or interventional therapy. *Langenbecks Arch Surg.* 2009;**394**:1093–1100.
12. Abbas MA, Fowl RJ, Stone WM, et al. Hepatic artery aneurysm: factors that predict complications. *J Vasc Surg.* 2003;**38**:41–45.
13. Stanley JC, Thompson NW, Fry WJ. Splanchnic artery aneurysms. *Arch Surg.* 1970;**101**:689–697.
14. Salo JA, Aarnio PT, Järvinen AA, et al. Aneurysms of the hepatic arteries. *Am Surg.* 1989;**55**:705–709.
15. Moore SW, Guida PM, Schumacher HW. Splenic artery aneurysm. *Bull Soc Int Chir.* 1970;**29**:210–218.
16. Reiter DA, Fischman AM, Shy BD. Hepatic artery pseudoaneurysm rupture: a case report and review of the literature. *J Emerg Med.* 2013;**44**:100–103.
17. Arneson MA, Smith RS. Ruptured hepatic artery aneurysm: case report and review of literature. *Ann Vasc Surg.* 2005;**19**:540–545.
18. Stone WM, Abbas M, Cherry KJ, et al. Superior mesenteric artery aneurysms: is presence an indication for intervention. *J Vasc Surg.* 2002;**36**:234–237.
19. Berceli SA. Hepatic and splenic artery aneurysms. *Semin Vasc Surg.* 2005;**18**:196–201.
20. Komori K, Mori E, Yamaoka T, et al. Successful resection of superior mesenteric artery aneurysm. A case report and review of the literature. *J Cardiovasc Surg (Torino).* 2000;**41**:475–478.
21. Graham LM, Stanley JC, Whitehouse WM Jr., et al. Celiac artery aneurysms: historic (1745–1949) versus contemporary (1950–1984) differences in etiology and clinical importance. *J Vasc Surg.* 1985;**5**:757–764.
22. Olcott C, Ehrenfeld WK. Endoaneurysmorrhaphy for visceral artery aneurysms. *Am J Surg.* 1977; **133**:636–639.

23. Jiang J, Ding X, Su Q, et al. Therapeutic management of superior mesenteric artery aneurysms. *J Vasc Surg.* 2011;**53**:1619–1624.

24. Stone WM, Abbas MA, Gloviczki P, et al. Celiac arterial aneurysms: a critical reappraisal of a rare entity. *Arch Surg.* 2002;**137**:670–674.

25. Lorelli DR, Cambria RA, Seabrook GR, et al. Diagnosis and management of aneurysms involving the superior mesenteric artery and its branches: a report of four cases. *Vasc Endovascular Surg.* 2003; **37**:59–66.

26. Leon LR Jr., Mills JL Sr., Jordan W, et al. The risks of celiac artery coverage during endoluminal repair of thoracic and thoracoabdominal aortic aneurysms. *Vasc Endovascular Surg.* 2009;**43**:51–60.

27. Kitaoka T, Deguchi J, Kamiya C, et al. Pancreaticoduodenal artery aneurysm formation with superior mesenteric artery stenosis. *Ann Vasc Dis.* 2014;**7**:312–315.

28. Chandran S, Parvaiz A, Karim A, et al. Ruptured left gastric artery aneurysm successfully treated by thrombin injection: case report and literature review. *ScientificWorldJournal.* 2005;**5**:20–23.

29. Klausner JQ, Lawrence PF, Harlander-Locke MP, et al. The contemporary management of renal artery aneurysms. *J Vasc Surg.* 2015;**61**:978–984.

Iliac vein stenting

ARJUN JAYARAJ AND SESHADRI RAJU

CONTENTS

INTRODUCTION

Endovascular interventions in the femoro-ilio-caval segment are usually performed for chronic venous insufficiency (CVI). CVI can be primary (nonthrombotic) or secondary (post-thrombotic). The latter is the responsible etiology in most patients who develop CVI. Post-thrombotic syndrome (PTS) can develop in up to 50% of patients who develop deep vein thrombosis.[1] Nonthrombotic conditions include May–Thurner syndrome, which is the most common form of primary CVI.[2–3]

Clinical manifestations of CVI include pain (pelvic, hip, thigh), claudication, swelling, skin changes (eczema, lipodermatosclerosis, dermatitis), and ulceration(s) of the involved limb.

Diagnostic testing should focus on determining the etiology of CVI, in addition to determining the inflow and outflow of the affected segment. Such testing includes venous duplex ultrasound (US), air plethysmography, cross-sectional imaging (computed tomography venography (CTV)/magnetic resonance venography (MRV)), and ascending venography. Duplex US serves as a screening tool and helps to determine the extent of femoro-ilio-caval narrowing or obstruction based on luminal diameters in addition to providing reflux data; 12, 14, and 16 mm are the normal luminal diameter cutoffs used for the common femoral vein (CFV), external iliac vein (EIV), and common iliac vein (CIV), respectively (**Table 16.1**). Air plethysmography provides information on calf muscle pump function. Cross-sectional imaging, including

CTV and MRV, elucidates venous anatomy, vein status *vis-à-vis* compression/occlusion, and collateral circulation. Abdominal and pelvic pathology, including malignancy, can also be evaluated by cross-sectional imaging. Ascending venography provides supplementary data on segmental inflow and outflow.

Conservative management of CVI involves frequent leg elevation, the use of graduated compressive stockings, and local wound care for ulceration(s). Patients unable to tolerate compressive stockings or those who have persistent disabling symptoms including claudication, swelling, and nonhealing/recurrent ulcers should be considered for endovascular treatment.

ENDOVASCULAR TREATMENT TECHNIQUE

Endovascular treatment of CVI involves stenting of the femoro-ilio-caval segment and is the most common modality of treatment for patients who fail compression/conservative treatment. Stenting is performed under general anesthesia secondary to significant pain/discomfort that occurs during venoplasty. With the patient in the supine position, access to the femoral vein at mid-thigh is obtained under US guidance. While this can be done with a micropuncture kit, the authors' preference is to use an 18-G needle. An 0.035-inch GLIDEWIRE® (Terumo Medical Corporation, Somerset, NJ, USA) is used to gain purchase into the inferior vena cava (IVC). An incision is made around the wire to enlarge the entry tract with a No. 11 blade scalpel, and a short (10-cm) 11-Fr sheath is placed. An ascending venogram is performed through the sheath to delineate the anatomy. The authors skip venography in patients with significantly compromised renal function. Intravascular US (IVUS) is then performed with an 0.035-inch probe (Volcano Corporation, San Diego, CA, USA). Using planimetry, the luminal areas in the CFV, EIV, and CIV are assessed (125 mm², 150 mm², and 200 mm² are used as normal luminal area cutoffs in the CFV, EIV, and CIV, respectively) (**Table 16.1**). Any decrease in a symptomatic patient is considered abnormal, thereby meriting angioplasty and stenting.

Pre-dilation is performed with an 18 × 60-mm Atlas® PTA Dilatation Catheter (BARD Peripheral Vascular, Inc., Tempe, AZ, USA), proceeding from the CFV to the distal IVC. This sequence is especially helpful for balloon retrieval

Table 16.1 Luminal diameter cutoffs used for the common femoral (CFV), external iliac (EIV), and common iliac (CIV) veins

Vein	Luminal area (mm²)	Diameter (mm)
CFV	125	12
EIV	150	14
CIV	200	16

if disruption of the balloon occurs during inflation. Stenting is then carried out with 20-mm WALLSTENT™ Endoprostheses (Boston Scientific Corporation, Marlborough, MA, USA) with landing zones determined by IVUS. The proximal landing zone is typically 1–2 cm above the iliac confluence, while the distal landing zone is an area of adequate inflow in the CFV. Rarely does one need to stent into the femoral vein or profunda femoris vein. Given the decreased radial strength of the WALLSTENT™ endoprosthesis, a Gianturco Z-stent® (Cook Medical Inc., Bloomington, IN, USA) is used to provide additional strength across the confluence. The authors typically have about 5 mm of extension of the Gianturco Z-stent® beyond the wall stent proximally into the IVC. An overlap of 3 cm between wall stents is required to compensate for foreshortening during angioplasty. Post-dilation is performed with the 18 × 60-mm Atlas® PTA Dilatation Catheter (BARD Peripheral Vascular, Inc.). Completion IVUS is performed to ensure adequacy of the luminal area. Any residual narrowing on IVUS interrogation is overcome by repeat dilation with a larger balloon (20 mm). Completion venography is then performed. The 11-Fr sheath is subsequently withdrawn to just outside the vein and a SURGICEL® FIBRILLAR™ Absorbable Hemostat (Ethicon US, LLC, Somerville, NJ, USA) is introduced via the sheath to aid local hemostasis. Manual pressure is then held to complement hemostasis and a pressure dressing is applied. The published institutional experience of the authors of 982 stents for chronic, nonmalignant, obstructive lesions of the femoro-ilio-caval vein with a 6-year follow-up demonstrated primary, primary-assisted, and secondary patency rates of 79%, 100%, and 100% for nonthrombotic lesions and 57%, 80%, and 86% for post-thrombotic lesions, respectively. Risk factors for restenosis/stent occlusion after venous stenting were the presence and severity of post-thrombotic disease.[4]

Anticoagulation

For perioperative thromboprophylaxis, the authors use enoxaparin sodium 40 mg given subcutaneously in the preoperative area, in addition to bivalirudin 75 mg given intravenously in the operating room before starting the procedure. Following iliocaval stenting, in patients with thrombophilia/PTS, the authors continue therapeutic anticoagulation. Those patients in whom the thrombophilia workup is negative and have nonthrombotic femoro-ilio-caval lesions, the authors use aspirin 81 mg with cilostazol 50 mg twice daily, unless contraindications exist. The latter is used for its suppressive effect on neointimal hyperplasia. Presence of significant in-stent restenosis, but lack of symptom recurrence is an indication to switch to low-dose warfarin (1 mg) or apixaban 2.5 mg daily. Recurrence of symptoms is an indication for repeat IVUS interrogation and possible angioplasty.

Follow-up

Venous duplex US is performed on postoperative day 1 to obtain baseline postprocedure metrics, including stent patency, and to assess stent compression or in-stent restenosis. These parameters are again evaluated by repeat duplex US in addition to assessing symptom relief at clinic visits 2 weeks and 4 weeks postprocedure. A 3–6-month follow-up is required subsequently, which is gradually changed to an annual follow-up depending on symptoms and stent status. More frequent follow-up is typically required for PTS and recanalization patients.

SPECIAL CONSIDERATIONS

Chronic total occlusion

Recanalization of chronic total occlusions (CTOs) uses the same principles described for normal stenting. An 0.035-inch GLIDECATH® Hydrophilic Coated Catheter (Terumo Medical Corporation) and 0.035-inch GLIDEWIRE® (Terumo Medical Corporation) are most commonly used to get across CTO lesions. Access from the right internal jugular vein is sometimes necessary to obtain through-and-through access, using a snare to capture the wire caudally, in the process creating a "body floss" wire. Other devices used for recanalization of CTO lesions include the Quick-Cross™ Support Catheter (Spectranetics Corporation, Colorado Springs, CO, USA), TriForce® Peripheral Crossing Set (Cook Medical Inc.), and reentry devices. More recently, the authors have used laser recanalization as a last resort in occluded stents with modest success. Sequential angioplasty may have to be performed to create an appropriate tract to enable recanalization. Once access across the occluded vein is obtained, then the procedure is carried out as noted previously. Angioplasty is carried out caudal-to-cranial (femoral access) or cranial-to-caudal (jugular access) because this enables easier retrieval of the angioplasty balloon if it disrupts. The likelihood of this happening is higher in CTOs than in stenotic lesions. Stent use, post-dilation, IVUS interrogation, and venography are all performed as described hitherto.

Stent compression or in-stent restenosis

For patients with stent compression or in-stent restenosis who are symptomatic, the authors perform repeat IVUS interrogation of the affected segment and *hyperdilation*. The latter involves the use of an angioplasty balloon larger than the size of the stent used. (For example, for a 20-mm stent, the authors use a 22-mm angioplasty balloon.) Sometimes, an even larger-caliber balloon needs to be used to obtain adequate luminal areas, as noted previously. The authors term this hyperdilation as opposed to *isodilation*, which is dilation using an angioplasty balloon

of the same diameter as the stent. Stent compression is unique to the venous system and results from perivenous fibrotic/scar tissue buildup.

Stent occlusion

Treatment of stent occlusion in patients depends on the acuteness of the occlusion. For acute/subacute occlusions, treatment is with pharmacomechanical thrombectomy with or without catheter-directed thrombolysis. For more chronic occlusions, recanalization can be pursued as described earlier. Acceptable results have been noted in both situations.

Endophlebectomy

The CFV can be compromised by post-thrombotic changes, thereby impacting inflow into the iliocaval segment. Endophlebectomy (excision of the fibrotic/scar tissue) with saphenous vein or bovine pericardium patch angioplasty can overcome this by enlarging the lumen. The procedure also helps overcome the problem of multiple lumens that can arise from partial recanalization of the thrombosed vein.

COMPLICATIONS AND THEIR MANAGEMENT

In general, iliac vein stenting is a procedure that can be performed with minimal mortality and low morbidity. However, the following complications can potentially be encountered.

Access site-related complication

This complication can be minimized by using US guidance to access the femoral vein at mid-thigh. The incidence of thigh hematoma is very low (<1%) and can be effectively managed with compression and delayed start of anticoagulation medication.

Vein injury/rupture

This is very rare due to the relatively low pressure and significant inflammation/periadventitial fibrosis around the vein. In the authors' experience, the incidence of clinical bleed has been 1 contained hematoma in over 3000 iliac stents, and this was managed conservatively. There are instances in the literature where a stent graft has been used to exclude the site of extravasation.

Thrombotic events

Layering of thrombus within the stent occurs because of poor inflow or outflow. Incidence of such events has been <2% in the authors' practice. Contributing factors include stent undersizing, understenting, and lack of perioperative use of anticoagulation/antiplatelet agents. Re-stenting after fracture of a previously placed undersized stent with large-caliber angioplasty balloons, or extending the stent stack proximally or distally, is required for undersized stents and understenting, respectively.

Contralateral iliac vein thrombosis

This is a rare event occurring from jailing of the contralateral CIV by an ipsilateral stent. It can be overcome with a WALLSTENT™ (Boston Scientific Corporation) and Gianturco Z-stent® (Cook Medical Inc.) combination and by limiting extension into the IVC.

Stent compression/in-stent restenosis

This has an incidence of approximately 25%. It occurs from extrinsic compression of the stent because of fibrotic tissue or robust neointimal hyperplasia buildup. It is sometimes difficult to distinguish neointimal hyperplasia from in-stent thrombus buildup. Hyperdilation, as previously described, is used to treat stent compression/in-stent restenosis with recurrent symptoms.

Stent migration

This occurs because of the "choke point" effect of the iliocaval confluence. It is imperative to extend the stent stack proximally to the iliocaval confluence to overcome this effect. Furthermore, use of the Gianturco Z-stent® (Cook Medical Inc.) helps provide additional radial force and checks migration.

Mortality

Mortality is extremely rare, with an incidence of 1 in over 3000 iliocaval stents in the authors' practice.

CASE EXAMPLE

A 67-year-old woman presented with a long-standing history of CVI of the bilateral lower extremities, including pain and swelling. Her left lower extremity was more symptomatic. The remainder of her clinical history was unremarkable, except for obstructive sleep apnea. Examination revealed an obese lady with bilateral lower extremity edema, worse on the left. There was bilateral lipodermatosclerosis involving the lower legs. Workup included venous duplex US of the lower extremities, air plethysmography, and CTV that confirmed luminal compromise of the femoro-ilio-caval segment, which was likely post-thrombotic in nature. Calf pump function was also compromised. Given her lack of improvement with conservative therapy, she was taken to the operating room for a left femoro-ilio-caval venogram, IVUS interrogation, and possible angioplasty and stenting.

The operative procedure followed these steps:

1. US-guided access of the left femoral vein at mid-thigh;
2. Ascending venogram of the left CFV, EIV, CIV, and the distal IVC via an 11-Fr sheath placed in the femoral vein (**Figure 16.1a**);
3. Intravascular US interrogation of the left CFV, EIV, CIV, and distal IVC (**Figure 16.2a–c**);
4. Pre-dilation with an 18 × 60-mm dilatation catheter of the left CFV, EIV, CIV, and distal IVC (**Figure 16.3a–d**);
5. Stenting of the left CFV, EIV, and distal IVC with two 20 × 18-mm WALLSTENT™ Endoprostheses and one 25 × 50-mm Gianturco Z-stent® (**Figure 16.4a–c**);

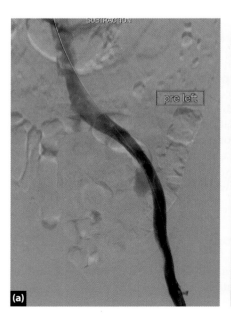
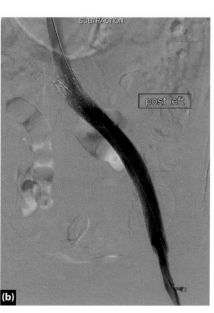

Figure 16.1 Ascending venogram. (**a**) Baseline. (**b**) Postangioplasty and stenting.

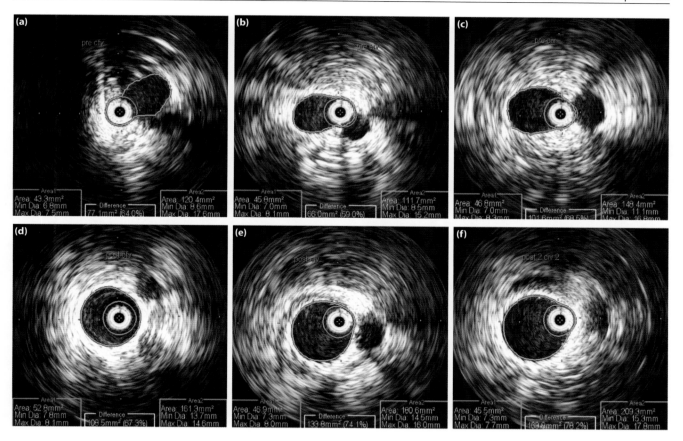

Figure 16.2 Intravascular ultrasound planimetry. Pre-dilation luminal areas of (**a**) common femoral (CFV), (**b**) external iliac (EIV), and (**c**) common iliac (CIV) veins. Postangioplasty and stenting luminal areas of (**d**) CFV, (**e**) EIV, and (**f**) CIV.

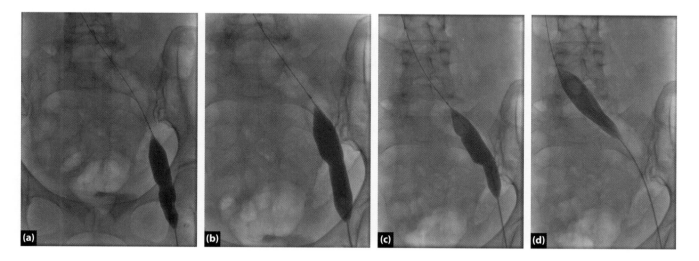

Figure 16.3 Sequential angioplasty of common femoral (CFV), external iliac (EIV), and common iliac (CIV) veins demonstrating multilevel disease suggestive of post-thrombotic syndrome. (**a**) CFV and EIV. (**b**) EIV. (**c**) EIV and distal CIV. (**d**) CIV.

6. Post-dilation with an 18×60-mm dilatation catheter of the stented left CFV, EIV, CIV, and distal IVC;

7. Completion venography (**Figure 16.1b**);

8. Completion intravascular US interrogation of the stented segments (**Figure 16.2d–f**).

Luminal areas obtained on IVUS interrogation

PRE-DILATION

These were: CFV 120 mm^2; EIV 112 mm^2; CIV 148 mm^2; and IVC 263 mm^2 (**Figure 16.2a–c**).

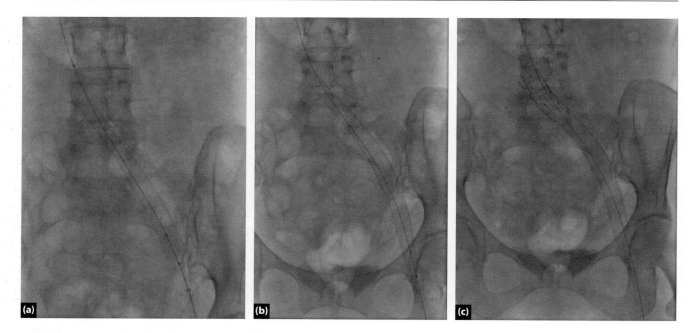

Figure 16.4 Stenting of the left distal femoro-ilio-caval tract. (**a**) Initial stent placement across iliocaval confluence. (**b**) Stent extension distally. (**c**) Stent stack postdeployment of Gianturco Z® stent across the confluence.

POST-STENTING AND DILATION USING 18 × 60-mm DILATATION CATHETER

These were: inflow 157 mm²; CFV 161 mm²; EIV 181 mm²; CIV 209 mm²; IVC in-stent 245 mm²; and IVC above the stent 172 mm² (**Figure 16.2d–f**).

Venography

Initial venography demonstrated some mild narrowing at the level of the CFV (**Figure 16.1a**). Postangioplasty and stenting, there was good luminal caliber throughout the stented segments with good inflow and outflow (**Figure 16.1b**).

The patient did well postoperatively and was discharged the day after the operation on aspirin and cilostazol. On follow-up, her symptoms had improved significantly and she had a patent stent with minimal in-stent restenosis.

REFERENCES

1. Kahn SR, Comerota AJ, Cushman M, et al. The postthrombotic syndrome: evidence-based prevention, diagnosis, and treatment strategies: a scientific statement from the American Heart Association. *Circulation.* 2014;**130**:1636–1661.
2. Cockett FB, Thomas ML, Negus D. Iliac vein compression. Its relation to iliofemoral thrombosis and the postthrombotic syndrome. *Br Med J*;1967;**2**:14–19.
3. Steinberg JB, Jacocks MA. May–Thurner syndrome: a previously unreported variant. *Ann Vasc Surg.* 1993;**7**:577–581.
4. Neglen P, Hollis KC, Olivier J, et al. Stenting of the venous outflow in chronic venous disease: long-term stent-related outcome, clinical, and hemodynamic result. *J Vasc Surg.* 2007;**46**:979–990.

17

Pharmacologic and pharmacomechanical thrombolysis for acute deep vein thrombosis

TODD M. GETZEN AND REHAN RIAZ

CONTENTS

INTRODUCTION

Despite the number of affected patients, and millions more at risk due to immobility, trauma, surgery, and hypercoagulable states, studies have only recently addressed invasive therapies for the treatment of venous thromboembolism (VTE). Published guidelines have focused on acute and chronic medical therapies but do not address the use of invasive, catheter-driven therapies and thrombolysis, which has been shown to reduce the incidence of post-thrombotic syndrome (PTS).[1] The most recent guidelines published by the American College of Chest Physicians proposed anticoagulant therapy alone over invasive therapy.[2] However, anticoagulants alone do not dissolve the occluding thrombus, decrease the venous outflow obstruction, or have any impact on the inflammatory reaction caused by persistent thrombus that is also believed to contribute to PTS. Removal of the thrombus alleviates the acute symptoms of VTE, improves venous patency, and reduces PTS rates.[3] This can be achieved much more reliably using catheter-directed thrombolysis (CDT) or pharmacomechanical CDT.

CDT uses fluoroscopy and image guidance to place a multihole catheter directly into the thrombosed venous segment to infuse thrombolytic agents (**Table 17.1**), allowing for a higher local drug concentration. The most commonly used fibrinolytic drug is recombinant tissue plasminogen activator (rtPA), infused continuously at a low dose (typically 0.5–1.0 mg/hour), along with intravenous (IV) infusion of unfractionated heparin at subtherapeutic levels, ideally infused into the affected venous segment(s). CDT has been shown to be more effective at restoring iliofemoral vein patency versus anticoagulation alone, with recent studies showing that CDT can also reduce the risk of PTS.[1] Reducing the thrombolytic dose decreases the risk of serious bleeding, but requires longer infusion times with the need for specialized monitoring in the intensive care unit (ICU), which add to the use of hospital resources. Pharmacomechanical CDT was developed to address these limitations by the addition of a mechanical device to break apart the thrombus and increase the surface area while delivering the thrombolytic agent. Several devices have come (and some, sadly, have gone) from the market over the last three decades, but the mechanisms of action remain the same: rotational or hydrodynamic thrombus fragmentation.

Rotational (or microfragmentation) thrombectomy devices employ a high-speed rotating basket or impeller to break apart the thrombus. Examples include Arrow-Trerotola™ Percutaneous Thrombolytic Device (Teleflex Medical Europe Ltd, Athlone, Ireland) and CLEANER15™ Rotational Thrombectomy System (Argon Medical Devices Inc., Plano, TX, USA). Hydrodynamic (or rheolytic) devices employ high-speed saline jets in a retrograde direction, using recirculation and the Venturi effect to fragment the thrombus. The most widely used example

Table 17.1 Commonly used thrombolytic agents in the treatment of acute deep vein thrombosis

Thrombolytic agent	Infusion dose
Tissue plasminogen activator (tPA)	0.5–1.0 mg/hour
Recombinant tPA	0.01 mg/kg/hour
Urokinase	120 000–180 000 IU/hour
Streptokinase	100 000 IU/hour

is AngioJet™ Peripheral Thrombectomy System (Boston Scientific Corporation, Marlborough, MA, USA). Balloon angioplasty can also be performed to macerate organized thrombus (**Figure 17.1**). The Indigo® Mechanical Thrombectomy System (Penumbra, Inc., Alameda, CA, USA), initially used in stroke treatment, has been adapted for use throughout the body and employs a catheter/guide-wire combined with a high-power aspiration pump. The EndoWave™ Infusion System drug delivery catheter (EKOS Corporation, Bothell, WA, USA) consists of an infusion catheter and a core wire with ultrasound (US) transducers. The US energy transmitted accelerates dispersion of the lytic agent and increases contact with thrombus-bound plasminogen receptors as it penetrates the clot.

PREPROCEDURE

There are no established criteria for which patients benefit most from CDT or pharmacomechanical CDT. Patients with limb-threatening phlegmasia cerulea dolens or young patients with significant symptoms from a proximal deep vein thrombosis (DVT) should be considered if they are not at an increased risk for bleeding complications. Additionally, involvement of the common femoral (CFV) or iliac veins should point toward endovascular therapy, because this level of involvement is associated with a much higher risk of PTS and recurrent DVT.[4] Otherwise, patient selection for intervention occurs on a case-by-case basis, with the clinical picture, concurrent medical conditions, individual risk of bleeding, patient desire, and ability to tolerate this procedure being the determining factors.

Patients on long-term oral anticoagulation should be managed with unfractionated or low-molecular-weight heparin (LMWH) for more reliable periprocedural control. If there are no contraindications to hydration, aggressive IV fluids should be administered to reduce the risk of contrast-induced nephropathy and the possibility of acute tubular necrosis from intravascular hemolysis. Duplex US of the other extremity should also be done to rule out

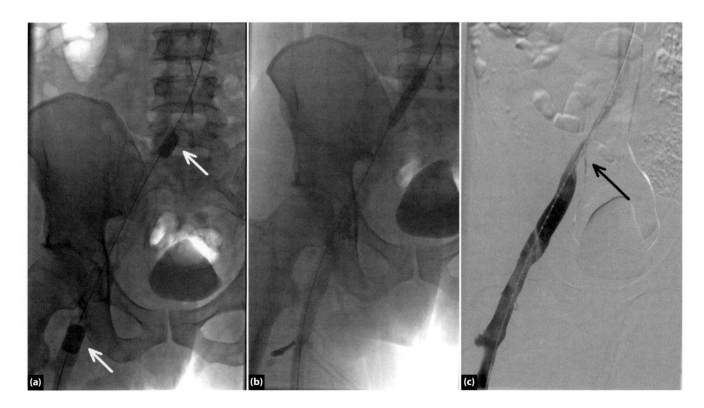

Figure 17.1 Mechanical thrombectomy device. (**a**) The Trellis thrombectomy system (Medtronic, Minneapolis, MN, USA) is positioned from the caval bifurcation to the left femoral vein. While this device is no longer available, current options use a similar mechanism to promote mechanical thrombectomy. Following balloon angioplasty (**b**), a digital subtraction angiogram (**c**) demonstrates the persistent area of stenosis.

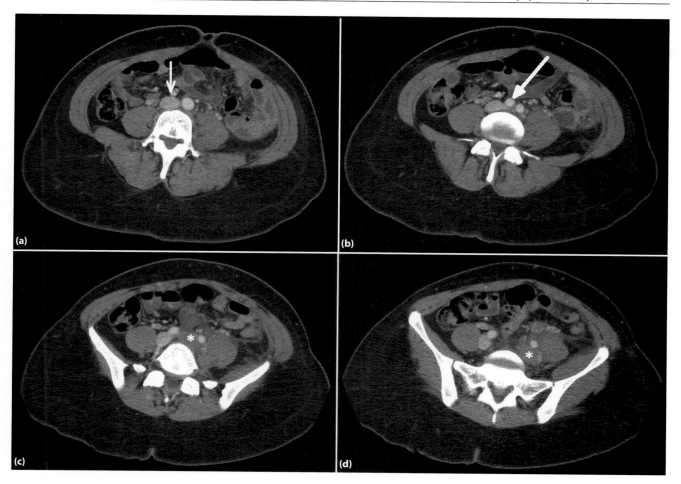

Figure 17.2 Computed tomography venogram of May–Thurner syndrome showing the inferior vena cava (IVC) (arrow, **a**) and aorta. The right common iliac artery (arrow, **b**) exerts mass effect on the IVC near the bifurcation, resulting in left common iliac vein thrombosis (*, **c,d**).

contralateral involvement. Computed tomography venography of the abdomen/pelvis should be considered in selected patients to assess proximal extension and associated anatomic pathologies (e.g., May–Thurner syndrome; **Figure 17.2**).

EQUIPMENT AND PROCEDURE

The preferred access site for iliofemoral lysis is the popliteal vein in the popliteal fossa. The patient is positioned prone, with standard sterile prepping and draping. If the popliteal vein is not patent, the tibial veins can be accessed if they are patent. In the authors' experience, a nonthrombosed point of access is a critical element for success in lower limb thrombolysis; this ensures that there is some blood flow cephalad to maintain patency once the affected venous segments start to lyse.

US-guided access skills are a must; if lytics are being administered, the goal should be single-wall access with a single puncture access to the vein. Blind puncture is not feasible and carries a high risk of subsequent hemorrhage.

A 21-G access system ("micropuncture set") should be used. The ability to image the tip of the needle inside the lumen of the vein is key; if the access point is thrombosed, the needle should be stabilized and a 0.018-inch guidewire (such as the stainless Cope Mandril Wire Guide (Cook Medical Inc., Bloomington, IN, USA) or a floppy tip nitinol wire) is carefully advanced under fluoroscopy. Once access has been obtained and the microwire has been upsized to a 0.035-inch J wire, a sheath should be placed. An 8-Fr sheath is typically used at the authors' institution because it allows follow-up contrast injection around any lysis catheter, accommodates most available mechanical devices and angioplasty balloon catheters, and allows coadministration of heparin (through the sheath) around the infusion catheter.

Imaging is then performed, with contrast injection in small amounts to outline the thrombus and determine the extent. Digital subtraction is not typically used at this point because of lack of flow. Images are saved for documentation. A 0.035-inch hydrophilic directional wire (e.g., stiff-angled GLIDEWIRE® Hydrophilic Coated Guidewire by the Terumo Medical Corporation, Somerset, NJ, USA) may be used along with an angled-tip 4- or 5-Fr catheter (the authors prefer the GLIDECATH® Hydrophilic Coated Catheter, Terumo Medical Corporation) to access the iliac veins and the inferior vena cava (IVC). Digital subtraction cavography should be performed using a flush catheter with graduated markers to ascertain the level of caval thrombosis. Typically, contrast is power-injected 15 mL/second for 2 seconds, at 500 psi through a flush catheter to study the IVC. Power injection of contrast should not be performed until after a test injection with a 10-mL syringe, to verify that the catheter tip is in a patent IVC segment. The hydrophilic wire and angled catheter combination is useful to cross anatomic lesions (e.g., a May–Thurner stenosis). Once such a lesion has been crossed, avoid uncrossing it for the duration of the treatment. For eventual placement of a lysis catheter, the authors recommend exchanging for a stiff, nonhydrophilic 0.035-inch guidewire such as an Amplatz Super Stiff™ Guidewire (Boston Scientific Corporation). A 180-cm wire or even a 260-cm wire (if using the EKOS delivery system) will be needed because of the length of the infusion catheters.

Once the extent of the thrombus is documented, the operator must decide on the method of lysis. The simplest technique is CDT, which only requires placement of a multisidehole catheter (e.g., the Cragg–McNamara® Valved Infusion Catheter (Medtronic, Minneapolis, MN, USA) or the Uni*Fuse™ infusion catheter (AngioDynamics, Latham, NY, USA)) with an infusion segment that spans all or at least most of the thrombosed segment. Avoid having too much infusion length of catheter in a patent vein segment; this will increase systemic administration of rtPA without benefit of thrombus lysis. In a thrombosed lower extremity, the typical length used is 50 cm, which may be too short to cover the entire thrombosed segment. The authors typically cover the distal part initially and leave the central thrombosed segment uncovered, changing the catheter out and placing the infusion segment more centrally once the distal thrombus is lysed. Lysing from distal to proximal is always a sound idea. Accelerated lysis is possible via bolus administration of rtPA into the infusion catheter, or a pulse spray technique. To accomplish this, the authors use rtPA in a concentration of 1 mg/mL of normal saline (the dose is dependent on the length of the thrombosed segment; up to 10 mg is typically used) administered by forceful pushes of a 1-mL syringe attached to a stopcock. This technique disperses rtPA into the thrombus, and fills the catheter dead space with lytic agent. After bolus administration, the stopcock should be closed until the rtPA pump infusion is ready. Infusion rates of 0.50–1.0 mg/hour of rtPA into the catheter are typically used, chosen by the operator with consideration of the amount of thrombus and individual patient risk factors for bleeding. In patients undergoing bilateral lower extremity and distal IVC lysis, the right- and left-sided catheters typically overlap in the IVC, resulting in a doubling of the rtPA dose in this largest venous segment. Another method of accelerating lysis is using a pharmacomechanical system such as the EndoWave™ system

(EKOS Corporation) (**Figure 17.3**). Use of the EndoWave™ system requires administration of a coolant fluid; the authors typically infuse normal saline at 35–70 mL/hour via the coolant port for this purpose. With any rtPA infusion system, concomitant infusion of heparin or other anticoagulant (**Table 17.2**) is usually performed via the access point sheath (popliteal, or in the case of an isolated iliac venous thrombus, a femoral sheath). The usual dose at the authors' institution is 500 IU/hour heparin in total, divided between one or two sheaths if both extremities are

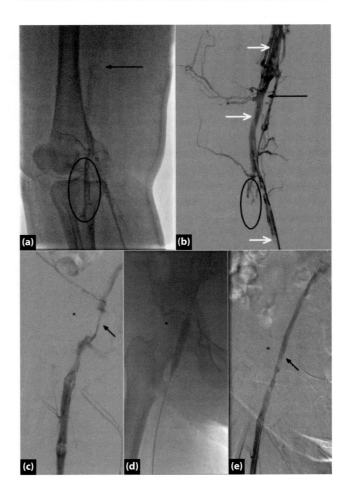

Figure 17.3 (**a**) Venogram performed through the left posterior tibial vein access shows occlusion of the popliteal vein (arrow) without any proximal filling. There is retrograde filling of the anterior tibial vein (circle). (**b**) Digital subtraction angiography (DSA) after 20 hours of continuous recombinant tissue plasminogen activator (rtPA) infusion shows patency of the popliteal vein (arrow) with the EKOS catheter (EKOS Corporation, Bothell, WA, USA) in place (open arrows). There is no longer backfilling of the anterior tibial vein (circle). (**c**) The DSA venography performed shows a large eccentric filling defect (arrow) in the common femoral vein (CFV). The superior margin of the femoral head is marked (*). (**d**) No significant change in the thrombus was seen after another 24 hours of treatment (not shown). The CFV and external iliac vein (EIV) underwent balloon angioplasty. (**e**) 48 hours after initial rtPA through the EKOS catheter, there is no significant thrombus in the CFV or EIV.

Table 17.2 Heparin and other anticoagulant drugs used concomitantly with a recombinant tissue plasminogen activator infusion system

Anticoagulant drug	Dosing
Unfractionated heparin	80 IU/kg bolus; 18 IU/kg/hour infusion for 5–7 days
Enoxaparin sodium	1 mg/kg twice daily or 1.5 mg/kg daily
Dalteparin sodium	100 IU/kg twice daily or 200 IU/kg daily
Argatroban monohydrate	2–10 μg/kg/minute infusion
Fondaparinux sodium	5 mg <50 kg, 7.5 mg 50–100 kg, 10 mg >100 kg

being lysed. In the case of documented heparin-induced thrombocytopenia, heparin should be switched to argatroban monohydrate, titrated to a low therapeutic partial thromboplastin time (PTT).[5]

Placement of a retrievable IVC filter in the infrarenal IVC is an important consideration. If the thrombosis is due to an IVC filter already in place, or an anatomic lesion such as May–Thurner, the likelihood of pulmonary embolism (PE) because of lysis is very low. If there is no identified anatomic lesion, the PE risk is higher and the operator should consider placing a filter. This should be of a retrievable variety, to be removed as soon as possible after the lysis procedure is complete and venous patency is restored

to reduce the risk of recurrent DVT or caval thrombosis. Before leaving the interventional suite, all patients should undergo placement of a peripherally inserted central catheter to aid in the frequent laboratory monitoring necessary for the safe conduct of CDT. Venipuncture and arterial lines should be avoided after rtPA is started.

Once thrombolysis is initiated, the patient should return for follow-up imaging every 12–24 hours. Laboratory monitoring is discussed later in the chapter. Lysis of extensive thrombus, such as bilateral or even unilateral lower extremities, is not a speedy procedure; it is not uncommon for the entire process to run for 48 or 72 hours. Follow-up procedures may consist of simple repeat imaging, with return to the ICU for continued rtPA administration if the thrombus is still present, or an additional endoluminal intervention if adequate clot lysis has been achieved. "Adequate" lysis is determined by the operator, with the knowledge that an older thrombus will likely result in slower and less complete lysis. The ability of the patient to tolerate a lengthy procedure, as well as bleeding and other problems, may limit the result that can be achieved.

Further interventions typically consist of balloon venoplasty to treat a significant stenosis or to macerate a thrombus that is resistant to rtPA after 24–48 hours of lysis. Lesions that demonstrate elastic recoil or otherwise inadequate response to venoplasty are stented with suitably sized metallic stents. May–Thurner lesions are primarily stented (**Figures 17.4** and **17.5**) (see Chapter 16). To avoid PE, use caution when treating stenoses if the thrombus is

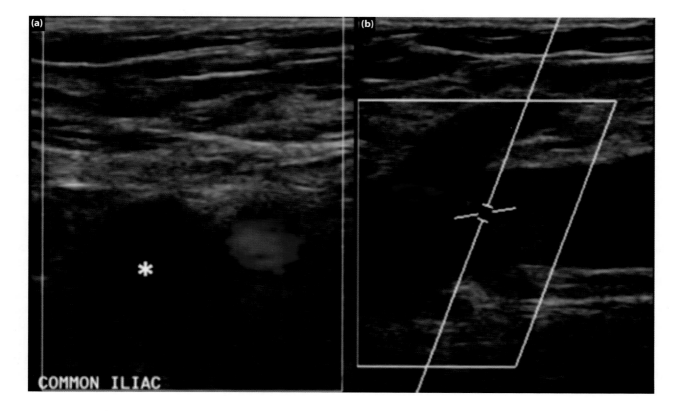

Figure 17.4 Transverse (**a**) and sagittal (**b**) ultrasounds of the left common iliac vein (*) and left common femoral vein demonstrate no color flow.

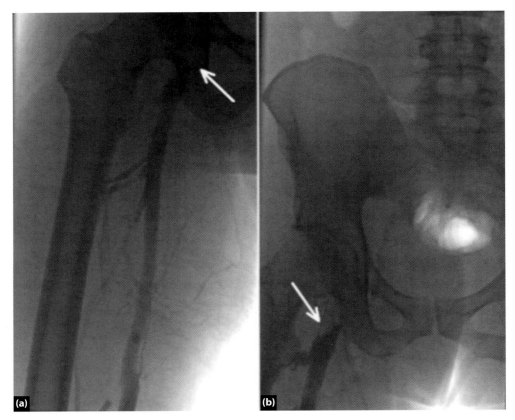

Figure 17.5 Venography of the left lower extremity (patient in a prone position) shows patency of the left femoral vein (**a**). The lack of flow on ultrasound was because of an occluding thrombus at the level of the femoral head (arrow). Contrast is seen outlining the thrombus in the left iliac vein (arrow, **b**) without any significant proximal opacification.

still present. The authors strongly recommend deferring treatment of anatomic lesions until the end of the entire lysis procedure to avoid this risk. For example, dilating a May–Thurner lesion on the first day of treatment, before thrombus clearance, is a critical mistake to be avoided.

TREATMENT DURING LYSIS

Postprocedural orders require ICU monitoring and include strict bed rest and a clear liquid diet, with consideration of sequential compression device (SCD) sleeves on the lower extremities. Frequent puncture site checks for bleeding/hematoma are crucial, with avoidance of all intramuscular/intra-arterial injections/punctures. Simultaneous heparin (or argatroban monohydrate) infusions through the access sheath(s) must be used to prevent the opened venous segment from immediately reoccluding. Fibrinogen and PTTs are measured every 4–6 hours, with goals at the authors' institution of >100–150 mg/dL and 45–60 seconds, respectively. Additional laboratory testing includes hemoglobin, prothrombin time, and platelet count, which will reveal any ongoing bleeding or risk thereof. If there are abnormal bleeding parameters, rtPA is either held or stopped and the infusion is replaced with a similar volume of normal saline; fibrinogen level correction is typically done with cryoprecipitate. Ideally, the lytic agent infusion should be reduced, not stopped,

while correction and laboratory retesting occurs. The authors reduce the rtPA infusion to half if fibrinogen falls below 150 mg/dL, and hold it if <100 mg/dL, while infusing cryoprecipitate to augment levels. Red cell transfusion should be considered if hemoglobin falls below 8 mg/dL or anemia is symptomatic. The authors cannot stress enough that any correction must be timely and aggressive. Stopping rtPA administration for even a short period can result in loss of all gains achieved up to that point.

POSTPROCEDURE

After thrombolysis has been achieved and anatomic lesions have been treated, all catheters and sheaths are pulled while the patient is still in the interventional suite. Hemostasis is achieved with manual compression; closure devices are never used. Full-dose anticoagulation with heparin is started without a bolus to maintain the PTT at 70–90 seconds. After 18–24 hours, the authors transition to warfarin with LMWH bridging. Patients are maintained on bed rest for 2 hours and then allowed to ambulate with assistance as needed. Thigh-high SCDs are used throughout this period to optimize venous flow through the previously occluded venous segments.

Following observation for clinical signs and symptoms of complications, patients are discharged on LMWH until therapeutic levels can be reached with oral anticoagulants.

Ambulation is encouraged once the patient's condition permits. Clinical and sonographic evaluation is performed at follow-up visits 1, 6, and 12 months after the procedure. Anticoagulation is maintained for a minimum of 3–6 months following thrombolysis in uncomplicated cases, with longer treatment regimens for those with a presumed hypercoagulable state.

COMPLICATIONS

The major complication with CDT is bleeding, with significant bleeding occurring in up to 9% of patients.[1] This is defined as intracranial bleeding, formation of a large hematoma requiring surgical evacuation, need for blood transfusion, and significant bleeding at the puncture site. Most bleeding is easily managed, although it may require cessation of the lysis procedure. Intracranial hemorrhage, while rare in the authors' experience, unfortunately may have devastating consequences. If significant bleeding occurs, the lytic agent should be stopped and hemostasis should be the goal with manual compression or sheath upsizing if at the access site. If major bleeding occurs elsewhere, thrombolysis should be stopped. Minor bleeding can manifest as pericatheter oozing, hematuria, or epistaxis. Physical inspection for bleeding and increased frequency of blood collection to monitor coagulation parameters are the reasons for patients requiring an ICU for periprocedure monitoring. The late complication of reocclusion can occur despite adequate anticoagulation therapy and compliance with DVT prevention strategies. In such cases, repeat thrombolysis can be considered.

CASE EXAMPLE

A man in his 30s with sudden onset of leg pain and swelling for one day presented to the clinic. His medical history was significant for spine surgery performed 1 month earlier. Doppler US showed an occluding thrombus of the left CFV and iliac veins (**Figure 17.6**). Venography demonstrated complete occlusion of the iliac vein extending to the caval bifurcation (**Figures 17.7 and 17.8**).

The patient returned for follow-up venography at 3 months (**Figure 17.9**), which showed no evidence of residual thrombus or narrowing. US performed at 6 months and 1 year following thrombolysis showed normal flow within the femoral vein. In consultation with the Hematology Department, oral anticoagulation was discontinued after 1 year.

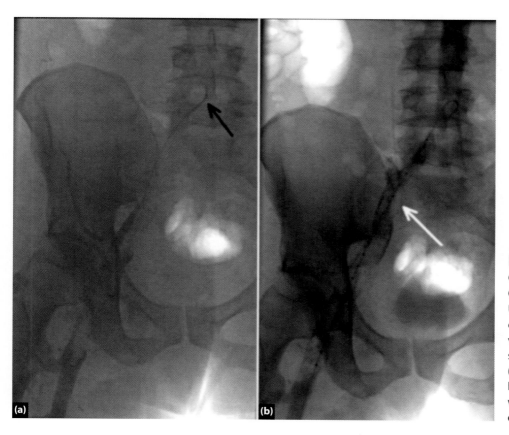

(a) (b)

Figure 17.6 A stiff Glidewire® (Terumo Medical Corporation, Somerset, NJ, USA) was needed to negotiate catheter (arrow) access to the vena cava (**a**). Contrast injection shows an area of stenosis (arrow, **b**) in the proximal left common iliac vein, with multiple filling defects extending to the caval junction.

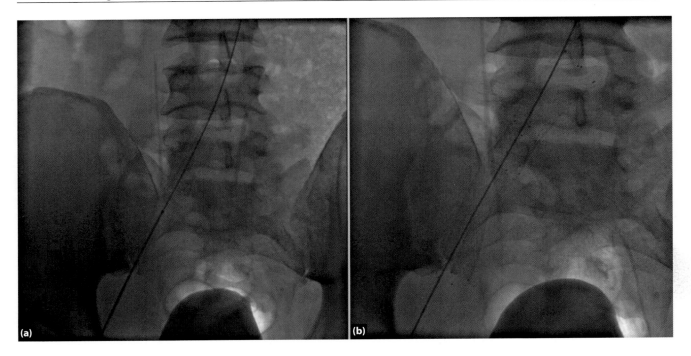

Figure 17.7 Following the completion of thrombolysis, two self-expanding nitinol stents were placed to cross the known area of stenosis (**a–b**).

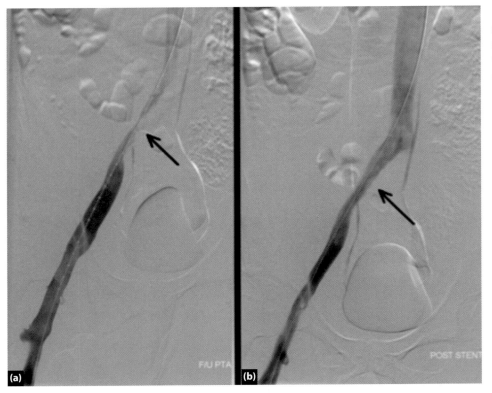

Figure 17.8 Digital subtraction angiograms show significantly improved venous flow following stenting of the anatomic stenosis (**a–b**).

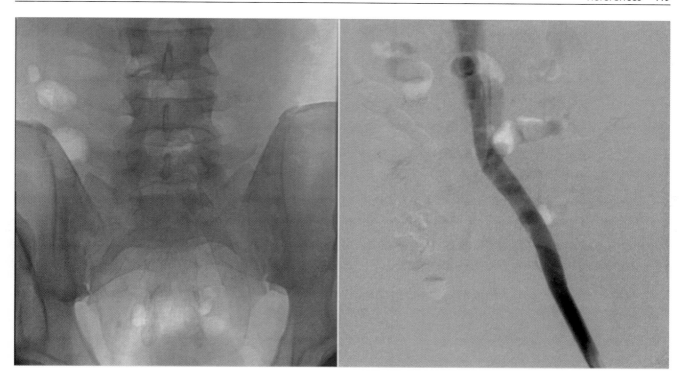

Figure 17.9 Images showing appropriate stent position with excellent opacification of the left iliac vein. The patient is now supine.

REFERENCES

1. Haig Y, Enden T, Grøtta O, et al. Post-thrombotic syndrome after catheter-directed thrombolysis for deep vein thrombosis (CaVenT): 5-year follow-up results of an open-label, randomised controlled trial. *Lancet Haematol.* 2016;**3**:e64–71.
2. Kearon C, Akl EA, Ornelas J, et al. Antithrombotic therapy for VTE disease: CHEST Guideline and Expert Panel Report. *Chest.* 2016;**149**:315–352.
3. Haig Y, Enden T, Slagsvold CE, et al. Determinants of early and long-term efficacy of catheter-directed thrombolysis in proximal deep vein thrombosis. *J Vasc Interv Radiol.* 2013;**24**:17–24.
4. Meissner MH, Manzo RA, Bergelin RO, et al. Deep venous insufficiency: the relationship between lysis and subsequent reflux. *J Vasc Surg.* 1993;**18**:596–605.
5. Sharifi M, Bay C, Nowroozi S, et al. Catheter-directed thrombolysis with argatroban and tPA for massive iliac and femoropopliteal vein thrombosis. *Cardiovasc Intervent Radiol.* 2013;**36**:1586–1590.

18

Endovenous catheter ablation of the saphenous vein

JUDITH C. LIN AND YASAMAN KAVOUSI

CONTENTS

INTRODUCTION

Endovenous catheter ablation can be performed using radiofrequency ablation (RFA) or endovenous laser treatment (EVLT) to deliver electromagnetic or laser energy, and obliterate the target vein in situ. Clinical trials using RFA and EVLT for the great saphenous vein (GSV) have shown excellent success rates with similar primary failure and recurrence rates between the two endovascular techniques compared to standard stripping surgery.[1] Advantages of catheter-based intervention over conventional surgical stripping include: shorter convalescence; less postoperative pain; and lower overall economic costs.[1,2]

PROCEDURE

Current vein practice has shifted from the hospital operating room to the outpatient procedure or office-based setting. In the authors' practice, patients take diazepam 5–10 mg by mouth an hour before the procedure. If needed, patients may also apply topical anesthetics (2.5% lidocaine, 2.5% prilocaine cream, 30-g tube) over the saphenous vein and bulging varicosities at home 2 hours before the procedure to minimize the pain perception of normal intact skin from needle injection of local anesthesia and tumescent anesthesia during the procedure. Ablation procedures may be performed on the GSV and any truncal veins, such as the small saphenous vein (SSV), anterior accessory saphenous vein, and intersaphenous vein.

The procedural table set-up requires the following: microaccess needle; 0.018-inch microaccess wire; 4-Fr or 7-Fr sheath; 25-G needle; 1% lidocaine for local anesthesia; syringes (5, 20, and 30 mL); normal saline; gauze; three mosquito clamps; tumescent tubing; acoustic coupling gel; marking pen; and labels (**Figure 18.1**). A portable ultrasound (US) system should be available in the room.

The patient's GSV is mapped the day before the procedure and any bulging tributary varicose veins are marked the same day with a skin marker. After obtaining informed consent, the patient is placed supine on the procedure table, which is positioned in reverse Trendelenburg to distend the veins in the lower extremities. The entire lower extremity is prepped and draped in sterile fashion. For veins <2 mm, nitroglycerine paste may be applied to the primary insertion site to dilate the vein and prevent venospasm before gaining intravascular access. Blood pressure, heart rate, and oxygen saturation are monitored intraoperatively.

A rapid US scan of the medial leg is performed to assess for areas of tortuosity and the location of tributaries and perforators. Under US guidance, 1% lidocaine is used to infiltrate the skin; percutaneous access to the GSV just below the knee is obtained with a micropuncture access needle (**Figure 18.2**). The authors use the VSI Micro-HV Introducer Kit (Vascular Solutions, Inc., Minneapolis, MN, USA) for RFA procedures or the VenaCure EVLT NeverTouch Direct Procedure Kit (AngioDynamics, Latham, NY, USA) for EVLT procedures. After needle cannulation of the GSV, a microaccess guidewire is introduced and the 7-Fr RFA or 4-Fr EVLT sheath is inserted (**Figure 18.3**). An endovenous radiofrequency or laser catheter is advanced under US up to the saphenofemoral junction (SFJ) and the tip is withdrawn approximately

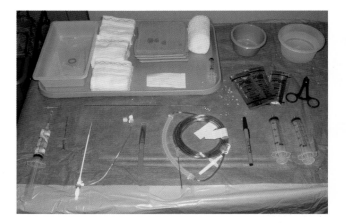

Figure 18.1 Procedural table set-up.

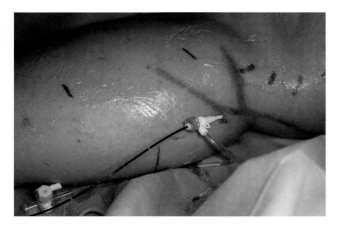

Figure 18.3 Insertion of sheath and catheter for radiofrequency ablation.

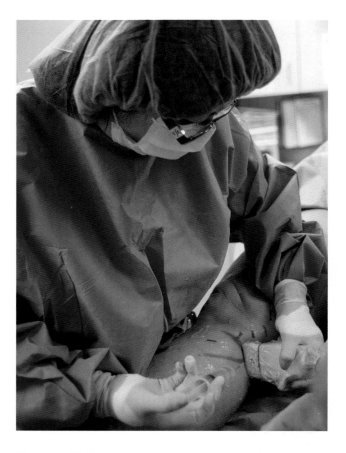

Figure 18.2 Ultrasound-guided percutaneous access of distal great saphenous vein.

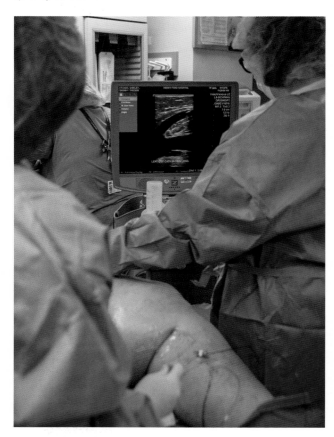

Figure 18.4 Confirmation of catheter tip placement via ultrasound.

2–3 cm below the SFJ (**Figure 18.4**). Good positioning of the endovenous catheter distal to the SFJ must be obtained under US to reduce the incidence of heat-induced thrombus formation. The GSV below the calf is not routinely treated with thermal energy because of the increased risk of paresthesia from thermal injury to the saphenous nerve, which lies near the GSV.

Tumescent anesthesia is then injected into the perivenous space in the saphenous compartment using a 21-G

spinal needle and tumescent pump under US guidance (**Figure 18.5**). The tumescent solution is composed of 1000 mL of 0.9% normal saline solution, 100 mL of 1% lidocaine with epinephrine, and 10 mL of 8.4% sodium bicarbonate. Tumescent anesthesia involves subcutaneous infiltration of this solution around the vein as a buffer from the thermal energy, deepening the truncal vein to >1 cm to reduce the risk of skin burn, and reducing GSV size so that vein ablation is more effective.

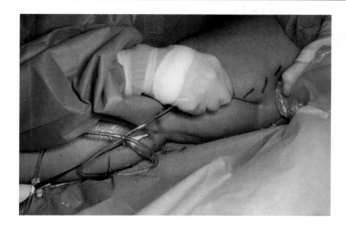

Figure 18.5 Ultrasound-guided injection of tumescent anesthesia.

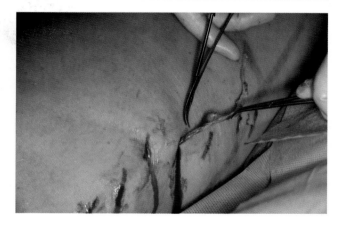

Figure 18.6 Extraction of varicosities for ambulatory phlebectomy.

Following satisfactory tumescent anesthesia, endovenous ablation of the GSV is started. For RFA, the authors use a radiofrequency catheter via a 7-Fr sheath. The ClosureFast™ Endovenous Radiofrequency Ablation (RFA) Catheter (Medtronic, Minneapolis, MN, USA) heats the vein in 7-cm segments with 20-second treatment cycles. For EVLT, the authors use the VenaCure EVLT NeverTouch Direct system (AngioDynamics) with laser wavelengths of 980, 810, and 1470 nm via a 4-Fr sheath. Hemoglobin absorption does not play a role when using a wavelength >1320 nm, and water absorption is the dominant mechanism. Thus, the vein wall is gently heated and shrunk without perforations, translating into less pain less frequently felt after EVLT at a higher wavelength. The choice of thermal ablation mechanism depends on the operator and patient preference. On US, the GSV should be fully thrombosed and closed, and there should be no evidence of thrombus extending into the common femoral vein. The catheter is then removed with the sheath and hemostasis is obtained.

Removal of associated varicosities may be done concomitantly or as a staged procedure. The decision is based on patient's choice and surgeon's preference. Based on the authors' experience, there is a slightly increased risk of endovenous heat-induced thrombus with concomitant phlebectomy of varicosities. To perform ambulatory phlebectomy of varicosities, the skin is anesthetized with 1% lidocaine and small skin incisions are made over the bulging veins. Varady or Mueller phlebectomy hooks are used to extract the veins. Gentle traction is used to extract vein segments with mosquito clamps. Additional tumescent anesthesia may be used to further numb the area (**Figure 18.6**).

Hemostasis is obtained with direct pressure over the incision sites, which are closed with gauze bandage rolls. Suture is not generally required; if needed, 4-0 nylon suture may be used to obtain hemostasis. Gauze bandage rolls and compression elastic wrap bandages are applied from the foot to the upper thigh. Patients can ambulate immediately after the procedure. After 2 days, they may remove the gauze and bandage, shower, and wear thigh-high, elastic compression stockings (30–40 mmHg compression level) for an additional 2 weeks. Patients are followed with a venous duplex US and clinic appointment within 1 week of the procedure.

HAZARDS AND ADVERSE EVENTS

Aside from technical difficulties with cannulation, guidewire placement, and catheter advancement, other recognized complications include: endovenous heat-induced thrombosis (EHIT); de novo deep vein thrombosis (DVT); superficial thrombophlebitis; nerve injury; ecchymosis; thermal skin burn; hematoma; persistent pain; and hyperpigmentation.

Thrombotic complications after endovenous catheter ablation can be classified into two main categories: de novo DVT and EHIT. In endovenous ablation, a thrombus can originate from the superficial vein and extend into the deep venous system. A study of National Surgical Quality Improvement Program data showed that patients undergoing endovenous ablation have higher odds of postoperative DVT.[3] The prevalence of DVT after RFA has been reported to be 0.2–1.2%.[4] Studies have shown that the risk of DVT after RFA is greater in patients with previous DVT. However, RFA in this subset of patients remains a safe approach, and preprocedural anticoagulation may be considered. Advanced age, female gender, and a history of superficial thrombophlebitis are significant predictors of DVT after EVLT.[4]

A vein diameter of >8 mm and operative time >40 minutes are predictive factors for EHIT following RFA.[4] However, successful treatment of veins >12 mm carries a slightly higher risk of EHIT formation after ablation of larger truncal veins. The frequency of EHIT has been reported as 0–8%.[1]

Superficial thrombophlebitis is a known complication of endovenous catheter ablation, often several days after the procedure. The risk of phlebitis is approximately 2.9%.[5]

This is often self-limiting and treated with conservative management, including compression and nonsteroidal anti-inflammatory drugs.

Nerve injury is another complication of endovenous catheter ablation. Although the potential for nerve injury is greatly reduced in endovenous ablation when compared to conventional surgery, the risk of neurologic damage remains a clinically important complication of thermal ablation. Paresthesia is seen in 19.6% of patients after surgery versus 9.7% after RFA and 4.8% after EVLA.[4] Nerve injury following endovenous ablation usually involves small cutaneous nerves in close anatomic proximity to the treated veins. The mechanism of nerve injury is through thermal effects radiating from the ablated venous segment into the surrounding structures. Complications of varicose vein treatment may be explained by the anatomy of the saphenous veins in relation to neural structures. The SSV courses closely with the sural nerve, whereas the GSV is associated with the saphenous nerve. Because of the very close proximity of SSV and sural nerve from the distal calf to the ankle, puncturing the SSV at mid-calf may decrease postoperative paresthesia.

Skin burns are another adverse event associated with endovenous ablation, with an incidence of around 1.2%,[6] and may occur if the administered energy is too high or the cooling effect of tumescent anesthesia is insufficient. In EVLT, optimization of the energy delivered and pullback speed, as well as administration of ample tumescent anesthesia, may reduce the frequency and intensity of skin burns and ecchymosis.

Ecchymosis and hematoma are other minor complications of endovenous ablation. Ecchymosis is self-limiting and can last approximately 10 days. The authors believe that the ecchymosis over the treated areas may be due to perforation of the vein wall during ablation, and the injury sustained from the spinal needle during tumescent infiltration. The rate of ecchymosis is unchanged between endovenous and conventional surgery groups. However, endovenous catheter ablation has shown reduced rates of hematoma by approximately 50–60% when compared to conventional surgery.[1,7]

Overall, endovenous ablation is a very safe, effective, and well-tolerated procedure; it is associated with lower postoperative complications, faster recovery time, and improved quality of life compared to standard surgery.

REFERENCES

1. Siribumrungwong B, Noorit P, Wilasrusmee C, et al. A systematic review and meta-analysis of randomised controlled trials comparing endovenous ablation and surgical intervention in patients with varicose vein. *Eur J Vasc Endovasc Surg.* 2012;**44**:214–223.
2. Lin JC, Nerenz DR, Migliore P, et al. Cost analysis of endovenous catheter ablation versus surgical stripping for treatment of superficial venous insufficiency and varicose vein disease. *J Vasc Surg Venous Lymphat Disord.* 2014;**2**:98–103.
3. Carruthers TN, Farber A, Rybin D, et al. Interventions on the superficial venous system for chronic venous insufficiency by surgeons in the modern era: an analysis of ACS-NSQIP. *Vasc Endovascular Surg.* 2014;**48**:482–490.
4. Boersma D, Kornmann VN, van Eekeren RR, et al. Treatment modalities for small saphenous vein insufficiency: systematic review and meta-analysis. *J Endovasc Ther.* 2016;**23**:199–211.
5. Merchant RF, Pichot O. Long-term outcomes of endovenous radiofrequency obliteration of saphenous reflux as a treatment for superficial venous insufficiency. *J Vasc Surg.* 2005;**42**: 502–509.
6. Chi YW, Woods TC. Clinical risk factors to predict deep venous thrombosis post-endovenous laser ablation of saphenous veins. *Phlebology.* 2014;**29**:150–153.
7. Christenson JT, Gueddi S, Gemayel G, et al. Prospective randomized trial comparing endovenous laser ablation and surgery for treatment of primary great saphenous varicose veins with a 2-year follow-up. *J Vasc Surg.* 2010;**52**:1234–1241.

19

Explantation of aortic endografts

WESLEY R. BARNES AND GRAHAM W. LONG

CONTENTS

INTRODUCTION

Since its first description in the early 1990s, endovascular aneurysm repair (EVAR) has transformed aortic surgery. Today, EVAR is the preferred treatment for an abdominal aortic aneurysm (AAA) with approximately 70% of infrarenal AAAs treated this way. Although EVAR has lower perioperative morbidity and mortality compared to traditional open repair, long-term survival is similar. However, the rate of secondary intervention is higher among those patients undergoing EVAR—up to 20% within 6 years. Thus, continued surveillance imaging is important to detect complications and ensure long-term success. Given the mounting number of endovascular grafts being placed, the vascular surgeon must be familiar with the mechanisms of device failure, as well as the techniques available to assist in their removal and conversion to open repair when necessary.

INDICATIONS

With advancements in endovascular techniques, most of the complications associated with EVAR are successfully managed with catheter-based means, but certain circumstances may arise that mandate explantation and conversion to open AAA repair. According to a recent meta-analysis, an average of 1.5% and 1.9% of patients undergoing EVAR require early (<30 days after EVAR) or late (>30 days after EVAR) conversion, respectively.[1] The most frequent reasons for early conversion are problems with access, technical failure of graft deployment, vessel rupture, inappropriate endograft placement, and graft kinking or thrombosis.

When considering late conversion, the most common indications are aneurysm growth with or without an identifiable endoleak (especially type I) and graft migration. Other indications for late explantation include aortic rupture, graft infection, aortoenteric fistula, and limb kinking or thrombosis. No endograft to date has been immune to these complications, and the risk seems to increase with time and longer follow-up. Conversion to open repair should be considered after failed endovascular intervention for all type I and III endoleaks, continued annual aneurysm growth of ≥5 mm on two consecutive imaging assessments, or aneurysm sac enlargement to >6 cm on minor axis measurement on computed tomography angiography. The improved outcomes associated with elective conversion to open repair compared to those seen under emergency conditions underscores the importance of close surveillance and timely intervention when indicated. Nevertheless, the decision for conversion to open repair must be made after considering the patient's comorbidities, life expectancy, the indication for conversion, and the extent of the proposed open procedure (i.e., complete or partial explantation or lumbar or inferior mesenteric branch ligation).

TECHNIQUE

Transabdominal and retroperitoneal approaches are the most commonly practiced for conversion to open repair. Because there is no strong evidence promoting one approach over the other, the type of incision used is often a matter of surgeon preference, but one should be familiar with both techniques. For most, a midline laparotomy is preferable, especially in the case of aortic rupture or immediate conversion to expedite the establishment of proximal control. A history of left-sided retroperitoneal surgery, intra-abdominal visceral arterial pathology, a left-sided inferior vena cava (IVC), non-ostial stenosis of the right renal artery (RRA), or an aneurysm of the right common iliac artery constitute additional relative indications for a transabdominal technique. Some relative indications for a retroperitoneal approach include: multiple previous transperitoneal operations; obesity; enteric or urinary stoma; inflammatory aneurysms; prior radiation; horseshoe kidney; and proximal endograft fixation problems. Exposure of the paravisceral aorta and left renal artery is facilitated by the retroperitoneal technique, but control and exposure of the RRA often proves difficult should the artery be damaged during explantation. A left-sided transperitoneal medial visceral rotation provides similar exposure to that obtained with a retroperitoneal approach.

Clamp placement

One of the most vital components for the safe removal of an endograft is control of the proximal aorta. Preoperative considerations in this regard include: the type of endograft previously implanted and associated suprarenal struts, hooks, and barbs; the integrity of proximal and distal fixation points; the presence of periaortic inflammation; prior secondary interventions using stents, cuffs, or coils; and dilation of the infrarenal neck with subsequent endograft distal migration. As a result, infrarenal aortic clamp placement is usually not feasible. Supraceliac aortic clamp placement gives the surgeon the maneuverability to remove any suprarenal struts but subjects the patient to hepatic, intestinal, and renal ischemia, as well as increased cardiac stress. Minimizing supraceliac aortic clamp time and stepwise movement of the clamp distally as the operation proceeds is essential to limiting ischemic and hemodynamic consequences. Attempts at suprarenal clamp placement across suprarenal struts are discouraged, since this may result in laceration of the paravisceral aorta by these struts; often, it does not result in adequate proximal control and interferes with endograft removal. If there is adequate distance between the renal ostia and the superior mesenteric artery, and there are no suprarenal struts

present, safe suprarenal clamp placement is possible but may be hampered by extensive endograft-induced periaortic inflammation at this level. Infrarenal cross-clamping is feasible when there is sufficient distance between the renal arteries and the stent graft, as may be seen following endograft distal migration, or when there is a good seal proximally and partial graft excision with preservation of the proximal attachment system is elected.

Another option for proximal control involves inflating an intraluminal aortic occlusion balloon proximal to the endograft within the suprarenal or supraceliac aorta; this maneuver can obviate the need for exposure of the paravisceral aorta and can reduce the time needed to obtain proximal aortic control. Insertion can be accomplished through the anterior wall of the stent graft after opening the aneurysm or, if opening the aneurysm sac before gaining proximal control is not advisable, via a femoral or brachial approach. When the balloon is placed retrograde, a large (12–14 Fr), long stiff sheath should be advanced along the balloon shaft up to the level of the balloon for support and prevention of caudal migration of the occlusion balloon. Once the endo graft is removed and a cross-clamp is placed across the infrarenal aneurysm neck, the balloon is deflated and removed to allow reperfusion of the viscera. Distal control is obtained by clamping the iliac arteries below the endograft distal to the site of any anticipated distal anastomoses, by clamping the iliac limbs of the graft once the aneurysm sac is opened, or less frequently, by Fogarty embolectomy catheter balloon occlusion (Edwards Lifesciences, Irvine, CA, USA).

Endograft removal

Endograft removal is the most challenging part of the procedure. The goal is to remove the segment responsible for the aneurysm sac's continued expansion while limiting renal and visceral ischemic time and preserving infrarenal aortic and common iliac segments for sewing new graft anastomoses. Complicating removal, the endograft is generally covered with various layers of mural debris/thrombus and is intimately attached to the arterial wall at the proximal and distal landing zones, even in the presence of extensive endoleaks. Careful preoperative review of imaging studies is performed to consider the design and fixation system of the endograft (e.g., suprarenal stents), the integrity of the seal zones, the extent of graft incorporation, current aneurysm morphology, the presence of periaortic inflammation that occurs with all EVARs, and the nature of any secondary interventions.

After the proximal and distal dissections are complete, the patient is given a standard dose of heparin, clamps are applied, and the aneurysm is opened with a longitudinal aortotomy. In the early EVAR era, the preferred operation was complete graft excision with open repair using undamaged, nonaneurysmal aorta and iliac or femoral arteries for reconstruction. Recent strategies have evolved to preserve intact components of the endovascular reconstruction (this is discussed in the *Partial endograft removal* and *Complete graft preservation* sections of this chapter, and in the case example), usually reserving complete removal only for infected endografts. To facilitate the latter strategy, the aortotomy is extended to just below the renal arteries and below the level of the aortic bifurcation. Back-bleeding lumbar and inferior mesenteric artery (IMA) branches are oversewn.

Suprarenal stents are a component of most devices with or without associated barbs. Each of these is designed to stabilize the endograft in the proximal neck of the aneurysm; however, in the explantation scenario, they present challenges to endograft removal and preservation of an intact aortic wall for creation of a proximal aortic anastomosis. Moreover, barbs and hooks penetrate the aortic wall; this not only enhances graft incorporation but also contributes to periaortic inflammation that distorts tissue planes and increases the risk of injury to adjacent structures (i.e., the duodenum, IVC, and left renal vein). Similarly, well-incorporated distal limbs can create issues with the iliac arteries in terms of endograft removal, subsequent anastomosis, and adjacent iliac vein or ureteral injury.

Endografts that are infected, poorly incorporated, have migrated, or employ passive fixation systems can often be completely removed atraumatically with simple traction ("clamp and pull"). With others, simple traction is frequently hazardous and usually does not permit graft explantation. A plaque elevator can be helpful in liberating the graft from areas of incorporation or fixation. There are two options for addressing suprarenal hardware: leaving it in situ with removal of the remaining skeleton and graft material, or complete excision. Leaving the suprarenal fixation component in place and trimming the endograft from it with wire cutters and scissors is the easier approach, though this complicates the subsequent graft-to-aorta anastomosis that must incorporate the remaining hardware.

Three approaches are used for complete excision. One technique involves pouring iced saline onto nitinol stents with thermal memory (incorporated into the Talent stent graft (Medtronic, Minneapolis, MN, USA), GORE® EXCLUDER® AAA Endoprosthesis (W. L. Gore & Associates, Flagstaff, AZ, USA), and Ovation® Abdominal Stent Graft Platform (Trivascular, Inc., Santa Rosa, CA)), which may ease removal from the aortic neck by decreasing device diameters closer to their predeployment state. Another technique, described by Koning and collaborators,[2] uses a sterile 20-mL syringe that is prepared by removing the plunger, cutting off the end of the barrel with a saw, and rounding the edges of the cylinder with a file. After obtaining supraceliac aortic control, the aneurysm sac is opened and the iliac endograft limbs are controlled with vascular clamps and removed from their connection with the main body. The syringe barrel is slid proximally over the main body and a Kelly clamp or umbilical tape is used to grasp the main body at the inferior end of the syringe. The syringe is advanced superiorly over the

main body with downward tension on the clamp or tape. Care is taken so that there is no superior or inferior net tension on the endograft during this maneuver; otherwise, the hooks and barbs will tear the aorta. The syringe barrel collapses the suprarenal struts and, more importantly, pulls the attached hooks away from the aortic wall. Once the hooks are detached, downward tension on the Kelly clamp brings the main body out of the aortic neck (**Figure 19.1**). This approach works with the Zenith® Flex (Cook Medical Inc., Bloomington, IN, USA) and Talent (Medtronic) stent grafts but not with the newer Endurant®

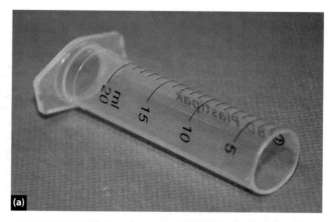

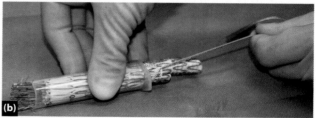

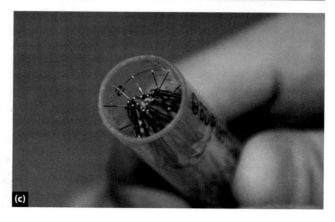

Figure 19.1 Explantation of the main body of an endograft. **(a)** Ex vivo demonstration of a prepared 20-mL syringe barrel used to explant the main body of an endograft. Umbilical tape or a clamp is used to pull the stent graft through the device. **(b)** Superior movement of the syringe barrel with downward traction on the umbilical tape. **(c)** Endograft compression and hook/barb retraction into the syringe barrel. (Reprinted with permission from Koning OH, Hinnen JW, van Baalen JM. Technique for safe removal of an aortic endograft with suprarenal fixation. *J Vasc Surg.* 2006;**43**:855–857. © Elsevier)

II AAA Stent Graft System (Medtronic) graft. This graft has reverse barbs on its suprarenal stents, making en bloc removal with this technique impossible. In this situation, only the third and final approach for complete excision is possible; this involves cutting the suprarenal struts away from the infrarenal portion of the main body of the graft with sterile wire cutters and removing them piecemeal from the paravisceral aorta, with a vertical aortotomy extending above the renal arteries. This technique is the most complicated option and is associated with the longest supravisceral/renal clamp times. After graft removal, the aorta is flushed and irrigated of any accumulated debris and the conventional proximal anastomosis is completed. Following complete excision of an Endurant® II AAA Stent Graft System, aortic reconstruction usually requires a beveled anastomosis to incorporate the suprarenal aortotomy. The aortic clamp is moved to an infrarenal location when possible.

Partial endograft removal

Although complete removal of the endograft is sometimes necessary, preservation of functional graft components is frequently possible (**Figure 19.2**). For example, if an uninfected graft is well-incorporated proximally via suprarenal fixation, one option is to transect the main body just below the renal arteries and sew a conventional graft to the

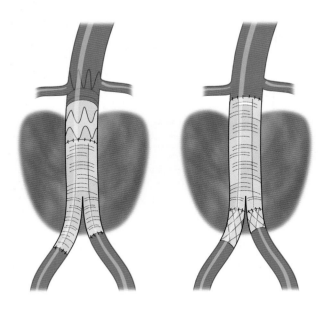

Figure 19.2 Partial endograft removal. Examples incorporating residual endografts into the aortic reconstruction. (**a**) Incorporated proximal Zenith® (Cook Medical Inc., Bloomington, IN, USA) endograft into distal aorto-bi-iliac repair. (**b**) Proximal polyethylene terephthalate graft with distal AneuRx® (Medtronic, Minneapolis, MN, USA) limbs. (Reprinted with permission from Kelso RL, Lyden SP, Butler B, et al. Late conversion of aortic stent grafts. *J Vasc Surg*. 2009;**49**:589–595. ©Elsevier)

endograft or to both the aorta and endograft at this level. The remaining main body is excised. Alternatively, the suprarenal struts above the graft material can be detached from the endograft with sterile wire cutters, and a conventional proximal anastomosis constructed without incorporating any stent graft material. With the Endurant® II AAA Stent Graft System, the authors use this technique routinely for the reasons outlined earlier. An analogous scenario to the first example is well-incorporated iliac limbs into the iliac landing zones. In the uninfected endograft situation, the limbs are not removed but are anastomosed to the limbs of the new conventional bifurcated bypass graft. Early concerns regarding an increased risk of pseudoaneurysm formation from partial graft removal have not been substantiated.[3–5]

Complete graft preservation

In cases of type II endoleaks, complete preservation of the endograft may be possible. The aneurysm sac is opened and back-bleeding lumbar and IMAs are oversewn after the mural thrombus is evacuated. This maneuver can be difficult if the endograft is near the side branch ostia, since the stiff endograft can be difficult to retract without disrupting proximal or distal attachment sites. There are reports of a laparoscopic approach to this maneuver, but the authors have no experience with this.[6] Lastly, in the situation of frank aneurysmal degeneration of the pararenal aorta, a tube graft can be sewn to the paravisceral aorta proximally and to the main body of the endograft distally, preserving the endograft and minimizing dissection, blood loss, and operative time.

Reconstruction

Assuming complete graft removal and absence of infection, aorto-bi-iliac or aortobifemoral reconstruction with a bifurcated woven polyester (Dacron) graft is preferred. With partial graft preservation, a bifurcated graft is used with anastomosis to the previous endograft main body proximally or to the endograft limbs distally. Construction of these distal graft-to-endograft anastomoses can be challenging. Care must be taken to avoid detaching the loose pseudointima (i.e., compacted fibrin layer) lining the stent graft limbs. This material can embolize or create a flap that can lead to subsequent narrowing. Also, the thin polyester graft material can tear as the anastomosis is created; the resulting suture line bleeding can be troublesome to control.

The aortic sac and retroperitoneum should be tightly closed around the repair to separate the graft from the overlying bowel. Omental interposition can also be used to help in this endeavor. The presence of infection or an aortoenteric fistula necessitates using either an extra-anatomic bypass (axillo-bifemoral) or an in-line aortic reconstruction using a rifampin-soaked prosthetic graft, autologous femoral vein graft, or cryopreserved allograft. Detailed descriptions of these reconstructions are found in Part 2 of this book.

OUTCOMES

Perioperative mortality reported for late conversion averages nearly 10% in patients presenting without rupture. Patients presenting with rupture, endograft infection, or aortoenteric fistula experience higher mortality rates (approximately 25%). The presence of an endograft is thought to be protective in the rupture situation, resulting in this lower mortality rate, compared with 75% in a previously untreated AAA.[3–5] These results underscore the importance of long-term surveillance imaging following EVAR to identify potential problems and allow elective, rather than urgent, surgical conversion.

Overall morbidity rates are as high as 50–70%, depending on the type of postoperative complications included in the analysis, with a lower morbidity rate (13%) shown for partial or complete graft preservation.[3–5] Prolonged supravisceral aortic clamping is associated with a higher incidence of hepatic, intestinal, and renal ischemia, metabolic derangements, and overall perioperative morbidity and mortality.

CONCLUSION

While the percentage of endografts requiring explantation remains low, the increasing numbers of aortoiliac endografts placed annually necessitate increasing application of the techniques described in this chapter. Except for infection, future technological advances will potentially address many of the current indications for explantation, allowing for effective treatment using catheter-based means. Until that time, and certainly for the foreseeable future, open explantation techniques remain applicable.

CASE EXAMPLE

A 75-year-old man underwent EVAR in 2007 with an AneuRx® stent graft (Medtronic) for an AAA. He subsequently underwent aortic cuff extension for a type I endoleak in 2009 and coil embolization for a type II endoleak in 2010 and 2012. In late 2012, he presented with rupture from a type Ia endoleak (**Figure 19.3**). He underwent emergent explantation via a midline laparotomy. Supraceliac control was obtained, the aneurysm was opened, the distal iliac graft limbs were controlled with vascular clamps, and the main body was divided. A bifurcated Dacron graft was used for the aorto-bi-iliac reconstruction. Proximal anastomosis to the infrarenal aorta was performed, and the clamp was moved down onto the main body of the graft. Because there was excellent overlap and incorporation of the graft distally, the iliac limbs of

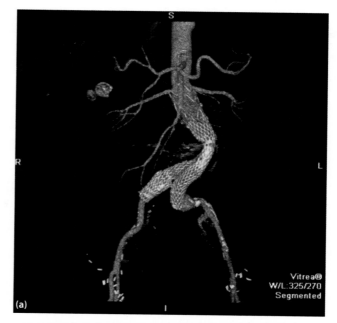

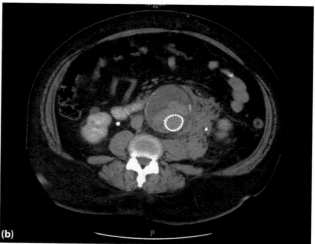

Figure 19.3 Patient presenting with rupture from a type Ia endoleak. (**a**) CT angiography three-dimensional reconstruction. (**b**) Axial view of the same patient with a large endoleak and retroperitoneal hemorrhage from rupture.

the graft were left in situ and included in the distal anastomoses. The patient survived 4 years after this repair. He ultimately died of a ruptured suprarenal AAA.

REFERENCES

1. Moulakakis KG, Dalainas I, Mylonas S, et al. Conversion to open repair after endografting for abdominal aortic aneurysm: a review of causes, incidence, results, and surgical techniques of reconstruction. *J Endovasc Ther.* 2010;**17**:694–702.
2. Koning OH, Hinnen JW, van Baalen JM. Technique for safe removal of an aortic endograft with suprarenal fixation. *J Vasc Surg.* 2006;**43**:855–857.

3. Chaar CI, Eid R, Park T, et al. Delayed open conversions after endovascular abdominal aortic aneurysm repair. *J Vasc Surg.* 2012;**55**:1562–1569.e1.

4. Kelso RL, Lyden SP, Butler B, et al. Late conversion of aortic stent grafts. *J Vasc Surg.* 2009;**49**:589–595.

5. Lipsitz EC, Ohki T, Veith FJ, et al. Delayed open conversion following endovascular aortoiliac aneurysm repair: partial (or complete) endograft preservation as a useful adjunct. *J Vasc Surg.* 2003;**38**:1191–1198.

6. Wisselink W, Cuesta MA, Berends FJ, et al. Retroperitoneal endoscopic ligation of lumbar and inferior mesenteric arteries as a treatment of persistent endoleak after endoluminal aortic aneurysm repair. *J Vasc Surg.* 2000;**31**:1240–1244.

20

Inferior vena cava filter placement and retrieval

EMILY ABBOTT AND GRAHAM W. LONG

CONTENTS

INTRODUCTION

Venous thromboembolic disease affects 900 000 people annually in the USA with a 15% mortality from pulmonary embolus (PE) involving 50 000–100 000 people.[1] First-line treatment for deep vein thrombosis (DVT) and PE is systemic anticoagulation with a variety of intravenous, subcutaneous, and oral medications. Length of treatment ranges between 3 and 12 months, depending on the extent and severity of the disease process. A small subset with significant risk factors for hypercoagulability require lifelong anticoagulation. Indications for inferior vena cava (IVC) filter placement, relevant anatomy, and algorithms for their placement and removal are discussed in this chapter.

INDICATIONS

Several guidelines set forth by the various vascular societies have somewhat differing indications for the placement of IVC filters. There are therapeutic indications for those with current DVT or PE and prophylactic indications for those without current venous thromboembolism (VTE). Absolute indications include patients with a significant bleeding complication or patients who have sustained a PE while on therapeutic anticoagulation. Relative indications include: iliofemoral DVT; a free-floating thrombus; an inability to achieve or maintain adequate anticoagulation; and propagation or progression of a DVT while on adequate anticoagulation. Prophylactic indications include: trauma patients with closed head or spinal cord injuries;

multiple long bone or pelvic fractures; or high-risk immobilized patients in intensive care units (ICUs). Suprarenal IVC filters have separate indications which include: presence of an IVC thrombus; filter placement during pregnancy or in women of childbearing age; a thrombus extending above a previously placed infrarenal IVC filter; gonadal vein thrombosis; certain venous anatomic variants (discussed in the next section); significant extrinsic IVC compression; intrinsic infrarenal IVC narrowing; and an intra-abdominal mass with planned IVC mobilization during resection. Contraindications to placing an IVC filter include bacteremia and severe coagulopathy.

ANATOMY

The IVC originates at the level of the fourth or fifth lumbar vertebral body where the common iliac veins (CIVs) converge. The renal veins join at the level of the first or second lumbar vertebral body and the hepatic veins join just below the diaphragm. The operator should be familiar with anatomic variants of the IVC to appropriately prevent PEs from all pelvic and lower extremity sources. Transposition of the IVC to the left side of the aorta occurs in 0.2–0.5%. The IVC drains into the left renal vein, which crosses over to the right side of the aorta and drains into a normal suprarenal IVC. Duplication of the IVC occurs in 0.2–0.3%.[2] Typical duplication anatomy includes a right-sided IVC draining the right iliac and renal vein and a left-sided IVC draining the left iliac vein, which extends along the left side of the aorta. The latter joins the left renal vein, which crosses the aorta to join the right IVC and continues as a normal suprarenal IVC. Finally, IVC agenesis is a very rare anatomic anomaly (0.0005%), although 5% of patients with acute DVTs under the age of 30 years have this condition.[3] There are multiple variants of IVC agenesis including infrarenal, suprarenal, and complete IVC agenesis. Infrarenal and complete IVC agenesis are very rare. In these anomalies, lower extremity venous return typically occurs via dilated ascending lumbar veins draining into the azygos-hemiazygos system. When the suprarenal IVC is affected, it involves the retrohepatic portion of the IVC. The renal segment of the IVC drains into the azygos system and into the right atrium through the superior vena cava.[3]

TECHNIQUES

IVC filters are placed either in an angiography suite with a fixed C-arm or in the operating room with a mobile C-arm. Periodically, they are placed in the ICU with a mobile C-arm. A 4- or 5-Fr sheath is placed using ultrasound (US) guidance, either in the common femoral (CFV) or internal jugular vein (IJV), usually on the right side. Certain IVC filters, such as the Simon Nitinol® (BARD Peripheral Vascular, Inc., Tempe, AZ, USA) and TRAPEASE® Permanent Vena Cava Filter and OPTEASE® Retrievable Vena Cava Filter (Cordis Corporation, Milpitas, CA, USA) can be placed through the brachial vein. A diagnostic iliocavogram is performed with a marked pigtail or other multisided catheter with 1-cm interval markings to outline the anatomy and accurately measure the IVC diameter. Alternatively, a sterile ruler is placed on the patient's back or abdomen to obtain similar measurements. However, these are somewhat less accurate, since they are not within the vessel lumen. A stiff wire is advanced into the IVC. The 5-Fr sheath is exchanged for a long delivery sheath that comes with each filter kit. It is flushed with heparinized saline, but usually the patient is not systemically anticoagulated. Filter placement is performed with either vertebral bodies, a sterile ruler, or roadmapping techniques for landmarks. It is typically placed with the apex just inferior to the more inferior renal vein origin with the base of the filter above the iliac vein confluence (**Figure 20.1**). Each filter has an IVC diameter limit for which it is approved; this is usually 28 mm. The exception is the Bird's Nest® Vena Cava Filter (Cook Medical Inc., Bloomington, IN, USA), which has a 40-mm diameter upper limit. Placing a filter in an IVC with a larger diameter than approved increases the risk for migration and embolization to the right atrium or ventricle. It is important to check the instructions for use to obtain this safe range before placement. Deployment systems consist of a simple "pinch-and-pull" technique or a sequence of buttons to be pressed. A completion cavogram is required to demonstrate placement in the infrarenal position with appropriate deployment of each limb.

Adjustments in technique are required when encountering anatomic variants. If the IVC is >28 mm in diameter,

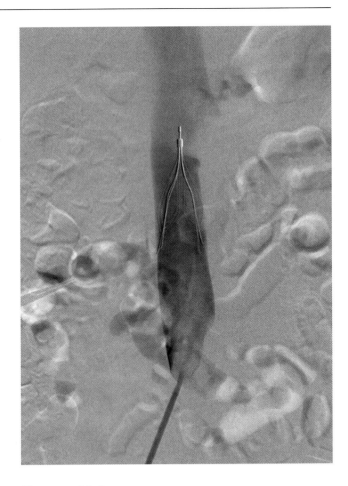

Figure 20.1 Iliocavogram demonstrating the correct placement of an inferior vena cava filter. Note the unopacified blood entering the IVC from the left renal vein at the apex of the filter.

either a Bird's Nest® Vena Cava Filter is placed or bilateral CIV filters are placed. If the IVC appears smaller than expected on the initial cavogram, US-guided puncture of the opposite CFV with cavography is indicated to determine if there is a duplicated IVC. If this is the case, bilateral IVC filters are indicated. When encountering IVC agenesis, the iliac veins empty into the azygous system and a filter is placed into the azygous vein.

Less frequently, filters are placed using transabdominal or even intravascular US (IVUS) guidance. This is usually done when a patient is too sick to be moved, has an anaphylactic allergy to contrast, or has severe renal insufficiency. Before placement, a venous duplex US is obtained to evaluate the femoral veins for patency, measure the caval diameter, and view the anatomy of the renal veins and iliac vein confluence. Transabdominal duplex US-guided placement is feasible only when the IVC and renal vein confluences can be adequately visualized. Under these conditions, femoral access is gained and the US probe is used to track the passage of the wire and sheath, and filter placement in the positions described previously. A plain abdominal X-ray is performed to confirm filter positioning and alignment.[4]

When using IVUS guidance, an 8- or 9-Fr sheath is placed to accommodate the IVUS probe. The probe is inserted to the level of the right atrium and the anatomy is assessed as the probe is pulled back toward the sheath. The IVC diameter is measured and the distance along the shaft of the probe from the access site to the renal vein confluence is determined. The IVC filter delivery sheath is advanced over the stiff guidewire so the tip is just inferior to the more inferior renal vein. The filter is advanced through the sheath to the tip and deployed in the manner described earlier. The IVUS probe is reinserted to check the position of the filter struts, but care needs to be taken not to dislodge or entangle the filter. A postprocedure abdominal X-ray is obtained to confirm filter position and alignment.

TYPES OF FILTERS

There are four major types of IVC filters: permanent, temporary, convertible, and retrievable.

Permanent filters are made to be left in place for the patient's lifespan. Permanent filters include the Greenfield™ Vena Cava Filter (Boston Scientific Corporation, Marlborough, MA, USA), Bird's Nest®, TRAPEASE® Permanent Vena Cava Filter, VenaTech LGM (B. Braun Melsungen AG, Hessen, Germany), and Simon Nitinol®. Each has a specific deployment mechanism and a required delivery sheath size ranging from 6 to 12 Fr. The majority are placed through the IJV or femoral vein, but a few can be inserted through the subclavian or antecubital (cephalic) veins, such as the Simon Nitinol® filter.

Temporary filters are not available in the USA, but are used in Europe and Japan. They have no attachment mechanism to the IVC; a wire connected to the filter traverses the skin for easy removal at the bedside. Guidelines for insertion are like those for filters currently used in the USA, but these filters are only for short-term use, usually a maximum of 2 weeks. One example of their utility is during thrombolytic therapy for DVT. However, one study described significant morbidity from these, including PE on filter removal, device infection and dislocation, and venous perforation.[5]

Convertible filters are placed percutaneously, but are designed to lose their filtration function when it is no longer needed. One example is the Sentry Bioconvertible Inferior Vena Cava Filter (Novate, Galway, Ireland), which recently completed clinical trial enrollment. It is designed to provide protection against PE for up to 60 days after placement. This nitinol device features a stabilizing cylindrical frame and a filter cone formed by six arms held together in the center of the IVC by means of a small bioabsorbable filament. The filament hydrolyzes over a fixed period, after which time the arms are released from the filtering cone and return toward the IVC wall where they are endothelialized, leaving an unobstructed lumen (**Figure 20.2a,b**).

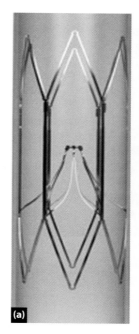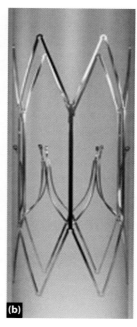

Figure 20.2 Photographs of the Sentry Bioconvertible Inferior Vena Cava Filter (Novate, Galway, Ireland) with (**a**) filter struts adjoined with a bioabsorbable filament, forming the filtering mechanism, and (**b**) after release of the struts from the hydrolyzed filament.

Retrievable filters are like permanent ones, but within a certain time interval can be removed once they are no longer needed. Many of these can be left in place permanently. Retrievable filters include: Denali® Vena Cava Filter (BARD Peripheral Vascular, Inc.); Günther Tulip® Vena Cava Filter (Cook Medical, Inc.); Celect™ Platinum Vena Cava Filter (Cook Medical, Inc.); OPTEASE® Retrievable Vena Cava Filter; Option™ ELITE Vena Caval Filter (Argon Medical Devices Inc., Plano, TX, USA); and ALN Vena Cava Filter (ALN, Ghisonaccia, France). The duration the filter has been in place must be considered before removal. The less time it has been in place, the easier it is to remove, because there is less endothelialization and incorporation into the IVC wall.

RETRIEVAL

Retrievable filters are generally removed through the IJV under fluoroscopic guidance using a coaxial system and snare catheter. After US-guided access and sheath placement, catheter and wire access to the IVC is gained. A cavogram is performed to determine IVC patency and lack of thrombus within the filter. If the IVC is thrombosed up to the filter, or if there is significant thrombus within the filter, attempts at removal should be abandoned. Systemic anticoagulation is continued and, in the case of thrombus within the filter, the patient is re-evaluated for clearance of this thrombus in 4–6 weeks. After obtaining the cavogram, the pigtail catheter is removed over a stiff wire.

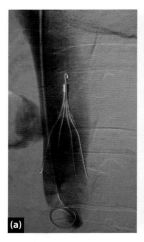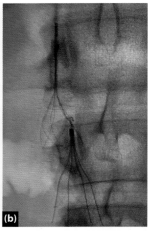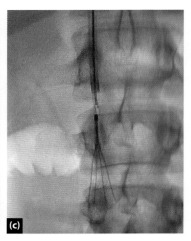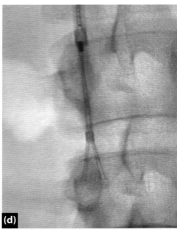

Figure 20.3 Images demonstrating the sequence for inferior vena cava (IVC) filter retrieval. (**a**) Cavogram demonstrating patent IVC without filter thrombus. (**b**) Snare capture of the filter apical hook. (**c**) Advancement of the sheath over the apex of the filter. (**d**) Release of the hooks from the IVC wall to complete recapture of the entire filter within the 12-Fr sheath.

A long, 12-Fr sheath is placed into the IVC over the stiff wire. A coaxial system with an inner sheath and snare is used to encircle the hook on the top of the filter. The filter is recaptured by keeping tension on the snare-filter combination while advancing the sheath over the filter. There should be no net upward or downward force during the recapture phase. The most difficult part of the procedure is the dislodgement of the hooks from the IVC wall (**Figure 20.3a–d**). Judgement is required as to how long to persist and how hard to pull on the retrieval system, since these factors influence the risk of caval tear and internal hemorrhage. No effort should be made to remove the coaxial system from the patient before the entire filter is within the sheath.

Additional endovascular devices and strategies for challenging cases include: the use of rigid forceps; modified loop snares; double loop techniques; balloon displacement; the Excimer laser; and open surgical removal. However, precise descriptions of these techniques are beyond the scope of this chapter.

COMPLICATIONS

Immediate complications after placement include: malpositioning in the gonadal, renal, or lumbar veins, in the upside-down position, or with the apex against the IVC wall (1.3%); hematoma (0.6%); air embolism (0.2%); arterial puncture (0.04%); arteriovenous fistula (0.02%); and pneumothorax (0.02%) (IJV access). Longer-term complications include migration (1%), infection, and death (<1%). IVC perforation and penetration of the IVC wall by the filter legs are rare but can lead to retroperitoneal hematoma or bowel injury.[6,7] There is a 2–5% risk of PE with an indwelling IVC filter and a long-term risk of IVC thrombosis, which can cause chronic severe bilateral leg edema. This latter risk is not known in the newer devices, but is approximately 5% at 10 years after implantation for the Greenfield™ Vena Cava filter and up to 20% with other devices.[2,6]

REFERENCES

1. Horlander KT, Mannino DM, Leeper KV. Pulmonary embolism mortality in the United States, 1979–1998: an analysis using multiple-cause mortality data. *Arch Intern Med*. 2003;**163**:1711–1717.
2. Passman MA. Vena cava interruption and pulmonary embolism. In: Cronenwett JL, Johnston KW, eds. *Rutherford's Vascular Surgery*. Philadelphia, PA: Saunders/Elsevier; 2010. pp. 811–832.
3. Lambert M, Marboeuf P, Midulla M, et al. Inferior vena cava agenesis and deep vein thrombosis: 10 patients and review of the literature. *Vasc Med*. 2010;**15**:451–459.
4. Fisher BT, Naslund TC. Ultrasound-guided cava filter placement. In: AbuRahma A, Bandyk D, eds. *Noninvasive Vascular Diagnosis*. London: Springer; 2010. pp. 519–528.
5. Wada H, Sakakura K, Kubo N, et al. Complications of temporary vena cava filter placement. *J Cardiol*. 2012;**60**:306–309.
6. Jaff M, McMurtry MS, Archer SL, et al. Management of massive and submassive pulmonary embolism, iliofemoral deep vein thrombosis, and chronic thromboembolic pulmonary hypertension: a scientific statement from the American Heart Association. *Circulation*. 2011;**123**:1788–1830.
7. Konstantinides S, Torbicki A, Agnelli G, et al. 2014 ESC guidelines on the diagnosis and management of acute pulmonary embolism. *Eur Heart J*. 2014;**35**:3033–3069.

SECTION II

Open Vascular Reconstructions

21

Carotid endarterectomy

SACHINDER SINGH HANS

CONTENTS

INTRODUCTION

Carotid endarterectomy (CEA) is one of the most common arterial reconstructions performed by vascular surgeons. Technical aspects of the operation and appropriate patient selection are keys to achieving satisfactory outcomes, because a slight technical imperfection may result in a serious postoperative complication, such as stroke. The primary indications for CEA are:

- patients with recent mild-to-moderate stroke in the distribution of the middle cerebral artery (MCA) (occasionally in the anterior cerebral artery) with good recovery;
- transient contralateral motor or sensory deficits or ipsilateral amaurosis fugax (transient loss of vision; this may be either partial or complete and usually lasts for <1 hour);

- symptomatic high-grade internal carotid artery (ICA) stenosis (>80% stenosis) in selected patients who are otherwise good risk and have at least 5 years of life expectancy.

Following clinical evaluation, carotid duplex imaging is performed. Imaging studies, such as computed tomography angiography (CTA) or catheter-directed, intra-arterial digital subtraction arteriography of the carotid artery, may be necessary in many instances to further evaluate the cervical carotid artery, for example, when the distal end of the plaque is not visualized by duplex scan, or when proximal and distal artery disease is suspected. CT scans or magnetic resonance imaging (MRI) and magnetic resonance angiography of the brain are performed in patients who exhibit focal neurologic symptoms and positive neurologic findings. Magnetic resonance angiography of the neck is not as helpful as CT angiography of the neck. Magnetic resonance angiography tends to overestimate the degree of stenosis by 15–20% in general.

Anesthetic choice (regional versus general) has been a matter of considerable debate over many years. Although the GALA (General Anaesthesia versus Local Anaesthesia for carotid surgery) trial showed no difference in the outcomes of patients undergoing CEA, either under cervical block anesthesia (CBA) or general anesthesia (GA), the author prefers CBA in most patients.[1] However, in patients whose plaque extends distally thereby requiring more extensive dissection (determined by preoperative imaging studies), those with extreme anxiety, and patients who are deaf and have poor command of the language, GA is preferred.

SHUNT PLACEMENT DURING CEA

Shunt use during CEA has been the subject of considerable controversy, with most surgeons favoring its routine or selective use based on intraoperative monitoring with stump pressure (SP) (back pressure), electroencephalography, or transcranial Doppler monitoring under GA or continuous neurologic assessment when CEA is performed in awake patients under CBA. There have been few case series reporting satisfactory outcomes without shunt placement under GA. The rate of shunt placement for CEA in awake patients is usually around 10% (8–12% under CBA and 15–18% under GA).[2–4] In the presence of contralateral ICA/common carotid artery (CCA) occlusion, the rate of shunt use increases up to 20% under CBA.[2]

POSITIONING

The neck is hyperextended by a roll behind the scapulae and an occipital support. The neck is turned toward the contralateral site. Incision options include a vertical, transverse, or oblique incision; the latter is often preferable because of better cosmetic results. If the plaque extends considerably distally into the ICA or proximally into the CCA, a transverse incision may not provide adequate exposure. In patients with short necks, adhesive tape is applied to the shoulder, pulled downward, and attached to the operating table to improve exposure in the space between the clavicle and mandible.

Duplex imaging with evaluation of carotid bifurcation in relation to the angle of the mandible and CTA (carotid bifurcation in relation to the level of the cervical vertebral body) are good guides for the length of the incision and its extension proximally or distally.

TECHNIQUE

An oblique incision is made, with the lower end of the incision 2 cm anterior to the anterior border of

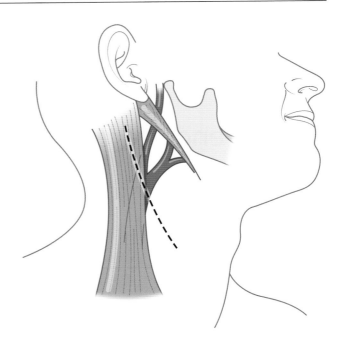

Figure 21.1 Line of skin incision.

sternocleidomastoid muscle (SCM) and the upper end of the incision 2-cm posterior to the anterior border of the SCM (**Figure 21.1**). The platysma muscle is incised, and the transverse cutaneous nerve is divided with scissors after infiltrating local anesthesia (LA); this is because when electrocautery is used to divide the nerve in awake patients, it leads to considerable discomfort. The external jugular vein and its branches are ligated and divided. The greater auricular nerve is seen in the upper portion of the incision; usually, it can be preserved.

Two toothed forceps are used to lift the skin (medial flap) superiorly. With Metzenbaum scissors, the dissection plane is developed along the anterior border of the SCM.

Two blunt Weitlaner retractors are placed superiorly and inferiorly and a dissection plane is developed along the medial border of the internal jugular vein (IJV), in the lower part of the exposure. As the dissection proceeds upward along the medial border of the IJV, the common facial vein is seen and may have several branches that are individually ligated and divided. Superior to the common facial vein, deep cervical lymph nodes and fascia are carefully dissected and mobilized posteriorly. In the lower portion of the incision, the middle thyroid vein is ligated and divided.

The carotid sheath is opened. The CCA is looped with a double silastic vessel loop. The entire premise of the dissection is that both CCAs and ICAs are left in their bed and the patient is dissected away from the artery rather than performing extensive mobilization of the carotid artery, which can lead to embolization with serious consequences.

The external carotid artery (ECA) is looped with a silastic loop; tension is put on the loop caudally with a straight hemostat to get better distal exposure of the ICA above the bifurcation. The ansa cervicalis is seen anteriorly in

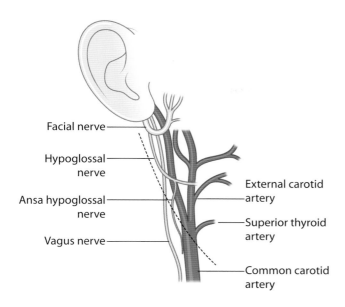

Figure 21.2 Anatomical relationship of the carotid bifurcation.

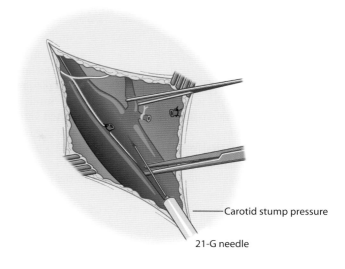

Figure 21.3 Measurement of carotid stump pressure.

the carotid sheath and is mobilized anteriorly. The vagus nerve is seen posteriorly between the IJV and the CCA; however, in the lower portion of the incision, the nerve can be seen lying more in an anterolateral plane and is carefully preserved (**Figure 21.2**). In the upper portion of the exposure, small veins joining the IJV are ligated and divided along with the region of the sternocleidomastoid branch (sometime two branches) of the occipital artery. The hypoglossal nerve (HGN) is visualized just below the posterior belly of the digastric muscle, with the upper end of the vagus nerve, which is closely approximating the HGN about 3–4 cm beyond the origin of the ICA. Lidocaine 1% is infiltrated into the carotid body to prevent bradycardia. Intravenous heparin (100 IU/kg) is given by the anesthesia personnel and the activated clotting time is monitored (250–300 seconds).

STUMP PRESSURE

An SP of 40 mmHg is considered a reasonable cutoff as a guide to shunt placement. In general, patients with SP ≥40 mmHg can tolerate carotid clamping provided systemic pressure does not decrease during the performance of CEA. Various types of shunts are available and include the Javid™ Peripheral Carotid Bypass Shunt (BARD Peripheral Vascular, Inc., Tempe, AZ, USA), the Argyle™ Carotid Artery Shunt (Medtronic, Minneapolis, MN, USA), the Pruitt-Inahara® Carotid Shunt (LeMaitre Vascular, Inc., Burlington, MA, USA), and the Sundt™ External Carotid Endarterectomy Shunt (Integra LifeSciences Corporation, Plainsboro, NJ, USA). Surgeons should use the shunt they are most familiar with during CEA. The author prefers the Sundt™ External Carotid Endarterectomy Shunt

because of its relative ease of insertion and its flexibility. SP is measured by inserting a 21-G needle into the CCA after the proximal CCA and ECA have been clamped, and pressure tubing is connected to a recording monitor (**Figure 21.3**).

A proximal vascular clamp is applied to the CCA and a distal clamp to the ICA. The double vessel loop is tightened and pulled caudally around the ECA and the arteriotomy incision is made in the distal CCA and ICA with angled Potts scissors (**Figure 21.4**).

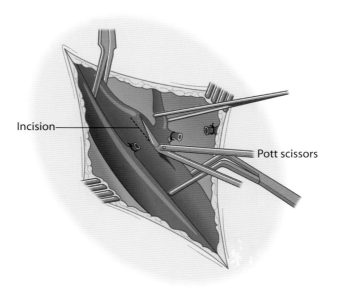

Figure 21.4 Arteriotomy incision in the distal common carotid artery and proximal internal carotid artery showing proximal and distal clamping.

TECHNIQUE OF SHUNT PLACEMENT

After applying the angled proximal vascular clamp to the CCA and a Micro Kitzmiller clamp (Scanlan International, Inc., St. Paul, MN, USA) distally to the ICA, an arteriotomy incision is made from the distal CCA over the plaque and extending into the ICA. The smaller end of the Sundt™ External Carotid Endarterectomy Shunt is inserted into the ICA, a smaller-size Javid clamp is applied, and retrograde bleeding occurs from the lower end of the shunt, which is inserted into the CCA and is then held in place by a large Javid clamp along with tightening of the double vessel loop so that the shunt does not come out accidentally from the lower end (**Figures 21.5–21.8**). In patients with soft plaque in the middle segment of the CCA, it may be preferable to insert the proximal end of the shunt to extrude any embolic plaque and then clamp the shunt with a Fogarty softjaw clamp before inserting the distal

end of the shunt into the ICA to prevent plaque emboli lodging into the brain. Shunt flow should be checked with a Doppler probe.

Plaque dissection is started with FREER-Type elevator at the thickest portion of the plaque and then continues distally into the ICA until the plaque tapers smoothly like onion peel. Plaque is removed from the ECA with the eversion technique and the carotid bifurcation plaque is then dissected proximally and sharply divided with Potts scissors (**Figure 21.8**). In patients undergoing CEA for stroke, the ICA is not clamped because a recent thrombus may be present in the distal ICA; clamping is not carried out because of retrograde bleeding from the ICA. Next, the distal vascular clamp is applied. Irrigation at the endarterectomy site is performed with heparinized saline, removing loose fibers of the media or any flimsy tissue particles. If the distal end of the plaque is not firmly attached to the intima, two 7-0 polypropylene tacking sutures

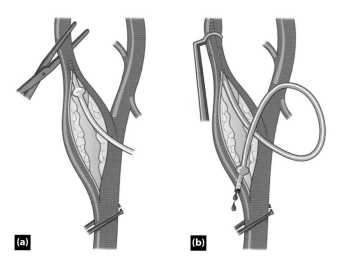

(a)   **(b)**

Figure 21.5 Endarterectomy technique. (**a**) Insertion at the distal end of the shunt. (**b**) Back-bleeding from the proximal end of the shunt.

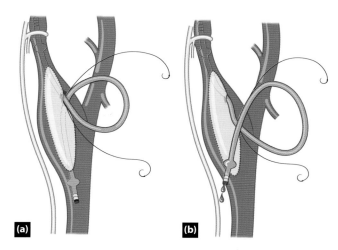

(a)   **(b)**

Figure 21.7 Endarterectomy technique. (**a**) Shunt with closure of endarterectomy with patch. (**b**) Removal of shunt from the common carotid artery.

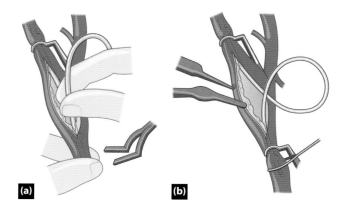

(a)   **(b)**

Figure 21.6 Endarterectomy technique. (**a**) Proximal insertion of the shunt into the common carotid artery. (**b**) Plaque dissection with the shunt in place.

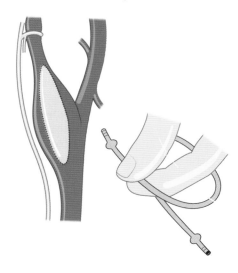

Figure 21.8 Removal of shunt patch (complete) closure.

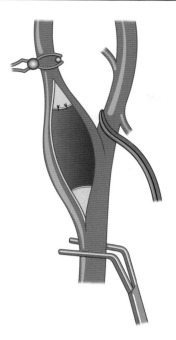

Figure 21.9 Removed plaque with tacking sutures.

(Ethicon US, LLC, Somerville, NJ, USA) are applied at the 5 o'clock and 7 o'clock positions (**Figure 21.9**). Except in patients whose ICA has a very large diameter (>5 mm), patch grafting (bovine pericardium, Dacron, or polytetrafluoroethylene patch) is performed. Suturing is started distally in the ICA with a continuous 7-0 polypropylene suture and continued proximally. At the lower end, the patch is divided and sutured to the CCA with a 6-0 polypropylene suture and the suturing is continued proximally. On the medial side, suturing is completed; on the lateral side of the arteriotomy, the shunt prevents further closure. The shunt is first removed from the CCA. A proximal vascular clamp is applied to and then removed from the ICA, and the ICA is clamped. The remaining suture line closure is completed. After the suture line closure is completed, blood is first allowed to perfuse the ECA before the clamp on the ICA is removed.

ANATOMICAL VARIATIONS

Venous anomalies

The IJV can be anatomically located anteriorly instead of laterally; in that situation, a retrojugular approach to CEA provides excellent exposure, a good plane of dissection, and only a few blood vessels need to be ligated and divided. Usually, the HGN is not seen in the operative area and is not in danger of injury.

Superior thyroid artery (STA)

The STA may arise from the CCA and may have to be controlled separately with a vessel loop.

Ascending pharyngeal artery

The ascending pharyngeal artery, which usually arises at the carotid bifurcation or as a first branch of the ECA, may arise from the ICA up to 2 cm from its origin and will cause retrograde bleeding with difficulty in visualizing the plaque. It must be controlled separately with a ligation using 3-0 silk tie.

Ansa cervicalis

There can be variations of the ansa cervicalis, with the superior root of the ansa coming from the vagus nerve. Division can result in paralysis of the infrahyoid muscles and hoarseness. If a large nerve connection is found, the author tends to preserve the variations of ansa cervicalis and perform the arteriotomy by passing the Potts scissors under the loop and then starting patch grafting. Patch grafting is performed in the ICA; the patch is then brought underneath the loop and continued toward the CCA (**Figure 21.10**). In addition, the HGN may occasionally be anatomically lower (close to the carotid bifurcation) and may be injured during ligation of the common facial vein.

COMPLICATIONS

Neck hematoma

Hematoma in the neck is usually secondary to venous bleeding, but can also result from unsatisfactory closure of the arteriotomy and may resolve in a few weeks' time.

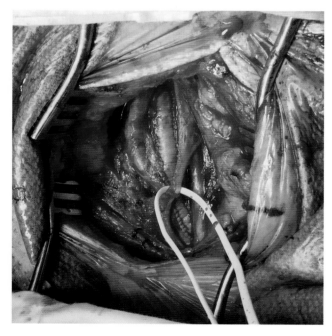

Figure 21.10 Variation of ansa cervicalis with sutured patch brought underneath the abnormal ansa cervicalis loop. Please note that below the cilastic loop encircling the abnormal ansa cervicalis loop, the Vagus nerve is seen.

However, large, tense hematomas can cause compression of the airway and esophagus. They are considered an emergency and should be evacuated in the operating room immediately. It can be difficult to perform oral tracheal intubation in a patient with a large neck hematoma; therefore, it is preferable to evacuate the hematoma by removing the sutures under LA, which relieves pressure on the airway, and continue the procedure either under LA or subsequent maintenance of airway by the anesthesiologist and GA, if necessary.

Hemodynamic instability

Patients undergoing CEA may develop hypotension associated with bradycardia during and in the first 6 hours after CEA. This is the result of carotid sinus nerve (CSN) stimulation and can be prevented in most instances by blocking the CSN during CEA with an injection of LA. Hypertension during and immediately after CEA occurs frequently and is more common in patients with uncontrolled blood pressure before the procedure. Hypertension during and following CEA needs immediate control with intravenous antihypertensive medication like labetalol hydrochloride, hydralazine hydrochloride, sodium nitroprusside, or nitroglycerine. The author and others have reported less hemodynamic lability in patients undergoing CEA under CBA.

Cranial nerve palsy

The HGN is the most common cranial nerve injured during CEA. Temporary HGN palsy (tongue deviation to the ipsilateral side) and vagal paresis (hoarseness) are not uncommon following CEA. Permanent nerve damage is suspected if there is no recovery in nerve function in 3 months. The transverse cutaneous nerve must be divided during neck incision resulting in temporary loss of sensation anterior to the incision. Glossopharyngeal nerve injuries are more common in patients undergoing CEA for high plaque. Injury to the ramus mandibularis (mandibular nerve) can occur if dissection is done too close to the angle of the mandible, resulting in flattening of the lower lip. If the patient develops hoarseness after CEA and contralateral CEA is planned, a vocal cord functional assessment by an ear, nose, and throat surgeon is necessary before the procedure is contemplated because bilateral vagal nerve injury may necessitate tracheostomy. Injury to the external laryngeal nerve resulting in loss of pitch of the voice can occur during mobilization of the STA. Injury to the spinal accessory nerve is uncommon.

Postoperative stroke

This is the most dreaded complication of CEA.[5] Most post-CEA strokes are embolic and in these patients further surgical intervention is not helpful. However, in patients with embolic occlusion of the main trunk of the MCA or its superior or inferior branches, neurovascular intervention with the Solitaire™ revascularization device (Medtronic), can achieve successful recanalization and neurologic recovery if performed within 8 hours of neurologic deficit. In patients, stroke can also develop secondary to cerebral ischemia because of lack of shunt placement, or the malfunction of a shunt in patients who do not tolerate carotid clamping. If a patient has a new neurologic deficit (minutes-to-hours) post-CEA, thrombosis should be suspected; the patient should undergo an immediate head CT and should be taken back to the operating room for carotid reexploration and thrombectomy. There may be a distal intimal flap causing the thrombosis. Flap removal, use of tacking sutures, and a complete arteriogram should be performed. Intracerebral hemorrhage may occur (usually between 2 and 5 days) occasionally in patients with uncontrolled hypertension and severe contralateral ICA stenosis or ICA occlusion; this is the result of hyperperfusion syndrome. Hyperperfusion syndrome in its mild form may manifest as post-CEA headache (common) that should resolve in a few days, or post-CEA seizures and intracerebral hemorrhage in its most severe form. Postoperative seizures are more common in patients undergoing CEA for stroke and usually respond well to antiseizure medication, but may be associated with postictal paralysis.

Postoperative myocardial infarction and cardiac arrhythmias

These may occur after CEA. They are usually diagnosed by serum troponin; an electrocardiogram assessment and cardiology consult should be obtained. The patient may not experience classic chest pain or the typical symptoms of myocardial infarction following CEA.

Patch graft infection

Synthetic patch graft infection, though rare, can be a very serious complication of CEA and often requires removal of the patch with autogenous reconstruction using saphenous vein graft interposition. If there is an extensive infection within the cutaneous sinus, a myocutaneous flap by a plastic reconstructive surgeon may become necessary.

Carotid pseudoaneurysm

This is an uncommon complication and can be treated with an endovascular technique or with open surgery depending on its location, presence or absence of infection, and the general condition of the patient.

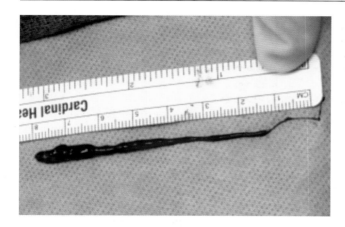

Figure 21.11 Thrombus removed at the time of carotid endarterectomy for recent stroke.

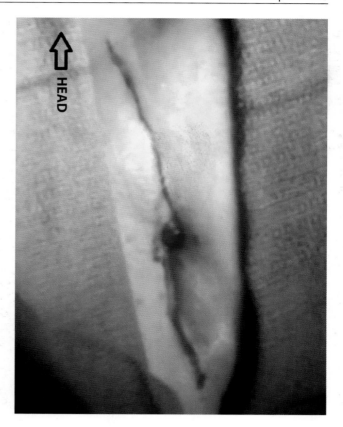

Figure 21.12 Neck sinus following carotid endarterectomy with synthetic Dacron patch grafting.

The patient underwent left CEA with patch grafting without any complications.

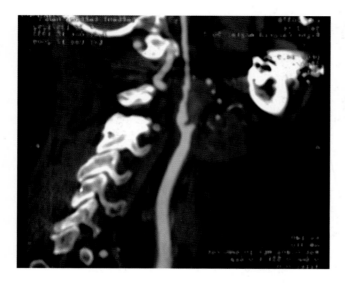

Figure 21.13 Computed tomography image showing soft tissue mass around the carotid bifurcation following carotid endarterectomy.

CASE EXAMPLES

Case example 1

A 61-year-old man presented with speech difficulty and right upper extremity weakness with good recovery (National Institutes of Health Stroke Scale score = 3). Carotid duplex and CTA showed 90% stenosis of the left ICA. Brain MRI showed ischemic changes and a small infarct in the distribution of the left MCA. The patient underwent left CEA with bovine pericardium patch graft placement under CBA. A long thrombus was removed from the ICA (**Figure 21.11**). The distal ICA was not clamped, and because of excellent back-flow from the distal ICA, the clot extruded itself.

Case example 2

A 78-year-old woman with a history of diabetes mellitus was referred because of persistent sinus in the neck, which appeared 2 months after undergoing right-sided CEA with Dacron patch graft for high-grade, asymptomatic (>80%) stenosis of the right ICA (**Figure 21.12**). The patient underwent CT evaluation of the neck, which showed a soft tissue mass around the carotid bifurcation (**Figure 21.13**). The patient underwent reexploration of the neck under GA and was found to have an unincorporated synthetic Dacron patch graft (**Figure 21.14**). The distal CCA and proximal ICA, including the unincorporated Dacron patch, were resected and vein graft interposition using the greater saphenous vein in a nonreversed fashion from the right CCA and the proximal ICA was used (5 cm), with healing of the sinus. However, 1 year later, the patient developed severe stenosis secondary to myointimal hyperplastic lesion in the interposition vein graft interposition and was treated with carotid stenting. One year later, the carotid stent thrombosed, yet the patient has remained asymptomatic.

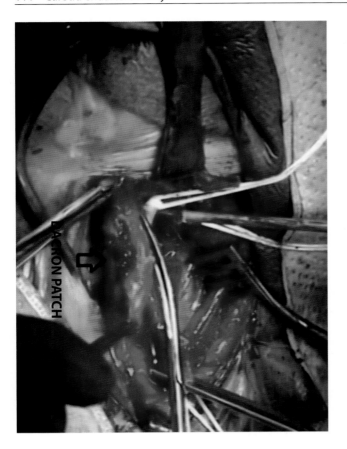

DACRON PATCH

Figure 21.14 Operative photograph showing unincorporated synthetic Dacron patch at the site of endarterectomy.

REFERENCES

1. Lewis SC, Warlow CP, Bodenham AR, et al. General anesthesia versus local anesthesia for carotid surgery (GALA): a multicentre, randomised controlled trial. *Lancet.* 2008;**372**:2132–2142.
2. Hans SS, Jareunpoon O. Prospective evaluation of electroencephalography, carotid artery stump pressure, and neurologic changes during 314 consecutive carotid endarterectomies performed in awake patients. *J Vasc Surg.* 2007;**45**:511–515.
3. Schneider JR, Droste JS, Schindler N, et al. Carotid endarterectomy with routine electroencephalography and selective shunting: influence of contralateral internal carotid artery occlusion and utility in prevention of perioperative strokes. *J Vasc Surg.* 2002;**35**:1114–1122.
4. Calligaro KD, Dougherty MJ. Correlation of carotid artery stump pressure and neurologic changes during 474 carotid endarterectomies performed in awake patients. *J Vasc Surg.* 2005;**42**:684–689.
5. Goodney PP, Likosky DS, Cronenwett JL. Factors associated with stroke or death after carotid endarterectomy in Northern New England. *J Vasc Surg.* 2008;**48**:1139–1145.

22

Eversion carotid endarterectomy

JUDITH C. LIN AND CONSTANTINE G. SAITES

CONTENTS

INTRODUCTION

Since its introduction nearly 75 years ago, there have been few modifications to the technical approach of carotid endarterectomy (CEA). As medical management of atherosclerotic risk factors and perioperative care improve, the outcome differences attributed to these small, but significant technical details embody the "holy grail" of carotid atherosclerosis surgery. Conventional CEA with patch angioplasty has been the most widely practiced technique and is the standard to which the approach of eversion CEA (ECEA) is compared. Contemporary ECEA is an alternative technique used to facilitate the removal of plaque isolated to the carotid bulb and proximal internal carotid artery (ICA). Advantages of eversion versus standard endarterectomy include: the ability to shorten a redundant ICA; better visualized end point and easier detection of intimal flaps; faster closure by simple anastomosis of the ICA to the carotid bulb; an all autogenous reconstruction; and decreased restenosis rates in women. In the authors' practice, most patients still undergo standard CEA with bovine or vein patch angioplasty; only a minority of selected patients undergo ECEA.

TECHNIQUE

Anesthetic choice, cerebral monitoring, and neuroprotection are identical for both methods of CEA. During the case, neurologic monitoring is routine. Electroencephalographic monitoring is used for patients under general anesthesia, while continuous neurologic assessment is used for patients undergoing CEA under cervical block anesthesia. Most patients undergoing CEA do not require intraoperative shunt placement. If shunting is needed during ECEA, shunt insertion is performed after everting and removing the bulk of the ICA plaque. The authors prefer to use the short Sundt™ internal shunt (Integra LifeSciences Corporation, Plainsboro, NJ, USA) with nonreinforced segment, 3 × 4 mm. Shunt insertion is performed distally into the ICA and held in place with a shunt clamp. An extension of the common carotid artery (CCA) arteriotomy may be needed to expose the open lumen before the shunt is inserted into the CCA. ECEA is the preferred procedure for ICA kinks or loops. After transection, the redundant ICA may be resected and anastomosis completed to a more distal portion of the ICA. Initial neck dissection and isolation of the carotid artery are similar to the conventional CEA technique. Dissection and mobilization of the carotid bulb and proximal ICA are more extensive with ECEA than standard CEA. The need for more extensive dissection for ECEA has not caused an increase in vagus nerve injury. Some surgeons mark the level of the carotid bulb with ultrasound before incising the skin to minimize the length of the incision.

The patient is placed supine on the operating table with a shoulder roll and the head rotated to the opposite side. The neck is prepped and draped to expose the mastoid process, angle of the mandible, sternal notch, and cervical incision. An incision is made along the anterior border of the sternocleidomastoid muscle (SCM) over the carotid bifurcation. The authors prefer a longitudinal over a transverse incision because of better exposure of the distal ICA. After the platysma muscle is divided, dissection is made along the anterior border of the SCM to identify the confluence of the internal jugular (IJV) and facial veins. The facial vein is suture-ligated and divided to expose the underlying carotid artery medially. The carotid artery is exposed circumferentially to isolate the ICA and the carotid bulb. Within the carotid sheath, the vagus nerve lies posteriorly between the CCA medially and IJV laterally. If sinus bradycardia occurs, 1–2 mL of 1% lidocaine without preservatives may be administered topically between the ICA and external carotid artery (ECA) to block nerve conduction to the carotid sinus.

After dissection of the CCA, ICA, and ECA, intravenous heparin is administered to achieve an activated clotting time >250 seconds. The ICA is clamped first, followed by the CCA, and finally the ECA. At this time, the ICA is transected obliquely by dividing the crotch of the carotid bulb from the carotid bifurcation to a point more proximal on the lateral side of the CCA. Generally, an opening of 10–15 mm can be obtained without extending the arteriotomy at either end, as long as the transection line is beveled enough. Otherwise, the arteriotomy on the lateral wall of the CCA may be extended caudally and the arteriotomy medial wall of the ICA extended cephalad to a similar length to facilitate later anastomosis of the arteries. An extended arteriotomy on the CCA also allows for removal of a more proximal plaque in the CCA.

ECEA is performed by circumferentially elevating the plaque with a Penfield elevator from the arterial wall to remove both the intima and media; the adventitia is grasped with two fine forceps while an assistant holds the plaque (**Figure 22.1**). The adventitia with its outer layer of media is everted and the atheromatous core is held away in tension until the end of the plaque is reached in the distal ICA. After removal of the plaque, the surgeon may inspect the entire circumference of the end point, remove loose fragments, and make sure the distal intima is adherent with no loose pieces (**Figure 22.2**). If a loose flap is found, it may be peeled off or alternatively "tacked" down using

7-0 double-armed polypropylene sutures from the luminal side and tied externally.

After the end point is secured, the ICA is unrolled and the luminal surface inspected for loose debris with irrigation of heparinized saline. Any loose fragments should be removed and the entire circumference of the end point inspected. Any persistent plaque or flap is identified and corrected before reanastomosis. To shorten an elongated or kinked ICA at the carotid bifurcation, the spatulated ICA is then pulled down to straighten the carotid kink (**Figure 22.3**). Once the endarterectomy of the ICA is completed, the distal CCA and the ECA are inspected for plaque removal. The plaque is elevated in the bulb and carried up the ECA and proximally into the CCA. Endarterectomy of the ECA and CCA may be performed with direct elevation of the exposed plaque and proximal eversion of a more extensive plaque.

The arteriotomy is irrigated with heparinized saline to remove loose fragments and with low-molecular-weight dextran to inhibit platelet adhesion (**Figure 22.4**).

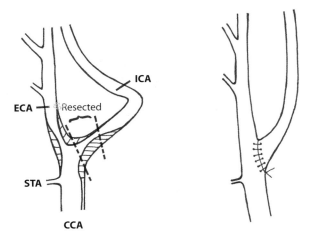

Figure 22.2 Inspection of distal intima end point.

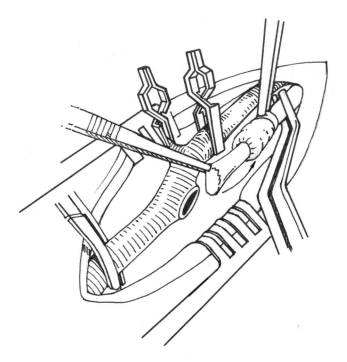

Figure 22.1 Circumferential elevation of plaque from the arterial wall.

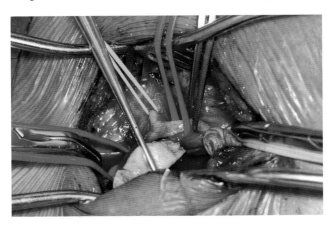

Figure 22.3 Shortening of an elongated internal carotid artery and straightening of carotid kink. CCA: common carotid artery; ECA: external carotid artery; ICA: internal carotid artery; STA: superior thyroid artery.

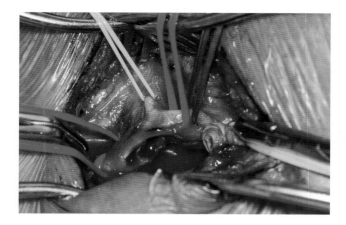

Figure 22.4 Irrigation to remove loose fragments and primary anastomosis.

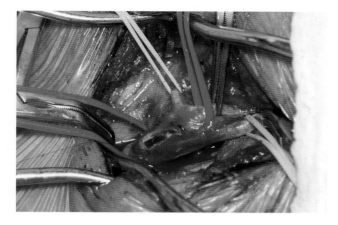

Figure 22.5 Continuous monofilament suture starting from the back wall and inside the artery.

Primary anastomosis between the ICA and CCA is performed with continuous 6-0 monofilament suture, starting at the most cephalad portion of the ICA arteriotomy. The back wall of the anastomosis is usually sewn from the inside of the artery, which provides the best visualization (**Figure 22.5**). The running suture is completed posteriorly then brought anteriorly where it is tied to the other end. After completion of the anastomosis, blood flow is restored in the usual sequence: (1) temporarily opening the ICA first to allow backfilling of the bulb; (2) unclamping the ECA to allow backfilling; (3) opening the CCA to allow forward blood flow into the ECA; and (4) finally opening the ICA. Hemostasis is then obtained (**Figure 22.6**).

Care must be taken to avoid beginning different planes of dissection for plaque removal. The distal end point of the plaque in the ICA is visualized and disengaged from the underlying media. Demonstration of the plaque shows a feathered end superficial to the internal elastic lamina. This natural transition and termination for plaque allows for a tapered end of the carotid occlusive disease (COD).

Postoperative care is routine, with blood pressure control and assessment of neurologic deficits. Postoperative complications of ECEA are similar as standard CEA: stroke; transient ischemic attack (TIA); cranial nerve injury; neck hematoma; and cardiac morbidity. Cranial nerve injury includes the hypoglossal, vagus, pharyngeal, and laryngeal branches of the vagus and glossopharyngeal nerves.

LITERATURE REVIEW

Results of the EVEREST (EVERsion carotid Endarterectomy versus Standard Trial) validated the short- and long-term safety and efficacy of ECEA for carotid atherosclerosis. This prospective, multicenter, randomized trial compared rates of carotid occlusion, restenosis, major stroke, and death among standard CEA (*n* = 675)

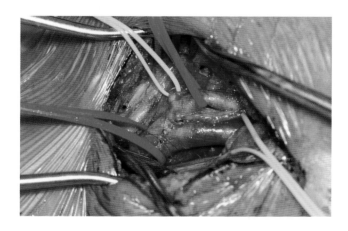

Figure 22.6 Completion of anastomosis and restoration of blood flow.

and ECEA (*n* = 678) patients. Long-term results showed a significantly lower restenosis rate in the eversion group (2.7 versus 5.6%; *p* = 0.01) at a mean follow-up of 33 months. Eversion CEA was an independent predictor of carotid patency, in that the eversion population of patients were three times less likely to have restenosis than patients who had standard CEA with either patch or primary closure.[1]

Several single-institution studies have provided a consensus that there is no significant difference between eversion and standard techniques in early (<30 days) postoperative complications.[2] Among its advantages, ECEA is associated with decreased operative times and shorter cross-clamp times due to a single anastomosis. Schneider and collaborators compared the results of 2635 ECEAs and 17 155 standard CEAs.[3] Early perioperative morbidity, including ipsilateral stroke and TIA, were equivalent although ECEA showed a significantly shorter operative time (median 99 versus 114 minutes; *p* <0.001) but a higher incidence of return to the operating room for bleeding (1.4 versus 8%; *p* = 0.002).

Antonopoulos and collaborators pooled randomized and nonrandomized studies in a meta-analysis that favored ECEA in both short- and long-term outcomes in 16 251 CEA procedures.[4] Eversion CEA was associated with a significant reduction in perioperative stroke (odds ratio (OR) = 0.46; 95% confidence interval (CI): 0.35–0.62; number needed to treat (NNT) = 68; 95% CI: 56–96), death (OR = 0.49; 95% CI: 0.34–0.69; NNT = 100; 95% CI: 85–185), and stroke-related death (OR = 0.40; 95% CI: 0.23–0.67; NNT = 147; 95% CI: 115–270). Regarding long-term outcomes, ECEA was associated with a significant reduction in late carotid artery occlusion (OR = 0.48; 95% CI: 0.25–0.90; NNT = 143; 95% CI: 100–769) and late mortality (OR = 0.76; 95% CI: 0.61–0.94; NNT = 40; 95% CI: 25–167); subanalysis of patched CEA replicated only the finding on late mortality.

In the longest follow-up published to date, Black and collaborators reported a restenosis rate of 4.1% (n = 20/534) within a mean follow-up period of 8.86 years (95% CI: 6.56–9.16).[5] The mean time to recurrence was 4.4 years, following no predilection for anatomic distribution, suggesting these occurrences represent systemic atherosclerotic disease rather than neointimal hyperplasia of the single eversion CEA suture line. Current level I evidence studies and meta-analyses comparing ECEA and standard CEA have validated excellent results with both techniques. Although the eversion method has not shown superior results conclusively, ECEA provides another reliable technique that should be in every vascular surgeon's armamentarium for the treatment of high-grade COD, particularly when associated with a kinked or highly redundant ICA.

REFERENCES

1. Cao P, Giordano G, De Rango P, et al. Eversion versus conventional carotid endarterectomy: late results of a prospective multicenter randomized trial. *J Vasc Surg.* 2000;**31(1 Pt 1)**:19–30.
2. Ben Ahmed S, Daniel G, Benezit M, et al. Eversion carotid endarterectomy without shunt: concerning 1385 consecutive cases. *J Cardiovasc Surg (Torino).* 2017;**58**:543–550.
3. Schneider JR, Helenowski IB, Jackson CR, et al. A comparison of results with eversion versus conventional carotid endarterectomy from the Vascular Quality Initiative and the Mid-America Vascular Study Group. *J Vasc Surg.* 2015;**61**:1216–1222.
4. Antonopoulos CN, Kakisis JD, Sergentanis TN, et al. Eversion versus conventional carotid endarterectomy: a meta-analysis of randomised and non-randomised studies. *Eur J Vasc Endovasc Surg.* 2011;**42**:751–765.
5. Black JH 3rd, Ricotta JJ, Jones CE. Long-term results of eversion carotid endarterectomy. *Ann Vasc Surg.* 2010;**24**:92–99.

23

Redo carotid endarterectomy

JEFFREY R. RUBIN

CONTENTS

INTRODUCTION

Carotid artery restenosis following both carotid endarterectomy (CEA) and stenting averages 4–10% nationally (ranging from 1 to 20%).[1–3] Restenosis poses a clinical dilemma for many physicians since they face several options: (1) redo endarterectomy; (2) carotid artery stenting; or (3) balloon angioplasty. There is currently no consensus as to what method of treatment provides the safest and best outcomes for treating recurrent carotid artery disease. This chapter summarizes the methods and results for performing redo CEA (RCEA) for restenosis following CEA.[4,5]

Very early on, recurrent carotid stenosis (RCS) is usually due to technical problems with the initial repair. Restenosis that develops within the first 24 months is most likely due to intimal hyperplasia. After 24 months, RCS is usually due to recurrent atherosclerosis. Restenosis may be asymptomatic or symptomatic. When patients are referred for RCS requiring intervention, it is the responsibility of the surgeon to determine the best treatment modality. Factors that enter the equation include: plaque morphology; anticipated neck "hostility;" level of the recurrent lesion; and the patient's overall health and anticipated life expectancy. Finally, the open and endovascular operative skill sets of the treating surgeon need to be weighed when determining the best approach. The author does not have adequate information from his own experience to determine whether stenting is appropriate for the treatment of RCS. However, the good long-term results for RCEA have led him to recommend this treatment for most of his patients.[6]

PREOPERATIVE EVALUATION

Indications for RCEA are similar to those for initial CEA and include: asymptomatic severe carotid artery stenosis (>70%); asymptomatic or symptomatic stenosis with large or multiple plaque ulcerations; symptomatic carotid stenosis >60%; crescendo transient ischemic attacks (TIAs) or stroke in evolution with high-grade carotid stenosis; >50% ipsilateral carotid artery stenosis associated with a contralateral occlusion.

Duplex scanning by an Intersocietal Accreditation Commission-approved vascular laboratory is the author's diagnostic modality of choice and is the only noninvasive test performed in most of his patients. The technician must pay attention to the level of the bifurcation, plaque morphology, and the presence of disease in the proximal common carotid artery (CCA). If duplex ultrasonography does not provide adequate information for operative planning, computed tomography angiography is also useful. Carotid angiography is rarely required.

PREPARATION

Indirect laryngoscopy should routinely be performed preoperatively to evaluate vocal fold function. This is especially important in patients who have had previous cranial nerve injury, preoperative neck radiation, previous neck surgery exclusive of CEA, and in patients with known head and neck cancers. Patients with a history of TIAs or stroke should undergo head CT scanning or magnetic resonance imaging to ascertain whether there is a pre-existing stroke, since this may affect the need for intraoperative shunting.

Patients should be well hydrated preoperatively. A minimal hemoglobin in the 8.0–8.5 g/dL range is desirable. Of critical importance is the patient's blood pressure (BP), which should be maintained at baseline or slightly higher perioperatively. If the patient is significantly hypertensive before the operation and emergent surgery is not required, the author prefers outpatient BP stabilization before intervention. It is not appropriate to aggressively reduce BP immediately before the operation, intraoperatively, or postoperatively. However, BP control is of paramount importance during the operation and wide fluctuations are to be avoided. The anesthesia team should have vasopressors and antihypertensive agents ready to be infused if there are issues. They should also have atropine available in case carotid bulb manipulation results in bradycardia and subsequent hypotension. The author prefers to inject the carotid sinus (Hering's nerve) at the carotid bulb with lidocaine 1% if problems arise during dissection in this area. The type of anesthesia used for RCEA depends on the comfort level of the patient, surgeon, and anesthesiologist; however, because RCEAs take longer than de novo CEAs, general anesthesia is generally preferred. For the same reason, a Foley catheter is inserted at the beginning of all cases.

PROCEDURE

Following intubation, the patient is positioned with a scapula roll and extension and rotation of the head to the side opposite the operative site. Excessive cervical spine extension and rotation should be avoided to prevent possible kinking of the vertebral arteries and muscle strain. The table is generally placed in a relaxed, semi-Fowler's position with slight head elevation. The author recommends prepping one of the groins and thighs for saphenous vein or superficial femoral artery (SFA) harvesting in cases where interposition grafting is anticipated.

The author prefers an oblique incision, anterior to the sternocleidomastoid muscle. Pre-existing transverse incisions are modified to gain more distal exposure; otherwise, the previous neck incision is reopened in its entirety. Dissection is deliberate if not tedious. Knowledge of normal anatomy and common variants is essential. Exposure of the internal carotid artery (ICA), external carotid artery (ECA) and CCA is usually begun either as far distal or as far proximal as possible, attempting to find an arterial segment that has not been previously dissected. The author avoids dissection around the area of recurrent disease (usually the carotid bulb) and obtains proximal and distal control at this time. Excessive "Weitlaner" retraction can cause a traction injury to the vagus nerve and should be avoided. Dissection should be carried out directly on the anterior surfaces of the arteries to avoid nerve injury. The vagus nerve and jugular vein are carefully dissected free from the carotid artery to avoid clamp and

retractor injury. Distal dissection of the ICA needs to proceed cautiously. The hypoglossal nerve is frequently indistinguishable from surrounding scar tissue crossing the ICA. Dissection in unusual planes and increased retraction for "better exposure" may result in nerve trauma. Vagal, superior laryngeal, glossopharyngeal, recurrent laryngeal, and other nerve injuries are more common following RCEA than primary CEA and are to be avoided.

Distal control of the ICA should be obtained above the previous endarterectomy site. It is not unusual to need to divide the digastric muscle, which is best accomplished with a right angle clamp and electrocautery. Dissection along the lateral aspect of the hypoglossal nerve may provide additional mobility and allow for gentle vessel loop retraction of the nerve. Strong retraction on the mandible is occasionally necessary and can result in a marginal mandibular nerve injury. Fortunately, this usually resolves within 6 months, but it is bothersome during recovery and quite often may be confused with an ischemic cerebral injury by ancillary staff. Removing the styloid process with a rongeur helps gain additional exposure of the distal ICA. If preoperative assessment suggests that distal exposure will be problematic, nasotracheal intubation should be used. Consultation with otolaryngology or oral and maxillofacial surgery personnel preoperatively, for mandibular subluxation, should also be considered.

Systemic heparinization takes place after all the arteries are controlled and dissection is completed. The author gives a bolus of unfractionated heparin sulfate (100 IU/kg) and redoses as necessary, routinely checking the activated clotting time after heparinization and every hour thereafter. In cases of known heparin sensitivity argatroban is used. The author also administers low-molecular-weight dextran 40 via a 50-mL intravenous bolus followed by a maintenance drip at 10 mL/hour overnight, or until the patient can receive oral medications.

After clamping the ICA, CCA, and ECA, an arteriotomy is made in the CCA and continued distally and proximally to a point above and below the recurrent disease. Shunting is at the surgeon's discretion. The author selectively shunts patients with: (1) previous ipsilateral stroke; (2) contralateral carotid artery occlusion; (3) carotid stump pressures <50 mmHg; and (4) crescendo TIAs or a stroke in evolution. Other methods for determining whether a shunt is required include electroencephalographic and transcranial Doppler monitoring. If regional anesthesia is used, communication with the patient during clamping determines the adequacy of cerebral perfusion. The author uses Sundt™ Carotid Endarterectomy Shunts (Integra LifeSciences Corporation, Plainsboro, NJ, USA) and prefers clamps to hold them in place proximally and distally; Rummel tourniquets can also be used. The shunt is inserted distally first, de-aired, and then placed proximally and secured. The surgeon needs to be aware of possible proximal CCA disease when inserting the shunt proximally to avoid embolization of atherosclerotic debris.

RCS may be hyperplastic, atherosclerotic, or most frequently a combination of the two. The author generally prefers "re-endarterectomy" and patching if technically possible. Occasionally, the author encounters a purely hyperplastic lesion that may be amenable to patch angioplasty alone. Otherwise, the author attempts to remove the recurrent lesion, which is frequently quite tedious and without an easy end point, in contrast to primary CEA. However, deep endarterectomy through both layers of media is to be avoided because the author feels this creates a very thrombogenic flow surface and weakens the arterial wall, making it susceptible to aneurysm formation. If prior patching with non-autogenous material was used, the author recommends excision of the entire patch including all old suture material.

The author does not routinely tack distal end points and "chases" plaque distally. The use of a Beaver® blade (Beaver-Visitec International, Inc., Waltham, MA, USA) is at times very helpful to establish a good distal end point. However, if there is any concern, the author recommends a running tacking suture between the intima and the endarterectomized arterial wall. Either a Gore-Tex® CV-8 (W. L. Gore & Associates, Inc., Flagstaff, AZ, USA) or an 8-0 polypropylene are the author's sutures of choice. A running suture eliminates scalloping of the transition area. Finally, when faced with loss of integrity of the arterial wall, interposition bypass grafting may be necessary; the author prefers autogenous grafts (saphenous vein or SFA) over prosthetic grafts. When SFA harvest is performed, it must be replaced with a polytetrafluoroethylene (PTFE) graft to avoid leg ischemia. If the SFA is occluded, no bypass is required; an eversion endarterectomy of the occluded SFA segment is performed before sewing it into place as a carotid interposition graft.

The author routinely patches all carotid artery closures unless the arteries are of extremely generous size where patching would result in a patulous artery. Patch selection is up to the individual surgeon, with no study demonstrating superiority of one material over another. Bovine pericardium, PTFE, Dacron, and vein are all acceptable materials. However, ankle saphenous vein should be avoided based on a Cleveland Clinic study that noted an increased rupture rate when using veins from this location.[7] The author routinely uses a Hemashield® "Dacron" patch (MAQUET Ltd., Sunderland, UK). The patch width should be tailored individually to prevent arterial narrowing while not making the artery diameter too large. The latter may result in mural thrombus formation in the patched area or low sheer stress predisposing to restenosis.

The author routinely performs completion angiography following all carotid operations. An 18-G angiocatheter is inserted through the ECA, aimed proximally, and contrast is gently injected under direct fluoroscopy. The author visualizes the entire operative site including portions of the intracranial circulation. More than one view may be required. The author does not hesitate to reexplore the operative site if there is a problem on the arteriogram. Intraoperative completion duplex scanning may also be performed if the clinician is more comfortable with this

modality, though duplex scanning cannot evaluate the intracranial circulation.

The author routinely drains the wound with a 10-mm, fully perforated, flat, Jackson–Pratt drain placed through a separate stab incision and connected to a standard bulb suction. Drains are generally removed the morning after surgery. Drains do not prevent neck hematomas nor do they decrease return rates to the operating room for bleeding. However, the author subjectively feels that neck edema is decreased when drains are used.

POSTOPERATIVE COMPLICATIONS

Complications following RCEA are similar to those following primary CEA. The only difference is an increased incidence of cranial nerve injuries in redo operations. Based on the author's review of 219 RCEAs, 25 (13%) patients experienced nerve injuries of which 4 had prolonged recovery and 1 had a permanent injury. This is significant when compared to a nerve injury rate of 4% (44/1105) following primary CEA.[5] Operative mortality and neurologic morbidity were similar in both cohorts.

Carotid duplex scans are obtained within 1 month postoperatively, at 6 months, 12 months, and then yearly. Restenosis (>60%) occurred in three patients (1.5%) over an average 2.1 years in the author's redo group compared to 0.4% (4/1105) over an average of 4.4 years in the author's primary CEA group.

CASE EXAMPLE

A 63-year-old asymptomatic man with a history of bilateral CEAs was referred after an ultrasound (US) demonstrated left RCS in the 80–99% range. His first CEA was in 2002 and he was unaware of any problems with the artery until his US in 2009. The patient underwent a RCEA in February 2009 where the patch was completely removed and redo endarterectomy was performed removing diffuse, irregular plaque in the area of the patch. Postoperative scanning revealed a well-healed endarterectomy site without evidence of stenosis. Seven years later, the patient re-presented with left hemispheric TIAs and was found to have a new recurrence in the 80–99% range. Risk factors included insulin-dependent diabetes mellitus and cigarette smoking. During repeat surgery, the carotid bifurcation was carefully dissected free from surrounding scar (**Figure 23.1**). On opening the artery, severe, diffuse plaque throughout the patch site with an area of "coral reef" plaque in the common carotid proximal to the patch was found (**Figure 23.2**). Re-endarterectomy with patching was performed and completion arteriography revealed a nice technical result (**Figure 23.3**). The patient went home within 24 hours. Postoperative scanning did not reveal new problems <6 months on. He has been maintained on a statin, aspirin, and clopidogrel combination regimen, and has stopped smoking.

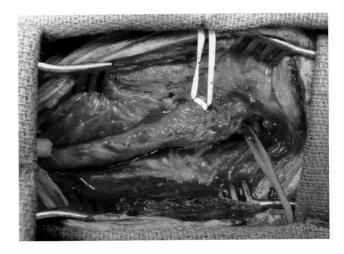

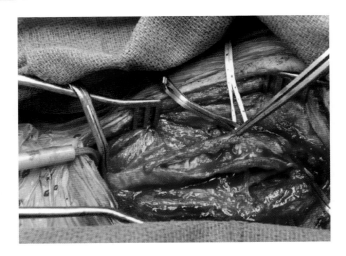

Figure 23.1 Photograph of carotid artery bifurcation at completion of dissection for a redo procedure in 63-year-old asymptomatic man with a history of bilateral carotid endarterectomy (case example). When the artery was opened, severe and diffuse plaque throughout the patch site was found, with an area of "coral reef" plaque in the common carotid artery (CCA) proximal to the patch. The CCA is to the left and the internal (ICA) and external (ECA) carotid arteries are to the right. White tape encircles the ECA while pink tape encircles the ICA.

Figure 23.2 Re-endarterectomy and patching of the 63-year-old patient. Operative photograph showing recurrent carotid stenosis after opening the artery. Orientation is the same as in **Figure 23.1**.

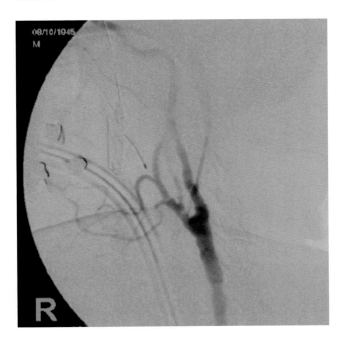

Figure 23.3 Completion angiogram of the same patient following redo endarterectomy and patching. Postoperative scanning has not revealed new problems <6 months on.

REFERENCES

1. Hertzer NR, Martinez BD, Benjamin SP, et al. Recurrent stenosis after carotid endarterectomy. *Surg Gynecol Obstet.* 1979;**149**:360–364.
2. Moore WS, Kempczinski RF, Nelson JJ, et al. Recurrent carotid stenosis: results of the asymptomatic carotid atherosclerosis study. *Stroke.* 1998;**29**:2018–2025.
3. Lal BK, Hobson RW 2nd, Goldstein J, et al. In-stent recurrent stenosis after carotid artery stenting: life table analysis and clinical relevance. *J Vasc Surg.* 2003;**38**:1162–1168.
4. Attigah N, Külkens S, Deyle C, et al. Redo surgery or carotid stenting for restenosis after carotid endarterectomy: results of two different treatment strategies. *Ann Vasc Surg.* 2010;**24**:190–195.
5. Akingba AG, Bojalian M, Shen C, et al. Managing recurrent carotid artery disease with redo carotid endarterectomy: a 10-year retrospective case series. *Ann Vasc Surg.* 2014;**28**:908–916.
6. de Borst GJ, Zanen P, de Vries JP, et al. Durability of surgery for restenosis after carotid endarterectomy. *J Vasc Surg.* 2008;**47**:363–371.
7. O'Hara PJ, Hertzer NR, Krajewski LP, et al. Saphenous vein patch rupture after carotid endarterectomy. *J Vasc Surg.* 1992;**15**:504–509.

24

Carotid interposition grafting

SACHINDER SINGH HANS AND MARIKA GASSNER

CONTENTS

INTRODUCTION

Compared to carotid endarterectomy (CEA), carotid interposition grafting (CIG) is infrequently performed. Main indications for CIG include: (1) failed endovascular therapy for restenosis following carotid artery stenting (CAS); (2) locally advanced head and neck cancer involving the carotid artery; (3) infected patch graft following CEA; (4) malignant carotid body tumor; (5) resection of a large extracranial carotid aneurysm; and (6) carotid artery trauma when local repair is not feasible.

For in-stent stenosis, repeat endovascular therapy or CEA should be the first option.[1] The patient who fails CAS because of heavy calcific burden at the carotid bifurcation, recurrent in-stent stenosis, or structural failure of the stent may need removal of the stent and CIG. Reconstruction with interposition greater saphenous vein graft or superficial femoral artery (SFA) can be used. The SFA as a conduit is evaluated by duplex scan and is often preferred in en bloc resection of head and neck malignancy invading the carotid artery.[2] In most patients undergoing CIG, an expanded polytetrafluoroethylene (PTFE) graft (tapered 7 × 5 mm) is preferred. Proximal anastomosis is usually end-to-end. However, if there is size discrepancy, end-to-side proximal anastomosis can be performed.[3] Distal anastomosis is usually performed end-to-end in this configuration.

Before selecting the operative technique, for in stent stenosis the stent must be imaged in situ. This can be best performed by computed tomography angiography (CTA). Duplex ultrasound can be used as a screening tool to follow the degree of in-stent stenosis, but it does not allow for adequate visualization of the extent of the stent and occlusive disease and their relation to bony structures. If the stent extends above the C2 vertebral body, additional maneuvers may be needed to facilitate distal control of the internal carotid artery (ICA) at the time of the surgical procedure (see Chapters 13 and 25).

OPERATIVE CONSIDERATIONS

This operation is preferably performed under general anesthesia (GA). It is important that any monitoring equipment does not obstruct potential fluoroscopic views of a stent and the ICA, should the stent extend higher than anticipated and intraoperative imaging is required. These operations frequently occur in the context of a previous CEA with subsequent stent placement, making the dissection tedious and higher-risk. One should be prepared to perform distal exposure of the ICA by dividing the occipital artery with cephalad mobilization or dividing the posterior belly of the digastric and stylohyoid muscles. An oblique skin incision extending from the base of the neck along the anterior border of the sternomastoid muscle to below and behind the ear lobe is necessary. With sharp dissection, mobilization is performed along the medial wall of the internal jugular vein and the common facial vein is ligated and divided. The carotid sheath is opened and silastic vessel loop are passed around the common carotid artery (CCA) just above the base of the neck, the origin of the external carotid (ECA) and superior thyroid (STA) arteries (**Figure 24.1**). Since the patient is under GA, electroencephalograph (EEG) monitoring and somatosensory evoked potential of the median nerve are performed

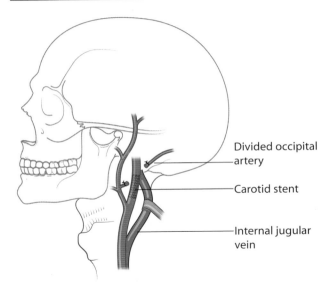

Figure 24.1 Anatomy overview with exposure of the neck and carotid stent.

after CCA clamping to determine the need for a shunt. Stump pressure (SP) is measured (see Chapter 21). In most patients, a shunt is not required unless there are ischemic changes in the EEG, significant decrease in somatosensory evoked potentials, or the SP is <40 mmHg.

INTERPOSITION GRAFT PLACEMENT WITHOUT SHUNT

If CTA imaging of the neck shows that the upper end of the stent is above the level of the middle of the C2 vertebral body, intraoperative balloon occlusion is helpful to control retrograde bleeding from the ICA. After systemic heparin administration (100 IU/kg), the CCA is punctured with a micropuncture needle. Using a microcatheter, a 7-Fr sheath is inserted into the CCA just above the base of the neck. A 0.014-mm guidewire (ChoICE™ PT, Boston Scientific Corporation, Marlborough, MA, USA) is advanced into the ICA near the base of the skull and an over-the-wire 3-Fr Fogarty catheter is placed. A 50% diluted contrast medium is used to inflate the balloon and allow fluoroscopic visualization of balloon placement (**Figure 24.2**).

If the upper end of the stent is at the lower portion of the C2 vertebral body or below, balloon occlusion of the distal ICA is not necessary. Distal clamping of the ICA can be performed by careful mobilization. SP is recorded with a 21-G needle placed below the proximal end of the stent. The ICA is opened transversely with a No. 15 blade scalpel a few millimeters below the upper end of the stent, which is then separated from the distal ICA with caudal retraction. The origin of the ECA is divided and the distal end is suture-ligated with running polypropylene suture; the proximal end of the CCA is divided. In patients with distal balloon occlusion, after the ICA has been circumferentially divided, it is further mobilized distally. The balloon is

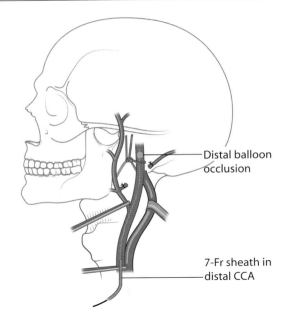

Figure 24.2 Balloon occlusion of the distal internal carotid artery.

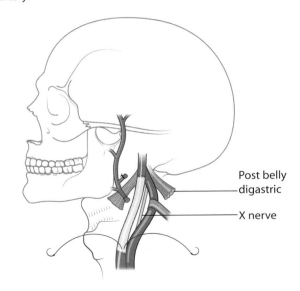

Figure 24.3 Interposition of common carotid-internal carotid artery graft.

deflated and removed, and an atraumatic vascular clamp or clip (Yasargil® aneurysm clip (Aesculap, Inc., Center Valley, PA, USA)) is applied. The specimen consisting of the distal CCA, proximal ICA, and stent is removed. A 5 × 7-mm tapered PTFE graft is selected (W. L. Gore & Associates, Inc., Flagstaff, AZ, USA) and distal anastomosis is performed with a 6-0 polypropylene suture. After completion of the distal anastomosis, blood is allowed to flow retrograde to remove any debris, the graft is flushed with heparin-saline solution, and the vascular clamp is moved just proximal to the distal anastomosis. Proximal anastomosis is performed with a 5-0 or 6-0 polypropylene suture (**Figure 24.3**). Appropriate antegrade and retrograde flushing and declamping is performed. The authors prefer PTFE as a graft conduit, although reversed great saphenous vein (GSV) harvested from the upper thigh or nonreversed GSV with valve lysis can be used as alternatives. Completion arteriogram is performed either with a 5-Fr sheath inserted into the CCA below the proximal anastomosis. Contrast with 50% dilution in amount of 5–7cc is injected to obtain images of the neck and brain.

If the completion arteriogram does not show any abnormalities, the opening in the common carotid artery after removal of the sheath is closed with 6-0 cardiovascular polypropylene suture. Subcutaneous tissue including the platysma muscle is sutured with a 3-0 absorbable suture and the skin is approximated with 3-0 nylon interrupted sutures and staples.

SHUNT PLACEMENT

If the EEG and somatosensory median nerve evoked potentials indicated cerebral ischemia, or the SP is <40 mmHg, an indwelling shunt is required. The distal end of the shunt is first advanced into the divided ICA; after back-bleeding fills the shunt, the proximal end of the shunt is inserted into the CCA. The interposition graft is then passed over another shunt (second shunt). The first shunt is removed and the second shunt with the interposition graft around it is inserted (**Figure 24.4**). Distal end-to-end anastomosis is performed first followed by proximal anastomosis to the divided CCA. Before proximal anastomosis is completed, the shunt is removed and suturing is completed.

COMPLICATIONS

Most complications after carotid interposition graft are like those after CEA (see Chapters 21–23). However, there

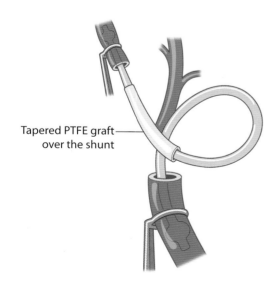

Tapered PTFE graft over the shunt

Figure 24.4 Polytetrafluoroethylene graft passed over the shunt with insertion of the distal and proximal ends of the shunt.

is a higher incidence of cranial nerve injury because of the more extensive higher dissection, especially the superior laryngeal and glossopharyngeal nerves.

CASE EXAMPLE

A 71-year-old woman underwent staged bilateral carotid stenting for high-grade, asymptomatic, bilateral ICA stenosis. Comorbidities included diabetes mellitus, diabetic neuropathy, retinopathy, hyperlipidemia, hypothyroidism, and significant coronary artery disease with previous coronary artery stenting. Review of records from an outside hospital showed that following pre-dilation, a 7 × 10-mm ACCULINK™ self-expanding carotid stent (Abbott Vascular, Abbott Park, IL, USA) was deployed and post-stent angioplasty was performed. A cerebral protection device (Emboshield® NAV⁶ Embolic Protection System, Abbott Vascular) was used. There was a 10% residual stenosis at the time of carotid stent placement. Six months later, recurrent asymptomatic carotid stenosis was detected on carotid duplex study with an ICA peak systolic velocity of 345 cm/second, end diastolic velocity of 126 cm/second, and CCA peak systolic velocity of 345 cm/second. CTA showed >80% bilateral ICA stenosis with surrounding heavy calcification (**Figure 24.5**). Because the upper end of the right carotid stent extended to the level of the C1-C2 intervertebral body, a distal balloon occlusion at the level of the base of the skull using a 0.014-mm guidewire with a 3-Fr Fogarty over-the-wire balloon catheter was inflated for distal control (**Figure 24.6**). The patient underwent CCA-ICA interposition graft placement with a

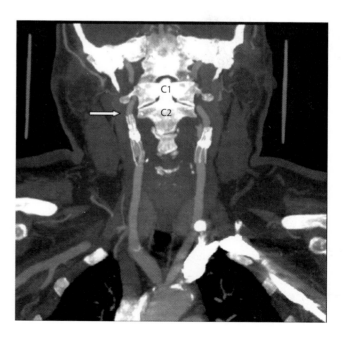

Figure 24.5 Computed tomography angiography demonstrating right carotid stent extending to the level of the C1-C2 disk (arrow).

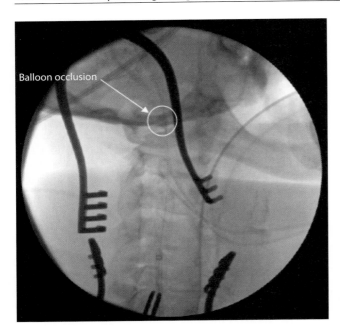

Balloon occlusion

Figure 24.6 Intraoperative imaging of distal balloon occlusion into the internal carotid artery at the base of the skull.

tapered 7 × 5-mm PTFE graft (W. L. Gore Associates, Inc.) under EEG and SP monitoring.

Postoperatively, the patient had no neurologic deficits. Follow-up duplex imaging at 6 months showed a peak systolic velocity of the ICA of 61 cm/second and CCA of 33 cm/second. She underwent an identical procedure on the left side 9 months later. The patient did not require distal balloon occlusion on the left side because the upper end of the stent was at the junction of the C2 and C3 vertebral bodies. The patient has done well for the past 18 months, with no evidence of recurrent stenosis.

REFERENCES

1. Gonzalez A, Drummond M, McCord S, et al. Carotid endarterectomy for treatment of in-stent restenosis. *J Vasc Surg.* 2011;**54**:1167–1169.
2. Jacobs JR, Korkmaz H, Marks HC, et al. One stage carotid artery resection: reconstruction in radiated head and neck carcinoma. *Am J Otolaryngol.* 2001;**22**,167–171.
3. Berguer R. *Function and Surgery of the Carotid and Vertebral Arteries.* Philadelphia, PA: Lippincott Williams & Wilkins Health; 2014. p. 109.

25

Carotid endarterectomy for high plaque

SACHINDER SINGH HANS

CONTENTS

INTRODUCTION

Carotid endarterectomy (CEA) for high plaque within the cervical internal carotid artery (ICA) that extends toward the base of the skull can be an extremely challenging operation for a vascular surgeon. In most patients, high plaque can be anticipated by imaging studies (carotid duplex exam, CT angiography (CTA) or conventional digital subtraction angiography, and carotid/cerebral arteriography). However, in some patients, distally extending plaque is an unexpected finding at the time of CEA. High plaque is defined as plaque within the ICA that extends up to or cephalad to the inferior border of the C2 vertebral body. Difficulty with CEA for high plaque is exacerbated in patients who have short necks or high carotid bifurcations. Exposure of the ICA in patients with high plaque is conceptualized by dividing the ICA in the neck into three zones, with carotid bifurcation being at the level of the disc space between the C3 and C4 vertebral bodies (**Figure 25.1**) in most patients. To surgically expose the ICA in the neck, the artery can be divided into three zones based on their relationship to the plane of the cervical vertebral bodies:[1]

- Zone 1 is where most plaques terminate; it corresponds to the upper end of the C3 vertebral body or the disc space between the C2 and C3 vertebral bodies.
- Zone 2 is plaque extending to the level of the C2 vertebral body (high plaque), but below the level of the C1 vertebral body.
- Zone 3 is plaque extending above the level of the C2 vertebral body. This is extremely uncommon.

In patients with plaque extending up to and distal to zone 2, carotid artery stenting (CAS) should be considered as an alternative option. However, in patients who are not good candidates for CAS, such as those with heavily calcified plaque, CEA performed with some modifications in the technique and exposure often remains a valuable treatment option. (The standard technique for CEA has been described in Chapter 21.)

SPECIAL OPERATIVE CONSIDERATIONS IN PATIENTS UNDERGOING CEA FOR HIGH PLAQUE

Additional exposure of the distal portion of the cervical ICA may be obtained by extending the skin incision cephalad and posteriorly behind the ear. Additional aids in exposure include removal of the carotid sinus nerve branches at the carotid bifurcation and placing a double vessel loop around the external carotid artery with which caudal traction may be applied. This can be held in place by clamping the vessel loop to the drape with a small mosquito clamp. As the dissection proceeds toward the base of the skull, the sternocleidomastoid branch of the occipital artery and the veins crossing the hypoglossal nerve are carefully ligated and divided. In some patients, the occipital artery may need to be divided. This helps in cephalad mobilization of the hypoglossal nerve, which can be looped carefully with a silastic loop. The posterior belly of the digastric muscle should be mobilized; if necessary, it can be divided. Similarly, the stylohyoid muscle may also be transected.

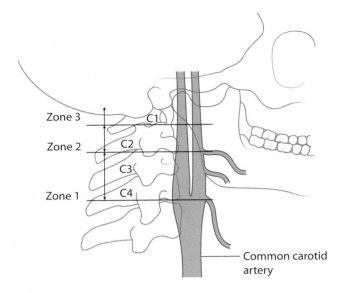

Figure 25.1 Carotid artery bifurcation with three zones corresponding to the extension of the upper end of the plaque. Zone 1 shows the upper end of the plaque below the C3 vertebral body.

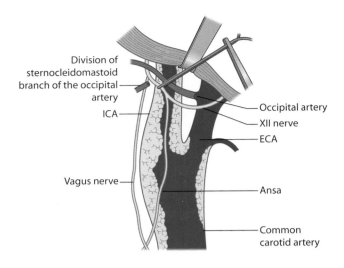

Figure 25.2 Exposure of common carotid artery and distal internal carotid artery for high plaque with upward retraction of the posterior belly of the digastric muscle and silastic loop around the hypoglossal nerve. Zone 2 shows the upper end of the plaque below the C2 vertebral body. Zone 3 shows the upper end of the plaque above the C2 vertebral body.

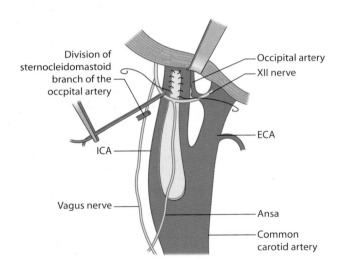

Figure 25.3 Upper end of the patch being sutured to the internal carotid artery above the hypoglossal nerve.

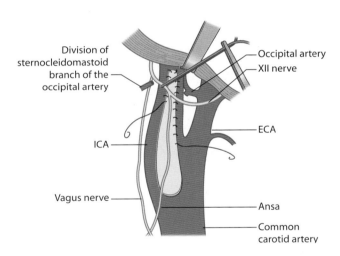

Figure 25.4 Exposure of the common carotid artery and distal internal carotid artery for high plaque with upward retraction of the posterior belly of the digastric muscle. The patch is being sutured below the hypoglossal nerve, which is retracted upward.

If further exposure is required, the styloid process can be carefully removed with a rongeur. In this maneuver, care should be taken to prevent injury to the glossopharyngeal nerve. In most instances, distal control can be obtained with a balloon occlusion catheter or 4 or 4.5-mm Pilling dilator. After removal of the plaque with an arterial dissector, patch grafting is started at the distal apex of the arteriotomy. Suturing is continued caudally on the artery; when the hypoglossal nerve is encountered, the patch and suture are passed under the nerve and suturing is completed in the standard fashion (**Figures 25.2–25.4**). When a perfectly feathered distal breakoff point of the plaque cannot be obtained, tacking stitches should be placed to prevent dissection of the distal artery. This can be accomplished with 7-0 polypropylene U-shaped stitches. The U-shaped stitches are placed parallel to the flow of blood in the artery, with one side of the stitch about 2 mm distal to the end point of the endarterectomy and one side 2 mm proximal to the end point. Stitches are placed across the back wall of the artery. The artery is then flushed with saline to ensure that the endarterectomy end point does not lift.

In rare instances, the ICA may have to be divided at its origin, the artery transposed anteriorly to the hypoglossal nerve, and the origin of the ICA carefully sutured to the transposed artery. This technique is preferred during eversion CEA if the end point of the plaque is higher than usual.[2] However, if the upper end of the plaque extends above the level of the C2 vertebral body (zone 3), mandibular subluxation carried out by an oral/maxillofacial surgeon with nasotracheal intubation should be considered. In rare instances, mandibular osteotomy or resection of the tip of the mastoid process are alternative choices to mandibular subluxation.[3]

In rare cases, the upper end of the posterior tongue of the plaque may reach at the junction of the C1 and C2 vertebral bodies (at the junction of zones 2 and 3). If the operating surgeon is not certain about the end point of the CEA, intraoperative carotid stenting should be considered.[4] Cephalad extension of the plaque into the upper end of zone 2 or the beginning of zone 3 may not have been anticipated preoperatively because many plaques at the upper end are thin and feathery. Intraoperative carotid stenting is performed by extending the lower end of the incision toward the base of the neck, dividing the inferior belly of the omohyoid muscle and the loop of the ansa cervicalis. Micropuncture of the common carotid artery (CCA) just above the base of the neck is performed and a 7-Fr sheath is inserted. Before that, arteriotomy incision with patch grafting has already been performed. A carotid/cerebral arteriogram is performed on the operating table by injecting 8–10 cc of diluted contrast through the 7-Fr sheath. Using a 0.014-mm guidewire (ChoICE™ PT, Boston Scientific Corporation, Marlborough, MA, USA) and advancing it under fluoroscopy into the intracranial portion of the ICA, a 6 × 4-cm long, self-expanding PRECISE PRO RX® Nitinol Stent System (Cordis Corporation, Baar, Switzerland) is deployed; postdeployment angioplasty is performed with a 5-mm angioplasty catheter at the upper end and a 6-mm balloon angioplasty catheter at the lower end of the stent.

SHUNT PLACEMENT

In most patients undergoing CEA (approximately 90%), intraoperative shunt placement is not necessary and may be quite cumbersome in patients with high plaque. When a shunt is required in patients with high plaque, one that uses balloon occlusion, such as the Pruitt-Inahara® Carotid Shunt (Lemaitre Vascular, Inc., Burlington, MA, USA), may be easier to successfully place than a carotid shunt requiring shunt clamps. Such a shunt is also useful for distal arterial control with balloon occlusion.

The author uses continuous neurologic assessment under cervical block anesthesia (usually not possible in patients with high plaque), stump pressure (SP) measurement, and electroencephalogram (EEG) monitoring in patients under general anesthesia. The author uses an SP cutoff at 40 mmHg and ischemic EEG changes in the brain as guides to shunt use.

COMPLICATIONS

Perioperative stroke, cranial nerve injury, neck hematoma, and myocardial infarction can occur after CEA for high plaque because these complications occur after CEA with plaque ending in zone 1. During exposure of the distal ICA, injury to the hypoglossal nerve, and the pharyngeal branch of the vagus and glossopharyngeal nerves may occur. These nerve injuries can cause tongue weakness and swallowing difficulty. More commonly, hypoglossal injury is transient. Glossopharyngeal nerve injury may necessitate placement of a percutaneous endoscopic gastrostomy tube.

CASE EXAMPLES

Case example 1

During performance of CEA in this patient, the posterior plaque was unexpectedly found to be extending into zone 2. CEA with patch grafting was performed. Completion arteriogram showed significant narrowing at the upper end of the arteriotomy. Through a 7-Fr sheath placed in the lower portion of the CCA (just above the base of the neck), intraoperative stent placement was performed with satisfactory results (**Figures 25.5 and 25.6**). This case illustrates a "bailout" procedure in patients where termination of the upper end of the plaque cannot be entirely satisfactory. Intraoperative stenting is necessary in only a few circumstances.

Case example 2

A 69-year-old man presented with high-grade stenosis of the right ICA with a history of amaurosis fugax (painless temporary loss of vision). The patient underwent CTA as well as carotid and cerebral arteriography and was found to have plaque extending to the junction of zones 2 and 3 (C1-C2 vertebral body junction) (**Figures 25.7 and 25.8**). In this patient, mandibular subluxation (**Figure 25.9**) was performed and CEA was carried out in the usual fashion with patch grafting. Because of the heavy calcification in the lesion, the patient was not a suitable candidate for CAS. With the help of unilateral subluxation of the mandible, an additional 1 cm of exposure near the base of the skull was obtained resulting in a satisfactory end point of the endarterectomy.

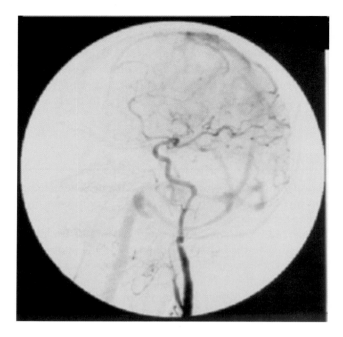

Figure 25.5 Completion arteriogram showing stenosis at the upper end of the endarterectomy site.

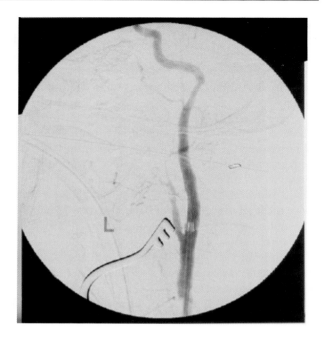

Figure 25.6 Intraoperative carotid stent placement through a 7-Fr sheath.

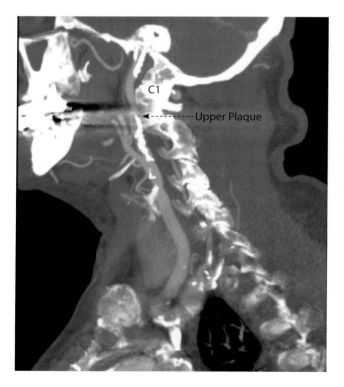

Figure 25.7 Upper end of the plaque at the C1-C2 vertebral body junction.

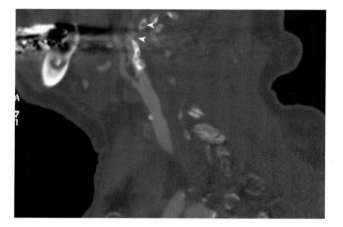

Figure 25.8 Upper end of the plaque at the C1-C2 vertebral body junction.

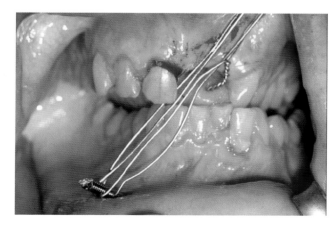

Figure 25.9 Intraoral wiring for subluxation of mandible.

REFERENCES

1. Hans SS, Shah S, Hans BA. Carotid endarterectomy for high plaques. *Am J Surg.* 1989;**157**:431–434.
2. Berguer R. Operations on the internal carotid artery. In: *Function and Surgery of the Carotid and Vertebral Arteries.* Philadelphia, PA: Lippincott, Williams & Wilkins; 2014. pp. 90–119.
3. Dossa C, Shepard AD, Wolford DG, et al. Distal internal carotid exposure: a simplified technique for temporary mandibular subluxation. *J Vasc Surg.* 1990;**12**:319–325.
4. Ross CB, Ranval TJ. Intraoperative use of stents for the management of unacceptable distal internal carotid artery end points during carotid endarterectomy: short-term and midterm results. *J Vasc Surg.* 2000;**32**:420–427.

26

Extracranial carotid aneurysm resection

SUNITA D. SRIVASTAVA

CONTENTS

INTRODUCTION

Surgical treatment for extracranial carotid aneurysm was first described by Sir Astley Cooper.[1] The first successful repair by common carotid artery (CCA) ligation proximal to a large pulsatile internal carotid aneurysm took place in a hypertensive patient whose course was complicated by wound infection.[1] However, this surgical technique had not been successful 2 years previously in another patient with a carotid aneurysm. Fortunately, sufficient posterior collaterals supplied the anterior circulation in the successful case and the patient lived for 14 years after the ligation procedure.

In 1926, Dr. Nathan Winslow and colleagues reviewed the early reported cases of carotid aneurysm and found that of the 124 patients treated, 82 were treated with carotid ligation, and operative mortality was 28%.[2] The untreated patient population had a mortality rate of 71%, which led to the recognition of the importance of prompt diagnosis and treatment. These patients often presented with erosion of the vessel wall to adjacent structures and their presentation mimicked ear or tonsillar infections.[3-9]

The current standard techniques of vein grafting and direct arterial repair became the optimal strategy in the 1970s, with several authors reporting technical success and low mortality.[3-9] Although less common than carotid endarterectomy (CEA), surgery for carotid aneurysms is a necessary tool to prevent complications such as thrombosis, embolization, and rupture. This chapter describes the surgical techniques used to repair carotid aneurysms.

ETIOLOGY

The incidence of carotid aneurysm in the literature is low (0.1–3.7%).[3-9] Aneurysms are classified into two categories: true and false. Atherosclerotic disease of the carotid artery is the most common cause of extracranial carotid aneurysms. Other less common etiologies are connective tissue disorders, fibromuscular dysplasia, irradiation, arteritis, and cystic medial necrosis. True aneurysms can also be described as fusiform or saccular. Fusiform carotid aneurysms tend to be bilateral, degenerative, and located near the carotid bifurcation. Saccular aneurysms are typically unilateral and occur in the internal carotid artery (ICA). False aneurysms, which are described by a discontinuous and dilated segment of the arterial wall, can occur anywhere. The most common causes of disrupted vessel wall occur in the suture lines of patch angioplasty, infections of previously placed prosthetic patches, and atherosclerotic degeneration of the endarterectomized carotid artery. Other less common causes of carotid pseudoaneurysms include arterial dissection, and blunt and penetrating traumatic injuries.

CLINICAL PRESENTATION

Extracranial carotid aneurysms are not detected until symptoms occur. The most common presentation is neurologic, with a transient ischemic attack or stroke due to embolization. They may also present as a cervical mass and may be mistaken for an abscess, lymphadenopathy, or malignancy. Larger aneurysms can produce symptoms of compression of adjacent structures and cranial nerves. Dysphagia, occipital and retro-orbital pain, and headaches have been described. Nerve compression may result in pain, Horner syndrome, hoarseness, and nerve palsy. Middle-ear and tonsillar abscesses may indicate a mycotic aneurysm. Rupture of carotid aneurysms is rare, but bleeding and cervical hematoma may lead to tracheal compression and airway compromise.

DIAGNOSIS

Physical examination may demonstrate a pulsatile cervical mass. In cases of presumed infection, rapidly expanding neck masses may be tender, fluctuant, and erythematous and may result in an incorrect diagnosis of abscess. Carotid duplex, computed tomography, or magnetic resonance imaging may assist in the diagnosis. While duplex imaging is efficient and fast, the other two modalities may assist in viewing the extent of the aneurysm, its location with respect to bony structures, and in surgical planning. Angiography has also been used to detail carotid aneurysms. However, embolization of aneurysm contents with sequelae of neurologic events is a risk that may not justify the benefit of anatomical detail. Balloon occlusion testing has been touted as an option with angiography in cases of high lesions for surgical ligation and to assess cross-filling from the contralateral side. The presence of collateral circulation and the status of the contralateral carotid and bilateral vertebral arteries are critical when contemplating surgical options.

SURGICAL TREATMENT

The goal of surgical treatment is to remove the aneurysm and restore vessel continuity. Aneurysm resection can be challenging depending on size, inflammation, and location. In addition, the contents are vulnerable to embolization and must be removed completely. There are several operative techniques, all of which involve the standard oblique surgical incision and can extend from the sternal notch to the mastoid process. The internal jugular vein (IJV) and its branches are mobilized. Identification and protection of the vagus, hypoglossal, and glossopharyngeal nerves are necessary. Division of the posterior belly of the digastric muscle can assist in mobilization of the ICA near the skull base. The fragile branches of the IJV anterior to the ICA must be ligated for additional exposure. Other maneuvers to assist in dissection of the distal ICA include mandibular subluxation. Nasotracheal intubation is essential for this technique. Further exposure and control can be obtained by dividing the stylohyoid ligament and removing the styloid process. This higher mobilization requires dividing the styloglossus, stylopharyngeus, and stylohyoid muscles and avoiding injuring the glossopharyngeal nerve. Manipulation of the ICA at this level should be limited to prevent nerve injury.

Intraoperative shunting remains operator- and skill-dependent as in CEA. Intraluminal shunting can be difficult to secure and the risks of distal embolization and dissection should be considered. Other adjuncts, such as electroencephalography monitoring or transcranial duplex can be used. Anticoagulation with heparin to keep an activated clotting time >250 seconds is performed; continuation of an antiplatelet regimen before surgery is essential to prevent thrombosis. Dissection and mobilization of the carotid aneurysm are typically performed after vascular occlusion of the proximal and distal vessels to reduce the risk of intraoperative embolization of the aneurysmal contents.

Ligation of the carotid artery was described as the treatment option for carotid aneurysms in early reports, but in the current surgical era, it is considered a last resort because of the high stroke risk and mortality rate. In challenging cases where distal control cannot be obtained, stump pressures and test occlusion may assist in determining the safety of carotid ligation. Carotid reconstruction is always recommended when possible.

Small or focal aneurysms may be resected and direct end-to-end anastomosis may be performed in continuous or interrupted fashion with monofilament suture. Mobilization of the proximal and distal vessel to prevent tension on the anastomosis is necessary. Spatulating or beveling both ends of the vessel preserves luminal diameter and prevents constriction of the vessel at the suture line.

Aneurysmorrhaphy or resection of the aneurysmal wall with patch angioplasty using prosthetic or native autologous tissue is another option that may be feasible, especially in anatomically challenging areas or high lesions. Care must be taken to remove all debris and aneurysmal contents. In addition, removal of the redundant and thin-walled vessel permits patch angioplasty on the healthier portion of the vessel wall and prevents aneurysmal degeneration later. Some practitioners advocate avoiding extensive posterior wall resection because this may result in higher cranial nerve injury.

Interposition grafting with synthetic graft or vein graft has also been described.[3–9] Choice of conduit classically depends on vessel size and operative field. In mycotic aneurysms, autologous arterial or venous conduit are the preferred options. Considerations for choice of conduit include length of bypass, diameter match, and availability. While prosthetic interposition patency is marginally inferior to vein interposition, the ease and timeliness of this technique, particularly in a challenging or high-risk patient, may be justified. Grafts with graduated diameters may also be suitable when transitioning from a large CCA to a small ICA. The appropriate length of the interposition bypass is critical to avoiding kinking and redundancy, especially given the extensive mobility and confines of the neck. Vein bypasses are vulnerable to such factors and distend both in diameter and length after flow is established. Carefully considering these factors assists in ensuring the patency and durability of the interposition graft.

Postreconstruction considerations include the placement of external drains and intraoperative imaging. The use of these adjuncts is dependent on surgeon preference and the availability of imaging systems, such as duplex scan and portable C-arm, or fixed imaging for angiography within the surgical suite.

The most common postoperative complication of carotid aneurysm repair remains cranial nerve injury with reports ranging from 3 to 17%.[3-9] The postoperative stroke-free rate is favorable with 80–87% of patients remaining symptom-free. The stroke rate of untreated carotid aneurysms has been reported at >50%.[1,3,6-9]

ENDOVASCULAR TREATMENT

With the use of carotid stenting for atherosclerotic lesions and the development of novel embolization protection devices, endovascular therapy for extracranial carotid aneurysms is a feasible option. Placement of a covered stent graft may be particularly expeditious in treating bleeding, rupture, and high lesions. In addition, unfavorable open surgical factors, such as an irradiated neck, previous cervical surgery, or tracheostomy and physiologic high risk play a role in determining optimal treatment strategies.

Embolization with coils and thrombosis of the aneurysm sac have also been reported with mixed results. The risk of intracranial embolization of the agent or components of the aneurysm sac may outweigh the complications of open surgery, including nerve injury and physiologic stress.

CONCLUSIONS

Long-term results are not available for open surgical reconstruction or endovascular exclusion of extracranial carotid aneurysms. Because of the low stroke rate and definitive repair achieved by open surgery, this remains preferable to endoluminal therapy in most cases. Anatomic constraints, presence of infection, bleeding, or rupture in select patients may require an endovascular option for efficiency and to permit transition to open repair when the patient is stabilized.

CASE EXAMPLES

Case example 1

A 52-year-old woman with dysphagia and pulsatile mass in her left neck presented to our institution. No neurologic symptoms were present and family history was not available. She had no history of smoking or hypertension. A CT scan (**Figure 26.1**) demonstrated a left ICA saccular aneurysm. Intraoperative exposure of the left ICA saccular aneurysm with redundant internal carotid loop was performed (**Figure 26.2**). Primary resection of the aneurysm and end-to-end repair was carried out after

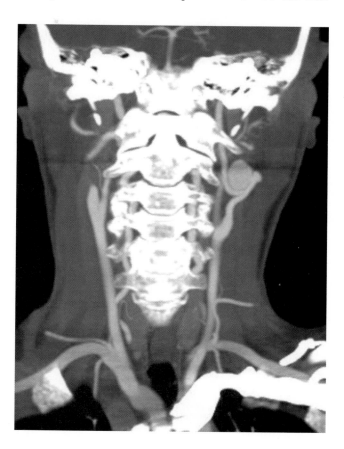

Figure 26.1 Computed tomography scan of 52-year-old woman demonstrating left internal carotid artery saccular aneurysm.

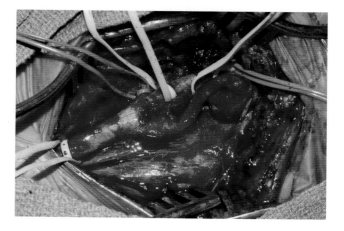

Figure 26.2 Intraoperative exposure of the left internal carotid artery (ICA) saccular aneurysm with redundant ICA loop.

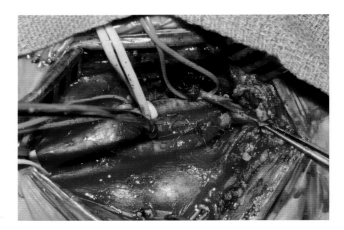

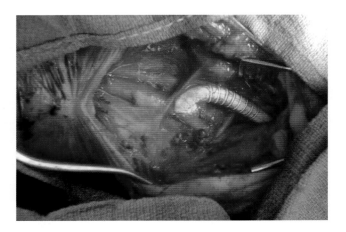

Figure 26.3 Primary resection of aneurysm and end-to-end repair after extensive mobilization. Interrupted repair with 6-0 monofilament suture.

Figure 26.5 Resection of carotid aneurysm with prosthetic common carotid artery to distal internal carotid artery interposition bypass.

extensive mobilization (**Figure 26.3**). Interrupted repair with 6-0 monofilament suture was chosen and performed.

Case example 2

A 31-year-old woman with Marfan syndrome presented with a symptomatic right carotid pseudoaneurysm (**Figure 26.4**). The carotid aneurysm was resected with a prosthetic CCA to distal ICA interposition bypass (**Figure 26.5**).

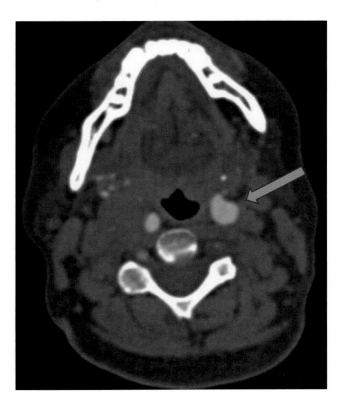

Figure 26.4 Computed tomography scan of 31-year-old woman with Marfan syndrome presenting with symptomatic right carotid artery pseudoaneurysm.

REFERENCES

1. Zwolak RM, Whitehouse WM Jr., Knake JE, et al. Atherosclerotic extracranial carotid artery aneurysms. *J Vasc Surg.* 1984;**1**:415–422.
2. Winslow N. Extracranial aneurysm of the internal carotid artery: history and analysis of the cases registered up to Aug. 1, 1925. *Arch Surg.* 1926;**13**:689–729.
3. Painter TA, Hertzer NR, Beven EG, et al. Extracranial carotid aneurysms: report of six cases and review of the literature. *J Vasc Surg.* 1985;**2**:312–318.
4. Moreau P, Albat B, Thévenet A. Surgical treatment of extracranial internal carotid artery aneurysm. *Ann Vasc Surg.* 1994;**8**:409–416.
5. El-Sabrout R, Cooley DA. Extracranial carotid artery aneurysms: Texas Heart Institute experience. *J Vasc Surg.* 2000;**31**:702–712.
6. Faggioli GL, Freyrie A, Stella A, et al. Extracranial internal carotid artery aneurysms: results of a surgical series with long term follow-up. *J Vasc Surg.* 1996;**23**:587–594.
7. Rosset E, Albertini JN, Magnan PE, et al. Surgical treatment of extracranial internal carotid artery aneurysms. *J Vasc Surg.* 2000;**31**:713–723.
8. Attigah N, Külkens S, Zausig N, et al. Surgical therapy of extracranial carotid artery aneurysms: long-term results over a 24-year period. *Eur J Vasc Endovasc Surg.* 2009;**37**:127–133.
9. Srivastava SD, Eagleton MJ, O'Hara P, et al. Surgical repair of carotid artery aneurysms: a 10-year, single-center experience. *Ann Vasc Surg.* 2010;**24**:100–105.

27

Resection of carotid body tumors

MITCHELL R. WEAVER AND DANIEL J. REDDY

CONTENTS

INTRODUCTION

Carotid body tumors (CBTs), also referred to as chemodectomas or carotid body paragangliomas, are the most common head and neck paragangliomas. These tumors arise from paraganglionic cells that migrate from the neural crest, near the sympathetic ganglia. Usually benign and indolent, they often go undetected until they are large enough to be visible or palpable. Less commonly, CBTs present with symptoms secondary to mass effect, such as cranial nerve dysfunction or dysphagia. In recent years, with the increased use of cross-sectional imaging, they are more commonly diagnosed as incidental findings. They are most prevalent in patients in their fourth to sixth decades of life, and are found in greater number in women than men.[1-3]

A common presentation is that of a painless, slow-growing, anterolateral neck mass that has been present from weeks to years. Because of tumor size, location, and pressure on neighboring structures, other symptoms may be reported, including: neck pain; dysphonia; dysphagia; hoarseness; stridor; jaw pain; sore throat; odynophagia; amaurosis fugax; facial droop; and Horner syndrome. Along with a CBT, initial differential diagnosis includes an enlarged lymph node, carotid artery aneurysm, branchial cleft cyst, and neurilemmoma.

Larger tumors, especially if >3 cm in size, are usually palpable on physical examination. They are identified as a neck mass anterior to the sternocleidomastoid muscle and overlying the carotid bifurcation. These tumors are usually nontender and often appear pulsatile because of proximity to the carotid artery. Typically, the tumor is mobile in a lateral or side-to-side fashion, but not in the vertical plane (Fontaine's sign).[2] A thorough examination of the oral and nasal pharynx should be performed. Cranial nerve examination with special attention to the function of the facial, glossopharyngeal, vagus, and hypoglossal nerves should be carefully documented.

Tumor biopsy to confirm the diagnosis is not recommended because of the significant vascularity of these tumors. CBTs rarely produce neuroendocrine secretions or catecholamine-related symptoms, thus routine screening of urine catecholamines is not indicated. However, such screening should be considered in the rare case that it is accompanied by paroxysmal hypertension, tachycardia, or palpitations. Likewise, metastatic disease is rare, but in those patients with additional systemic symptoms of weight loss and malaise, further workup should be considered.[2,3]

Though they are usually benign and indolent, once identified in acceptable-risk patients, tumor resection is indicated. If allowed to grow large enough to cause symptoms, such as a palpable mass or cranial nerve dysfunction, because of its significant vascularity and adherence to neurovascular structures, a CBT will present significantly greater technical challenges during surgical resection.

IMAGING AND PREOPERATIVE PLANNING

Several imaging studies are available to confirm the diagnosis and provide adequate information for surgical planning. These studies include color-flow duplex ultrasound, computed tomography (CT), magnetic resonance imaging (MRI), conventional catheter-directed angiography with digital subtraction imaging, and positron emission tomography. Spiral CT technology with multiplanar reformatting has become the authors' diagnostic test of choice.

The diagnostic finding is that of a vascular mass at the carotid bifurcation displacing the internal (ICA) and external carotid (ECA) arteries. Adequate preoperative imaging must define the extent of the tumor, the presence of any synchronous ipsilateral or contralateral tumors, and any associated carotid artery occlusive disease. This information allows the surgeon to plan the most appropriate surgical approach, being prepared for extended distal exposures and arterial reconstructions. In cases of bilateral disease, the surgeon can determine the appropriate order of staged resections.

Traditionally, catheter-directed angiography has been the gold standard for the diagnosis of CBTs. However, this invasive imaging study is not necessary in most cases. In certain situations, angiography may provide clearer information regarding the blood supply to the tumor that may be of value in planning resection; in the same setting, this modality also offers the opportunity for embolization of the tumor when felt appropriate with the hope of reducing perioperative blood loss.[4] In an effort to reduce intraoperative blood loss during the resection of these tumors, highly selective embolization of these tumors was introduced with reports of reduced blood loss; however, other series failed to demonstrate any significant benefit of this technique and questioned whether the benefits outweigh the risks, namely stroke or transient ischemic attack, and the additional cost of the procedure.[5,6] Consideration of performing preoperative embolization would typically be reserved for those tumors >5 cm that appear to pose a significant technical challenge. When embolization is performed, surgical resection is recommended within the next 24–48 hours to avoid a postembolization inflammatory response in the surrounding tissue. Tumors <5 cm likely do not benefit from preoperative embolization.

If the need for distal ICA exposure for tumors extending cranially is anticipated by preoperative imaging, nasal intubation and mandibular subluxation should be strongly considered. Mandibular subluxation is performed by the authors' ear, nose, and throat colleagues after induction of anesthesia, but before prepping and draping for tumor resection. The desired result is that the ramus of the mandible is displaced forward; with this altered position of the mandible, the normal narrow triangular field is converted to a rectangular field. This increased width provides additional distal ICA exposure. However, the local anatomy becomes slightly distorted with this positioning. The posterior belly of the digastric muscle and the hypoglossal nerve are displaced anteriorly and superiorly, and the carotid bifurcation and ICA and ECA are rotated medially.

Other preparations for operation include: the availability of autotransfusion for larger tumors; intraoperative cerebral monitoring with electroencephalography in cases that may require carotid artery clamping or reconstruction;

vein mapping and preparation of a saphenous vein harvest site; and use of bipolar cautery to avoid heat conduction injury to adjacent nerves.

SURGICAL MANAGEMENT

The procedure is performed under general anesthesia and once induced, if mandibular subluxation is planned, it is performed at this time. A roll is placed under the patient's shoulders and the neck is extended and rotated slightly to the contralateral side, before performing sterile prepping and draping of the skin. The authors' standard approach is through a longitudinal anterior sternocleidomastoid incision, like that for a carotid endarterectomy. Once the tumor is visualized, assessment of the carotid artery is performed and dissection is typically directed to achieve control of the common carotid artery (CCA) proximally and then the ECA and ICA distal to the tumor. The vagus nerve should be identified proximally along the CCA and followed distally. The vagus nerve and adjacent noninvolved cranial nerves are separated from the tumor and protected by dissecting through the tumor pseudocapsule. Distal exposure can be facilitated with standard techniques, such as division of the posterior belly of the digastric muscle, taking care not to injure the glossopharyngeal nerve that is then mobilized. Ligation and division of the occipital artery will assist with this. The next maneuver is division of the stylohyoid muscle groups. If further exposure is required, styloidectomy and mastoidectomy are described but carry with them an increased risk of morbidity with cranial nerve injury. During dissection of the ECA, one needs to be aware of the hypoglossal nerve anteriorly and the superior laryngeal nerve posteriorly. In exposing the ICA, one must be aware of several nerves, including the mandibular branch of the facial nerve, proximal hypoglossal nerve, distal vagus nerve, pharyngeal branch of the vagus nerve, spinal accessory nerve, and glossopharyngeal nerve.

Having completed proximal and distal exposure of the arterial structures, further intervention is based on the extent of the tumor as described by the Shamblin classification system.[7] This classifies tumors in relation to their involvement with the carotid artery and the subsequent difficulty in surgical resection. Group I tumors can be resected without significant trauma to the vessel wall or tumor capsule. Those in group II are more adherent to the adventitia and partially surround the artery, making their dissection more difficult, but can be excised without sacrificing the vessel. In group III, the artery is completely encased in the tumor and is best treated by resection of the involved artery with the tumor. Thus, for less advanced tumors, attempt is made to create a periadventitial dissection plane between the tumor and the artery (white line of Gordon-Taylor), and resect the tumor in a caudal-to-cranial fashion, leaving the artery intact. The typical blood supply originates from the ECA and these multiple feeding branches are sequentially ligated and divided. It is not unusual to also find branches originating from the ICA. For larger tumors, the ECA may be ligated and divided to assist with mobilization and resection. A minority of cases will require some type of arterial repair, such as lateral arteriorrhaphy, patch angioplasty, or bypass. In cases where the tumor completely encases the artery, the tumor and artery are resected en bloc, followed by arterial reconstruction, usually with the saphenous vein. When carotid artery clamping and reconstruction are required, the authors recommend monitored anticoagulation, along with selective shunting, depending on the intraoperative electroencephalography findings. Attempt should be made to remove the whole tumor, since incomplete excision is associated with a high likelihood of local recurrence.[5] If suspicious lymph nodes are encountered, biopsy should be performed; if nodal metastasis is present, a modified neck dissection should be performed. A closed suction drain is placed before closure and usually removed on postoperative day 1 or 2.

OUTCOMES

Most current series report mortality for surgical resection of CBTs at <3%; however, it has been reported as high as 8.8% in more complex resections requiring arterial reconstruction.[4,5,8,9] Postoperative cranial nerve dysfunction remains significant, with an incidence of up to 40%, and permanent cranial nerve injuries occur in about 20% of patients with a range from 8 to 39%.[2,4,9,10] Perioperative stroke occurs in 0–16% of patients.[1,4,11] Mortality and morbidity have been reported more frequently in cases of advanced tumors and those requiring arterial reconstruction. Complete resection of CBTs can be accomplished in most patients; those patients with complete resection can expect a survival rate like that of their peers. Recurrence is rare, but does occur, suggesting the need for continued surveillance.[1,3,4]

CASE EXAMPLES

Case example 1

A 32-year-old woman presented with a left neck mass she had had for over 1 year that was increasing in size but otherwise asymptomatic. Cross-sectional imaging with MRI (**Figure 27.1**) and catheter-based digital subtraction angiography (**Figure 27.2**) demonstrated a vascular mass at the carotid bifurcation displacing the ICA and ECA, consistent with a CBT. At the time of surgical resection, the tumor completely encased the ICA (Shamblin classification group III) (**Figures 27.3** and **27.4**). The tumor and involved ICA and ECA were excised en bloc. Arterial reconstruction was performed with a reversed great saphenous vein from the CCA to the ICA (**Figure 27.5**). The patient recovered uneventfully.

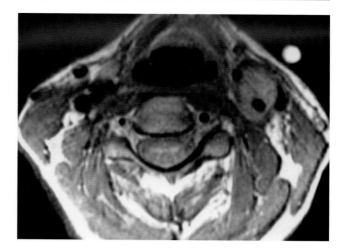

Figure 27.1 Magnetic resonance imaging of a 32-year-old woman revealed a left carotid body tumor. The external marker overlies the mass.

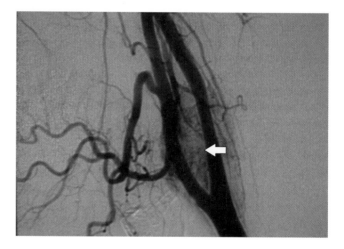

Figure 27.2 Digital subtraction angiography demonstrated significant vascularity of the carotid body tumor (arrow), which splayed the internal and external carotid arteries.

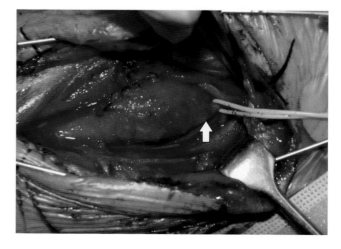

Figure 27.3 Operative finding of carotid body tumor completely encasing the internal carotid artery (arrow).

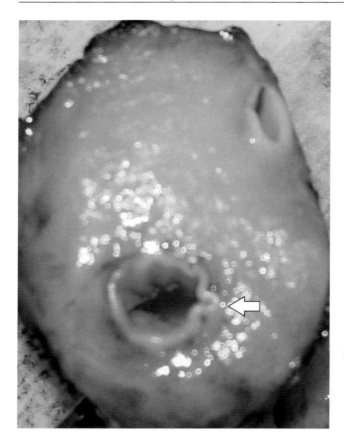

Figure 27.4 Transected gross specimen of a carotid body tumor shown completely encasing the internal carotid artery (arrow).

Case example 2

A 67-year-old woman presented with a 2-cm mass at the bifurcation of the CCA, consistent with a CBT (**Figure 27.6**). In this case, the tumor could be completely resected from the artery (**Figures 27.7** and **27.8**). The patient recovered uneventfully. Pathology confirmed completely excised CBT.

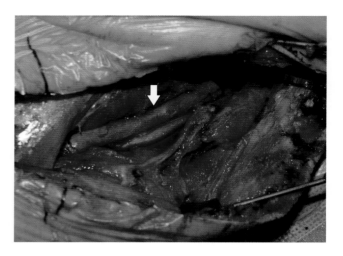

Figure 27.5 Common carotid-to-internal carotid artery reconstruction with reversed great saphenous vein conduit (arrow).

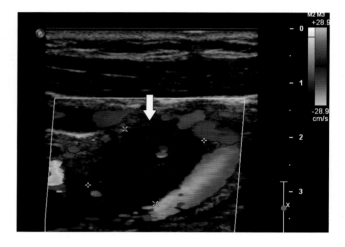

Figure 27.6 Carotid bifurcation duplex ultrasound demonstrating carotid body tumor splaying the carotid bifurcation (arrow) in a 67-year-old woman.

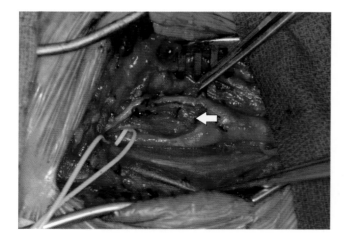

Figure 27.7 Intraoperative image of Shamblin classification group I tumor (arrow) with several of the feeding branches ligated.

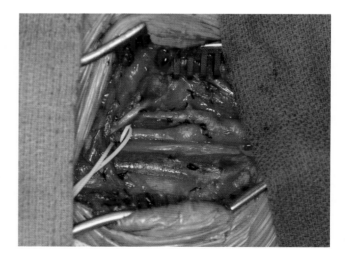

Figure 27.8 Operative image of carotid bifurcation following complete resection of carotid body tumor.

REFERENCES

1. Paris J, Facon F, Thomassin JM, et al. Cervical paragangliomas: neurovascular surgical risk and therapeutic management. *Eur Arch Otorhinolaryngol.* 2006;263:860–865.

2. Patetsios P, Gable DR, Garrett WV, et al. Management of carotid body paragangliomas and review of a 30-year experience. *Ann Vasc Surg.* 2002;16:331–338.

3. Papaspyrou K, Mann WJ, Amedee RG. Management of head and neck paragangliomas: review of 120 patients. *Head Neck.* 2009;31:381–387.

4. Kakkos SK, Reddy DJ, Shepard AD, et al. Contemporary presentation and evolution of management of neck paragangliomas. *J Vasc Surg.* 2009;49:1365–1373.

5. Plukker JT, Brongers EP, Vermey A, et al. Outcome of surgical treatment for carotid body paraganglioma. *Br J Surg.* 2001;88:1382–1386.

6. Smith RF, Shetty PC, Reddy DJ. Surgical treatment of carotid paragangliomas presenting unusual technical difficulties. The value of preoperative embolization. *J Vasc Surg.* 1988;7:631–637.

7. Shamblin WR, ReMine WH, Sheps SG, et al. Carotid body tumor (chemodectoma). Clinicopathologic analysis of ninety cases. *Am J Surg.* 1971;122:732–739.

8. Wang SJ, Wang MB, Barauskas TM, et al. Surgical management of carotid body tumors. *Otolaryngol Head Neck Surg.* 2000;123:202–206.

9. Maxwell JG, Jones SW, Wilson E, et al. Carotid body tumor excisions: adverse outcomes of adding carotid endarterectomy. *J Am Coll Surg.* 2004;198:36–41.

10. Sajid MS, Hamilton G, Baker DM, et al. A multicenter review of carotid body tumour management. *Eur J Vasc Endovasc Surg.* 2007;34:127–130.

11. Hallett JW Jr., Nora JD, Hollier LH, et al. Trends in neurovascular complications of surgical management for carotid body and cervical paragangliomas: a fifty-year experience with 153 tumors. *J Vasc Surg.* 1988;7:284–291.

28

Carotid-subclavian bypass and carotid-subclavian transposition

MITCHELL R. WEAVER

CONTENTS

INTRODUCTION

Traditionally, nonanatomic arterial reconstructions between the major vessels of the aortic arch, such as carotid-subclavian bypass or transposition, have been performed for the treatment of symptomatic, proximal, occlusive disease in one of these vessels when there is a nondiseased vessel to serve as a donor. The most typical lesions treated have been those of the proximal left subclavian artery (SCA). More recently, the maturation of endovascular techniques has led to a decrease in the number of open arterial reconstructions required for this indication. However, the advent of endovascular means to treat aortic arch pathology, has led to an increase in the number of these procedures being performed in the author's practice to "debranch" the aortic arch and thereby create a satisfactory proximal landing zone for a thoracic stent graft.

PREOPERATIVE CONSIDERATIONS

Carotid-subclavian transposition is technically more difficult than carotid-subclavian bypass because it requires a more extensive dissection, including identifying and isolating the internal thoracic and vertebral arteries, but has the advantage of avoiding the use of a prosthetic graft.

OPERATION

The operation is performed under general anesthesia with the patient in a supine, semi-Fowler's position with the head and torso raised approximately 30 degrees. A rolled-up sheet is placed underneath the patient's shoulder. The neck is extended and rotated slightly to the contralateral side. The ipsilateral arm is adducted with slight downward pull to depress the shoulder. Perioperative antibiotics, typically a first-generation cephalosporin, are administered before skin incision. The neck and chest are prepped in a sterile fashion.

A transverse incision is then made, starting approximately 1 cm lateral to the midline and 1–2 cm above the clavicle. The incision is continued laterally approximately 6–8 cm. The platysma muscle is divided with cautery and flaps are developed superiorly, approximately 5 cm, and inferiorly to the clavicle. The sternocleidomastoid muscle (SCM) is mobilized along its lateral border and if necessary, more often in the case of SCA transposition, the clavicular head of the SCM is freed at the clavicle to allow for extended medial exposure.

Once the SCM has been mobilized medially and anteriorly, the carotid sheath is identified and incised, taking care not to injure the structures within it. The common carotid artery (CCA) is approached posteriorly, by mobilizing the internal jugular vein (IJV) and vagus nerve running parallel with it anteriorly and medially. This is also the pathway through which the transposed SCA or bypass graft will traverse. Approximately 5–6 cm of the CCA is exposed to allow for clamping and to create the anastomosis. In cases where the goal of the operation is to treat proximal disease of the left CCA (carotid-subclavian transposition), the artery is dissected proximally as far as possible to allow for adequate length to transpose to the SCA. If a concomitant procedure is planned for the more distal carotid artery (e.g., carotid endarterectomy (CEA)), this portion of the artery may be exposed through a separate incision along the anterior border of the SCM.

Continuing exposure of the SCA, the omohyoid muscle is encountered and divided, furthering exposure of the anterior scalene fat pad. Starting on the medial edge of the anterior scalene, it is separated from the IJV; then, its inferior border is mobilized. This allows for it to be retracted laterally and superiorly. During this dissection, all lymphatics are carefully ligated as they are divided. On the left side, care is taken not to injure the thoracic duct; however, if injured or divided, it is meticulously oversewn with fine monofilament polypropylene suture.

The anterior scalene muscle (ASM) is then exposed along with the phrenic nerve that runs lateral-to-medial, anterior to, and within the investing fascia of the muscle (**Figure 28.1**). The nerve is carefully mobilized off the muscle, by incising the fascia a few millimeters either side of it. The edges of the ASM are then freed and the muscle is divided exposing the SCA (**Figure 28.2**) and brachial plexus. For cases in which carotid to SCA bypass is planned, only enough of the SCA needs to be exposed to allow for the application of vascular clamps for proximal and distal control, and to allow for an area to perform the anastomosis. When carotid-subclavian transposition is planned more proximal dissection of the SCA is required. Dissection is continued medially, identifying and mobilizing the internal mammary and vertebral arteries. An adequate length of SCA proximal to the vertebral artery to allow for safe clamping and oversewing of the proximal

stump, as well as sufficient length to reach the CCA, needs to be exposed. Consideration may be made to ligating the internal mammary artery to allow for increased mobilization of the SCA.

Having completed dissection, the artery is palpated and assessed to ensure that it can be successfully clamped and oversewn, while still leaving adequate length for transposition to the carotid artery. If there is uncertainty, carotid-subclavian transposition should be abandoned in favor of performing a carotid-subclavian bypass.

Having made the decision to proceed with carotid-subclavian transposition, the patient is systemically anticoagulated with heparin (100 IU/kg) with its effect monitored using activated clotting time. After adequate anticoagulation is achieved, vascular clamps are applied to the SCA and its branches. The SCA is divided proximal to the vertebral artery, and the proximal stump is carefully oversewn with monofilament polypropylene suture. Before cutting the suture, the clamp is slowly released and the arterial closure is inspected for hemostasis. Once hemostasis is ensured with the clamp completely removed, the sutures are cut. This is a critical point because loss of control of the SCA as it retracts back into the chest after ligation may lead to catastrophic bleeding that is very difficult to control.

Having controlled the proximal stump, the distal end of the divided SCA is swung over to the adjacent CCA. The carotid artery is clamped proximally and distally with atraumatic vascular clamps. A No. 11 blade knife is used to create an arteriotomy that is lengthened in a longitudinal fashion on the lateral aspect of the carotid artery with Potts scissors to a size that will accept the SCA. An end of SCA to side of carotid artery anastomosis is then performed typically with running 5-0 or 6-0 monofilament

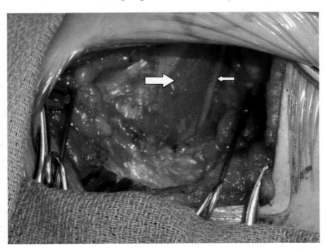

Figure 28.1 Reflection of the anterior scalene fat pad exposes the anterior scalene muscle (large arrow) and overlying phrenic nerve (small arrow).

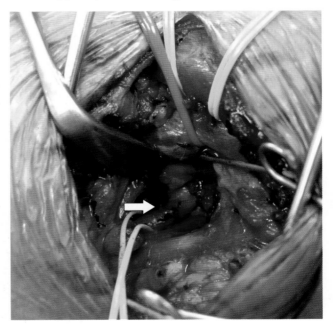

Figure 28.2 Division of the anterior scalene muscle reveals the subclavian artery (arrow).

polypropylene suture. Just before completion of the anastomosis, the vessels are vented. The anastomosis is completed and flow is restored. Distal perfusion is assessed with pulse examination and continuous wave Doppler interrogation. If found to be satisfactory, the heparin effect is reversed with protamine sulfate. The author does not routinely monitor cerebral perfusion with electroencephalography during this procedure.

The wound is inspected for bleeding and any sign of lymphatic leak. Having ensured hemostasis and ligation of any possible lymphatic leaks, the anterior scalene fat pad is reapproximated to its original position. A closed suction drain is placed within the wound and taken out through the skin via a separate inferior stab incision. The platysma muscle is closed with interrupted 3-0 braided polyglactin suture and the skin is closed with running 4-0 braided polyglactin suture. The drain is removed only after the patient has resumed normal oral intake without signs of lymphatic leak.

When carotid-subclavian bypass is planned, having completed adequate dissection and initiated anticoagulation as described previously, one is ready to proceed with the bypass operation. Typically, a prosthetic graft is chosen. The author prefers a Dacron graft because of ease of handling and reduced needle hole bleeding. While the size of the graft is ultimately determined by the size of the donor and recipient vessels, a graft 6–8 mm in diameter is typically chosen.

Technically, it is easier to perform the SCA anastomosis first, followed by the carotid artery anastomosis. The mid and most apical portion of the SCA is typically the site chosen for the anastomosis. Atraumatic clamps are applied proximally and distally while allowing adequate space for the anastomosis. One should be aware that the SCA is more fragile than the typically encountered common femoral artery. Manipulation should be minimized, including clamping and unclamping of the artery; significant caution should be exercised if considering arterial endarterectomy. Clamps should be applied in a deliberate and gentle manner. Once the artery is controlled, an arteriotomy is created with a No. 11 blade scalpel and extended appropriately with Potts scissors. The end of the graft is cut in a beveled fashion and sewn end-to-side to the artery with running 5-0 or 6-0 monofilament polypropylene suture. Once the anastomosis is completed, the proximal and distal arteries are vented through the graft and the anastomosis is tested for hemostasis. After ensuring hemostasis, the graft is brought over to the carotid artery. Typically, the graft will lie over, as opposed to being taken under, the phrenic nerve. Either way, documentation of its course in the operative note is beneficial, should any remedial operation be required in the future. The graft is then cut so as not to be redundant or under tension when anastomosed to the carotid artery (**Figure 28.3**). The anastomosis is performed as described previously for the carotid-subclavian transposition as is closure of the wound.

In operations when the carotid artery is transposed to the SCA, obtaining adequate proximal length of the CCA is essential. Also, the same care is required when ligating

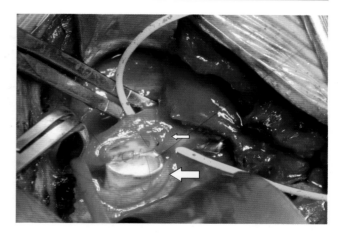

Figure 28.3 An arteriotomy is created in the lateral aspect of the common carotid artery (small arrow). An end of the prosthetic graft tunneled under the jugular vein (large arrow) to the side of the artery anastomosis is performed with a running suture.

the proximal stump. When additional carotid intervention is planned, such as CEA, the graft to the SCA anastomosis is performed first, followed by the endarterectomy. If a carotid shunt is required during the endarterectomy, it may be placed. The endarterectomy is then performed, and prior to patch closure of the artery, a second arteriotomy is created on the lateral aspect of the CCA for the bypass anastomosis. Once completed, patch closure of the artery may be performed and the shunt removed just before completion.

Both carotid-subclavian bypass and carotid-subclavian transposition have low morbidity and excellent long-term patency (75–80% at 5 years for carotid-subclavian bypass and almost 100% for carotid-subclavian transposition).[1–5] Complications include injury to adjacent nerves (brachial plexus, phrenic nerve, and sympathetic chain) and lymphatic structures (thoracic and accessory thoracic ducts). Nerve injuries are usually self-limited. Lymphatic injuries can be problematic and, if drainage is significant or persistent, early reexploration and thoracic duct ligation are advised.

CASE EXAMPLES

Case example 1

An 83-year-old man with a history of hypertension presented with back pain and was found to have an intramural hematoma of the thoracic aorta. He was initially managed medically with anti-impulse therapy; however, short-term surveillance computed tomography imaging demonstrated aneurysmal degeneration of the proximal descending thoracic aorta up to 6.7 cm at the greatest diameter. The patient was offered thoracic endografting to treat this aneurysm. Coverage of the left SCA was required to secure an adequate length for the proximal landing zone. This was performed in a staged fashion. First, a carotid-subclavian bypass was performed. Two days later, the patient underwent endografting of his proximal descending thoracic aorta (**Figures 28.4** and **28.5**). The patient has done well in the long-term follow-up with a patent bypass (**Figure 28.6**).

Case example 2

A 72-year-old man presented with recurrent left hemispheric transient ischemic attacks. Workup revealed findings of right

internal carotid artery (ICA) occlusion and severe proximal left CCA stenosis, but a patent left carotid bulb and ICA. The patient's left SCA was disease-free and the patient was offered left carotid-subclavian bypass versus transposition. At the time of the operation, the length of the normal carotid artery allowed it to be easily transposed to the SCA (**Figure 28.7**). The patient did well postoperatively with no recurrent neurologic symptoms.

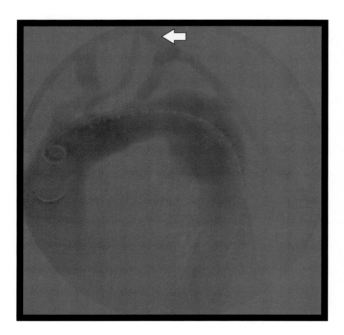

Figure 28.4 Left carotid-subclavian bypass before thoracic endografting (arrow) to treat a descending thoracic aortic aneurysm.

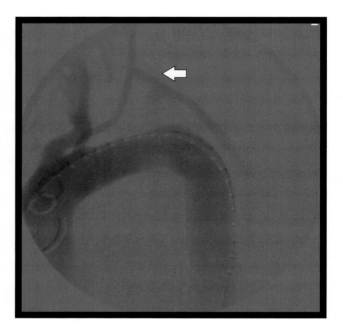

Figure 28.5 Angiogram following thoracic aortic endografting demonstrating the exclusion of the aneurysm and distal arterial flow maintained in the subclavian artery via carotid-subclavian bypass (arrow).

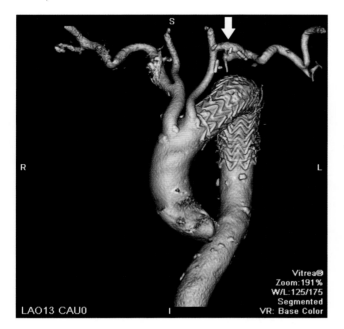

Figure 28.6 A three-dimensional reconstruction computed tomography scan obtained 7 years postoperatively demonstrating patent bypass (arrow) and exclusion of aneurysm.

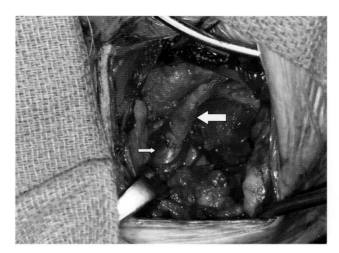

Figure 28.7 Operative image demonstrating a completed end of carotid artery (large arrow) to side of subclavian artery transposition (small arrow).

REFERENCES

1. Aziz F, Gravett MH, Comerota AJ. Endovascular and open surgical treatment of brachiocephalic arteries. *Ann Vasc Surg.* 2011;**25**:569–581.

2. Aiello F, Morrissey NJ. Open and endovascular management of subclavian and innominate arterial pathology. *Semin Vasc Surg.* 2011;**24**:31–35.

3. Ziomek S, Quiñones-Baldrich WJ, Busuttil RW, et al. The superiority of synthetic arterial grafts over autologous veins in carotid-subclavian bypass. *J Vasc Surg.* 1986;**3**:140–145.

4. AbuRahma AF, Robinson PA, Jennings TG. Carotid-subclavian bypass grafting with polytetrafluoro-ethylene grafts for symptomatic subclavian artery stenosis or occlusion: a 20-year experience. *J Vasc Surg.* 2000;**32**:411–418.

5. Law MM, Colburn MD, Moore WS, et al. Carotid-subclavian bypass for brachiocephalic occlusive disease. Choice of conduit and long-term follow-up. *Stroke.* 1995:**26**:1565–1571.

29

Vertebral artery reconstruction

MARK D. MORASCH

CONTENTS

INTRODUCTION

Atherosclerosis is the most common disease affecting the vertebral artery. Uncommon pathologic processes include trauma, fibromuscular dysplasia, Takayasu's arteritis, osteophyte compression, dissections, and aneurysms,[1,2] all of which can lead to symptoms of posterior circulation ischemia. Approximately 25% of all ischemic strokes occur in the vertebrobasilar territory; 50% of patients present initially with stroke and 26% of patients present with transient ischemic symptoms rapidly followed by stroke.[3] For patients who experience vertebrobasilar transient ischemic attacks, disease in the vertebral arteries indicates a 22–35% risk of stroke over 5 years.[4–6] The mortality associated with a posterior circulation stroke is 20–30%; this is higher than that for an anterior circulation event.[7–9]

Ischemia affecting the temporo-occipital areas of the cerebral hemispheres or segments of the brain stem and cerebellum characteristically produces bilateral symptoms. The classic symptoms of vertebrobasilar ischemia are: dizziness; vertigo; drop attacks; diplopia; perioral numbness; alternating paresthesia; tinnitus; dysphasia; dysarthria; and ataxia.

In general, the ischemic mechanisms can be broken down into those that are hemodynamic and those that are embolic. Hemodynamic symptoms occur because of transient "end organ" (brain stem, cerebellum, occipital lobes) hypoperfusion and rarely result in infarction. Symptoms tend to be transient, repetitive, and more of a nuisance than a danger. For hemodynamic symptoms to occur, occlusive pathology must be present in both paired vertebral vessels or in the basilar artery. In addition, compensatory contribution from the carotid circulation via the circle of Willis must be incomplete. Alternatively, hemodynamic ischemic symptoms may follow proximal subclavian artery (SCA) occlusion and SCA/vertebral artery steal syndrome.

Up to one-third of vertebrobasilar ischemic episodes are caused by embolization from plaques or mural lesions of the SCA, vertebral, or basilar arteries.[10] Actual infarctions in the vertebrobasilar distribution are most often the result of embolic events.

Surgical reconstruction is not indicated in an asymptomatic patient with stenotic or occlusive vertebral lesions because these patients are well compensated from the carotid circulation through the posterior communicating vessels. The minimal anatomic requirement to justify vertebral artery reconstruction for patients with true hemodynamic symptoms is stenosis >60% diameter in both vertebral arteries if both are patent and complete, or the same degree of stenosis in the dominant vertebral artery if the opposite vertebral artery is hypoplastic, ends in a posteroinferior cerebellar artery, or is occluded. A single, normal vertebral artery is sufficient to adequately perfuse the basilar artery, regardless of the patency status of the contralateral vertebral artery. Conversely, patients with symptomatic vertebrobasilar ischemia due to emboli are candidates for surgical revascularization regardless of the condition of the contralateral vertebral artery.

Surgical intervention is not indicated in asymptomatic patients who harbor suspicious radiographic findings.

Duplex ultrasound (US) is an excellent tool for detecting lesions in the carotid artery, but it has significant limitations when used to detect vertebral artery pathology. The usefulness of duplex US lies in its ability to confirm reversal of flow within the vertebral arteries and detect flow velocity changes consistent with a proximal stenosis.[11]

Contrast-enhanced magnetic resonance angiography (MRA) with three-dimensional reconstruction and maximum image intensity techniques provide full imaging of the vessels including the supra-aortic trunks and the carotid and vertebral arteries. Better than computed tomography, transaxial magnetic resonance imaging can readily diagnose both acute and chronic posterior fossa infarcts.

The most common site of disease, the vertebral artery origin, may not be well imaged with US or MRA and often can only be displayed with catheter-based angiography that employs oblique projections, which may not be part of standard arch evaluation. Patients with suspected vertebral artery compression should also undergo dynamic angiography, which incorporates provocative positioning. Finally, delayed imaging should be performed to demonstrate reconstitution of the extracranial vertebral arteries through cervical collaterals, such as the occipital artery, or via collaterals from the ipsilateral SCA, such as branches of the thyrocervical trunk (**Figure 29.1**).[12]

OPERATIVE STRATEGY AND TECHNIQUE

Surgical anatomy of the vertebral artery

The surgical anatomy of the paired vertebral arteries is divided into four segments: (1) the V1 segment, the origin of the vertebral artery arising from the SCA to the point at which it enters the C6 transverse process; (2) V2, the segment of the artery buried deep within the intertransversarium muscle and the C6–C2 cervical transverse processes; (3) V3, the surgically accessible extracranial segment between the C2 transverse process and the base of the skull before it enters the foramen magnum; and (4) V4, the intracranial portion beginning at the atlanto-occipital membrane and terminating as the two vertebral arteries converge to form the basilar artery (**Figure 29.2**). Disease location dictates the type of surgical reconstruction that is required. With rare exceptions, most reconstructions of the vertebral artery are performed to relieve either an orificial stenosis (V1 segment), or stenosis, dissection, or occlusion of its intraspinal component (V2 and V3 segments).

Stenosing ostial lesions in the V1 segment[13] are best managed surgically with transposition of the proximal vertebral artery onto the adjacent carotid artery. More distal pathology usually requires bypass from the common carotid artery (CCA) to the V3 segment vertebral artery between C1 and C2.

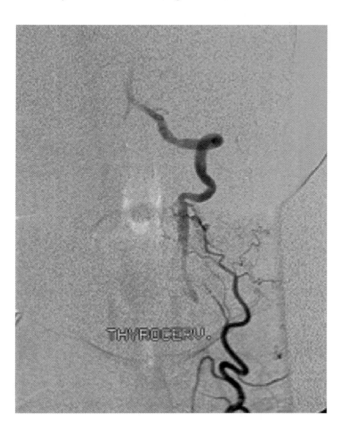

Figure 29.1 V3 segment reconstitution via thyrocervical collateral.

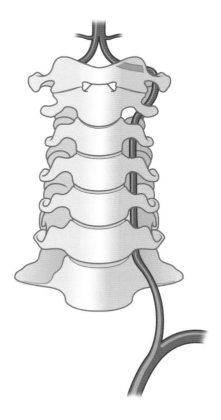

Figure 29.2 Vertebral artery anatomy: V1–V4 segments.

Exposure and transposition of the vertebral artery into the CCA

The approach to the proximal vertebral artery is the same as the approach for a SCA-carotid transposition. The patient is positioned in a slight chair position to decrease venous pressure. The incision is made transversely just above the clavicle and directly over the two heads of the sternocleidomastoid muscle. Subplatysmal skin flaps are created to provide adequate exposure. Dissection follows between the two bellies of the sternocleidomastoid muscle after the omohyoid muscle is divided. The jugular vein is retracted laterally, and the carotid sheath is entered. The vagus nerve is retracted medially with the CCA (**Figure 29.3**). The remainder of the dissection is carried out between the jugular vein and the carotid artery in the base of the neck.

On the left side, the thoracic duct is encircled with a right-angled clamp and then divided between ligatures. Accessory lymph ducts, often seen on the right side of the neck, are also identified, ligated, and divided. The entire dissection is confined medial to the prescalene fat pad that covers the scalenus anticus muscle and phrenic nerve. These structures are left unexposed lateral to the field. The inferior thyroid artery runs transversely across the field, and it is ligated and divided.

The vertebral vein should be identified as it emerges from the angle formed by the longus colli and scalenus anticus muscles. The vein invariably overlies the proximal vertebral artery and, at the bottom of the field, the SCA. It is ligated and divided. The vertebral and subclavian vessels lie immediately deep to the vein. It is important to identify and avoid injury to the adjacent sympathetic chain. The vertebral artery is exposed from its origin at

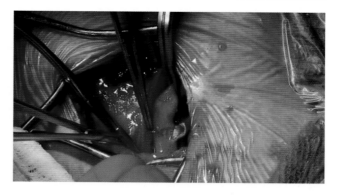

Figure 29.4 Surgical approach to the V1 segment of the vertebral artery. The distal portion of the V1 segment is clamped, and the proximal vertebral artery is ligated immediately above its origin. The artery is then divided, pulled from under the sympathetic chain, and brought over the common carotid artery. The free end is spatulated for anastomosis.

the posteromedial aspect of the SCA distally to the tendon of the longus colli muscle where it enters the transverse foramen of C6. The vertebral artery is freed from the sympathetic trunk resting on its anterior surface without damaging the trunk or the ganglionic rami.

Once the artery is fully exposed, an appropriate site for carotid reimplantation is identified. The patient is given systemic heparin. The distal portion of the V1 segment of the vertebral artery is clamped below the edge of the longus colli muscle with a microclip, avoiding any axial twisting. The proximal vertebral artery is ligated with a 5-0 polypropylene transfixion suture immediately above its origin. The artery is divided, pulled from under the sympathetic chain, and brought over to the CCA. The free end is spatulated for anastomosis (**Figure 29.4**). The carotid artery is cross-clamped. An elliptical 5–7-mm arteriotomy is created in the posterolateral wall of the CCA with an aortic punch. The anastomosis is performed in parachute fashion with continuous 7-0 polypropylene suture. On completion of the anastomosis, the suture slack is tightened, standard flushing maneuvers are performed, the suture is tied, the clamps are removed, and flow is reestablished (**Figure 29.5**). A drain is placed. This can be removed the following morning provided there is no chylous leak. The incision is then closed by reapproximating the platysma and closing the skin with a subcuticular stitch.

V3 segment exposure and distal vertebral artery reconstruction

Saphenous vein bypass from the CCA or SCA to the V3 vertebral segment is the technique most commonly used to perform a distal reconstruction.[12] Alternatively, the radial artery can be used as conduit in the absence of a suitable vein. The distal portion of the reconstruction is generally completed at the C1–C2 spinal level.

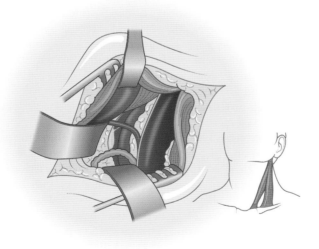

Figure 29.3 Surgical approach to the V1 segment of the vertebral artery. The jugular vein is retracted laterally and the carotid sheet is entered. The vagus nerve is retracted medially with the common carotid artery.

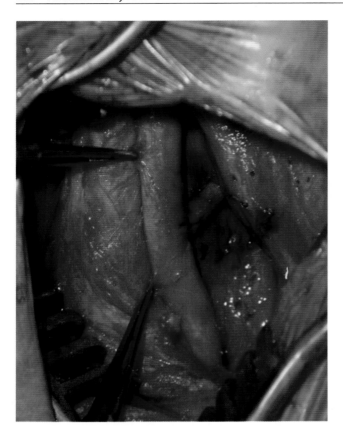

Figure 29.5 Completed proximal vertebral-to-common carotid artery bypass.

The skin incision is placed anterior to the sternocleidomastoid muscle, the same as in a carotid operation, and is carried superiorly to immediately below the earlobe. The dissection proceeds in a retrojugular plane between the vein and the anterior edge of the sternocleidomastoid muscle. The spinal accessory nerve will be encountered and should be dissected gently over a 5-cm length so that it can be retracted safely. The nerve is followed proximally as it crosses in front of the jugular vein and the C1 transverse process. The first cervical vertebrae can be easily felt with finger palpation.

The levator scapulae muscle is exposed by removing the fibroadipose tissue overlying it. Once the anterior edge of the levator scapulae muscle is identified, the anterior ramus of C2 becomes visible. With the ramus as a guide, a right-angle clamp is slid under the levator scapulae muscle and then divided. The C2 ramus divides into three branches after crossing the vertebral artery. The ramus should be cut (**Figure 29.6**) before it branches. This exposes the V3 segment of the vertebral artery that can then be freed from the surrounding venous plexus over a 1–2-cm length.

Once the vertebral artery is adequately exposed, the distal CCA should be prepared as inflow for the bypass graft. There is no need to dissect the carotid bifurcation;

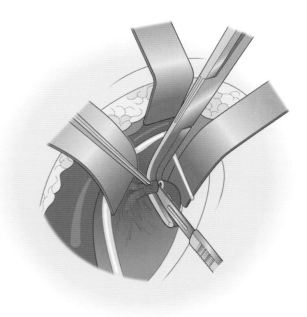

Figure 29.6 Transection of the C2 nerve root and the V3 segment of the vertebral artery, which lies just deep to this structure. The C2 ramus should be cut before it branches.

the location selected for the proximal anastomosis should not be too close to the bifurcation because cross-clamping at this level may fracture an underlying atheroma.

A suitable conduit of appropriate length is harvested and prepared. A valveless segment of vein facilitates back-bleeding of the vertebral artery after completion of the distal anastomosis. The patient is given intravenous heparin. The vertebral artery is elevated by gently pulling on an encircling vessel loop and is occluded with a small J clamp. This isolates a short segment for an end-to-side anastomosis. The vertebral artery is opened longitudinally over a short length adequate to accommodate the spatulated end of the vein graft. The end-to-side anastomosis is done with continuous 7-0 polypropylene suture and fine needles. A vascular clamp is placed in the vein graft proximal to the anastomosis and the vertebral J clamp is removed.

The proximal end of the graft is passed behind the jugular vein and in proximity to the side of the CCA. The CCA is then cross-clamped, an elliptical arteriotomy is made in its posterior wall with an aortic punch, and the proximal vein graft is anastomosed end-to-side to the CCA (**Figure 29.7**). Before the anastomosis is completed, standard flushing maneuvers are performed, the suture is tied, and flow is reestablished. The vertebral artery is occluded with a clip placed immediately below the anastomosis to create a functional end-to-end anastomosis and avoid competitive flow or the potential for recurrent emboli. The wound is closed without a drain,

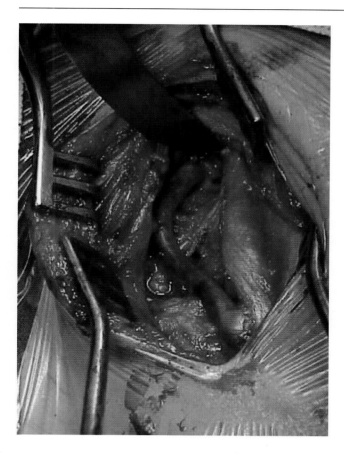

Figure 29.7 Completed common carotid artery-to-V3 segment vertebral artery bypass using reverse great saphenous vein as conduit.

by reapproximating the platysma muscle and closing the skin with a subcuticular stitch.

Intraoperative completion imaging with digital angiography is useful and should be considered for all types of vertebral artery reconstruction. Reparable technical flaws may be identified and repair can prevent reconstruction failure.

POTENTIAL POSTOPERATIVE COMPLICATIONS

The perioperative complication rates differ for proximal versus distal vertebral artery repairs. Perioperative complications that can follow any reconstruction include stroke, bleeding, thrombosis, and nerve injury.

Stroke is usually the result of prolonged clamp time or immediate postoperative thrombosis of vertebral arteries or conduits. Completion angiography may be helpful in preventing these complications. Distal reconstructions have a combined stroke and death rate of 3–4% and have higher stroke and death rates than operations on the proximal vertebral artery.[12]

Nerve injury

Complications that are specific to proximal reconstruction include vagus and recurrent laryngeal nerve palsy (2%) and Horner syndrome (8.4–28%). Complications that may follow distal reconstruction include vagus (1%) and spinal accessory nerve (2%) injuries. Most patients who undergo proximal vertebral reconstruction experience at least a short-lived Horner syndrome. Often, it is not noticeable to the patient but can be seen by other observers. The treatment is expectant. Most, if not all, resolve in time. Vagus nerve injuries manifest as hoarseness and are most often the result of traction on the vagus nerve itself during exposure of the deep neck structures during proximal vertebral transposition or during mobilization of the CCA in a distal bypass. Because this is rarely the result of cutting the recurrent nerve, usually time and patience are all that are required. If vocal cord palsy persists beyond 3 months, cord medialization may be warranted. A spinal accessory nerve injury results from undo traction. Most neuropraxia-type injuries resolve in time.

Conservative management is appropriate initially for a chylous or significant lymphatic leak as most resolve in time. This includes local compression, dietary manipulation, and administration of octreotide. Leaks that persist beyond 3 days require reexploration of the surgical wound; direct suture repair should be attempted. Purse-string placement of a small-gauge monofilament suture works best to control a large lymphatic or thoracic duct leak. If all else fails, ligation of the thoracic duct with video-assisted thoracotomy surgery can be considered.

CASE EXAMPLE

A 69-year-old man initially presented to an academic institution with symptoms of hemodynamic posterior circulation ischemia including vertigo, tinnitus, diplopia, and perioral numbness. An MRA demonstrated chronically occluded right internal carotid (ICA) and right vertebral arteries, a high-grade stenosis of the left vertebral artery, a patent left ICA, but an incomplete circle of Willis. He was managed at this institution with a left proximal vertebral angioplasty with stent placement. His symptoms resolved transiently, but after 8 months he was referred to the author with recurrent symptoms. Angiography demonstrated vertebral stent fracture and recurrent high-grade vertebral artery stenosis at the site of the stent damage (**Figure 29.8a,b**). Because the stent extended the full length of the V1 segment, proximal vertebral-carotid transposition was not feasible. Instead, he underwent left CCA-to-V3 segment vertebral artery bypass. Six years later, he remains symptom-free.

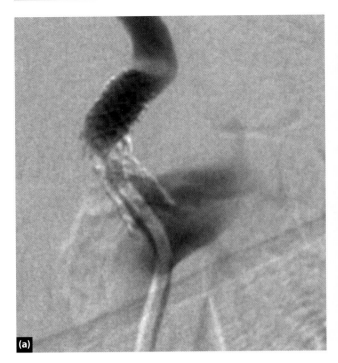
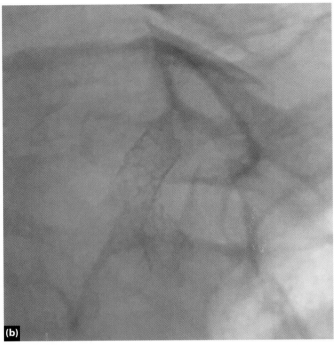

Figure 29.8 Angiography of 69-year-old man (case example) showing vertebral stent fracture and recurrent high-grade vertebral artery stenosis at the site of the stent damage. (**a,b**) V1 segment stent fracture with symptomatic in-stent restenosis.

REFERENCES

1. Morasch MD, Phade SV, Naughton P, et al. Primary extracranial vertebral artery aneurysms. *Ann Vasc Surg.* 2013;**27**:418–423.

2. Sultan S, Morasch M, Colgan MP, et al. Operative and endovascular management of extracranial vertebral artery aneurysm in Ehlers–Danlos syndrome: a clinical dilemma. Case report and literature review. *Vasc Endovascular Surg.* 2002;**36**:389–392.

3. Wityk RJ, Chang HM, Rosengart A, et al. Proximal extracranial vertebral artery disease in the New England Medical Center Posterior Circulation Registry. *Arch Neurol.* 1998;**55**:470–478.

4. Cartlidge NE, Whisnant JP, Elveback LR. Carotid and vertebral-basilar transient cerebral ischemic attacks. A community study, Rochester, Minnesota. *Mayo Clin Proc.* 1977;**52**:117–120.

5. Heyman A, Wilkinson WE, Hurwitz BJ, et al. Clinical and epidemiologic aspects of vertebrobasilar and non-focal cerebral ischemia. In: Berguer R, Bauer RB, eds. *Vertebrobasilar Arterial Occlusive Disease. Medical and Surgical Management.* New York, NY: Raven Press; 1984. pp. 27–36.

6. Whisnant JP, Cartlidge NE, Elveback LR. Carotid and vertebral-basilar transient ischemic attacks: effect of anticoagulants, hypertension, and cardiac disorders on survival and stroke occurrence. A population study. *Ann Neurol.* 1978;**3**:107–115.

7. Jones HR Jr., Millikan CH, Sandok BA. Temporal profile (clinical course) of acute vertebrobasilar system cerebral infarction. *Stroke.* 1980;**11**:173–177.

8. McDowell FH, Potes J, Groch S. The natural history of internal carotid and vertebral-basilar artery occlusion. *Neurology.* 1961;**11(Pt2)**:153–157.

9. Patrick BK, Ramirez-Lassepas M, Synder BD. Temporal profile of vertebrobasilar territory infarction. Prognostic implications. *Stroke.* 1980;**11**:643–648.

10. Caplan LR, Wityk RJ, Glass TA, et al. New England Medical Center Posterior Circulation registry. *Ann Neurol.* 2004;**56**:389–398.

11. Berguer R, Higgins R, Nelson R. Noninvasive diagnosis of reversal of vertebral-artery blood flow. *N Engl J Med.* 1980;**302**:1349–1351.

12. Berguer R. Distal vertebral artery bypass: technique, the "occipital connection," and potential uses. *J Vasc Surg.* 1985;**2**:621–626.

13. Edwards WH, Mulherin JL Jr. The surgical approach to significant stenosis of vertebral and subclavian arteries. *Surgery.* 1980;**87**:20–28.

30

Brachiocephalic artery reconstruction

JAMIL BORGI AND MITCHELL R. WEAVER

CONTENTS

INTRODUCTION

Symptomatic arterial occlusive disease of the branches of the aortic arch is not frequently encountered. When present, it is manifested by ischemia as the result of low flow or atheroembolism. Brachiocephalic artery (BCA) disease may present with upper extremity tissue loss or effort fatigue, or in the cerebral hemispheres with stroke, transient ischemic attack, or vertebrobasilar insufficiency. Patients with prior coronary artery bypass via an internal mammary artery may present with symptoms of coronary insufficiency. Atherosclerosis is the leading cause of BCA occlusive disease. However, other etiologies exist including: arteritis; congenital anomalies; and mechanical or radiation-induced trauma. All may lead to symptoms and the need for intervention.

Advances in endovascular technology, along with its minimally invasive nature, have led to endovascular therapy becoming the first-line treatment for most proximal aortic arch lesions. A second option is extra-anatomic (cervical) revascularization, which is often ideal for isolated, single-vessel disease. Both interventions are discussed in other chapters. In patients with multivessel disease, or in situations where complete arch debranching is indicated for aortic arch endografting, anatomic (transthoracic) revascularization may be the preferred or only option and is the topic of this chapter.

The vascular surgeon should be fluent in the approaches needed to treat such lesions. This may require collaboration with a cardiac surgeon; sometimes, it may require cardiopulmonary bypass, but rarely hypothermic circulatory arrest.

PREOPERATIVE CONSIDERATIONS

Noninvasive vascular laboratory studies, such as upper extremity segmental pressures, may reveal reduced distal extremity pressures or abnormal Doppler waveforms; carotid duplex imaging may document reduced flow velocities suggestive of proximal BCA occlusive disease. However, cross-sectional imaging with computed tomography angiography (CTA) (**Figure 30.1**) or magnetic resonance angiography are the studies of choice for confirming the diagnosis and planning surgical intervention. It is important to image not only the aortic arch, but also the outflow, including the entire cervical and intracranial vasculature. Imaging is reviewed to determine the appropriate disease-free clamping sites for the proximal ascending aortic anastomosis and the distal targets for bypass, whether the distal BCA, the right subclavian artery (RSA), or either/both carotid arteries. Assessment for carotid bifurcation occlusive disease is made to determine the need for concomitant carotid endarterectomy (CEA). Conventional catheter-based angiography may be of value in assessing aortic arch branch vessel disease, especially when heavily calcified walls make it difficult to truly determine the degree of stenosis on cross-sectional imaging (**Figure 30.2a,b**).

Preoperative cardiopulmonary assessment is important before aortic arch reconstruction. The presence of any cardiac dysfunction, valvular heart disease, or coronary ischemia should be carefully ruled out. Noninvasive studies, such as echocardiography and myocardial perfusion scans, are useful in this evaluation. However, because these reconstructive procedures are performed via a median sternotomy, to ensure no other cardiac intervention is indicated, one should have a low threshold for obtaining catheter-based coronary angiography before proceeding with aortic arch surgery. Severe cardiopulmonary disease, a heavily calcified aortic arch, or prior sternotomy places patients at higher risk, makes the operation more difficult, and may occasionally preclude direct arch branch reconstruction.

PROCEDURE

Preparation

Procedures are performed under general anesthesia (GA). Appropriate preoperative antibiotics are administered within 1 hour before incision. Preoperative discussion with the anesthesiology team regarding arterial line placement and venous access is important. Considerations include which arteries are diseased, which arteries are going to be clamped, and the plans for any concomitant procedures (i.e., CEA). The authors generally avoid electroencephalography monitoring unless carotid bifurcation clamping is planned. The patient is placed in a supine position with a posterior shoulder roll to extend the neck and elevate the sternal notch after GA is induced. The midline is marked with a pen before prepping and draping. A chlorhexidine-based solution is used for prepping the skin. The field should be large enough to incorporate the neck should extension of the skin incision be needed to expose the proximal carotid arteries (**Figure 30.3**). The field should also include both groins, in case emergency access to the femoral vessels is needed for cardiopulmonary bypass.

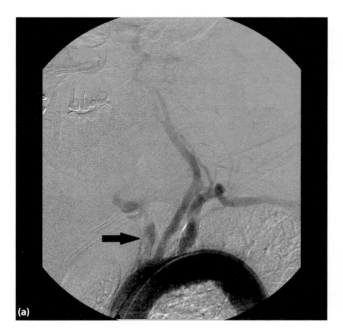

Figure 30.1 Reformatted computed tomography angiogram of aortic arch with heavily calcified brachiocephalic artery (arrow).

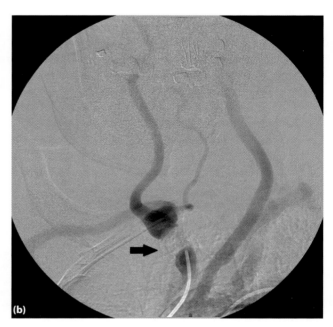

Figure 30.2 Nonselective aortic arch angiogram in a patient with right upper extremity effort fatigue and an ulcer on the little finger. (**a**) Severe calcified arterial occlusive disease is noted in the brachiocephalic artery (BCA) (arrow). (**b**) Selective angiogram of the BCA demonstrating severe stenosis of the BCA (arrow).

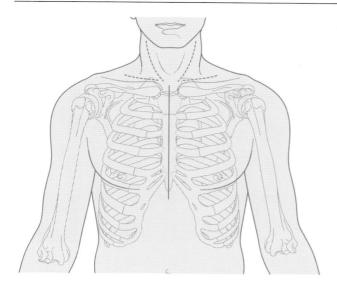

Figure 30.3 Incision for median sternotomy (solid line) and optional cervical extensions (dotted lines).

Exposure

Median sternotomy is performed by incising the skin from the sternal notch to the xiphoid process with a No. 10 blade scalpel. Electrocautery is then used to divide the subcutaneous tissues until the sternum is reached. The interclavicular ligament is then split and the midline of the sternum is marked from the sternal notch to the xiphoid process. After having the anesthesiologist suspend ventilation, a standard pneumatic saw is used to divide the sternum in the midline. The saw can be used from cranial-to-caudal or caudal-to-cranial depending on surgeon preference. After controlling any periosteal bleeding points, a sternal retractor is placed on the mid-to-lower aspect of the sternal edges.

A ministernotomy or upper hemisternotomy is another slightly less invasive option that can provide adequate exposure of the aortic arch and great vessels. This exposure is performed by limiting the incision to just below the angle of Louis (sternal angle). The sternotomy is performed from the sternal notch to the level of the third intercostal space. The saw is then turned at a right angle to "T-off" the sternotomy into the right or left intercostal space. Care must be taken not to injure the underlying internal mammary artery.

After placing a sternal retractor, the pericardium is divided in the midline and three heavy silk stay sutures are placed on both edges of the pericardium to elevate the mediastinal structures and create a pericardial well. The thymic fat that typically covers the aortic arch and proximal arch vessels is either divided in the middle or excised until the left brachiocephalic vein (BCV) is identified. This vein is dissected circumferentially and encircled with a vessel loop that is used to retract the vein superiorly or inferiorly to provide exposure of the underlying structures (**Figure 30.4**). The ascending aorta may be dissected free

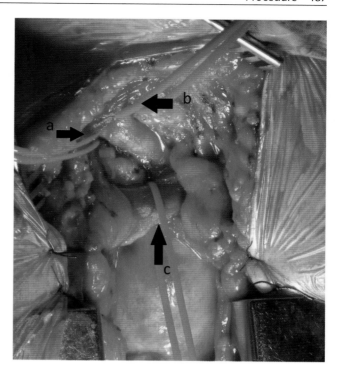

Figure 30.4 Intraoperative photograph demonstrating exposure of the brachiocephalic artery. Proximal right subclavian artery (a arrow). Proximal right common carotid artery (b arrow). Left brachiocephalic vein (c arrow). Both arteries and vein have been encircled with vessel loops.

from the main pulmonary trunk laterally and the right pulmonary artery inferiorly to provide additional mobility and excellent proximal control.

The arch is then further exposed by dividing the pericardial reflection. The BCA, left carotid artery (LCA), and as needed, left subclavian artery (LSA) are then dissected and encircled with vessel loops. In case of BCA reconstruction, the BCA is dissected distally until a soft spot is identified to clamp or, more commonly, the proximalmost right common carotid artery (CCA) and RSA are exposed and controlled. When controlling the RSA, care should be exercised to avoid injury to the vagus and recurrent laryngeal nerves. While BCA endarterectomy can occasionally be performed on a very focal mid-BCA stenosis, most brachiocephalic lesions are best served with a bypass originating from the ascending aorta.

After completing dissection, heparin is given intravenously to achieve an activated clotting time of 200–250 seconds. An appropriately sized graft is then brought to the field (typically 8–12 mm). After lowering the mean blood pressure (BP) to <70 mmHg, a deep and strong side-biting clamp is then applied to the ascending aorta slightly lateral and to the right (**Figure 30.5**). The authors prefer a LEMOLE-STRONG aortic clamp (Becton, Dickinson and Company, Franklin Lakes, NJ, USA) for this (**Figure 30.6**). The graft is beveled appropriately to lay comfortably on the anterolateral (right) side of the ascending aorta. An aortotomy is performed with a No. 11 blade scalpel

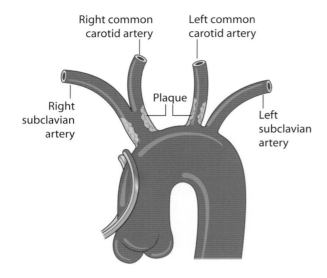

Figure 30.5 Placement of side-biting aortic clamp on the ascending aorta in preparation for performance of proximal anastomosis.

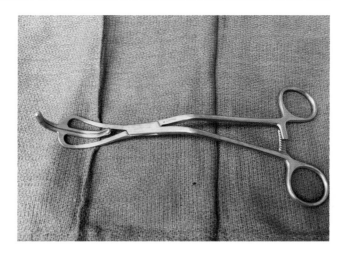

Figure 30.6 LEMOLE-STRONG aortic clamp (Becton, Dickinson and Company, Franklin Lakes, NJ, USA) used for partial (side-biting) clamping of the ascending aorta.

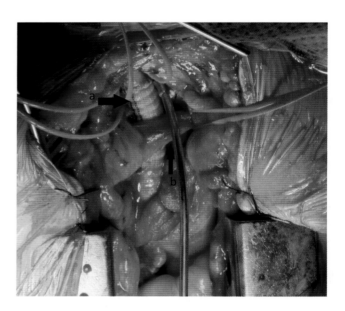

Figure 30.7 Intraoperative photograph demonstrating aorta-to-brachiocephalic artery (BCA) bypass. End-to-end anastomosis to BCA (a arrow). Bypass graft passes beneath the left brachiocephalic vein (b arrow).

and extended with Potts scissors; if the aorta is dilated, the authors frequently remove a small ellipse of aortic wall. The proximal anastomosis is performed with 4-0 polypropylene running suture. After assuring hemostasis, attention is directed distally to the BCA.

While it is sometimes possible to clamp a disease-free segment of the distal BCA, in most situations it is necessary to clamp the RSA and CCA separately. Clamp application on calcified vessels should be avoided because of the risk of embolization. After clamping these arteries, the proximal BCA needs to be ligated and a segment resected to provide more room. A stapler works nicely for this purpose if the vessel is not calcified. Otherwise, it needs to be clamped and oversewn in two layers with 4-0 polypropylene suture. A distal cuff of BCA is prepared for anastomosis; limited plaque at the BCA bifurcation can be endarterectomized. The graft is tunneled distally, usually under the BCV to avoid compression; it is pressurized and cut to length to reach the distal anastomosis site. This anastomosis is usually performed under slight tension because of the tendency for the field to collapse after removal of the sternal retractor predisposing to graft redundancy. If there is any doubt, the sternal retractor should be temporarily loosened before graft transection. The distal anastomosis is then performed with a 5-0 polypropylene running suture (**Figure 30.7**). When the disease extends beyond the BCA bifurcation, the authors prefer to perform the distal anastomosis to the right CCA after sewing a sidearm on for RSA bypass. While a tempting option, bifurcated aortic grafts should be avoided because of their increased bulk, which can lead to compression following removal of the sternal retractor.

The same technique can be applied to bypass the LCA or LSA when they are involved. A side branch graft can be anastomosed to the larger main graft, ideally after performing the aortic anastomosis and checking the lay of the graft (**Figure 30.8**). Branded grafts are commercially available that are designed for bypassing more than one arch vessel. Bypass to the LCA should be performed only after BCA flow has been restored. Again, the proximal vessel can be stapled or oversewn. Depending on the anatomy of the LSA, specifically how laterally and posteriorly it is positioned, adequate exposure for performing arterial reconstruction via a median sternotomy may not be possible. If revascularization of this vessel is required, an extra-anatomic reconstruction (i.e., carotid-subclavian bypass or carotid-subclavian transposition) may be considered after revascularization of the LCA.

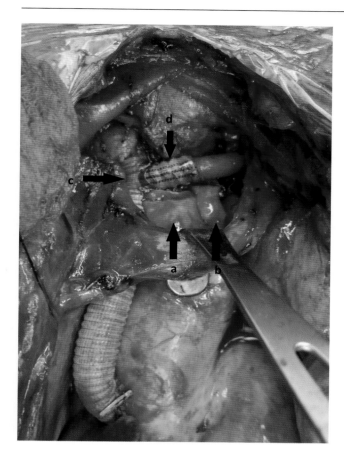

Figure 30.8 Intraoperative photograph demonstrating ligated (stapled) brachiocephalic artery (BCA) (a arrow). Ligated (stapled) left carotid artery (b arrow). Ascending aorta-to-BCA bypass (c arrow), with side branch bypass to the left common carotid artery (d arrow).

Closure

Having completed the bypass, heparin is reversed with protamine sulfate and hemostasis is ensured with cautery and hemostatic agents as needed. Typically, one large-bore (36-Fr) drainage tube is used to drain the mediastinum. It is exteriorized inferiorly and sutured to the skin. The sternum is closed with interrupted sternal wires. Soft tissues and skin are then closed with absorbable suture in a layered fashion.

POSTOPERATIVE MANAGEMENT

The patient usually remains intubated on mechanical ventilation at the end of the surgery and is transferred to the intensive care unit. The patient is then gradually weaned off sedation and extubated when fully awake typically within a few hours of the procedure. Hemodynamic monitoring is provided to maintain normal-range BP. Severe fluctuations in hemodynamics are not typically seen when the procedure is completed without the use of cardiopulmonary bypass. Mediastinal drainage should be minimal and any sudden increase in drainage should prompt consideration for return to the operating room.

OUTCOMES

Outcomes are generally very satisfactory when performed for BCA occlusive disease. Early complications typically involve cardiopulmonary events or stroke. Mortality rates range from 2.7 to 8%. Stroke rates from 2.7 to 8%, and myocardial infarction rates from 1.5 to 3%, have been reported. Survival rates at 5 and 10 years are 77.5–87% and 51.9–81%, respectively. Graft patency at 5 and 10 years is reported from 94 to 98% and 88 to 96%, respectively.[1–3]

CASE EXAMPLE

A 69-year-old woman with a history significant for tobacco abuse, hypertension, dyslipidemia, peripheral arterial disease, and stroke was referred for a painful, nonhealing ulcer on her right little finger and an abnormal pulse examination. Questioning revealed a history of easy fatigability in the right arm. The BP in her right upper extremity was 70 mmHg systolic compared to 154 mmHg on her left side. Noninvasive vascular studies revealed monophasic Doppler signals in the right brachial and radial arteries. A carotid duplex demonstrated a >80% stenosis at the right carotid artery (RCA) bifurcation and a 60% stenosis at the LCA bifurcation. A CTA demonstrated calcific atheromatous changes involving the great vessel origins (**Figure 30.1**). Catheter-based angiography documented severe stenosis of the BCA (**Figure 30.2a,b**). Given the patient's nonhealing ulcer and concern that it was secondary to atheroembolism, the patient was advised to undergo BCA bypass, along with concomitant RCA endarterectomy.

The operation was performed through an upper hemisternotomy, with an 8-mm Dacron graft bypass from the ascending aorta to the BCA bifurcation (**Figure 30.7**). Following this bypass, a RCA endarterectomy was performed via a standard incision along the anterior border of the sternocleidomastoid muscle, which was not contiguous with the hemisternotomy incision. The patient had an uneventful postoperative course. Her finger ulcer healed and she has remained asymptomatic over 7 years of follow-up.

REFERENCES

1. Kieffer E, Sabatier J, Koskas F, et al. Atherosclerotic innominate artery occlusive disease: early and long-term results of surgical reconstruction. *J Vasc Surg.* 1995;**21**:326–336.
2. Berguer R, Morasch MD, Kline RA. Transthoracic repair of innominate and common carotid artery disease: immediate and long-term outcome for 100 consecutive surgical reconstructions. *J Vasc Surg.* 1998;**27**:34–41.
3. Takach TJ, Reul GJ, Cooley DA, et al. Brachiocephalic reconstruction I: operative and long-term results for complex disease. *J Vasc Surg.* 2005,**42**:47–54.

31

Upper extremity arterial occlusive disease

HISHAM BASSIOUNY

CONTENTS

INTRODUCTION

This chapter addresses the revascularization techniques required to relieve upper extremity critical ischemia. In contrast to the lower extremities, atherosclerotic occlusive disease is less common in the upper extremities and develops preferentially in the distal arterial bed of patients with diabetes and end-stage renal disease.

Upper extremity critical ischemia may develop from a host of pathologic conditions that involve the axillary artery and beyond,[1] including: embolism from a cardiac source; blunt or penetrating trauma; and in situ thrombosis following arterial cannulation. High-volume hemodialysis arteriovenous fistulae or grafts may siphon significant arterial flow from the hand, inducing an ischemic steal syndrome. Less frequently, arterial pathology is due to repetitive extrinsic trauma to the axillary artery in high-performance baseball pitchers and to the ulnar artery in workers who use the heel of their hands as a "hammer" (hypothenar hammer syndrome) (**Figure 31.1**). A proximal arterial aneurysm or an ulcerative plaque may also present as a source of distal embolization. Radiation and giant-cell arteritis, while uncommon, can result in diffuse stenosis of the axillobrachial axis.

Other causes of digital ischemia include vasospastic (ergotism, Raynaud syndrome) and autoimmune arteriopathies (connective tissue and myeloproliferative disorders). Such entities are unsuitable for open or endovascular revascularization techniques (**Figure 31.2**) and respond better to vasodilators or sympathectomy.[2]

CLINICAL EVALUATION

At the outset, one must determine if the clinical scenario presents as acute or chronic limb ischemia. In most instances, an accurate history and physical examination can identify the arterial segment involved and the degree of forearm and hand ischemia. The presence of classic signs and symptoms of acute ischemia, namely the six Ps (pulselessness, pallor, paralysis, paresthesia, pain, and poikilothermia), indicate that revascularization should be undertaken as an emergency during the golden 6-hour period from the onset of ischemia. Delay in reperfusion risks permanent extremity neurologic impairment. In acute thromboembolic occlusion, systemic anticoagulation is promptly started to minimize thrombus propagation. In patients suffering from joint or fracture

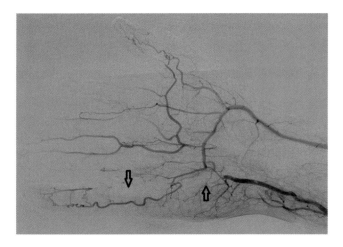

Figure 31.1 Angiography of hypothenar hammer syndrome of the right hand. The upward arrow points to distal ulnar artery occlusion as it traverses through the hypothenar region. The downward arrow points to embolic occlusion of one of the digital arteries of the little finger, resulting from clot in the thrombosed ulnar artery.

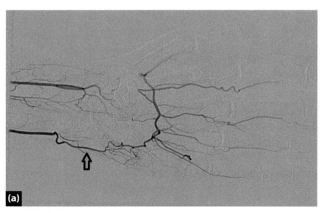

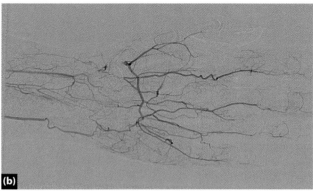

Figure 31.2 Angiography of nonreconstructible small artery occlusive disease of the left hand. (**a**) Early phase demonstrating occlusion of the distal radial and ulnar arteries. The arrow points to a large collateral around the occluded ulnar artery. (**b**) Later phase demonstrating occlusion of multiple digital arteries.

dislocations, reduction of the orthopedic injury may restore distal arterial perfusion; however, the proximate artery should be subjected to close surveillance by duplex ultrasound (US) or computed tomography (CT) angiography to identify a silent intimal injury, nonocclusive thrombus, or pseudoaneurysm.

Digital ischemia due to radial artery thrombosis from an indwelling catheter is commonly encountered in the intensive care unit setting. Initial management entails line removal, anticoagulation if feasible, and weaning of vasopressors to improve digital flow. Most of these patients are high-risk and unfit for thrombectomy or lytic therapy.

NONINVASIVE VASCULAR TESTING

As with the lower extremities, segmental pressure testing including selected digits is useful in occlusive disease to assess the degree of ischemia and the level of any detected obstructive lesions. Digital pressure measurements are useful to diagnose vasospastic disorders with cold immersion. Improvement in digital pressures during arteriovenous access compression helps substantiate the diagnosis of ischemic steal syndrome.[3] Duplex US is invaluable as a first-line, noninvasive test to define the nature and extent of arterial pathology. The examination should include imaging of the arterial tree from the proximal axillary artery to the wrist. High-resolution B-mode imaging can readily distinguish acute thromboembolism, diffuse radiation-induced fibrotic stenosis or autoimmune vasculitis, aneurysmal degeneration, and any associated venous pathology. In suspected athletic injuries, positional shoulder maneuvers assist in detecting muscular entrapment of the axillobrachial artery or humeral head compression. In cases of isolated digital ischemia, patency of the palmar arch can be evaluated with duplex imaging; however, selective arteriography provides a more comprehensive assessment of palmar arch integrity and digital artery patency.

INDICATIONS FOR UPPER EXTREMITY ARTERIOGRAPHY

In acute ischemic conditions, preoperative conventional or CT arteriography may add little to the physical examination and a high-quality arterial duplex evaluation. That said, intraoperative arteriography is essential to confirm outflow patency beyond the site of the arterial reconstruction. In the case of extensive forearm and hand arterial thrombosis, arteriography helps guide decision-making for thrombolysis and catheter placement for optimum drug delivery. In chronic arterial ischemia, CT arteriography provides sufficient information in many situations to formulate an intervention strategy for correcting the ischemic condition. Suboptimal visualization of distal runoff arteries in the distal forearm and hand by CT arteriography should prompt further selective conventional arteriography to determine the feasibility of planned revascularization procedures.

OPEN SURGICAL REVASCULARIZATION

The revascularization technique is selected according to the arterial pathology encountered. **Figure 31.3** illustrates the preferred incisions for the operative exposure of various arterial segments.

Thromboembolectomy

Emboli of cardiac origin can be readily removed by exposure of the distal brachial artery and its bifurcation via a longitudinal skin incision just distal to the elbow crease in the proximal forearm. The median nerve is in close proximity and should be kept out of harm's way. Division of the bicipital aponeurosis facilitates exposure. An adequate length (2–3 cm) of the artery is dissected and the vessel is looped to allow for proximal and distal control.

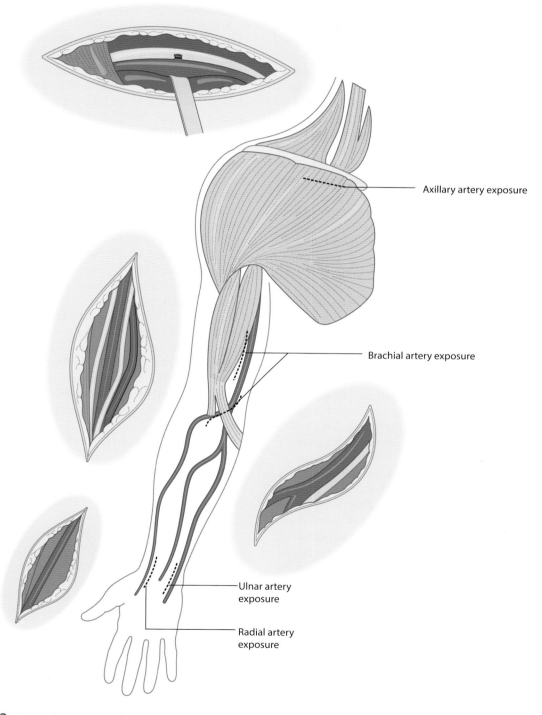

Axillary artery exposure

Brachial artery exposure

Ulnar artery exposure

Radial artery exposure

Figure 31.3 Surgical exposures of the axillary, brachial, and ulnar and radial arteries.

Before clamping, systemic anticoagulation with heparin is augmented to achieve an activated clotting time >200 seconds. Fine bulldog or pediatric arterial clamps are used for proximal and distal clamping. A 3-mm transverse arteriotomy is performed with a No. 11 scalpel blade on the brachial artery, just above its bifurcation, to allow selective catheterization of the radial and ulnar arteries as necessary. The thromboembolus is extracted with a 3- or 4-Fr Fogarty catheter introduced proximally and a 2- or 3-Fr catheter distally. The catheter is advanced proximally to the subclavian artery to extract any residual proximal thrombus and to achieve brisk arterial inflow. While retrieving the thrombus from the distal arterial bed, it is crucial to avoid balloon overinflation and iatrogenic injury of the forearm outflow vessels. Complete removal of the occluding thromboembolus may require several catheter passages to accomplish satisfactory pulsatile inflow and back-bleeding. Completion arteriography is performed to document clearance of the all-important thrombus. The arteriotomy is repaired with an interrupted 6-0 polypropylene suture to avoid purse stringing and narrowing of the artery lumen. The artery is fore- and back-bled before complete arteriotomy closure.

Restoration of palpable radial and ulnar pulses indicates successful thromboembolectomy. Lack of a palpable distal pulse should prompt evaluation of the distal arterial tree with arteriography, if not already performed. Intraoperative fluoroscopy with roadmapping assists in the guidance of over-the-wire thrombectomy catheters in the forearm arteries. When available, over-the-wire coronary suction thrombectomy catheters assist in thrombus retrieval. Should arteriography demonstrate segmental vasospasm, intra-arterial infusion of a vasodilator (e.g., 30–60 mg of dilute papaverine or 100 μg aliquots of nitroglycerin diluted in normal saline) should be considered. Additional cutdown on the distal radial and ulnar arteries at the wrist may be necessary to extract residual thrombus. In the forearm arteries, longitudinal vein patch closure may minimize the risk of iatrogenic stenosis with primary repair.

Intraoperative, catheter-directed thrombolysis is rarely necessary but should be considered to clear residual thrombus distal to the wrist. No more than 5 mg of tissue plasminogen activator should be given intraoperatively; the infusion can be continued at 1–2 mg per hour postoperatively. In this instance, the catheter is removed in the operating room following a satisfactory completion arteriogram.

Arterial reconstruction

Autogenous conduits, namely the greater saphenous vein and more recently the radial artery,[4] are the conduits of choice for reconstruction of the axillary artery and beyond. The greater saphenous vein is preferred over the cephalic or basilic vein because of ease of handling and

length requirements. The cephalic and basilic veins, however, should be preserved in traumatic injuries associated with deep vein injury to avoid venous hypertension and possible resulting compartment syndrome.

Interposition bypass grafting

Interposition bypass grafting is the technique of choice for traumatic injuries and aneurysmal degeneration of the axillary and brachial arteries (**Figure 31.4**). Transmural or significant intimal damage related to repetitive athletic or occupational trauma, orthopedic traction injury, and penetrating or blast injuries should be resected to healthy margins. While it is sometimes possible to mobilize the artery and perform an end-to-end arterial anastomosis in limited injuries, caution should be exercised to avoid undue tension or kinking because this may lead to subsequent suture line disruption or in situ thrombosis. With interposition bypass grafting, the proximal and distal anastomoses are performed in an end-to-end fashion with anterior and posterior spatulation of the artery and vein, respectively, to avoid suture line stenosis. For the upper arm arteries, a running suture starting from both corners of the anastomosis is used, while interrupted sutures are advised for forearm anastomoses.

Careful attention is paid to conduit course and length to avoid musculofascial entrapment or repetitive trauma by a bony prominence. A subcutaneous course is preferred to facilitate conduit access for postoperative clinical and duplex surveillance and for redo procedures. Conduits traversing the elbow joint should be of sufficient length to avoid tension on the anastomotic suture lines when the joint is fully extended. Reduction and fixation of fracture dislocation(s) in the arm and forearm may inadvertently alter conduit course or orientation. Hence, conduit integrity and patency must be verified before exiting the operating room after orthopedic manipulation and fixation.

For distal ulnar artery bypass, the conduit of choice is the contralateral radial artery because of a better size match and superior long-term performance. Continuity of the palmar arch is evaluated by an Allen test and duplex imaging before the radial artery is harvested.

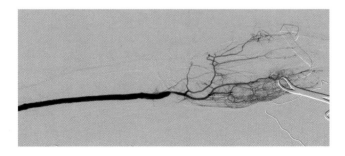

Figure 31.4 Upper extremity arterial interposition bypass graft from brachial artery to distal radial artery with a reversed greater saphenous vein conduit.

Either end-to-side or end-to-end anastomosis is performed with an interrupted or running 7-0 polypropylene suture.

Endarterectomy and vein patch angioplasty

Endarterectomy is used rarely. The sole indication might be a focal stenosis at a joint line where balloon angioplasty has failed.

Distal revascularization and interval ligation

Patients with ischemic steal syndrome due to high-flow brachial arteriovenous conduits are candidates for a distal revascularization and interval ligation (DRIL) procedure (**Figure 31.5**). A disease-free brachial artery proximal to the arterial anastomosis, an adequate saphenous vein conduit, and reasonable forearm outflow are essential for a successful DRIL procedure.[5]

Initially, the brachial artery is ligated just distal to the arteriovenous anastomosis above the elbow crease. This is followed by distal revascularization to restore arterial perfusion to the forearm and hand. The location of the proximal anastomosis of the distal revascularization bypass is the key variable for hemodynamic efficacy of the procedure. The anastomosis must be created 5–10 cm proximal to the arteriovenous anastomosis where there is normal systemic pressure to drive blood flow into the bypass and the arteriovenous communication. Intra-arterial pressure measurements help to select the optimum region for the proximal anastomosis. Distally, the bypass is anastomosed

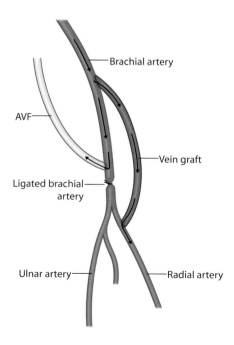

Figure 31.5 Distal revascularization and interval ligation procedure for steal syndrome in patients with upper extremity arteriovenous fistulae.

in an end-to-side fashion to the brachial artery, below the elbow, or to the proximal radial or ulnar arteries.

Endovascular interventions: Indications and techniques

Indications for catheter-directed interventions include: thrombolysis[6] for acute thrombotic occlusions that are inaccessible with surgical techniques; focal or diffuse stenosis; and aneurysmal disease. Access site depends on the location of the lesion. Axillary or proximal brachial artery pathology requires either a transfemoral or retrograde transbrachial route. For forearm arterial pathology, antegrade brachial access is used. Access with low-profile sheaths (5 and 6 Fr) is advised. It remains debatable whether a percutaneous or open cutdown technique is safest. If a percutaneous technique is used, US-guided puncture is advised. The author prefers the open cutdown technique for several reasons: (1) relative ease in exposing the upper arm vessels with a limited incision; (2) direct closure of the puncture site, which avoids hematoma formation and allows for continuing systemic anticoagulation; and (3) primary closure, which minimizes the risk of in situ thrombosis from compression of the puncture site after percutaneous sheath removal.

For stenotic lesions, plain balloon angioplasty is used. Because the advantage of drug-eluting balloons in upper extremity atherosclerotic or vasculitic stenosis is unknown, such balloons may be considered for off-label use in restenotic lesions. Stenting across joint lines is ill-advised to avoid stent compression and fracture. Treating the rare case of an axillobrachial artery aneurysm with a covered (self-expanding or balloon-mounted) stent is a reasonable option in patients deemed at high risk for surgery.

Catheter-directed interventions[7] may be more frequently employed as experience evolves; however, further studies examining the long-term efficacy of such interventions for upper extremity arterial occlusive disease are needed.

COMPLICATIONS

Because most patients who suffer from upper extremity acute thromboembolic occlusion have disease-free arteries, it is not uncommon to encounter segmental vasospasm of the forearm and hand arteries on completion arteriography after Fogarty catheter thrombus retrieval. The dictum "spasm is CLOT until proven otherwise" should be exercised with caution. Repeat arteriography after intra-arterial administration of papaverine or nitroglycerine should be undertaken to resolve this quandary. The operator must consider the risk of intimal damage with repetitive catheter passage. If there is adequate arterial continuity to the entire palmar arch, it is unnecessary to persist in recanalizing all forearm arteries to minimize the risk of iatrogenic arterial injury. In this scenario "the enemy of good is better."

Another potential complication is clamp injury to the forearm and hand vessels, which can be heavily calcified in patients with diabetes and those undergoing dialysis. Use of a tourniquet is highly advised to avoid clamping while creating an anastomosis to such a vessel, though sometimes proximal vessels are too calcified to be successfully occluded even in this fashion. Alternatively, intraluminal balloons can be used for control.

REFERENCES

1. Longo GM, Pearce WH, Sumner DS. Evaluation of upper extremity ischemia. In: Rutherford RB, ed. *Vascular Surgery*. 6th ed. Philadelphia, PA: Elsevier/ Saunders; 2005. pp. 1274–1293.
2. Herrick AL. Management of Raynaud's phenomenon and digital ischemia. *Curr Rheumatol Rep.* 2013;**15**:303.
3. Grasu BL, Jones CM, Murphy MS. Use of diagnostic modalities for assessing upper extremity vascular pathology. *Hand Clin.* 2015;**31**:1–12.
4. Masden DL, Seruya M, Higgins JP. A systematic review of the outcomes of distal upper extremity bypass surgery with arterial and venous conduits. *J Hand Surg Am.* 2012;**37**:2362–2367.
5. Aimaq R, Katz SG. Using distal revascularization with interval ligation as the primary treatment of hand ischemia after dialysis access creation. *J Vasc Surg.* 2013;**57**:1073–1078.
6. Schrijver AM, De Borst GJ, Van Herwaarden JA, et al. Catheter-directed thrombolysis for acute upper extremity ischemia. *J Cardiovasc Surg (Torino).* 2015;**56**:433–439.
7. Tomoi Y, Soga Y, Fujihara M, et al. Outcomes of endovascular therapy for upper extremity peripheral artery disease with critical hand ischemia. *J Endovasc Ther.* 2016;**23**:717–722.

32

Open nonruptured infrarenal aortic aneurysm repair

ALEXANDER D. SHEPARD

CONTENTS

INTRODUCTION

In the endovascular era, open repair of infrarenal abdominal aortic aneurysms (AAAs) is infrequently performed and is usually done only for aneurysms with complex anatomy not amenable to stent grafting. The surgeon needs a thorough understanding of the various open techniques to provide optimal care for such patients. Different approaches are available with distinct advantages and disadvantages.

APPROACHES

Transperitoneal exposure remains the standard. When performed through a midline incision, it is the most versatile approach allowing unlimited exposure of the infrarenal aorta (IRA) and its branches (**Figure 32.1**). No special positioning is required, so it is faster than a left flank retroperitoneal approach and hence more suitable for emergencies. When combined with medial visceral rotation, it also provides exposure of the suprarenal aorta to the level of the aortic hiatus. The biggest problem with this approach is the high incidence (20–25%) of postoperative incisional hernia. Transverse incisions are less prone to hernias and less painful; hence, they are of value in patients with pulmonary compromise. A supraumbilical transverse (frown) incision is particularly helpful when contemplating concomitant distal renal artery reconstruction, while an infraumbilical transverse (smile) incision is useful when good pelvic exposure for large iliac/hypogastric aneurysms is needed. Exposure beyond the iliac bifurcation is

harder with a supraumbilical incision, while exposure of the pararenal aorta is difficult through an infraumbilical incision.

A left flank retroperitoneal approach is increasingly useful for complex open repair of AAAs. The entire abdominal aorta, from hiatus to bifurcation, can be exposed with this approach. The only limitations are the visualization of the distal right iliac artery (RIA) system and the nonostial right renal artery. Situations in which this approach is helpful include: need to expose the aorta proximal to the renal arteries; redo aortic surgery; AAAs associated with horseshoe kidney; large (>8 cm) or inflammatory AAAs; "hostile" abdomen (multiple prior celiotomies or ostomies); morbid obesity; diastasis of the abdominal wall; and, because of less pain than midline incisions, pulmonary compromise.

PREPARATION FOR SURGERY

Careful review of preoperative computed tomography angiography (CTA) is necessary to identify concomitant intra-abdominal pathology and venous anomalies (e.g., retroaortic left renal vein (LRV)), determine clamp sites, and plan the type of reconstruction. An epidural catheter is useful for postoperative analgesia to decrease the surgical stress response and reduce pulmonary complications. Central line, arterial line, Foley catheter, and large-bore intravenous lines are routine; the author rarely places pulmonary artery catheters anymore and relies on transesophageal echocardiography for cardiac

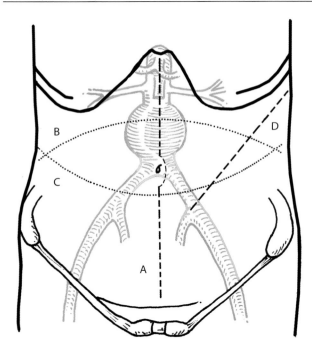

Figure 32.1 Different incisions available for performance of infrarenal abdominal aortic aneurysm repair. (A) Midline. (B) Supraumbilical transverse (frown). (C) Infraumbilical transverse (smile). (D) Left flank.

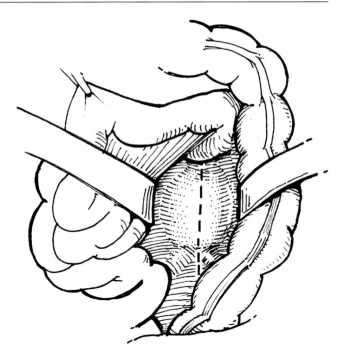

Figure 32.2 Initial inframesocolic exposure of infrarenal abdominal aortic aneurysm with transverse colon reflected superiorly, small bowel retracted to the right, and descending/sigmoid colon retracted to the left.

monitoring when necessary. Cell savers (autologous blood recovery systems), body warmers, and lower extremity sequential compression sleeves are also standard.

TRANSPERITONEAL APPROACH

The abdomen is opened through a long xiphoid-to-pubis midline incision. Complete exploration of the abdomen is rarely undertaken today because of the frequency and accuracy of preoperative CTA. Use of a large mechanical retraction system (e.g., Integra® Omni-Tract, Integra LifeSciences Corporation, Plainsboro, NJ, USA; Thompson retractor, Thompson Surgical Instruments, Traverse City, MI, USA) eliminates the need for personnel other than a single assistant. The IRA is exposed through an inframesocolic approach. The greater omentum and transverse colon are reflected superiorly out of the abdomen, while the small bowel is retracted to the right (**Figure 32.2**). The author prefers to pack the small bowel into the right side of the abdomen rather than retracting it out of the abdomen, because the latter leads to compression of the vasculature and creates more bowel swelling by the end of the procedure. The ligament of Treitz is divided to mobilize the duodenum off the aortic neck and to allow full mobilization of the small bowel.

The midline retroperitoneum overlying the aneurysm is incised longitudinally from the proximal neck to the bifurcation; the overlying lymphoareolar tissue is divided. The dissection is carried proximally looking for the LRV, which for most infrarenal aneurysms marks the proximal extent of the necessary exposure (**Figure 32.3**).

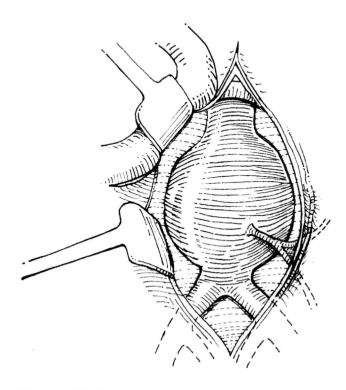

Figure 32.3 Incision through the retroperitoneum to expose an infrarenal aneurysm from the crossing left renal vein superiorly to the bifurcation distally. The inferior mesenteric artery is the only major branch originating anteriorly.

During this dissection, the inferior mesenteric vein is frequently encountered in a more superficial plane. Ligation and division of this vein can be performed to improve exposure. The LRV is cleaned off for a short distance to improve visualization of the underlying aorta. Lymphatics along the inferior margin of the vein require careful ligation to avoid a chyle leak; an ultrasonic scalpel is helpful in this regard. Once the aorta is identified, dissection stays on the aorta and the neck (nonaneurysmal aorta) is cleared off anteriorly and on either side down to the lumbar spine, enough to allow the application of a vertically oriented cross-clamp. Circumferential dissection of the proximal aorta is unnecessary. When exposing the proximal neck, one must watch out for the posteriorly coursing lumbar branch of the LRV, which may need to be ligated and divided to avoid injury.

If more proximal aortic exposure is required, the LRV may be either mobilized or ligated and divided. Mobilization involves freeing up the vein from entry into the inferior vena cava (IVC) back toward the hilum of the kidney with division of all the major branches distal to the kidney (lumbar branch, and gonadal and adrenal veins) (**Figure 32.4**). It is important to decide which technique (mobilization or division) to use because preservation of these branches is critical to providing collateral outflow to the kidney if LRV division is chosen. To avoid damage to these distal tributaries, the LRV should be divided as close to the IVC as possible.

As dissection is carried distally down the aorta, the origin of the inferior mesenteric artery (IMA) should be

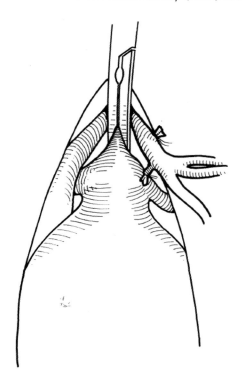

Figure 32.4 Mobilization of the left renal vein following division of the adrenal and lumbar branches to expose the pararenal aorta and allow placement of a suprarenal aortic cross-clamp.

identified and protected. The aortic bifurcation is identified and special attention is paid to the parasympathetic nerve chain passing over the origin of the left common iliac artery (CIA), which is carefully preserved. Great care is exercised when mobilizing the proximal CIAs for fear of injuring the caval confluence or iliac veins posteriorly. These venous structures can be adherent to the iliac arteries secondary to aneurysm- or atherosclerosis-induced inflammation. Clamping the iliac arteries slightly more distally may be safer. Venous injuries in this area can be quite challenging to repair; sometimes, they require aortic clamping and iliac artery division for adequate visualization. The midline retroperitoneal incision can be extended down over the RIA to expose it at any point along its course. Alternatively, if only distal RIA (bifurcation or beyond) exposure is necessary, a second short retroperitoneal incision over the artery can be made taking care to identify, mobilize, and protect the ureter as necessary. The proximal left CIA can be exposed from the midline incision in the retroperitoneum. For distal left iliac artery (LIA) exposure, the sigmoid colon is mobilized after dividing the lateral peritoneal reflection. If necessary because of iliac occlusive disease, the femoral arteries can be exposed through standard groin incisions, though the author prefers to avoid distal anastomoses at the femoral level whenever possible because of the associated increased risk of wound complications.

Before aortic clamping, patients are heparinized (100 IU/kg to maintain an activated clotting time >250 seconds). This test is repeated every 30 minutes during clamping, and additional heparin is administered as necessary. Lower body warmers and lower extremity sequential compression sleeves are turned off before clamping. Distal arteries are usually clamped before proximal arteries. The proximal aortic clamp site is chosen carefully. It is important to avoid multiple clamp applications, particularly with a diseased or calcified aorta or when clamping above the renal arteries. Clamp nondiseased aorta when possible; sometimes, this requires clamping the supraceliac aorta, which is reliably the least diseased segment of the abdominal aorta. The CHERRY clamp (Becton, Dickinson and Company, Franklin Lakes, NJ, USA) is our preferred clamp.

Standard repair is accomplished with an intraluminal technique, from within the aneurysm sac. Resection of the entire aneurysm sac and grafting is occasionally still used for very small or infected AAAs, but has been supplanted by intraluminal repair because of reduced blood loss, less injury to adjacent structures, speed, and because leaving the aneurysm sac in place provides better coverage of the aortic graft. Before clamping, a graft sizer can be helpful in deciding which size graft to use; the author's experience suggests that choosing a graft one size smaller than measured by the sizer on the pressurized aorta (e.g., 18 mm when the sizer suggests 20 mm) usually gives the best match when sewing to a nonpressurized undistended aorta. The author prefers Dacron to polytetrafluoroethylene (PTFE), unless there is significant iliac occlusive disease, because of concerns for perigraft seromas when using PTFE. After clamping, the aneurysm sac is opened longitudinally from a point just distal to the planned proximal anastomotic suture line to just above the aortic bifurcation, taking care to go to the right of the IMA and to avoid the autonomic nerves crossing the left iliac origin. The intraluminal mural thrombus is bluntly removed and back-bleeding lumbar arteries are identified and oversewn with 3-0 polypropylene suture (**Figure 32.5**). If the back wall is heavily calcified, it is frequently easier to perform an endarterectomy around the lumbar arteries that allows transfixing stitches to secure down appropriately. If the IMA demonstrates good back-bleeding, it can be suture-ligated from the inside; if back-bleeding from a patent IMA appears questionable, then the IMA can be controlled by either placing a small clamp across its origin or inserting and inflating a 3-Fr balloon catheter.

Reconstruction proceeds with a tube or bifurcated graft. A tube graft is faster and is suitable when there is no significant iliac occlusive disease and the CIAs are ≤16 mm in diameter, unless the patient is very young or has a known connective tissue disorder. Tube grafts are avoided when preservation of sexual function is a concern because it is difficult not to injure the parasympathetic plexus that courses over the LIA when trying to create a distal sewing ring. In younger patients, avoiding injury to these "sex" nerves is sometimes most easily accomplished by tunneling the limbs of a bifurcated graft through the origins of the iliac arteries, leaving the aortic bifurcation intact. When sewing to the iliac arteries, always try to get beyond all aneurysmal disease and preserve flow to at least one hypogastric artery (HGA).

A proximal sewing ring is created by "T-ing" off the aortotomy at the junction between the normal aorta and the aneurysm sac, and incising the lateral walls of the aorta to leave only the posterior third of the wall intact (**Figure 32.6**). Avoid sewing to aneurysmal aorta except in extenuating circumstances. Extensive, full-thickness endarterectomy of calcified aorta is also avoided because of the risk of further weakening an already abnormal aortic wall. If a bifurcated graft is chosen, the main shaft is trimmed to leave no more than a few centimeters. The proximal anastomosis is created with a running 3-0 polypropylene suture on a medium half needle (e.g. SH) beginning at one corner or the other of the posterior wall and incorporating double-thickness stitches of the back wall before transitioning to single-layer bites for the remainder of the anastomosis. After securing and testing this anastomosis, attention is directed to the distal anastomosis or anastomoses. A distal aortic sewing ring can be created at the bifurcation by T-ing off the aorta in identical fashion to proximally. After pressurizing the graft, it is trimmed to an appropriate length and the distal anastomosis is performed similar to the proximal. The posterior wall just above the bifurcation can be quite calcified making needle passage challenging. Local endarterectomy is usually not possible without the risk of creating a flap in one or both iliac arteries. Creating a track for needle passage with a penetrating towel clip is a useful maneuver for traversing a short segment of such a calcified wall. Iliac anastomoses are usually easier because there is less disease. When constructing an iliac end-to-end anastomosis, the author

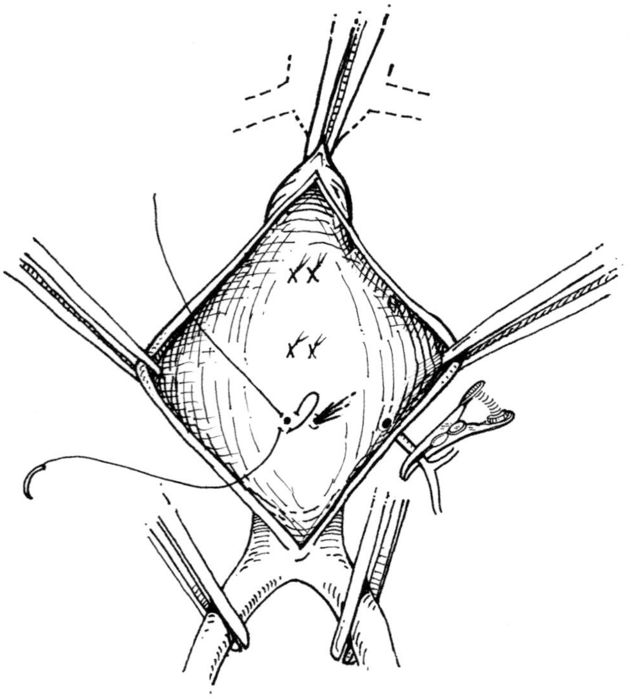

Figure 32.5 Aneurysm sac opened with oversewing of back-bleeding lumbar arteries. Inferior mesenteric artery controlled with small bulldog clamp.

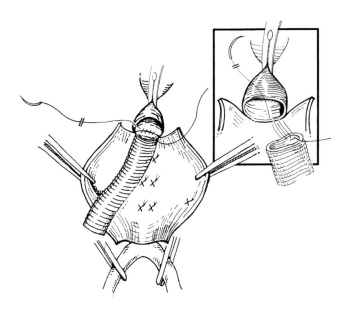

Figure 32.6 Aorta "T-d off" proximally and distally to create sewing rings for tube graft anastomoses. The inset shows proximal aorta-to-graft anastomosis constructed via a "parachute" technique with double-thickness bites through the nontransected posterior wall (Creech maneuver).

usually transects the artery completely after dissecting the posterior wall off the adjacent vein, which is much easier with a nonpressurized artery. It is important to get full-thickness bites because the adventitia tends to peel away from the media on the iliac arteries.

With CIA aneurysms, it is sometimes difficult to preserve flow into the HGAs if the origins of the external iliac artery (EIA) and HGA are splayed apart. In this situation, it is impossible to create a distal anastomosis incorporating both vessels. A variety of reconstruction techniques are available for this situation, but the easiest for the author has been to perform an end-to-end anastomosis of the graft limb to the HGA and then sew the EIA end-to-side to the graft limb, if there is enough redundancy in this vessel, or perform an interposition jump graft to the EIA if there is not (**Figure 32.7**). This is much easier than trying to reimplant the HGA into the side of a graft limb that has already been sewn into the EIA. After reconstructing one HGA in this fashion, the contralateral one may be safely ligated. When going to the iliac arteries, it is important to tunnel the graft limbs posterior to the ureters to avoid entrapping them in the scar tissue that occurs when the graft is tunneled superficial to them.

Before completing a distal anastomosis, the graft and distal vessel(s) should be vented to remove any athero-thrombotic material that could embolize into the distal circulation. Once the anastomosis is secured, flow is restored to the lower extremity(ies); this requires careful communication with the anesthesia team. One leg at a time is unclamped and the femoral artery on that side is compressed to direct any loose debris into the HGAs and to reduce the severity of the hemodynamic alterations caused by reperfusion. A drop in pressure of at least 20 mmHg is expected when the first leg is opened; anything less may be a sign of inadequate restoration of flow to that extremity. Following restoration of flow to both legs, distal perfusion is verified by palpating pedal pulses or checking pedal Doppler flow signals. If there was concern over IMA back-bleeding previously, it should be rechecked at this point, making sure to remove any retractor blades that may be inadvertently compressing the meandering mesenteric or other collaterals. If back-bleeding remains poor, implanting the IMA into the graft may be necessary. The IMA is excised along with a small button of adjacent aorta. It is usually necessary to endarterectomize this button and great care should be taken to avoid raising a flap into the proximal IMA. While it is possible to place a deep, partially occluding clamp on an aortic tube graft, the author has found it much easier to implant the IMA into the left limb of a bifurcated graft after occluding it proximally and distally (**Figure 32.8**). In this situation, it is important to anticipate this eventuality so that the main shaft of the graft is not left too long. A small disc of graft wall is excised

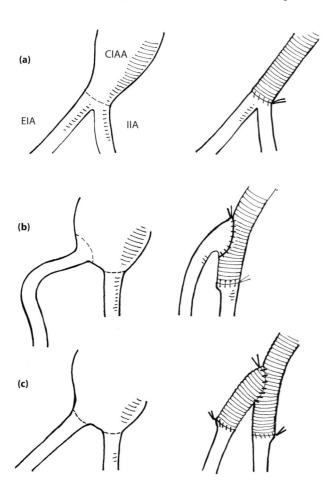

Figure 32.7 Iliac artery bifurcation reconstruction techniques. (**a**) Limb sewn to bifurcation. (**b**) Limb sewn to hypogastric artery with reimplantation of end of redundant external iliac artery (EIA) into the side of the graft. (**c**) Limb sewn to the internal iliac artery with jump graft to the EIA. CIAA: common iliac artery aneurysm; IIA: internal iliac (or hypogastric) artery.

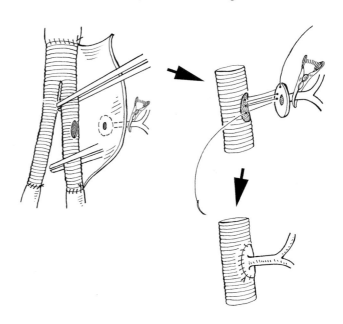

Figure 32.8 Inferior mesenteric artery reconstruction. Left limb of an aortoiliac graft occluded proximally and distally with creation of a small graftotomy to which a Carrel patch containing the inferior mesenteric artery is sewn.

to allow an end-to-side anastomosis with 5-0 or 6-0 polypropylene suture. After restoration of IMA flow, heparin anticoagulation is reversed and the hemostatic profile is corrected as necessary. Following hemostasis, the aneurysm sac is closed over the graft with absorbable suture and the edges of the retroperitoneal incision are reapproximated (**Figure 32.9**). Great care should be taken during

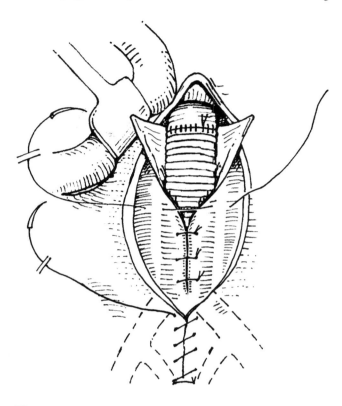

Figure 32.9 The aneurysm sac wall is closed over the graft, followed by reapproximation of edges of the retroperitoneal opening to prevent bowel adhesion to the prosthetic graft.

fascial closure because of the documented high incidence of incisional hernias in this population.

RETROPERITONEAL APPROACH

Proper patient positioning is key to this approach. The patient is placed in a modified right lateral decubitus position with the shoulders positioned at 70 degrees to the table and the hips rotated as far posteriorly as possible. Such axial rotation is important when groin incisions for femoral exposure are anticipated (**Figure 32.10**). A vacuum "beanbag" is helpful in maintaining this alignment. The midpoint between the patient's right costal margin and right iliac crest is centered over the break in the table and the table can be "jackknifed" to open the left flank as needed. The primary operator stands on the patient's left and the table is rotated to the right during incision and intra-abdominal exposure, and all the way back to the left to flatten out the hips as much as possible if a groin or right-lower-quadrant counterincision is required.

For infrarenal aortic procedures, the standard flank incision extends from the lateral margin of the left rectus sheath, midway between the umbilicus and symphysis pubis, laterally into the 11th intercostal space (ICS) for 8–10 cm. When exposure of the pararenal aorta is necessary, a 10th ICS incision is more suitable. The abdominal wall and intercostal musculature are divided in the line of the incision and the extraperitoneal space is entered at the tip of the 12th rib. The peritoneum, often with the overlying transversalis fascia, is stripped away from the abdominal wall musculature anteriorly as far as the rectus sheath. Posterolaterally, the plane of the flank and psoas musculature are followed as the peritoneal sac and its contents are retracted anteriorly. This plane is developed superficial to the lumbodorsal fascia (the posterior

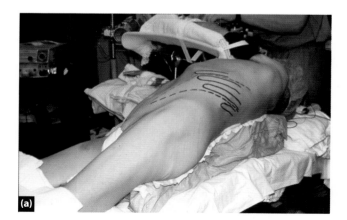
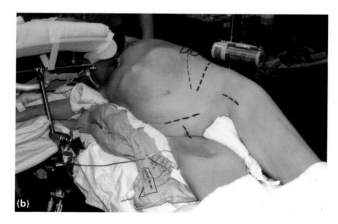

Figure 32.10 Patient positioning for left flank retroperitoneal approach. (**a**) View from the left (surgeon's) side of table showing vacuum "beanbag." Chest is at 70 degrees to the table while the hips are rotated posteriorly. A lower-most incision in the 11th intercostal space (ICS) is typically used for infrarenal abdominal aortic aneurysm, while an upper incision in the 9th ICS is most useful for extent IV thoracoabdominal aortic aneurysms. The 10th ICS incision (not shown) is most commonly used for pararenal AAAs. (**b**) View from the right side of the table demonstrating bilateral vertical groin incisions and right-lower-quadrant counterincision sometimes used to expose the right external iliac artery extraperitoneally.

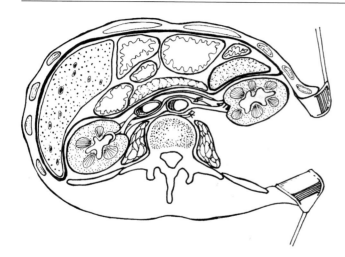

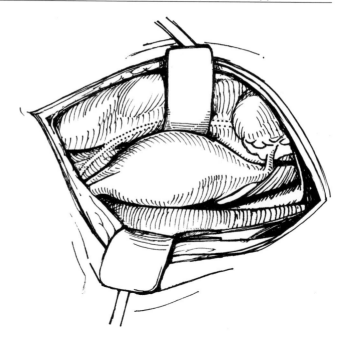

Figure 32.11 Cross-sectional view demonstrating the standard dissection plane posterior to the left kidney used with left flank retroperitoneal exposure. The lumbar branch of the left renal vein has been ligated and divided.

Figure 32.12 Left flank retroperitoneal exposure of infrarenal aorta from crus crossing over aorta just above left renal artery to aortic bifurcation. The dotted line is the course of left ureter.

extension of the transversalis fascia), behind the left kidney, so that the left ureter and kidney are also reflected anteriorly (**Figure 32.11**). Small bridging veins can cause troublesome bleeding and should be carefully cauterized when identified before division. The abdominal aorta and, more caudally, the LIA are exposed in the base of the wound. The left renal artery (LRA) is the only significant structure that can now be injured; it is therefore critical to identify and protect this vessel during the early stages of dissection. In thin patients, this artery is usually easy to palpate as it courses anteriorly off the left lateral wall of the aorta to the retracted left kidney. In individuals with more abundant retroperitoneal fat, some dissection is usually necessary. The lumbar branch of the LRV crossing over the aorta proximally is a reliable landmark, with the artery identifiable just above and proximally. This vein must be carefully ligated and divided to provide adequate exposure of the infrarenal aortic neck. If the lumbar branch is much larger than normal, then the preoperative CTA should be reexamined to ensure that the patient does not have a retroaortic LRV. In this situation, it may be necessary to leave the kidney "down" in its normal anatomic position and expose the aorta anterior to the kidney to avoid ligating the LRV. Once the LRA has been identified, the left posterolateral wall of the aorta can be safely exposed by dividing the overlying lymphatics and periaortic fat; an ultrasonic scalpel can be quite useful for this step as dissection is carried distally toward the bifurcation (**Figure 32.12**).

Following definition of the neck of the aneurysm, dissection anterior and posterior to the aorta establishes a plane for placement of a cross-clamp; no attempt is made to dissect the aorta circumferentially as long as the clamp arms can pass beyond its far wall. The vena cava is not immediately adjacent to the aorta at this level, so caval injury is not a concern. When suprarenal aortic control

is necessary, dissection proceeds cephalad along the aorta toward the left diaphragmatic crus, which is identified as a firm tendinous band crossing the aorta just proximal to the origin of the LRA. The crural fibers are divided 2–3 cm along the axis of the aorta and the underlying aortic wall is exposed. The origin of the LRA is cleared off and finger dissection anterior and posterior to the aorta creates a plane for clamp placement. A pair of lumbar arteries at this level should be carefully watched for and avoided. For supraceliac aortic control, the crural fibers are divided an additional 5 cm and the fascia investing the aorta is incised to allow fingertip dissection anterior and posterior to the aorta. Supraceliac aortic control is in fact easier to obtain with this approach than is suprarenal aortic control because of the relative absence of retroperitoneal fat and lymphatics at this level. When anticipating the need for supraceliac aortic control preoperatively, access can be improved by a 10th ICS incision.

After obtaining proximal control, the peritoneal sac is stripped out of the left iliac fossa to expose the iliac arteries. Care should be taken to mobilize the left ureter along with the peritoneal sac. The left CIA can be readily visualized and controlled along its entire length, but only the proximal-most right CIA can be exposed from this approach, particularly in the presence of a large aortic aneurysm. Division of the IMA (if this can be done safely) and further mobilization of the peritoneal sac to the patient's right can be helpful. A useful alternative is to obtain endoluminal control of the RIA with a balloon occlusion catheter or a small Foley catheter inserted into the proximal artery after clamping the aorta and

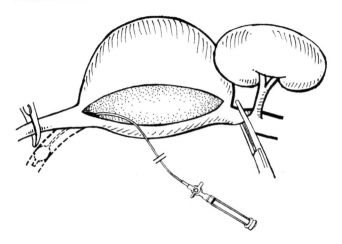

Figure 32.13 Balloon occlusion catheter controlling the right common iliac artery in a patient with a large infrarenal abdominal aortic aneurysm (AAA). The figure also demonstrates the ease of clamping the infrarenal neck of a large AAA from this approach as opposed to a transperitoneal, midline approach.

opening the aneurysm (**Figure 32.13**). More distal RIA exposure is also facilitated by bringing the flank incision all the way to the midline (linea alba), though even in this circumstance exposure beyond the iliac bifurcation is usually not possible. When more distal exposure is required, a small right-lower-quadrant incision a few centimeters above the inguinal ligament with extraperitoneal exposure of the right EIA can be performed (in nonobese patients) after the table has been rotated to the left as far as possible. If femoral anastomoses are necessary because of occlusive disease, groin incisions can be performed, again after posterior rotation of the table. In this circumstance, the location of the femoral arteries should be marked out preoperatively after the patient has been positioned because the required incisions will be shifted further to the patient's left than with routine supine exposure. In obese patients, the right groin may be somewhat obscured by an overhanging panniculus, but it can usually be exposed with sufficient retraction.

It is important to note that the right RA (RRA) is relatively inaccessible with this approach. Endarterectomy of a short, discrete ostial lesion is possible as is bypass to the very proximal RRA, though this latter maneuver can be challenging. The LRA is accessible along its entire course allowing

easy bypass grafting. Lumbar branches are also more easily visualized than with a traditional transperitoneal approach allowing ligation before opening the aneurysm sac, a step that can reduce blood loss considerably.

After appropriate exposure, aneurysm repair with this approach is identical to transperitoneal midline repair. Following hemostasis, the aneurysm sac is closed around the graft, but there is no need for reperitonealization. Wound closure is facilitated by flattening the table out of the jackknife position (if used). Any incision made in the left diaphragm is oversewn during wound closure and pleural air is evacuated through a temporary 16-Fr red rubber catheter following lung insufflation. Rib reapproximation is carried out with a looped No. 1 polydioxanone (PDS) suture on a blunt needle. The three muscle layers of the abdominal wall are closed separately with running 0 or 2-0 PDS suture.

Besides the limited exposure of the RIA and RRA, disadvantages of this approach compared to midline transperitoneal exposure include the slightly longer amount of time required for patient positioning and wound opening/closure, and the inability to fully explore the entire abdomen. Advantages include reduced evaporative fluid losses, reduced ileus, and reduced incisional pain. Given the complex nature of most open infrarenal AAA repairs being performed today, left flank retroperitoneal exposure is currently the author's approach of choice.

SUGGESTED READING

Chaikof EL, Brewster DC, Dalman RL, et al. The care of patients with an abdominal aortic aneurysm: the Society for Vascular Surgery practice guidelines. *J Vasc Surg.* 2009;**50(4 Suppl)**:S2–49.

Conrad MF, Crawford RS, Pedraza JD, et al. Long-term durability of open abdominal aortic aneurysm repair. *J Vasc Surg.* 2007;**46**:669–675.

Creech OJ Jr. Endo-aneurysmorrhaphy and treatment of aortic aneurysm. *Ann Surg.* 1966;**164**:935–946.

Shepard AD, Tollefson DF, Reddy DJ, et al. Left flank retroperitoneal exposure: a technical aid to complex aortic reconstruction. *J Vasc Surg.* 1991;**14**:283–291.

Sicard GA, Reilly JM, Rubin BG, et al. Transabdominal versus retroperitoneal incision for abdominal aortic surgery: report of a prospective randomized trial. *J Vasc Surg.* 1995;**21**:174–181.

33

Open ruptured abdominal aortic aneurysm repair

SACHINDER SINGH HANS

CONTENTS

INTRODUCTION

Most patients with ruptured abdominal aortic aneurysms (RAAAs) present with sudden onset of back pain or flank pain with associated diaphoresis secondary to low blood pressure (BP). Because of severe pain, BP may be temporarily elevated, which is detrimental for the expansion of retroperitoneal hematoma. Pain may be located in the periumbilical area and rarely in the inguinal area, masquerading as an incarcerated inguinal hernia. The location of pain depends on the site of rupture. Most ruptures occur in the posterolateral wall of the aneurysm and patients may remain hemodynamically stable for a few hours because of contained hematoma in the retroperitoneal space. On the other hand, anterior rupture is usually associated with free rupture into the peritoneal cavity, with severe shock secondary to massive blood loss. Rarely, an AAA may develop a "chronic" contained rupture because of a linear opening in the posterior wall of the aneurysm sealed by the anterior spinal ligament. These patients have persistent low back pain and are hemodynamically stable because there is no accompanying retroperitoneal hematoma.

Early transportation to an emergency department, prompt diagnosis (ultrasound/computed tomography angiography (CTA)) and resuscitation, preferably in the operating room, keeping the systolic BP between 80 and 100 mmHg, and immediate operation with proximal control of the aorta have a significant impact on the outcome of patients with RAAAs.[1-6] In most patients, there is time to obtain an emergency CTA of the abdomen and pelvis with 1-mm cuts. This not only confirms the diagnosis, but also helps to evaluate the patient for definitive treatment in the form of endovascular versus open repair, based on anatomic criteria from the imaging. Although endovascular repair of RAAAs is used, some patients do not have suitable anatomy for endovascular aneurysm repair (EVAR); therefore, open surgical repair is the only option. In patients with free rupture, obtaining a CTA may not be possible and immediate transfer to the operating room for aortic control is the best option.

OPERATIVE TECHNIQUE

How and how quickly proximal control of the aorta is obtained may help in determining the outcome of patients with RAAAs. If the patient's condition suggests free rupture in the form of persistent hypotension, that is, the patient needs large-volume resuscitation fluid and presents with increasing abdominal distention, obtaining rapid proximal control is of paramount significance. The patient is prepped from the nipple line to mid-thigh. To avoid cardiovascular collapse, close communication with the anesthesia team is very important because anesthetic introduction/intubation should be withheld until the surgeon is ready to make the incision. Induction of general anesthesia relieves pain, relaxes the abdominal wall musculature, and completely releases sympathetic tone, that is, all the protective mechanisms that serve to maintain BP in a patient with an RAAA. A rapid transfusion protocol with blood products in the room, cell saver (autologous blood recovery system), and body warmers should all be available. In most patients, a midline transabdominal incision from xiphoid process to symphysis pubis is performed. In selected patients with ileostomy/urinary stoma, or in patients with contained hematoma from leaking type IV thoracoabdominal aortic aneurysm, a left flank incision through the 10th intercostal space may be helpful. This incision is extended toward the lateral border of the rectus abdominis muscle between the symphysis pubis and the umbilicus.

Proximal control

Proximal aortic control is best achieved at the supraceliac level (near the diaphragm) in patients with extensive retroperitoneal hematoma and shock. In most patients with small-to-moderate retroperitoneal hematoma, blunt finger dissection of the infrarenal neck is performed after mobilizing the ligament of Treitz. The left renal vein (LRV) is mobilized and reflected upward and a vascular clamp is applied to the aorta just below the renal arteries (**Figures 33.1** and **33.2**). In some patients with acute decompensation during proximal dissection, two fingers (index and middle) or the thumb can be inserted into the aortic neck (**Figure 33.3**), and a No. 28 Foley catheter with 30-cc balloon (or a Pruitt® Aortic Occlusion Catheter, LeMaitre Vascular, Inc., Burlington, MA, USA) is guided into the lower thoracic aorta. Proximal control is obtained by inflating the catheter through the side port.

Exposure of the supraceliac aorta

The left lobe of the liver is retracted toward the right following division of the left triangular ligament. Dissection is done through the gastrohepatic omentum. The esophagus with the nasogastric tube is retracted toward the left; the author finds that encircling it with a Penrose drain can be helpful. Deep blades of a surgical retraction system (e.g., the Bookwalter III Retractor System, Symmetry Surgical, Antioch, TN, USA or the Thompson retractor, Thompson Surgical Instruments, Traverse City, MI, USA)

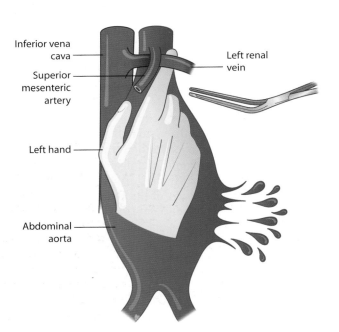

Figure 33.1 Mobilization of the pararenal aorta with right index finger under the left renal vein.

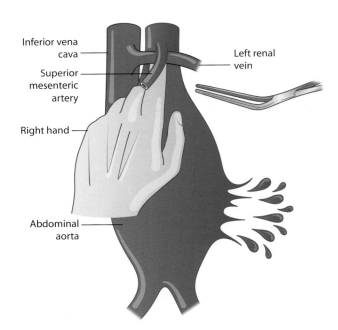

Figure 33.2 Mobilization of the pararenal aorta with left index finger under the left renal vein.

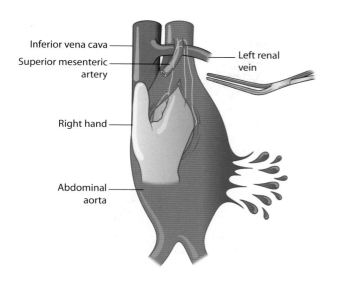

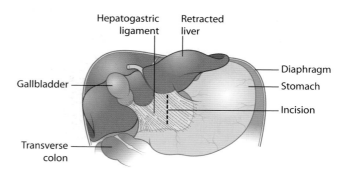

Figure 33.3 Insertion of right index and middle fingers into the neck of an abdominal aortic aneurysm to obtain proximal control.

Figure 33.4 Supraceliac control via the right crus of diaphragm. An incision is made into the gastrohepatic omentum to control the supraceliac aorta.

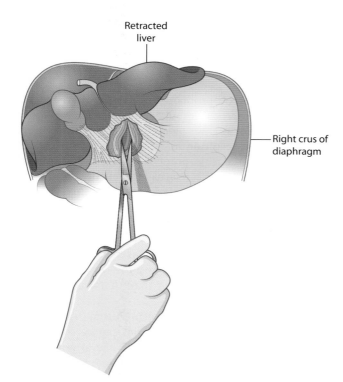

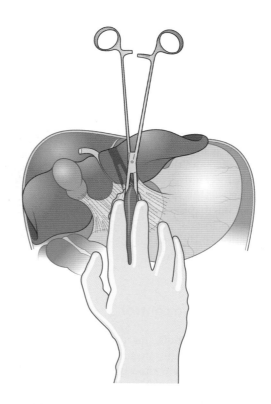

Figure 33.6 Supraceliac control via the right crus of the diaphragm. Application of proximal vascular clamp to the supraceliac aorta.

Figure 33.5 Supraceliac control via the right crus of the diaphragm. Scissors splitting the muscular fibers of the right crus of the diaphragm.

are inserted to expose the right crus of the diaphragm. The muscular fibers of the right crus are separated with the help of long Metzenbaum scissors, and a 5–6-cm opening is made in the crus. The index and middle fingers of the right hand are introduced through the opening, and the fascia surrounding the lower thoracic aorta is divided. With the help of the index and middle fingers of the right hand through the opening in the right crus, a long aortic clamp is guided into place with the left hand to clamp the lower thoracic aorta (**Figures 33.4–33.6**). The advantage of this approach is that the celiac artery and inferior phrenic vessels are relatively protected from iatrogenic trauma during this exposure.

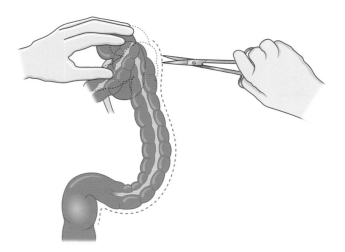

Figure 33.7 Medial visceral rotation started by incising the descending mesocolon, splenic flexure, tail of the pancreas, and outer border of the spleen.

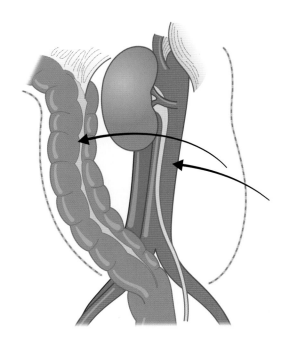

Figure 33.8 Medial visceral rotation started by incising the descending mesocolon, splenic flexure, tail of the pancreas, and outer border of the spleen. The top arrow shows the plane in front of the kidney. The bottom arrow shows the plane behind the kidney.

In some patients with ruptured proximal AAAs, medial visceral rotation (by mobilizing the spleen, tail of the pancreas, and splenic flexure) is necessary to obtain adequate proximal aortic exposure. The peritoneal reflection of the colon is divided and the viscera and left kidney are mobilized medially (**Figures 33.7** and **33.8**). With this maneuver, exposure of the suprarenal aorta is obtained and the left crus of the diaphragm is partially divided. Following control of the aorta at the supraceliac level, the clamp can then be moved distally to just below the renal arteries to reduce the visceral ischemic time.

Balloon occlusion control

An alternative technique for proximal control involves the insertion of a 12-Fr sheath into the femoral artery under local anesthesia to allow passage of a large-diameter occlusion balloon (e.g., 28–32-mm Z-MED™; B. Braun Interventional Systems Inc., Bethlehem, PA, USA), which can be inflated in the distal thoracic aorta to gain proximal control. A 12-Fr sheath tends to slip out; therefore, manual pressure by an assistant to keep the 12-Fr sheath in place may be necessary. Aortography to determine the suitability of EVAR can be undertaken after proximal balloon aortic occlusion is obtained (see Chapter 10). If the patient is not a suitable candidate for EVAR, open repair is continued. A left thoracotomy for proximal control of the thoracic aorta for RAAA repair is rarely necessary. In patients with better hemodynamic stability, proximal control at the pararenal level, as previously described, is usually preferred.

After obtaining proximal control, it is usually recommended to have the anesthesia team catch up with the fluids and blood products for resuscitation, even if the BP has improved. Without adequate fluid and blood resuscitation, any further blood loss can result in acute decompensation resulting in cardiac arrest. A decision should be made at this point whether to administer heparin. In patients with relatively stable BP and small-to-moderate retroperitoneal hematoma, intravenous heparin (75 IU/kg) is administered by the anesthesia team and serial monitoring with activated clotting time is necessary. In patients with shock and very large retroperitoneal hematoma, intravenous heparin is administered after proximal anastomosis is completed. The dose of heparin used is smaller than that used for elective open repair of AAAs.

Following proximal aortic control, distal exposure is obtained. Both common iliac arteries can be controlled if they are not aneurysmal; otherwise, the origin of the external and hypogastric arteries (HGAs) are clamped separately. The author does not recommend circumferential mobilization of the aortic neck and iliac arteries or passage of vessel loops or tapes because this maneuver can result in injury to adjacent venous structures (e.g., the LRV, posterior lumbar vein, and iliac vein). Iatrogenic major venous injury results in high morbidity and mortality. It is better to perform anterior and lateral dissection of the aortic neck and of the iliac arteries and place vascular clamps on the aortic neck and iliac arteries after compression between the index and middle fingers. The inferior mesenteric artery (IMA) is dissected and controlled with a silastic vessel loop close to its origin from the aorta. In patients with a small retroperitoneal hematoma following proximal aortic control, the operation should flow in a careful and deliberative manner similar to elective open AAA repair.

After ensuring adequate volume resuscitation and proximal and distal occlusion, the anterior wall of the aneurysm sac is opened to the right of the IMA origin with electrocautery and scissors and the intraluminal thrombus is removed. Lumbar arteries are carefully controlled by figure-of-eight 2-0 silk suture. Because of heavy calcified plaque, local endarterectomy of the origin of the lumbar artery may be necessary to achieve hemostasis. The infrarenal/juxtarenal aorta is prepared for proximal anastomosis by dividing the aorta wall. A transverse incision distal to the origins of the renal arteries is made and joins the longitudinal aortotomy incision in a "T"-shaped manner. After lateral division of the aortic neck, the posterior wall of the aortic neck is divided a few millimeters longer than the anterior wall. Sometimes, the posterior wall of the aortic neck is not divided and is used as a double layer for proximal anastomosis. In most patients with RAAAs, an aorto-bi-iliac graft (18 × 9 mm or 20 × 10 mm) is required. In some situations, a straight tube graft may be quite appropriate if the distal abdominal aorta above the origin of the iliac arteries is of suitable quality. A tube graft in a patient with suitable anatomy decreases operative time, fluid requirements, and postoperative ileus. Rarely, an aortounifemoral or aortobifemoral graft is necessary. The author prefers knitted Dacron grafts.

The proximal anastomosis of the main body of the Dacron graft to the aortic neck is first completed using a 3-0 or 4-0 cardiovascular polypropylene running suture (Ethicon US, LLC, Somerville, NJ, USA). In some patients with a dilated, friable aortic neck, a first layer of interrupted horizontal mattress suture on pledgets is used to suture the Dacron graft, then a second layer of continuous suture is performed. The use of BioGlue® surgical adhesive (CryoLife Inc., Kennesaw, GA, USA) or FLOSEAL hemostatic matrix (Baxter International Inc., Deerfield, IL, USA), following completion of proximal anastomosis may help in obtaining hemostasis. Once hemostasis of the proximal anastomosis is secured, attention is turned to the distal anastomosis.

In preparation for distal anastomosis, posterior circumferential dissection of the iliac arteries can now be undertaken. Graft limb-to-iliac artery anastomosis is done with a 4-0 cardiovascular polypropylene suture; retrograde and antegrade flushing are carried out. With poor back-bleeding from one or both iliac arteries, consideration should be given to the distal passage of a moderate-diameter (5-Fr) Fogarty balloon catheter before completing the anastomosis, particularly if the patient was not heparinized before clamping. Following completion of the anastomosis, flow is gradually restored to the lower

extremity to prevent declamping shock, which can be particularly severe in patients with RAAAs. Declamping shock results from redistribution of blood volume below the clamp, falling cardiac output, and release of vasodilators. Volume loading and correction of metabolic acidosis should be undertaken aggressively by the anesthesia team with monitoring of blood gases, electrolytes, and cardiac output. After restoration of flow to one iliac artery, there can be significant retrograde bleeding from the lumbar arteries that must be controlled with figure-of-eight 2-0 silk suture. Distal pulses/Doppler signals should be carefully checked at this point and consideration given to further interventions (e.g., passage of Fogarty balloon embolectomy catheters) if distal flow is absent.

Once adequate distal flow has been documented, all efforts should be directed to obtaining hemostasis. This is best accomplished with protamine sulfate reversal of heparin (if given) and administration of clotting factors as necessary. Once hemostasis has been achieved, the retroperitoneum is closed, carefully separating the duodenum and small bowel from any contact with the Dacron graft by suturing the remaining right lateral wall of the AAA to the descending mesocolon; the lower portion of the small bowel mesentery is sutured to the sigmoid mesocolon. The abdomen is closed with a single layer of No. 1 Maxon™ running monofilament absorbable suture (Medtronic, Minneapolis, MN, USA). If there is significant tension secondary to bowel edema or hematoma, delayed closure of the abdomen is planned in 3–5 days.

COMPLICATIONS

Bleeding

After open repair of an RAAA, postoperative bleeding may occur and is usually caused by coagulopathy associated with shock, hypothermia, and large-volume fluid resuscitation. For patients with a large retroperitoneal hematoma and associated shock, proactive transfusion encompassing two pooled buffy-coat platelet concentrates immediately and again 30 minutes before aortic unclamping together with fresh frozen plasma administered in a 1:1 ratio to the amount of red blood cells, should be instituted.[7] In a significant number of patients, coagulopathy is dilutional and can be corrected by administering appropriate blood products like fresh frozen plasma, cryoprecipitate, and in some instances factor VII. However, disseminated intravascular coagulation is a very serious complication of RAAA repair and is associated with very high mortality.

Acute lower extremity ischemia

This is usually the result of in situ thrombosis of the distal vascular bed because of hypotension and inadequate anticoagulation. Occasionally, it may be the result of embolic occlusion of mural thrombus from the aneurysmal sac. Lower extremity ischemia is a serious complication and should be investigated and treated before leaving the operating room. If a femoral pulse is absent, the iliac anastomosis should be checked; if the patient has good pulse distal to the anastomosis, the femoral artery should be opened via a groin incision and a Fogarty balloon catheter passed proximally and distally. If femoral pulses are palpable but no posterior tibial or dorsalis pedis flow is demonstrated by Doppler, the feet should be warmed; if distal flow is not reestablished soon, a No. 3 or 4 Fogarty embolectomy catheter is passed distally. If the patient is unstable and in shock, further interventions to improve lower extremity arterial flow should be postponed.

Colon ischemia

Colon ischemia is a very serious complication of RAAA repair and should be suspected in any patient with postoperative diarrhea that is usually not bloody. Flexible sigmoidoscopy should be performed as soon as the diagnosis is entertained. If colon ischemia is mild (confined to the mucosa or showing superficial muscular involvement), improvement with general supportive care (intravenous antibiotics directed against gut flora, nothing by mouth, and total parenteral nutrition) is expected. However, if there is progression to full-thickness necrosis and gangrene of the bowel, patients should undergo emergency laparotomy and colectomy with colostomy. In those patients, mortality is very high. At the time of RAAA repair, the IMA should be ligated close to its origin to preserve collateral flow. Should the sigmoid colon appear to be ischemic, and if there is a large liquefied hematoma involving the sigmoid mesocolon, consideration should be given to draining the hematoma to relieve compression of the branches of the IMA. If colon ischemia does not improve, then consideration should be given to reimplanting the original IMA into the Dacron graft using a Carrel patch. In the vast majority of patients, implantation of the IMA into the Dacron graft is usually not necessary. In a personal series of 125 consecutive RAAAs treated with open repair by the author, only one patient had revascularization of the IMA at the time of RAAA repair.

Spinal cord ischemia

Spinal cord ischemia in the form of paraplegia and paraparesis is more common after open RAAA repair than elective open AAA repair and is usually related to prolonged hypotension. It can also result from interruption of the blood supply to the spinal cord due to occlusion of an abnormally low origin (between L1 and L3) of the anterior spinal artery (artery of Adamkiewicz) or embolization into the HGAs. Recovery of neurologic function is usually poor.

Abdominal compartment syndrome

Abdominal compartment syndrome is not an uncommon complication of RAAA repair and occurs because of massive fluid resuscitation and prolonged aortic clamping. Using intra-abdominal pressure (IAP) measurements from an indwelling Foley catheter, 50% of patients had an IAP >20 mmHg after open repair of RAAAs; of those, approximately 20% developed multiple organ dysfunction or failure.[8] Medical therapy includes neuromuscular blockade, positive end-expiratory pressure, albumin, and furosemide. The abdomen should be kept open, avoiding adhesions between the intestines and the abdominal wall. Vacuum-assisted wound closure followed by delayed primary fascial closure is often necessary. Care should be taken to prevent a small bowel fistula with proper coverage of the exposed intestines.

Other complications

Cardiac arrhythmias, myocardial infarction, respiratory failure, acute renal failure, prolonged ileus, acute pancreatitis, and hepatic failure may occur following emergent RAAA repair; consultation with appropriate specialists may be helpful. Multiorgan failure following open repair of RAAAs is associated with high morbidity and mortality.

CASE EXAMPLES

Case example 1

A 68-year-old man presented with severe abdominal pain and shock. He was found to have a ruptured juxtarenal AAA with associated large bilateral iliac aneurysms. The patient underwent emergent RAAA repair with aortobifemoral graft because the iliac arteries were not suitable for distal anastomosis (**Figures 33.9** and **33.10**). On the third postoperative day, the patient developed left lower extremity ischemia secondary to thrombosed popliteal aneurysm. Repair of the thrombosed popliteal aneurysm was attempted; however, left above-knee amputation had to be performed because of irreversible ischemia. The patient developed right-sided weakness (stroke) and was found to have 90% stenosis of the left internal carotid artery (ICA) with contralateral ICA occlusion. He underwent left carotid endarterectomy and had a postoperative seizure that responded to antiseizure medication. The patient is ambulatory with above-knee prosthesis and is doing well 6 years after AAA repair.

Case example 2

A 68-year-old man with a family history of AAA presented to the emergency room with abdominal pain, back pain, and hypotension. A CT scan of the abdomen showed an infrarenal RAAA. After obtaining proximal control

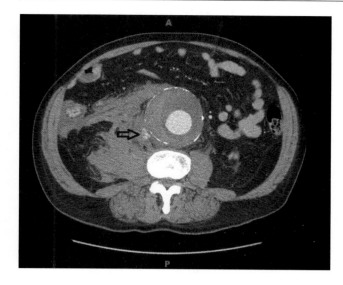

Figure 33.9 Computed tomography angiography of abdomen and pelvis showing a ruptured abdominal aortic aneurysm.

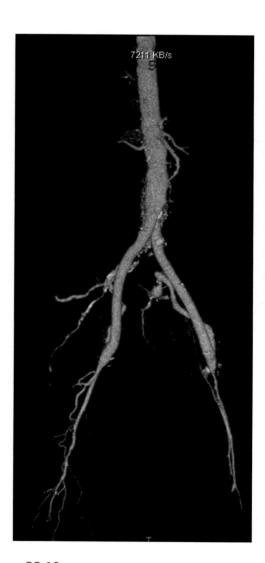

Figure 33.10 Repair of ruptured abdominal aortic aneurysm with aortobifemoral graft.

below the renal arteries, repair of the AAA with aorto-right femoral and left iliac Dacron graft (18 × 9 mm) was performed. At completion of the operation, the sigmoid colon was found to be ischemic; therefore, a vein graft was performed from the aortic Dacron graft to the main trunk of the IMA before its bifurcation because the proximal IMA was injured during the AAA repair. However, on the fifth postoperative day, the patient was found to be septic and developed high-output renal failure. He underwent sigmoidoscopy, which showed sigmoid colon infarction. He underwent reexploration of the abdomen and was found to have infarction of the left colon and ischemia of the right colon; he underwent total colectomy and ileostomy. Following prolonged hospital stay, the patient was discharged with ileostomy. He presented 3 years later with fever and sepsis and was found to have a small bowel-to-left iliac Dacron graft limb anastomotic fistula. The fistula was resected, the ileum was repaired, and the left limb of the Dacron graft was excised; a femorofemoral crossover graft was performed. After a protracted course, the patient was discharged; however, the patient died from bile duct cancer 2 years later.

REFERENCES

1. Robinson WP, Schanzer A, Li Y, et al. Derivation and validation of a practical risk score for prediction of mortality after open repair of ruptured abdominal aortic aneurysm in a US regional cohort and comparison to existing scoring systems. *J Vasc Surg.* 2013;**57**:354–361.

2. Gupta PK, Ramanan B, Englebert TL, et al. Comparison of open surgery versus endovascular repair of unstable ruptured abdominal aortic aneurysms. *J Vasc Surg.* 2014;**60**:1439–1445.

3. Hans SS, Huang RR. Results of 101 ruptured abdominal aortic aneurysm repairs from a single surgical practice. *Arch Surg.* 2003;**138**:898–901.

4. Noel AA, Gloviczki P, Cherry KJ Jr., et al. Ruptured abdominal aortic aneurysms: the excessive mortality rate of conventional repair. *J Vasc Surg.* 2001;**34**:41–46.

5. Eslami MH, Messina LM. Ruptured AAA: open surgical management. *Semin Vasc Surg.* 2010;**23**:200–205.

6. Cho JS, Kim JY, Rhee RY, et al. Contemporary results of open repair of ruptured abdominal aortoiliac aneurysm: effect of surgeon volume on mortality. *J Vasc Surg.* 2008;**48**:10–17.

7. Johansson PI, Stensballe J, Rosenberg I, et al. Proactive administration of platelets and plasma for patients with a ruptured abdominal aortic aneurysm: evaluating a change in transfusion practice. *Transfusion.* 2007;**47**:593–598.

8. Björck M. Management of the tense or difficult abdominal closure after operation for ruptured abdominal aortic aneurysms. *Semin Vasc Surg.* 2012;**25**:35–38.

34

Proximal abdominal aortic aneurysm repair

ALEXANDER D. SHEPARD

CONTENTS

INTRODUCTION

The proximal abdominal aorta is defined as the aorta running from the aortic hiatus to the renal arteries. Aneurysms of this segment present unique challenges in management compared to those of the infrarenal aorta (IRA). Operative exposure is more extensive and unfamiliar, leading to longer procedure times and increased risk of injury to adjacent organs (e.g., spleen, pancreas). Proximal aortic clamping leads to obligatory periods of renal/visceral ischemia and increased cardiac strain compared to IRA clamping. Finally, aortic reconstruction techniques are much more complicated than the simple end-to-end anastomoses of IRA repair.

Assessment of cardiac, pulmonary, and renal function is essential to stratify risk. Good, high-quality (thin-cut) computed tomography angiography (CTA) is also critical in preoperative evaluation; it allows the surgeon to plan the approach, identify a suitable proximal aortic clamp site, and devise an appropriate and expeditious reconstruction. Careful preoperative planning is the key to good outcomes with this operation. Intraoperative monitoring with an arterial line, central line, and Foley catheter is routine, supplemented by transesophageal echocardiography as needed.

OPERATIVE APPROACH

A standard transperitoneal, inframesocolic exposure is suitable only for juxtarenal abdominal aortic aneurysms (AAAs). Exposure of the more proximal abdominal aorta can be done through a midline incision using medial visceral rotation (MVR) or through a left flank approach (thoracoretroperitoneal or thoracoabdominal). With MVR, the abdomen is opened with a long midline incision in the standard fashion and the peritoneal reflection lateral to the left colon and spleen is incised from the sigmoid colon cephalad to the aortic hiatus. A retrorenal plane is developed and the spleen, pancreas, and left kidney are retracted medially to provide exposure of the entire abdominal aorta from hiatus to bifurcation. If required, access to the right renal artery (RRA) and distal right iliac artery can be obtained through standard transperitoneal exposure techniques. The major disadvantages of this approach are lack of access to the distal descending thoracic aorta, a high incidence of splenic injury (approximately 20%), and complications of excessive visceral retraction (e.g., bowel ischemia and pancreatitis).[1]

For these and other reasons, the author has favored a left flank approach through a 9th or 10th intercostal space (ICS) incision, 9th for paravisceral extent IV thoracoabdominal aortic aneurysms (TAAAs) and 10th for pararenal AAAs. Positioning of the patient in a modified left thoracotomy position is key (see **Figure 32.10** in Chapter 32). When grafting to the aortic bifurcation, the author leaves the patient in an almost pure lateral position, rotating the hips posteriorly only when iliac/femoral exposure is required. The incision is begun just below the umbilicus at the lateral margin of the left rectus sheath and carried obliquely into the appropriate ICS entering the left chest. More proximal aortic exposure can be gained by taking the incision further posteriorly (as far as the paraspinal muscles, if necessary), while more distal exposure is facilitated by extending the incision to the midline. The diaphragm is divided circumferentially, beginning at the costal margin approximately 2 cm from its lateral attachments, to avoid injury to the branches of the phrenic nerve. As much diaphragm as necessary is divided to avoid tearing it during subsequent rib retraction. The author has avoided radial division of the diaphragm because a 2001 review of his experience revealed that this was the most important factor associated with postoperative respiratory failure with this operation.[2]

A standard mechanical retraction system (e.g., the Integra® Omni-Tract, Integra LifeSciences Corporation, Plainsboro, NJ, USA or the Thompson retractor, Thompson Surgical Instruments, Traverse City, MI, USA) is key to good exposure. As described previously in Chapter 32, a retroperitoneal plane posterior to the left kidney is developed and the left kidney and the peritoneal sac and its contents are retracted to the patient's right. The lumbar branch of the left renal vein (LRV) is carefully sought as it crosses over the aorta and is divided, providing a guide to the location of the left renal artery (LRA). The left diaphragmatic crus is divided along the long axis of the aorta; this maneuver is facilitated by the surgeon inserting his/her left index finger under the crus (on top of the aorta) and dividing the muscle with electrocautery (**Figure 34.1**). This step is critical for exposure of the supraceliac aorta and the origins of the celiac artery and superior mesenteric artery (SMA). The LRA usually originates from the aorta just below the lowermost edge of the left crus. For juxtarenal AAAs, it is unnecessary to dissect out more than the LRA and potentially the supraceliac aorta, depending on the desired clamp level. For suprarenal AAAs, control of the LRA, SMA, and sometimes the celiac artery can be beneficial, while for more proximal AAAs, control of all three vessels is helpful. Lymphoareolar tissue overlying the proximal abdominal aorta is divided. The author has found the use of an ultrasonic scalpel quite helpful in this regard.

Control of the supraceliac aorta is relatively simple to obtain through a left flank approach; the investing fascia is divided and the surgeon's index finger is passed just anterior to and posterior to the aorta at this level to allow passage of the blades of a cross-clamp. There is no need to circumferentially control the aorta at this level. Care should be taken when developing the plane posterior to the aorta to avoid injury to any intervening segmental arteries. Supramesenteric aortic control is more tedious to obtain because of the presence of a vascular nerve plexus lying on the anterior surface of the aorta between the celiac artery and SMA. Suprarenal control is easier than supramesenteric control because of the absence of any tissue adherent to the aorta at this level. Once proximal aortic control has been obtained, the origins of the LRA, SMA, and celiac artery axes are dissected free as necessary. Though slightly more time-consuming, control of the celiac artery and SMA is associated with much less blood loss than simply allowing these vessels to back-bleed with a proximal aortic clamp on. Extraluminal control is also less cumbersome than intraluminal control with balloon occlusion catheters.

Next, the infrarenal component of the AAA is exposed by dividing the overlying tissues. Care should be taken to identify the left ureter and ensure that it is retracted along with the peritoneal sac out of harm's way. Iliac control is obtained as previously described in Chapter 32. Lumbar arteries that can be preserved at either the proximal or distal anastomotic sites are controlled, while those originating from the aneurysmal sac and easily accessible are routinely ligated to reduce blood loss after the aneurysm is opened.

AORTIC CLAMP LEVEL

Choosing an appropriate proximal clamp level is one of the most important determinants of operative success with proximal AAA repair. Anatomy and aortic disease dictate the clamp level, which is chosen based on a careful review of the preoperative CTA. The more proximally the aorta is clamped, the greater the cardiac strain and the greater the renal/visceral ischemic burden; in general, therefore, the most distal feasible clamp site is preferred. It is also important not to clamp diseased aorta with the consequent risk of renal/visceral and lower extremity atheroembolism. With suprarenal clamping, the relationship between the renal arteries and SMA needs to be carefully assessed; when the SMA originates too close to the renal arteries, suprarenal clamping may not be possible without risking injury to one of these vessels. One must also guard against injuring the unseen origin of the RRA when it arises more proximally off the aorta than the LRA.

When more proximal aortic clamping is required, the author has favored a supraceliac level over a supramesenteric one because the supraceliac aorta is reliably the least diseased segment of the abdominal aorta and because supraceliac aortic exposure is fast and easy to perform

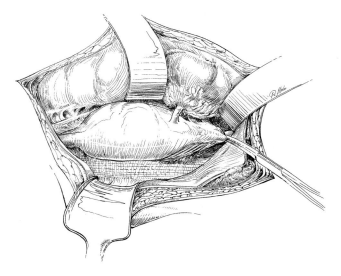

Figure 34.1 Exposure of a proximal abdominal aortic aneurysm through a left flank retroperitoneal approach. Divided left diaphragmatic crus is demonstrated just distal to the supraceliac aortic clamp.

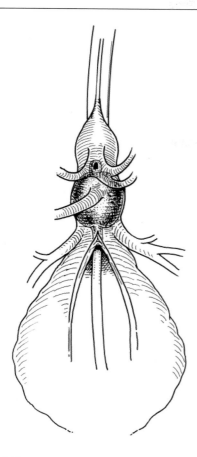

Figure 34.2 Foley balloon control of back-bleeding arteries (lumbar, renal, and visceral) originating from the proximal abdominal aorta below the aortic clamp site.

from this approach. Control at the supramesenteric level has the advantage of less cardiac stress and maintenance of visceral perfusion through the celiac artery; however, this exposure is more tedious than supraceliac exposure and can be associated with significant SMA back-bleeding if the SMA is not concomitantly controlled. With supraceliac clamping, 15 minutes before clamping, a bicarbonate drip (0.05 mEq/kg/min) is started to minimize the associated acidosis. Before proximal aortic clamping, the author always considers preliminary infrarenal clamping, if the aorta at this level is not too aneurysmal or diseased; this maneuver allows control of any back-bleeding lumbar arteries and the inferior mesenteric artery without wasting valuable visceral/renal ischemia time. When performing juxtarenal AAA repair with supraceliac clamping, back-bleeding from uncontrolled visceral and segmental branches can be controlled by inflating a 10-cc Foley balloon catheter in the paravisceral aorta (**Figure 34.2**).

PROTECTION AGAINST VITAL ORGAN ISCHEMIA

With proximal abdominal aorta clamping comes an obligatory period of renal ischemia with or without visceral and occasional spinal cord ischemia (SCI). Acute kidney injury

(AKI) is one of the most commonly reported complications of these repairs.[3] Minimizing clamp time is obviously critical. Before clamping, it is important to optimize hemodynamics; mannitol (25 gm) is administered 15–20 minutes before anticipated aortic clamping. Selecting an appropriate clamp site reduces the risk of embolizing debris into the renal arteries. When using a left flank approach, the RRA is particularly vulnerable to this complication because of its dependent position in the operative field. Inflation of a small (4 or 5-Fr) balloon-tipped occlusion catheter in to the origin of this vessel can block the passage of such debris. When prolonged (>30 minutes) renal ischemia times are anticipated or patients have pre-existing chronic kidney disease, the author routinely uses cold renal perfusion to reduce renal metabolic demands; 250 mL of 1°C Ringer's lactate solution (plus methylprednisolone, mannitol, and heparin) is infused into each kidney followed by 50 mL every 10–15 minutes for the duration of clamping. Infusion is accomplished through balloon-tipped Pruitt (LeMaitre Vascular, Inc., Burlington, MA, USA) perfusion catheters (9-Fr) for large renal arteries, or 4 or 5-Fr irrigating balloon catheters for smaller or diseased renal arteries (LeMaitre Vascular, Inc.). Several papers have demonstrated the value of this technique in the prevention of AKI.[3,4] Although unproven, the author has used a similar approach for visceral protection by infusing the SMA (400–500 mL initially followed by 75 mL every 10–15 minutes) during supraceliac clamping. Using this technique, the author has noted less coagulopathy and fewer hemodynamic changes with unclamping.

SCI is uncommon with proximal AAA repair, but frequent enough that protective steps should be taken in higher-risk situations, defined in the author's experience as all extent IV TAAAs and whenever supraceliac clamp times are anticipated to exceed 30 minutes. A lumbar drain is placed preoperatively and cerebrospinal fluid is drained to maintain an intrathecal pressure ≤10 cm H_2O. Other adjuncts include moderate passive hypothermia (allowing the patient to cool to 33 degrees) and avoidance of high-dose vasodilators during cross-clamping.

AORTIC RECONSTRUCTION

Before aortic clamping, the author routinely heparinizes, believing that microvascular thrombosis is a major determinant of multisystem organ failure when it occurs. Careful communication with the anesthesia team is necessary during clamping and blood should always be immediately available when opening the aneurysm sac.

Construction of the proximal aortic anastomosis differs from infrarenal repairs because of the need to maintain flow to the renal and visceral arteries. Repair of juxtarenal AAAs (defined as aneurysms with no infrarenal neck suitable for clamping and anastomosis) is the simplest. Although the author performs most of these AAA repairs through a left flank approach, they can also be done through a transperitoneal approach after full mobilization of the LRV. This maneuver allows full visualization of the juxtarenal aorta for both clamping and construction of the proximal anastomosis. The ostia of the two renal arteries are frequently incorporated into the proximal anastomotic suture line (**Figure 34.3**).

Reconstruction of more proximal AAAs is more complicated and usually requires a beveled, end-to-end anastomosis of some type incorporating the renal and visceral artery origins. How this is performed depends on the relationship of the renal arteries to the aorta. If both RAs originate anteriorly, with most of the aneurysmal wall extending posteriorly, a posterior bevel is possible. With this reconstruction, the aorta is trimmed to leave the two renal arteries, the SMA, and if necessary the celiac artery on an anterior tongue of the aorta while the graft is cut to leave a corresponding posterior bevel (**Figure 34.4**). Unfortunately, although simplest, this type of reconstruction is usually not possible.

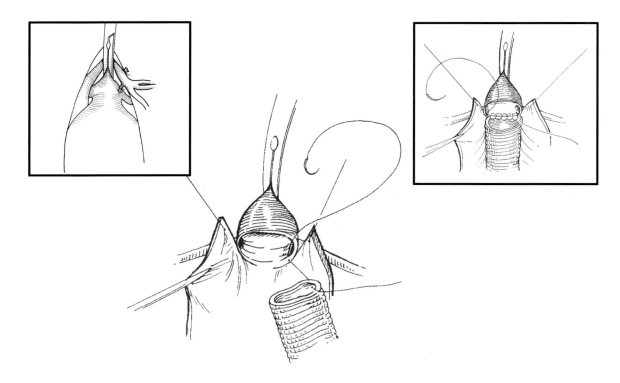

Figure 34.3 Construction of proximal aortic anastomosis during juxtarenal abdominal aortic aneurysm repair demonstrating incorporation of renal artery ostia into the suture line.

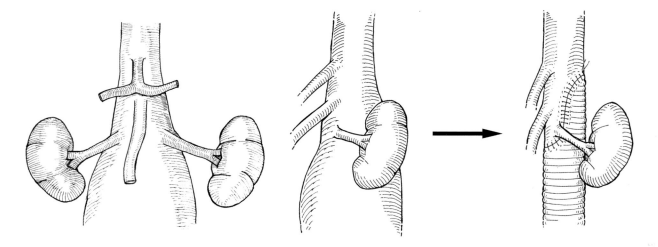

Figure 34.4 Proximal aortic reconstruction with a posterior beveled anastomosis leaving the celiac, superior mesenteric, and both renal arteries on an anterior tongue of aorta (arrow). This reconstruction is only appropriate when renal arteries arise near each other anteriorly as demonstrated in the drawings of a suprarenal aneurysm to the left and center (anterior–posterior perspective to far left and lateral perspective in center).

More commonly, the proximal reconstruction is a laterally based, beveled anastomosis that is used when the renal arteries are separated by a significant amount of aneurysmal aortic wall. This technique incorporates the RRA, SMA, and celiac artery (as necessary) on a tongue of the aorta, while the LRA is either reimplanted into the graft or more frequently bypassed with a small-caliber sidearm graft previously sewn onto the aortic graft (**Figure 34.5**). When using a renal graft, it is imperative to carefully rotate/trim the aortic graft so that the sidearm is appropriately positioned; the author has found the 2 o'clock position (SMA at 12 o'clock) to be the most satisfactory position to prevent subsequent sidearm kinking. The graft-to-aorta anastomosis is performed with the inclusion technique, taking the first suture bites at the level of the dependent RRA and then carrying the suture line up the posterior wall of the aorta, taking double-thickness bites until the transected edge of the aorta is encountered (**Figure 34.6a**). Single-thickness aortic wall stitches bring the suture line up to the level of the SMA or celiac artery, and then down the transected anterior wall. The anastomosis is completed by bringing the other suture along the anterior aortic wall (double-thickness transitioning to single-thickness

bites) to the level of the first suture line (**Figure 34.6b**). When performing a beveled anastomosis of any type, it is important to leave as little aortic wall behind as possible to reduce the risk of future aortic wall degeneration and recurrent aneurysm formation. Following appropriate flushing maneuvers, the perfusion catheters are removed and the suture line is secured allowing sequential restoration of flow to the RRA, the celiac, and finally the SMA.

A decision must be made at this point whether to proceed next with revascularization of the left kidney or the lower extremities. The author has usually chosen to proceed with the distal anastomosis first to restore hypogastric flow and reduce the SCI risk. In addition, performance of the distal anastomosis after left renal revascularization increases the risk that the left renal revascularization could be disrupted during performance of the distal aortic/iliac anastomoses. Continued cold perfusion of the left kidney can be carried out during the distal anastomosis; alternatively, the left kidney can be shunted using a Pruitt Carotid Shunt (LeMaitre Vascular, Inc.) with one end placed in the renal sidearm and the other in the LRA (**Figure 34.7**). Once the distal anastomosis (or if to the iliac arteries, the right iliac

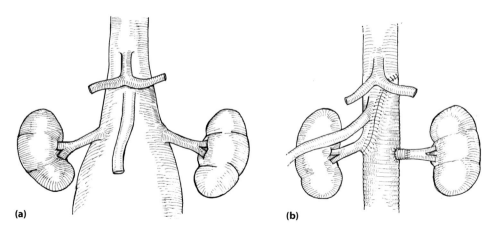

(a)   (b)

Figure 34.5 Proximal aortic reconstruction with a lateral beveled anastomosis, incorporating celiac, superior mesenteric, and right renal artery on a tongue of the aorta with either bypass to or reimplantation of the left renal artery. This is the most commonly performed proximal reconstruction and is used when there is significant aortic wall between the two renal arteries. (**a**) Aneurysm suitable for this type of reconstruction. (**b**) Postreconstruction.

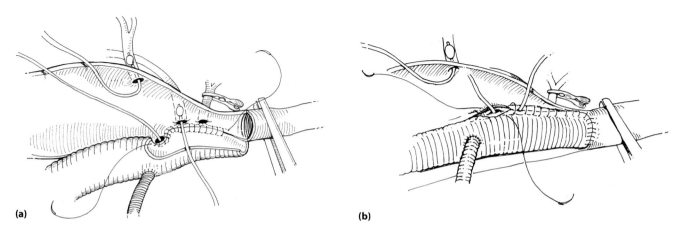

(a)   (b)

Figure 34.6 Lateral beveled proximal anastomosis to repair an extent IV thoracoabdominal aneurysm. (**a**) Demonstrating placement of perfusion catheters in the superior mesenteric artery and both renal arteries with construction of aortic suture line along the posterior wall. Bulldog clamp on the celiac artery. (**b**) Completion of anterior wall suture line.

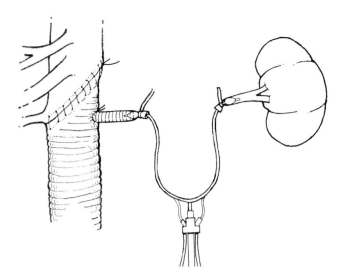

Figure 34.7 Pruitt Carotid Shunt (LeMaitre Vascular, Inc., Burlington, MA, USA) between sidearm graft and left renal artery allowing left kidney perfusion during construction of distal aortic/iliac anastomosis.

anastomosis) has been performed, attention is directed to the LRA. It is imperative that this anastomosis is performed under tension because there is invariably redundancy in the graft/artery that can lead to postoperative kinking when the left kidney is returned to its normal anatomic location. Reimplantation of the LRA along with a cuff of the aorta avoids this problem, but requires placement of a partially occluding clamp on the graft, frequently at the level of the visceral/RRA patch, which can sometimes lead to disruption of this fresh suture line. If distal flow has been restored before this reconstruction, the author usually checks for pedal Doppler flow and, if adequate, reverses heparin anticoagulation before completing the LRA bypass/reimplantation.

Sometimes, the aneurysm extends well above the origin of the celiac artery mandating an end-to-end anastomosis between the graft and the aorta with reimplantation of the celiac artery, SMA, and LRA as a separate inclusion patch (**Figure 34.8**). In patients with the origins of the celiac artery, SMA, and RRA widely spaced apart, constructing an inclusion patch with all three artery origins is simply not possible without leaving significant amounts of abnormal aortic wall behind. In this situation and in patients with documented connective tissue abnormalities, the author has used a graft with prefabricated sidearms for reconstruction (Vascutek® Gelweave™ Coselli Thoracoabdominal Graft, Terumo Medical Corporation, Somerset, NJ, USA) (**Figure 34.9**). Use of this graft requires significant attention to detail to ensure that the graft limbs line up with their respective branches. When using this graft, the author performs the proximal aortic anastomosis followed by the RRA graft anastomosis, which is the key graft limb to line up appropriately. Once the right kidney is perfused, flow is restored to the SMA and LRA through shunts or perfusion catheters placed into the graft limbs. This technique reduces renal/visceral ischemia time while giving priority to the restoration of hypogastric flow and reduction in SCI. After the distal anastomosis is done, the SMA and celiac grafts are performed, saving the LRA for last. Doing the left renal graft before the viscerals constrains exposure and risks disruption of this bypass during visceral reconstruction. In most situations, the Vascutek® Gelweave™ Coselli Thoracoabdominal Graft limbs are cut very short (no more than 10–15 mm) to avoid kinking.

Following completion of all anastomoses and assurance of good Doppler flow in all reconstructed vascular territories, heparin anticoagulation is reversed and the hemostatic profile is corrected as necessary. The left chest is drained with a small posterobasal pleural tube, the diaphragm is closed with 0 or 2-0 polypropylene suture, the ribs are reapproximated with looped No. 1 polydioxanone (PDS) suture, and the wound is closed in layers with 0 or

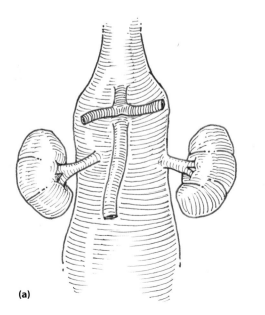

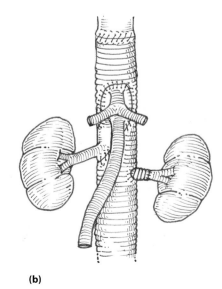

Figure 34.8 Extent IV thoracoabdominal aortic aneurysm showing end-to-end proximal aortic anastomosis with reimplantation of celiac, superior mesenteric, and right renal artery as a single patch and bypass of the left RA. (**a**) Aneurysm suitable for this type of reconstruction. (**b**) Postreconstruction.

(a)

(b)

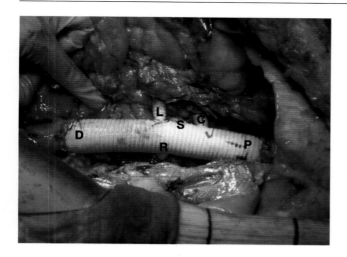

Figure 34.9 Branched (Vascutek® Gelweave™ Coselli, Terumo Medical Corporation, Somerset, NJ, USA) thoracoabdominal graft reconstruction of an extent IV thoracoabdominal aortic aneurysm. Proximal aortic anastomosis (P) to the right of the photo, distal aortic anastomosis (D) to the left of the photo. C: celiac limb; L: left renal artery; R: right renal artery; S: superior mesenteric artery.

2-0 PDS suture. Postoperatively, a spinal cord protection protocol is maintained for at least 24 hours in all patients who were treated with a lumbar drain. A postischemic renal diuresis occurs commonly when suprarenal clamp times exceed 30 minutes and is best treated by replacing urinary losses >100 cc/hour with Ringer's lactate solution 0.5 cc to replace every 1.0 cc of urine output for the first 12 hours postoperatively.

The key to this operation is reducing blood loss, which can be minimized by avoiding venous injuries, ligating lumbar arteries before opening the sac, and reducing the coagulopathy associated with gut/liver ischemia/reperfusion by cold SMA perfusion and expeditious visceral revascularization.[5] Cold renal perfusion reduces the risk of AKI. In experienced hands, the mortality and morbidity of open proximal AAA repair approaches that of infrarenal AAA repair and remains the standard approach for managing these complex AAAs.[3]

REFERENCES

1. Reilly LM, Ramos TK, Murray SP, et al. Optimal exposure of the proximal abdominal aorta: a critical appraisal of transabdominal medial visceral rotation. *J Vasc Surg.* 1994;**19**:375–389.
2. Anagnostopolous PV, Shepard AD, Pipinos II, et al. Factors affecting outcome in proximal abdominal aortic aneurysm repair. *Ann Vasc Surg.* 2001; **15**:511–519.
3. Kabbani LS, West CA, Viau D, et al. Survival after repair of pararenal and paravisceral abdominal aortic aneurysms. *J Vasc Surg.* 2014;**59**:1488–1494.
4. Köksoy C, LeMaire SA, Curling PE, et al. Renal perfusion during thoracoabdominal aortic operations: cold crystalloid is superior to normothermic blood. *Ann Thorac Surg.* 2002;**73**:730–738.
5. Anagnostopoulos PV, Shepard AD, Pipinos II, et al. Hemostatic alterations associated with supraceliac aortic cross-clamping. *J Vasc Surg.* 2002;**35**:100–108.

35

Thoracoabdominal aortic aneurysm repair

MARK F. CONRAD

CONTENTS

INTRODUCTION

Aneurysms that simultaneously involve the thoracic and abdominal aorta are referred to as thoracoabdominal aortic aneurysms (TAAAs). Such aneurysms are uncommon when compared to isolated AAAs and comprise no more than 2–5% of the total spectrum of degenerative aortic aneurysms.[1] The modern era in the surgical management of TAAAs began with the pioneering work of Ernest Stanley Crawford, who described a simplified operative approach involving the reconstruction of the aneurysmal aorta with direct anastomoses of the aortic origin of visceral and intercostal vessels to the main Dacron graft. This approach inherently leads to some degree of ischemia to the spinal cord, visceral vessels, and lower extremities, with the potential for significant morbidity from end organ damage. Indeed, several surgical and nonsurgical adjuncts intended to minimize distal ischemia and improve outcomes have been investigated and the author's approach to these complex aneurysms has evolved over time. Despite improvements in operative strategies, open repair of TAAAs still carries a 5–10% risk of perioperative morbidity and mortality in the form of renal, respiratory, and spinal cord ischemic complications.[2] Endovascular repair of TAAAs using modular grafts with branched and fenestrated technologies is continuing to gain favor in high-risk patients, but issues of long-term durability and a high rate of spinal cord ischemia (SCI) need to be addressed before it will supplant open repair as the standard of care.

CLASSIFICATION AND NATURAL HISTORY

Anatomy

TAAAs are classified according to the scheme originally devised by Crawford (**Figure 35.1**). This classification is especially useful in patients requiring operative repair because it has direct implications for both the technical conduct of the operation and the incidence of operative complications, in particular SCI. There is considerable variation in the operative approach required to manage different TAAA lesions; this chapter focuses on extent I–III TAAAs.

Natural history

The expected natural history of TAAAs is progressive enlargement and eventual rupture, regardless of etiology or location. The mean rate of growth for TAAAs is 0.2 cm/year and is accelerated in patients with dissections and connective tissue disorders. The 5-year survival of patients with TAAAs is 13%, and aneurysm rupture is the cause of death in nearly 75% of untreated patients. Factors associated with rupture include: aneurysm diameter; rapid expansion; chronic obstructive pulmonary disease (COPD); steroid use; female gender; advanced age; and renal insufficiency. Contemporary series indicate that the rupture risk increases substantially at aneurysm diameters >6 cm or growth rates of >10 mm per year, that is, 6 cm is the surgical threshold for consideration of intervention in patients with degenerative TAAAs. For patients with a TAAA secondary to chronic dissection or those with Marfan syndrome, a 5-cm threshold is used.[1]

DIAGNOSTIC IMAGING

Accurate radiographic evaluation is essential for precise operative planning, with no equivocation in the surgeon's mind as to the proximal and distal extent of aortic resection. In contemporary practice, a dynamic, fine-cut, contrast-enhanced computed tomography angiogram provides the physician with the following information: (1) location and qualitative assessment of the aorta in the region of the proximal cross-clamp; (2) patency of the visceral vessels; (3) topography of renal artery origin/kidney size and adequacy of perfusion; (4) relationship of left renal vein to the aorta; (5) distal extent of the resection; and (6) aneurysmal status of the iliac vessels and possible occlusive disease in the pelvis (important if retrograde transfemoral aortic perfusion is to be used).

PATIENT SELECTION AND PREOPERATIVE EVALUATION

Since most patients seen in consideration for TAAA resection are those with degenerative aneurysms, demographic and clinical features typical of a patient population with diffuse atherosclerosis are the rule. Patients treated for degenerative aneurysms average 70 years of age and a history of hypertension is nearly universal. Cigarette smoking or significant COPD are frequently encountered, with 25% of patients having significant COPD with a predicted forced expiratory volume 1 of <50%.[1] The coexistence of renovascular disease and some degree of renal insufficiency is commonplace in TAAA patients and has important implications for the accurate assessment of perioperative risk and long-term preservation of renal function.

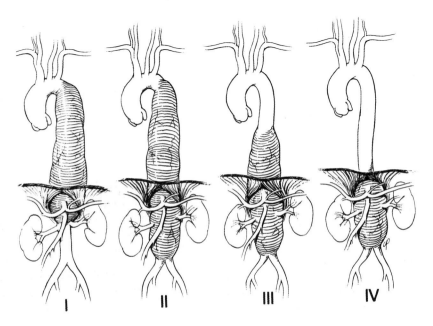

Figure 35.1 Crawford classification of the extent of thoracoabdominal aortic aneurysms (TAAAs). A type I TAAA begins just distal to the left subclavian artery (LSA) and extends to the diaphragm just above the celiac artery. A type II TAAA is the most extensive. It begins just distal to the LSA and extends beyond the celiac artery, often to the aortic bifurcation. A type III TAAA begins at the mid-descending thoracic aorta and extends to the aortic bifurcation. A type IV TAAA extends from the celiac artery to the aortic bifurcation.

I   II   III   IV

SURGICAL TREATMENT

Treatment options

Graft replacement by direct surgical approach is the current standard of care for TAAAs. The hybrid approach that combines visceral artery debranching with endovascular exclusion of the TAAA has allowed surgeons who lack the resources to perform distal perfusion to offer TAAA repair to their complex patients; however, the reported results compare poorly with open repair at high-volume centers. Medical therapy with aggressive blood pressure (BP) control is appropriate in patients who are frail, have prohibitive associated comorbid conditions, or small aneurysms.

Many adjuncts have been championed to minimize SCI after TAAA repair. However, only cerebrospinal fluid (CSF) drainage is appropriately evidence-based and used by most surgeons. Other adjuncts aimed at preserving spinal cord blood flow, such as intercostal reconstruction have been routinely practiced despite an evidence base that is limited to retrospective studies. The alternative position referable to intercostal vessel reconstruction is that it is unnecessary (related to the collateral network) and expends cross-clamping time and blood turnover. Distal aortic perfusion via left atrial femoral bypass, used in conjunction with motor evoked potential (MEP) monitoring to dynamically assess SCI during the operation, has replaced epidural cooling as the author's principal cord protective strategy in patients with type I–III TAAAs. This is based on a series of studies showing that individual intercostal vessels were typically not critical for cord preservation and most collateral support originates from the pelvis (i.e., hypogastric arteries); thus, preservation of continuous perfusion of the pelvis is logical and prudent. The addition of MEP monitoring affords the surgeon objective criteria to direct selective intercostal reconstruction and replaces the subjective application of intercostal reimplantation.

TECHNICAL COMPONENTS

Operative exposure

The key to operative success remains the provision of broad, continuous exposure of the entire left posterolateral aspect of the thoracoabdominal aorta. The patient is positioned in the right lateral decubitus position. The location of the thoracic portion of the incision is determined by the proximal extent of the aneurysm because the posterior portion of a standard posterolateral thoracotomy incision is only necessary for type I–II aneurysms. The author keeps the thoracic portion of the incision low and has found that the fifth or sixth intercostal space (ICS) with posterior division of the sixth or seventh rib provides adequate exposure for most aneurysms. The costal margin is divided at the sixth ICS and a self-retaining retractor is placed. The abdominal portion

of the incision is kept well lateral on the abdominal wall along the edge of the rectus.

Exposure of the abdominal aorta is obtained by entering the plane posterior to the spleen, left kidney, and colon. The abdominal contents are reflected to the patient's right and the left ureter is preserved under laparotomy pads (**Figure 35.2**). The retroperitoneal tissues overlying the aorta are transected with electrocautery and the renal lumbar vein is identified and divided. The left renal artery (LRA) is topographically close to this vein and is dissected toward its origin on the aorta. This serves as a point to initiate the division of the retroperitoneal tissues over the aorta inferiorly and the median arcuate ligament and diaphragmatic crura superiorly.

There are several methods by which the incision in the diaphragm may be managed. The simplest method that affords excellent exposure is direct radial division of the diaphragm from underneath the costal margin to the aortic hiatus. This approach, however, irrevocably paralyzes the left hemidiaphragm and ultimately contributes to postoperative respiratory embarrassment. Alternatively, circumferential division of the diaphragm through its muscular portion, leaving a few centimeters attached laterally to the chest wall, preserves the phrenic innervation to the left hemidiaphragm. A large Penrose drain can be passed around the diaphragm pedicle and is used to retract superiorly and inferiorly as needed. The author has applied this method liberally, particularly in patients with evidence of preoperative pulmonary compromise.

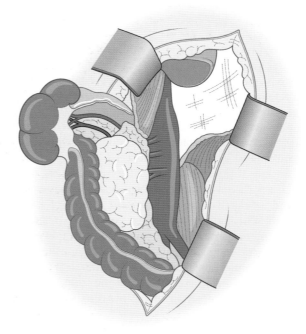

Figure 35.2 Schematic of exposure for thoracoabdominal aneurysm repair. Exposure of the left chest and abdomen through a thoracoabdominal incision with the left kidney, spleen, pancreas, and left colon reflected up. This exposes the entire left posterolateral aspect of the thoracoabdominal aorta.

Dissection of left pleural space

After deflation of the left lung, the thoracic component of the dissection is straightforward. Electrocautery is used to divide the mediastinal pleura over the aneurysm and proximal aorta. For type I–II aneurysms, proximal control of the aorta near the left subclavian artery (LSA) origin is necessary. The vagus nerve is mobilized by dividing it distal to the origin of the left recurrent nerve, which should be identified and preserved. Should more proximal control be necessary, the ligamentum arteriosum is divided on the underside of the aortic arch. Care must be taken to keep the dissection directly on the aortic arch to avoid injuring the left main pulmonary artery. In patients with chronic dissection, inflammation from the dissecting process makes exposure of the arch more difficult. The aorta is surrounded with a vessel tape on either side of the LSA, depending on the proximal extent of the aneurysm. Blunt dissection on the posterior aspect of the aorta is used to clear sufficient normal aorta to allow clamp application while maintaining an adequate length of aorta for an accurate proximal anastomosis. External control of the LSA is desirable but not mandatory because intraluminal balloon control can be obtained if necessary. The left inferior pulmonary vein (IPV) is isolated for atrial femoral bypass and a 4-0 polypropylene purse-string suture is used to introduce the venous cannula, which need not be larger than 19 Fr.

Atriofemoral bypass

Distal perfusion through atriofemoral bypass via a centripetal, motorized pump is simple and requires low doses of systemic heparin. Conversely, cardiopulmonary bypass with a femoral vein/artery technique requires an in-line oxygenator and full pump doses of heparin, making it less desirable given the extensive dissection required to complete TAAA repair. The author has adopted the liberal use of atriofemoral bypass for extent I–III TAAAs based on the concept of the spinal cord collateral network, which emphasizes the importance of the pelvic/hypogastric vessels and a selective approach toward intercostal reconstruction. The author prefers to continuously perfuse the mesenteric circulation during reconstruction of the visceral aortic segment. This can be accomplished with either a Y-connection from the atriofemoral bypass circuit, or with in-line mesenteric shunting from the proximal graft after completion of the proximal anastomosis (**Figure 35.3**).

Clamping sequence and proximal anastomosis

The aortic prosthesis is prepared by attaching a 6-mm polytetrafluoroethylene (PTFE) sidearm graft that will serve as the conduit for LRA reconstruction. For most

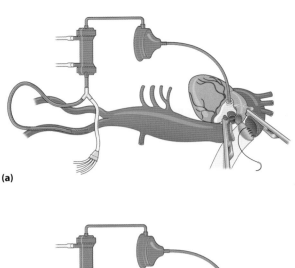

(a)

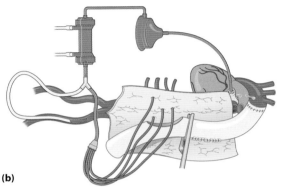

(b)

Figure 35.3 Approach to operative conduct of thoracoabdominal aneurysm repair. (**a**) Distal perfusion (via left heart bypass) with the heparin-impregnated Biomedicus 560 Centrifugal Pump (Medtronic, Minneapolis, MN, USA), where perfusion distal to the proximal cross-clamp is initially maintained via the femoral artery. (**b**) Perfusion is then maintained by multiple perfusion catheters once reconstruction proceeds distally.

aneurysms, a Dacron prosthesis is the preferred conduit. However, PTFE is used to repair mycotic aneurysms because of its decreased susceptibility to infection.

Atriofemoral bypass is initiated by cannulation of the left IPV and the arterial return is via the left common femoral artery. Flows are adjusted to maintain distal mean perfusion pressures of at least 60–70 mmHg; any deterioration in MEP should prompt an increase in stimulus intensity or an increase in distal perfusion pressures. A sudden drop in MEP amplitude (within 2–10 minutes) or a sustained progressive drop (within 10–40 minutes) of >75% from baseline is considered significant and should be addressed. Efforts are made to place the first sequential clamp to allow retrograde perfusion of the lower intercostals and renal/viscerals via atriofemoral bypass (**Figure 35.3**).

The orifices of the proximal intercostal vessel from T4 to T8 typically vigorously back-bleed and are rapidly oversewn. Intercostal vessels in the T9–L1 segments are evaluated for potential reimplantation based on MEP signals. These vessels are controlled with balloon occlusion catheters to prevent ongoing back-bleeding and prevent the negative "sump" effect on net spinal cord perfusion that can result from exposure to atmospheric pressure. Unless there are significant MEP changes, the author defers intercostal reconstruction to the later stages of the operation. The proximal neck is prepared for reconstruction. Circumferential division of the aorta avoids late suture line esophageal erosion, and permits the use of a circumferential PTFE felt wrap if the aorta is fragile. After completion of the proximal anastomosis, the clamp is moved to the graft and the distal clamp is moved below the visceral aortic segment.

Renal/visceral artery reconstruction

The superior mesenteric (SMA) and celiac arteries are controlled with bulldog clamps, while the renal arteries are gently cannulated with 6-Fr Pruitt® perfusion catheters (LeMaitre Vascular, Burlington, MA, USA) under direct vision. The LRA is transected at its origin from the aorta. The author uses direct installation of renal preservation fluid (4 °C Ringer's lactate solution with 25 g mannitol/L and 1 g/L methylprednisolone) into the renal ostia before the start of visceral reconstruction. Orificial endarterectomy should be performed when significant occlusive lesions of the right renal artery (RRA) and SMA exist. In cases where aortic endarterectomy is required, the SMA and celiac artery should be dissected sufficiently to facilitate countertraction from the external side of the vessel, if necessary. This is not possible with the RRA and sharp excision under direct vision is the best way to end an endarterectomy plane that does not feather.

The author uses a single inclusion button that encompasses the origins of the celiac artery, SMA, and RRA (**Figure 35.4a**). If there is wide separation of the visceral/renal ostia, individual anastomoses to each vessel may be necessary. Alternatively, the SMA and RRA can be reimplanted as a single inclusion button. The aortic graft is placed under tension and an elliptical side island is excised. This usually begins on the lateral aspect of the graft and spirals posteriorly toward the origin of the RRA. With the graft under tension, it is possible to complete the posterior portion of the anastomosis with single stitches of suture passing through both the aorta and the Dacron graft. As the posterior aspect of this suture line continues around the inferior border of the RRA, the author exchanges the 6-Fr perfusion catheter for a 12-Fr perfusion catheter to temporarily stent the origin of the RRA. The catheter is gently agitated up and down as the suture line moves around the orifice to ensure that it is not compromised by generous suture stitches as they pass outside of the aorta. Recently, the author has used a 6 × 5 or 6 × 18 balloon-expandable stent to ensure that the suture line does not compromise RRA flow. The stent is placed under direct vision after the proximal suture line is beyond the orifice of the artery (**Figure 35.4b**). The anterior suture line is completed and it is important to take stitches near the origin of the SMA and celiac artery to avoid leaving aneurysmal tissue behind. Just before completion of this suture line, back-bleeding and patency of the celiac artery, SMA, and RRA are verified and a single flush of the proximal aortic cross-clamp is performed to ensure that no clot or debris has built up in the graft.

Reconstruction of the LRA is accomplished with a separate sidearm graft of 6-mm PTFE. This provides a direct and

Right renal artery orifice

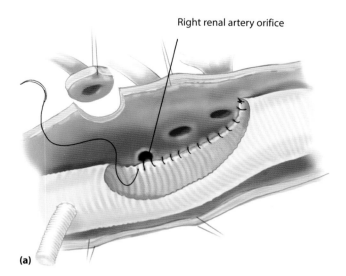

(a)

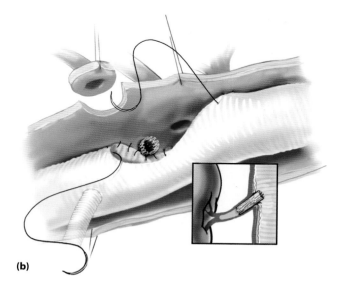

(b)

Figure 35.4 (a) Creation of visceral button inclusion anastomosis of the celiac axis, SMA, and right renal artery (RRA) and 6-mm polytetrafluoroethylene sidearm bypass for left renal artery reconstruction. When performing this, the author uses a 12-Fr perfusion catheter as a stent of sorts in the RRA to prevent compromise of its orifice as the anastomosis is carried around these arterial origins. (b) Deployment of balloon-expandable stent into the right renal orifice to either treat occlusive lesions or prevent encroachment by the suture line, which should be placed immediately at or into the vessel ostia.

deliberate anastomosis in end-to-end fashion while allowing flexibility to deal with the spectrum of occlusive lesions, multiple renal arteries, and other wrinkles that may be encountered. It is important to orient this sidearm graft so that it does not kink when the LRA is returned to its anatomic position.

Reconstruction of intercostal vessels

Next, the intercostal vessels in the T9–L1 segments are addressed. If there has been no change in MEP during the operation, the occlusion balloons are removed and the vessels are oversewn with silk suture. If reconstruction is desired, it can usually be accomplished through an inclusion button anastomosis. Intercostal arteries in the region

of a proximal or distal aortic anastomosis can be reconstructed using a long, beveled suture line. Other methods of revascularization include attaching additional short sidearm grafts to the main aortic graft; in cases where the vessel origin is rotated superiorly and to the patient's left side, implantation to the main aortic graft with Carrel patches of the aorta that contain the intercostal vessels may be feasible (**Figure 35.5**).

Distal anastomosis

The author makes every effort to perform tube reconstructions to the aortic bifurcation unless there is gross aneurysmal disease of the common iliac arteries.

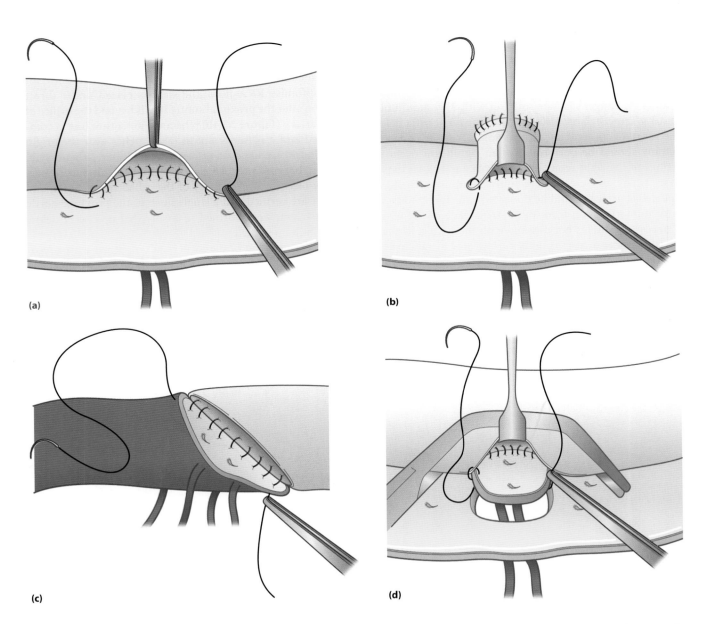

(a)

(b)

(c)

(d)

Figure 35.5 Methods of managing critical intercostal arteries. (**a**) Inclusion button anastomosis. (**b**) Separate sidearm graft. (**c**) Beveled anastomosis preservation, when possible. (**d**) Carrel patch mobilization and direct reimplantation into the graft.

Extending the reconstruction to the iliac or femoral arteries is only performed when no other technical alternative exists. After reestablishment of flow to the lower extremities and verification of adequate lower extremity perfusion by intraoperative pulse volume recordings, Doppler signals in the LRA, celiac artery, and SMA are checked and the SMA pulse in the root of the mesentery is palpated.

Hemostasis is usually adequate on completion of the distal anastomosis, but infusions of platelets and fresh frozen plasma (FFP) are typically increased at this point in the operation when a final check for surgical hemorrhage is made. Indeed, careful attention to hemostasis from the beginning of the operation, combined with minimal heparin use, is an important component of care. Careful inspection of the inferior aspect of the entire aneurysm sac is necessary to detect back-bleeding lumbar/intercostal vessels that can be a source of significant postoperative hemorrhage. The redundant aneurysm sac is sutured over the aortic prosthesis in the abdomen and chest. Before closure, renal artery reconstructions are interrogated one final time. As the left kidney is returned to its anatomic position, the perinephric fat usually suffices to provide adequate coverage of the aortic graft in the region of the visceral aortic segment. A single pleural tube is placed and a closed suction drain may be left in the retroperitoneum if hemostasis is in question. Closure of extensive incisions typically takes an hour.

Postoperative care

Postoperatively, patients should be monitored in an intensive care unit setting. It is important to limit hemodynamic shifts because these can lead to renal failure and SCI. BP parameters should be tailored to the patient with the goal of maintaining adequate perfusion to preserve urine output, cardiac function, and spinal cord perfusion. Oxygen delivery is important in the early phase of recovery and the author rarely extubates patients in the early postoperative period. If patients have stabilized overnight, the tube is pulled in the morning. It is important to monitor the hematocrit for signs of ongoing bleeding and all coagulation disorders should be aggressively corrected. The author typically supports intravascular volume with FFP infusions for the initial 12 hours after the operation. CSF drainage is arbitrarily continued for 48 hours postoperatively and the drain is then capped for 24 hours of observation before removal.

RESULTS OF TREATMENT AND COMPLICATIONS

Operative mortality

The operative mortality after TAAA repair ranges from 8 to 16%; however, in the author's experience, the 30-day mortality is 4.4% for elective TAAA repaired with atriofemoral bypass.[2] As the number of comorbid conditions increases, so does the overall operative risk. Individual series have reported that preoperative coronary artery disease, COPD, and renal insufficiency increase mortality. In addition, the extent of TAAA has a dominant effect on SCI.

Renal failure

Minimizing renal ischemic times, using cold perfusate, avoiding intraoperative hypotension, and treating stenotic lesions aggressively with either bypass or open stent placement reduce renal injury. Most cases are self-limited. The author reserves dialysis for specific clinical indications like volume overload, hyperkalemia, or acidosis. When needed, continuous venovenous hemodialysis is preferred because it provides for a smoother hemodynamic course than conventional hemodialysis. Preoperative renal insufficiency is the most powerful predictor of postoperative renal failure; postoperative renal dysfunction negatively affects short- and long-term survival.

Respiratory complications

Respiratory failure is the most common complication after TAAA repair. Indeed, if strict criteria are used, some 40% of patients suffer a respiratory complication. Contributing factors include paralysis of the left hemidiaphragm and pain from the extensive chest wall incision that impedes pulmonary hygiene. Accordingly, a diaphragm-sparing technique is applied when possible. For patients who fail extubation, the author favors early placement of a tracheostomy (required in <10% of patients).

Spinal cord ischemia

SCI is the most devastating nonfatal complication associated with TAAA reconstruction. Although advances such as epidural cooling, distal perfusion, and intraoperative monitoring of MEP have improved outcomes, this remains an unsolved problem. The pathogenesis of SCI after aortic replacement is likely multifactorial, but ultimately results from an ischemic insult caused by temporary or permanent interruption of the spinal cord blood supply. SCI manifests along a clinical spectrum from complete flaccid paraplegia to varying degrees of paraparesis; the degree of SCI directly predicts long-term survival after TAAA repair (**Table 35.1**). Patients with incomplete deficits typically recover reasonable function and have a long-term survival that is like those without SCI. However, patients with an SCI Deficit Scale score of I (flaccid paralysis) rarely live beyond the first year. The most common predictors of SCI after TAAA repair include extent I and II aneurysms and urgency of operation.

Table 35.1 Short- and long-term survival of 576 patients undergoing open TAAA repair at the Massachusetts General Hospital stratified by Spinal Cord Ischemic Deficit (SCID)

SCID category	Survival (%)		
	30-day	**1-year**	**5-year**
SCID 0[a]	92	73	51
SCID I[b]	54	21	41
SCID II[c]	87	70	41
SCID III[d]	100	73	45

[a] No SCI.
[b] Flaccid paralysis.
[c] Average neurologic muscle grade <50% function.
[d] Average neurologic muscle grade >50% function.
TAAA: thoracoabdominal aortic aneurysm.

Late outcomes

Late survival after TAAA repair is identical to that of patients who undergo elective AAA repair. In addition, late aortic events occur in about 10% of patients, but few of these are graft-related. Graft-related complications include occlusion of visceral vessel reconstructions, graft infections (including aortoesophageal fistulas), and the appearance of inclusion patch aneurysms; these are rare in the author's experience. Most late aortic events are the result of native aneurysmal disease in remote (or noncontiguous) aortic segments. With improvement of perioperative outcomes, the focus of long-term follow-up has shifted to examination of the impact of TAAA repair on functional outcome. Several reports have emerged validating that most operative survivors return to their preoperative independent living status.[3]

REFERENCES

1. Cambria RP. Thoracoabdominal aortic aneurysm repair: how I do it. *Cardiovasc Surg.* 1999;7:597–606.
2. Conrad MF, Cambria RP. Contemporary management of descending thoracic and thoracoabdominal aortic aneurysms: endovascular versus open. *Circulation.* 2008;**117**:841–852.
3. Lancaster RT, Conrad MF, Patel VI, et al. Further experience with distal aortic perfusion and motor-evoked potential monitoring in the management of extent I–III thoracoabdominal aortic aneurysms. *J Vasc Surg.* 2013;**58**:283–290.

36

Open inflammatory aortic aneurysm repair

CHARLES A. WEST Jr.

CONTENTS

INTRODUCTION

Inflammatory aortic aneurysms are uncommon vascular lesions ranging in frequency from 3 to 10% of surgically repaired abdominal aortic aneurysms (AAAs). They represent unique additional challenges to the vascular surgeon, compared with those seen during open repair of routine degenerative AAAs. The likelihood of these technical difficulties increases as the extent of the aneurysm and size of the inflammatory mass increase.

Inflammatory aortic aneurysms occur at a younger age, have a stronger familial tendency, and occur more predominantly in men compared to noninflammatory aneurysms. These patients are almost uniformly smokers. The majority are symptomatic at presentation with abdominal or back pain, weight loss, and elevated erythrocyte sedimentation rate as common clinical findings. The diagnosis is made preoperatively with 90% sensitivity using computed tomography angiography or magnetic resonance angiography. Inflammatory aortic aneurysms are usually isolated to the infrarenal segment of the abdominal aorta. A characteristic inflammatory cuff of periaortitis and perianeurysmal fibrosis encasing the aneurysm wall, which enhances with contrast, is the classic radiographic feature (**Figure 36.1**). At surgical exploration, the presence of a pearly white, glistening aortic wall with dense adhesions of retroperitoneal structures to its surface is the *sine qua non* of the inflammatory aortic aneurysm (**Figure 36.2**). The aortic wall is 3–4 times thicker and more rigid than degenerative aneurysms, and the inflammatory process is limited to the anterior and lateral aortic wall. These features increase the incidence of injury to both vascular and visceral retroperitoneal structures during aneurysm repair.

Endovascular aneurysm repair (EVAR) has been used in the treatment of inflammatory aortic aneurysms with success and some have demonstrated regression of the fibrosis. Results from EVAR are similar to those for noninflammatory AAAs. However, controversy exists regarding the resolution of symptoms from the perianeurysmal fibrosis and inflammation after EVAR, and this technique may not sufficiently address proximal aneurysms with pararenal extent. For complex AAAs, advanced endovascular techniques using branched and fenestrated endografts or aortic debranching may provide better alternatives; however, at this juncture, these are still investigational and have not been widely applied to the treatment of inflammatory aneurysms. As a result, the special considerations in the open reconstruction for inflammatory aortic aneurysms are still worthy of study and review for both vascular surgeons and trainees.

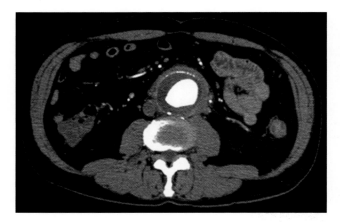

Figure 36.1 Computed tomography angiography axial image of an inflammatory abdominal aortic aneurysm with classic thickened and fibrotic aneurysm wall.

OPERATIVE MANAGEMENT

Exposures

The abdominal aorta can be approached from two sectors, anteriorly or laterally. The anterior, via a midline celiotomy using a xipho-pubic incision, affords specific advantages in treating aneurysmal and occlusive disease. The lateral approach can be from a thoracoabdominal incision involving two body cavities or a direct left lateral approach from a flank incision with the patient turned in a 90-degree position. The anterior approach offers the advantage of ease and facility in addressing the aorta and its branches from the renal artery level to beyond the femoral bifurcation in those with juxtarenal or infrarenal aortic aneurysms. Operating room preparation is simpler and easily reproducible for emergent procedures.

ANTERIOR EXPOSURE
Infracolic aortic exposure

The patient is placed in a supine position with both arms tucked and protected. The skin is sterilized from just above the nipple level to the knees. Fluorescent ureteral stents are placed before skin incision to prevent injury in the event of ureteral adhesion to the inflammatory aneurysm. A midline incision that extends from the xiphoid process to just above the pubis creates the space required to safely expose the proximal aorta at the renal and mesenteric level down to the iliac bifurcations. For added exposure, the xiphoid process may be resected and the skin incision carried further cephalad. An Omni-Tract Wishbone Retractor System (Integra LifeSciences Corporation, Plainsboro, NJ, USA) is placed to provide the required upward and lateral retraction. As the exposure is created, shallow blades are transitioned to longer blades for retraction of the posterior peritoneal tissues, the abdominal wall, and the lower chest wall. The retractor system must be properly placed to achieve lateral and superior retraction of the upper abdominal cavity. The retractor's central lock hinge

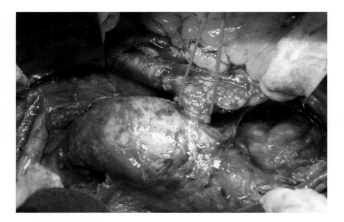

Figure 36.2 Intraoperative image of an inflammatory abdominal aortic aneurysm with its characteristic pearly white, glistening appearance.

is positioned in the midsternal region with the wishbone arms spread wide several centimeters lateral to the midaxillary line. The hinge lock mechanism and arms are elevated 15–20 cm above the horizontal surface of the chest and abdomen. The wishbone arms are kept parallel and slightly abducted. This allows the force vector generated by the retractors to be at a 45-degree angle from the horizontal plane of the anterior abdominal wall directed upward and outward.

After the abdomen has been opened, the nasogastric tube placement has been confirmed, and the abdomen has been explored, the falciform ligament is taken down between heavy ties. This is followed by division of the triangular ligament toward the dome of the diaphragm. The right side of the transverse colon is tucked above the liver. The mid-transverse colon and splenic flexure are pulled up and over the stomach and placed under the diaphragm with dry laparotomy pads. A longitudinal posterior peritoneal incision is made over the aneurysm from the base of the pancreas to the aortic bifurcation and biased toward the right iliac artery, as the small intestinal contents are manually retracted to the right with the surgeon's left hand or a handheld deep retractor.

In the setting of an inflammatory aneurysm, the duodenum is generally adherent to the anterior right lateral aneurysm wall. This segment should be left undisturbed until the proximal dissection is complete. The ligament of Treitz is mobilized completely before completing the full length of the posterior retroperitoneal incision. The small bowel and the third and fourth portions of the duodenum are wrapped in a moist towel and kept intracavitary; they are retracted with a wide malleable or Fence solid blade to the right. The duodenum adherent to the aneurysm is allowed to escape the enclosed towel; the remaining duodenum and small bowel are held.

At this juncture, the inferior mesenteric vein is divided between heavy ties. The long retractor blades are advanced deeper and the posterior peritoneal structures are hooked by the blades and retracted to the right and left.

The upper abdominal wall and lower rib cage are spread widely apart. Proximally, a transverse posterior peritoneal incision is made at the base of the pancreas in the avascular plain perpendicular to the longitudinal incision over the aneurysm. This incision is carried laterally above the left renal vein (LRV) and toward the inferior vena cava (IVC) on the right side. A Harrington blade is placed in the midline over the central mesenteric root for proximal gentle retraction of the body of the pancreas.

Deep to the pancreas, the LRV is either dissected in a comprehensive manner or divided. If the renal vein is densely adherent to the aneurysm, it is transected and closed with monofilament suture or a vascular stapler near the IVC and just to the left of the aorta, preserving the critical branches. Preserving the branches of the LRV during this process is important for kidney viability, and the decision should be made early to avoid undesirable bleeding. In smaller inflammatory aneurysms, the LRV is managed more easily, and preservation and mobilization of the vein may be possible. The branches are taken down sequentially between 3-0 silk ties, to include the adrenal vein, accessory renal branches, and the lumbar-renal vein. A renal vein retractor may be placed anterior to the pararenal aorta to retract the vein superiorly by several centimeters.

At this point, both renal arteries are dissected out sharply and encircled with silastic vessel loops. The diaphragmatic crura on either side of the aorta in the space above the renal arteries are visible. These are divided posteriorly down to the spine. These maneuvers liberate the aorta anteriorly and permit safe clamping of the suprarenal aorta after gentle circumferential digital exploration to ensure complete tissue clearance. The superior mesenteric artery can be dissected out sharply, excising lymphatic tissue if needed, and looped for a supramesenteric aortic clamp position, if necessary. This is the maximum proximal limit of aortic exposure with the infracolic approach.

The inferior abdominal wall retraction is expanded by dividing the inferior mesenteric artery and placing a deep retractor blade lateral to the left side of the midportion of the aneurysm, sweeping the posterior peritoneal structures laterally, including the mesentery of the sigmoid colon. The iliac arteries are sharply dissected out as needed down to the iliac artery bifurcations.

LATERAL APPROACHES

Thoracoabdominal and flank exposures

A thoracoabdominal or flank approach may be adopted to avoid structures that adhere to the inflammatory aneurysm, such as the duodenum and LRV. The thoracoabdominal approach involves a two-body cavity exposure with the patient turned 60 degrees at the chest and 45 degrees at the hip, with an "S" incision through the eighth intercostal space from a left-side up position. The dissection can be retroperitoneal or the parietal peritoneum can be opened, followed by an extended left medial visceral rotation. The author's preference is to open the abdomen and chest and divide the diaphragm circumferentially toward the hiatus, before embarking on the medial visceral rotation (MVR).

Generally, complete diaphragm division is not required. Once retractors are placed, the MVR begins by taking down the white line of Toldt from the left lower quadrant extending superiorly and medially. The kidney is brought anteriorly, to avoid the adherent LRV, and the crura on the left are divided. The mesenteric vessels are exposed with sharp dissection after dividing the crura and releasing the medial arcuate ligament. Location of the proximal clamp is established, and iliac vessel control is obtained via sharp dissection with COOLEY vascular scissors (Becton, Dickinson and Company, Franklin Lakes, NJ, USA). The iliolumbar vein is divided and care is taken to avoid injury to the left ureter.

The lateral flank approach is described in Chapter 34 and performed from a 90-degree right lateral decubitus position. The incision is begun at the lower costal margin and is transversely oriented toward the umbilicus. The dissection is kept in a true retroperitoneal plane. The 12th rib is often removed and the diaphragm is partially incised. This approach avoids the anatomic hazards encountered anteriorly. One disadvantage is the extreme posterior displacement of the right iliofemoral vessels, but this may be favored based on surgeon preference and experience.

Reconstruction

The reconstructive phases are like traditional methods of open degenerative aortic aneurysm repair. After systemic heparin administration (100 IU/kg), an activated clotting time >250 seconds is achieved before aortic clamping. Curved, heavy iliac clamps are placed first, followed by a curved aortic clamp placed suprarenal for the juxtarenal repair. The renal arteries are clamped with coarctation clamps. The aneurysm is opened, the thrombus is removed, lumbar bleeding is controlled, and a graft is sewn end-to-end in a standard fashion. A bifurcated graft is preferred and this is sewn end-to-end to the non-diseased appropriate iliofemoral vessels in a sequential manner (**Figure 36.3**). After declamping is accomplished

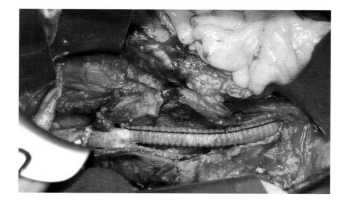

Figure 36.3 Intraoperative image of a completed aorto-bi-iliac bypass graft. Note the markedly thickened anterior aneurysm wall.

and hemostasis is achieved, enough of the inflammatory aneurysm sac is resected to allow for graft coverage by the remaining aneurysm wall. The posterior peritoneum is closed, followed by abdominal wall closure.

TECHNICAL KEYS

Inflammatory aortic aneurysms

The primary key to the operation is wide exposure. This permits the surgeon to reliably control the aorta and its surrounding structures, preventing injury to vascular and visceral structures.

Preincisional placement of ureteral stents is used in all cases. Appropriate retractor set-up is fundamental to the exposure process and ultimate safety and success. Adequate lateral and superior retraction of the upper abdominal wall and lower rib cage with sequential advancement of deep self-retaining retractor blades is needed. Early division of the LRV in the setting of anterior aortic wall adherence prevents undesired bleeding during renal vein dissection and provides better exposure.

Attempts at duodenal dissection of the inflammatory aneurysm risks injury and perforation of the duodenum. It should be left intact until the proximal and distal dissections are complete and preferably until after the aneurysm is clamped and opened. If necessary for adequate exposure, the duodenum can be dissected off the aneurysm wall with a No. 15 blade, leaving 1–2 mm of aneurysm wall on the duodenum as it is mobilized.

CONCLUSION

Open aortic reconstruction for complex aneurysms is becoming an infrequently applied skill set in contemporary vascular surgery. As a result, the anatomic nuances of inflammatory aortic aneurysms are even less frequently encountered than in the past. Familiarity with these and their impact on the risk of open repair of inflammatory aortic aneurysms continues to be worthy of study and review by vascular surgeons.

SUGGESTED READING

Crawford JL, Stowe CL, Safi HJ, et al. Inflammatory aneurysms of the aorta. *J Vasc Surg.* 1985;**2**:113–124.

Goldstone J, Malone JM, Moore WS. Inflammatory aneurysms of the abdominal aorta. *Surgery.* 1978;**83**:425–430.

Hill J, Charlesworth D. Inflammatory abdominal aortic aneurysms: a report of thirty-seven cases. *Ann Vasc Surg.* 1988;**2**:352–357.

Pennell RC, Hollier LH, Lie JT, et al. Inflammatory abdominal aortic aneurysms: a thirty-year review. *J Vasc Surg.* 1985;**2**:859–869.

Rasmussen TE, Hallett JW Jr. Inflammatory aortic aneurysms. A clinical review with new perspectives in pathogenesis. *Ann Surg.* 1997;**225**:155–164.

Tang T, Boyle JR, Dixon AK, et al. Inflammatory abdominal aortic aneurysms. *Eur J Vasc Endovasc Surg.* 2005;**29**:353–362.

Walker DI, Bloor K, Williams G, et al. Inflammatory aneurysms of the abdominal aorta. *Br J Surg.* 1972;**59**:609–614.

37

Open splanchnic artery aneurysm repair

R. JASON VONDERHAAR, AAMIR SHAH, AND BRUCE GEWERTZ

CONTENTS

INTRODUCTION

Splanchnic artery aneurysms are rare with a reported incidence of <2%.[1-3] While most patients with splanchnic artery aneurysms are asymptomatic, rupture does occur in 10–25% of patients and these patients have a significant mortality that ranges from 25% to as high as 70%.[4,5] Splenic artery aneurysms (SAAs) account for about 60% of reported visceral aneurysms; an additional 20% arise from the hepatic artery.[6]

Because of the limited insights into their natural history, size criteria for intervention are not clear. Most agree that "true" aneurysms should be treated only if symptomatic or if their size exceeds 2 cm; in contrast, most pseudoaneurysms merit treatment unless very small and stable.[7,8] While treatment by open surgery or catheter-based interventions is generally considered only in larger aneurysms,[3,9,10] aneurysms <2 cm can rupture. This is especially true in the jejunal, ileal, or colic distributions. SAAs, irrespective of size, are also particularly prone to rupture during pregnancy.

Before treating any aneurysm, adequate imaging is essential. In the past, this was accomplished by conventional angiography, although presently computed tomography angiography (CTA) or magnetic resonance angiography predominate. An important advantage of axial imaging over angiography is that it allows examination of adjacent intra-abdominal organs.

General treatment options of all splanchnic artery aneurysms include open surgical repair or endovascular treatment. The objective of treatment is to exclude the aneurysm from the circulation and to preserve adequate perfusion to the organs. With open repair, the aneurysm may be ligated or resected with distal organ revascularization. The preferred approach depends on the degree of collateral flow. Ligation is most often chosen for ruptured aneurysms with good collateral flow. Arteries that lack adequate collateral flow require revascularization. When revascularization is performed, a direct arterio-arterial anastomosis or aortic reimplantation may be performed. An autologous vein or prosthetic conduit may be used. In saccular aneurysms, aneurysmorrhaphy with excision of the diseased portion of the vessel wall can be performed, although recurrence is higher.

RELEVANT VASCULAR ANATOMY

A thorough knowledge of the anatomy and important collateral vessels involving the splanchnic arteries is required to determine the appropriate exposure and operative treatment of visceral artery aneurysms (**Figure 37.1**). The celiac axis originates from the anterior surface of the proximal abdominal aorta as it passes between the diaphragmatic crura at the level of the 12th thoracic vertebra. Most commonly, the artery divides into three major

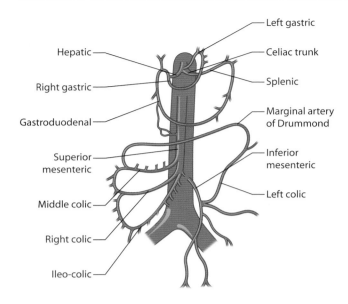

Figure 37.1 Mesenteric circulation. Reproduced from Gewertz BL, Schwartz LB, Brewster DC, et al. eds. *Surgery of the Aorta and Its Branches*. Philadelphia, PA: Saunders; 2000. p. 329.

branches within 2 cm of its origin: the common hepatic artery (CHA); splenic artery; and left gastric artery (LGA). These branches and their tributaries provide the blood supply for the stomach, liver, spleen, portions of the pancreas, and the proximal duodenum. The CHA gives rise to the superior pancreaticoduodenal arteries (PDAs), the cystic artery, and the right gastric artery (RGA) in addition to the left and right hepatic arteries. The splenic artery gives off the dorsal pancreatic artery, left gastroepiploic artery, and short gastric arteries before completing its tortuous course toward the spleen. The LGA supplies the gastric cardia and fundus before anastomosing with the RGA.

The next branch of the aorta, the superior mesenteric artery (SMA), provides the major arterial supply to the mid and distal small bowel, and the ascending and transverse colon. The SMA typically arises about 1 cm distal to the celiac axis, just inferior to the diaphragmatic hiatus at the level of the first lumbar vertebra. It travels behind the neck of the pancreas, in front of the uncinate process and over the third portion of the duodenum. It gives rise to the inferior PDA, which anastomoses with the corresponding superior branch from the celiac circulation, and to the middle colic artery just before entering the base of the mesentery of the small bowel.

SPLENIC ARTERY ANEURYSMS

SAAs are most often saccular; 80% are in the distal third of the splenic artery or at bifurcations.[11] Splenic artery pseudoaneurysms can be associated with blunt splenic trauma and pancreatitis, including the mechanism of erosion of pancreatic pseudocysts into the

splenic artery.[12] Rupture occurs in <2% of all SAAs, but they have a mortality rate of about 25%. Rupture of an SAA during pregnancy most commonly occurs in the third trimester, with maternal and fetal mortality rates of 70 and 95%, respectively.[13]

Ruptured aneurysms can either bleed freely into the peritoneal cavity, causing shock and death, or into the lesser sac, providing temporary containment and a chance for intervention. If undetected, such lesser sac hematomas eventually rupture into the peritoneal cavity and can cause fatal bleeding.[13] SAAs can also rupture into the gastrointestinal (GI) tract or pancreatic duct.[14,15] Treatment is recommended for all ruptured and symptomatic SAAs, all SAAs in pregnant women or those of childbearing age, and all pseudoaneurysms. Treatment of patients with asymptomatic aneurysms >2 cm in diameter is indicated if the procedural risk is acceptable.

Operative treatment varies with location of the aneurysm. Proximal or midportion aneurysms are treated with resection or ligation; revascularization is generally not required because the distal splenic artery fills through collaterals from the short gastric arteries. Distal aneurysms adjacent to the splenic hilum may require splenectomy, especially when the aneurysm involves distal branches within the splenic parenchyma (**Figure 37.2**). When distal aneurysms are located within the pancreatic parenchyma, distal pancreatectomy may be necessary.[16] Pseudoaneurysms associated with pancreatitis are best managed with endovascular treatment because of the elevated operative risk and the possibility of aggravating the pancreatitis. In a retrospective series from Pulli and collaborators,[9] 30 patients with SAAs underwent operative repair. The SAA was completely resected in 27 patients (including 22 patients with end-to-end splenic

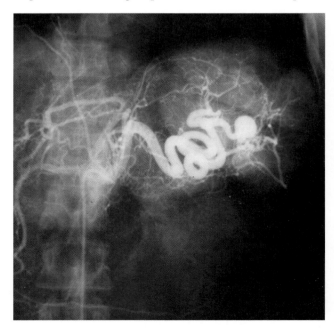

Figure 37.2 Distal splenic artery aneurysm (courtesy of James C. Stanley).

artery anastomotic reconstruction and 5 with distal pancreatectomy).

Proximal SAAs are best approached through the lesser sac after dividing the gastrohepatic ligament (GHL). The afferent and efferent vessels from the aneurysm are ligated to exclude blood flow from the sac. The aneurysm itself can be excised unless it is embedded in the parenchyma of the pancreas or adherent to other structures. If the aneurysm sac is not excised, it should be opened to ensure that all connected branches have been ligated. In either case, reconstruction of the splenic artery is generally not required.

Aneurysms of the mid-to-distal splenic artery are better approached by taking down the gastrocolic ligament (GCL) to enter the lesser sac. The pancreas may also need to be mobilized to better expose the splenic artery coursing just superior and posterior to its body and tail. Recurrent episodes of pancreatitis, especially with formation of pseudocysts, which can erode into the artery, can produce pseudoaneurysms in this location. These can be especially difficult to dissect. Often it is easier to ligate the orifice to each branch from inside the aneurysm sac rather than dissect out each branch separately. Clamping the splenic artery proximal and distal to the aneurysm before opening it will decrease blood loss and allow easier visualization of each orifice once the sac is opened. Each vessel is then suture-ligated from within the sac with monofilament polypropylene suture. Adjacent pseudocysts may need to be addressed with internal or external drainage. When cysts involve the distal body or tail of the pancreas, it may be preferable to perform a distal pancreatectomy, removing the diseased pancreas, pseudocyst, and aneurysmal artery all at once.

Historically, aneurysms near the hilum of the spleen have been treated with splenectomy. To provide better exposure, the spleen may need to be mobilized by taking down some of its ligamentous attachments to the diaphragm, colon, or kidney. If technically feasible, aneurysmorrhaphy, ligation exclusion, or aneurysm excision are all preferred methods of treatment over splenectomy.

Laparoscopic ligation of an SAA is a minimally invasive surgical option that was first reported in 1997 by Matsumoto and collaborators.[17] SAAs are laparoscopically accessible by dividing the GCL. If the aneurysm is saccular, a vascular stapler may be applied across its base, although this may leave behind a part of the aneurysmal wall as a source for recurrence.[17] For aneurysms in the hilum of the spleen, laparoscopic splenectomy can be performed. Laparoscopic ultrasonography is useful to localize the aneurysm and identify its tributaries. Such precise localization minimizes dissection near the pancreas and pancreatitis.

HEPATIC ARTERY ANEURYSMS

Hepatic artery aneurysms (HAAs) are the second most common visceral artery aneurysm.[18,19] A recent literature

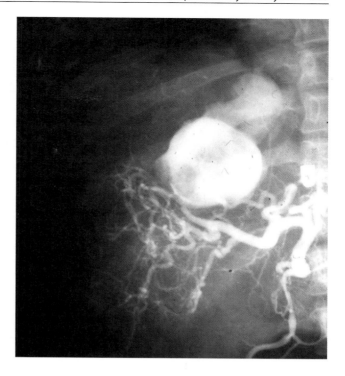

Figure 37.3 Hepatic artery aneurysm (courtesy of James C. Stanley).

review suggested that two-thirds of true HAAs are extrahepatic, while intraparenchymal lesions are much more commonly pseudoaneurysms arising from either blunt trauma or interventional procedures on the biliary tract (**Figure 37.3**). Approximately 90% of HAAs are solitary and degenerative in nature.[18] HAAs have one of the highest rates of rupture of all visceral artery aneurysms and have a high mortality rate of 40% when presenting with rupture.[20]

HAAs can rupture into the GI or biliary tract as well as the peritoneal cavity. The classic triad of abdominal pain, hemobilia, and obstructive jaundice, reflecting a ruptured intrahepatic aneurysm, is seen in less than one-third of cases.[21] Because of the high rupture rate and absence of prodromal symptoms, many authors have advocated more aggressive treatment of HAAs.

Current management recommendations include treatment of all symptomatic aneurysms and, in good operative candidates, all true aneurysms >2 cm or with rapid growth. Pseudoaneurysms should be treated regardless of size. HAAs in patients with polyarteritis nodosa and fibromuscular dysplasia also appear to be at increased risk for rupture and should be repaired if >2 cm.[20]

Precise preoperative evaluation of the arterial anatomy is especially important for HAAs given the relatively high rate of anatomic variations (replaced right or left hepatic arteries originating from the SMA in 18% or LGA in 12% of humans, respectively). Surgical exposure is obtained through either a right subcostal or upper midline laparotomy incision. Proximal aneurysms near the celiac trunk may be exposed by dividing the GHL and entering the lesser sac. More distal lesions can be found within the portal triad running in the hepatoduodenal ligament.

Most common HAAs can be treated by ligation without reconstruction or coil embolization. Retrograde flow through the gastroduodenal artery (GDA) into the proper hepatic artery (PHA) can almost always adequately perfuse the liver. Similarly, collaterals can also allow retrograde flow through the RGA into the PHA. An intraoperative trial of clamping the CHA for 5–10 minutes may be performed to assess for adequate collateral circulation. If there is concern about adequate blood flow to the liver, hepatic artery reconstruction with an interposition vein graft should be performed. CHA ligation is not recommended in the setting of cirrhosis or other liver disease, because even minimal decreases in blood flow may cause ischemic necrosis. In these cases and those in which the GDA has inadequate caliber, vein graft reconstruction should be strongly considered.[19]

Aneurysms in the PHA and its branches nearly always require revascularization to prevent liver ischemia. The PHA courses along the left side of the hepatoduodenal ligament and care must be taken during its dissection so as not to injure the other elements of the portal triad that are near; the common bile duct is usually to the right of the artery while the portal vein is more posterior. Exposure can be especially challenging when treating aneurysms associated with significant inflammation. If the dissection proves too difficult, the aneurysm sac can be opened and any vessels that have not yet been isolated can be controlled from within the sac using balloon catheters.

Saccular aneurysms involving less than half of the vessel circumference can be resected and the resulting arteriotomy closed either primarily or with a vein patch. For larger saccular or fusiform aneurysms, it is preferable to fully excise the aneurysm and then perform arterial reconstruction.

Arterial reconstruction can often be performed with an interposition graft between the remaining proximal and distal portions of the hepatic artery. The ends of the graft as well as the artery should be spatulated so as not to cause a narrowing in the lumen at the anastomosis. Alternatively, a bypass graft with inflow from the aorta or right renal artery to the remaining distal hepatic artery can also be performed. Autogenous saphenous vein is generally the preferred conduit for arterial reconstruction, but if the vein is not available because of prior use or inadequate size, a synthetic graft can be used.

Intrahepatic aneurysms are most commonly treated by endovascular means with coil or particle embolization. Embolization carries a risk of liver necrosis, abscess formation, and sepsis. For this reason, patients with liver dysfunction or with proximal intrahepatic aneurysms, where the aneurysmal artery supplies a large amount of the liver parenchyma, are not good candidates for intrahepatic embolization and are better managed with operative care.[19] Open treatment includes proximal and distal ligation, with or without liver resection, depending on the amount of parenchyma at risk for ischemia.

CELIAC ARTERY ANEURYSMS

Celiac artery aneurysms (CAAs) are rare and account for <5% of all visceral artery aneurysms. CAAs may be associated with other visceral artery aneurysms in about 40% of patients and with aortic aneurysms in 20%. The most common etiology of CAAs is atherosclerosis in 27%, followed by medial degeneration in 17%.[22] Other causes of CAAs include pseudoaneurysms from penetrating trauma, saccular mycotic aneurysms, collagen vascular disease, and aneurysms secondary to anomalous splanchnic circulation. The most common anatomic predistribution involves the flow disturbances associated with the common celiacomesenteric trunk, seen in 0.25% of the population.[1]

Because of the low incidence of CAA, it is difficult to reliably identify risk factors for rupture. Size as well as comorbid conditions including hypertension, calcification, etiology of aneurysm, and sex do not accurately predict rupture risk.[22,23] In reports, ruptured CAAs have ranged in size from 2 to 6 cm and were not different in size from unruptured CAAs.[22] With increasing use of axial imaging, most CAAs discovered today are asymptomatic at diagnosis. If symptomatic, they can cause epigastric abdominal pain or rarely obstructive jaundice from compression of the common bile duct. The lifetime risk of rupture of CAAs appears to be between 5 and 15%, with a mortality of approximately 50%.[13,22,23] As with SAAs, a "double rupture" phenomenon can occur, with initial contained lesser sac bleeding followed, in variable time intervals, by extension into the peritoneal cavity through the foramen of Winslow.

Because of the significant mortality associated with rupture, treatment of asymptomatic CAA >2 cm should be strongly considered.[23] Preoperative planning includes: CTA to examine the location of the aneurysm within the celiac artery; evaluation of atherosclerotic burden to determine if revascularization is required; and examination of collateral circulation through the GDA.

The preferred open surgical treatment of CAAs is aneurysm resection with revascularization. The celiac trunk and supraceliac aorta are best exposed by performing a left medial visceral rotation or by exposure through the lesser sac. The esophagus and lesser curvature of the stomach are identified and retracted to the patient's left after division of the GHL. The triangular ligament of the left lobe of the liver is divided (**Figure 37.4**), and the left lateral segment of the liver is gently retracted to the right. The right crus of the diaphragm is divided and the underlying median arcuate ligament incised, often through dense lymphatic and neural tissue. The posterior peritoneum may then be incised and the supraceliac aorta visualized and evaluated for its suitability for proximal anastomosis (**Figure 37.5**). Dissection in an inferior direction will expose the origin of the celiac axis and its primary branches. If the pancreas can be anteriorly retracted, the celiac origin and a limited portion of the origin of the SMA can be accessed. If bypass to the celiac axis is planned, adequate exposure will be available to perform a distal anastomosis to

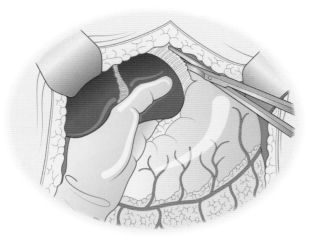

Figure 37.4 Incision of the triangular ligament of the liver, which will be gently retracted to the right in preparation for supraceliac aortic exposure. Reproduced from Zarins CK, Gewertz, BL eds. *Atlas of Vascular Surgery.* 2nd ed. Philadelphia, PA: Churchill Livingstone; 2005. p. 181.

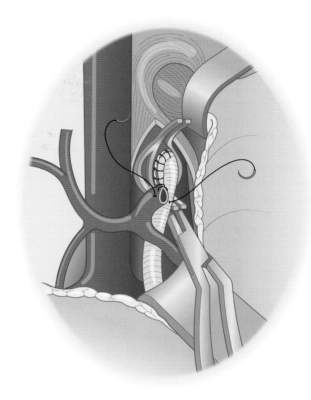

Figure 37.6 Anastomosis to the cut end of the celiac trunk. Reproduced from Zarins CK, Gewertz, BL eds. *Atlas of Vascular Surgery.* 2nd ed. Philadelphia, PA: Churchill Livingstone; 2005. p. 183.

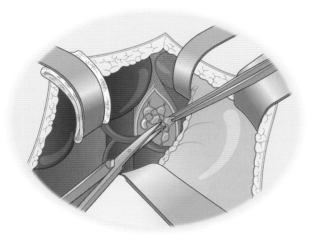

Figure 37.5 Incision of posterior peritoneum and celiac plexus to expose the celiac axis and the origin of the superior mesenteric artery. Reproduced from Zarins CK, Gewertz, BL eds. *Atlas of Vascular Surgery.* 2nd ed. Philadelphia, PA: Churchill Livingstone; 2005. p. 181.

either the CHA or to the cut end of the main celiac trunk (**Figure 37.6**). Reconstruction can be performed with autologous saphenous vein or prosthetic graft. On occasion, aortic reimplantation of the celiac artery is possible. An aortic punch is useful to create a circular opening in the aorta (often at the transected origin of the vessel) and the artery is anastomosed at a 90-degree angle without spatulation.

Ligation alone has been performed in about one-third of reported cases and is safe only when adequate collateral circulation is noted through the SMA. Ligation can pose a risk of intestinal or hepatic ischemia and should not be undertaken with liver dysfunction or with an inadequate caliber GDA. Aneurysmorrhaphy has been employed in <10% of cases for saccular aneurysms involving a small part of the arterial circumference.[22] If there is adequate length and mobility of the remaining proximal and distal ends, it may be possible to reconstruct the celiac artery with primary reanastomosis. Otherwise, an aortoceliac bypass from the supraceliac aorta can be performed with an autogenous or synthetic graft.

SMA ANEURYSMS

SMA aneurysms (SMAAs) account for 5% of all visceral artery aneurysms and are usually located in the first 5 cm of the SMA.[24,25] Complications include rupture, thrombosis, or embolization, all of which can cause intestinal ischemia. Etiologies of SMAAs include true degenerative aneurysms and pseudoaneurysms secondary to pancreatitis. In the past century, over half of all reported SMAAs were mycotic, often through embolization from bacterial endocarditis.[24]

Other than trivial fusiform dilations, most SMAAs should be repaired regardless of size or symptoms. The sequelae of thrombosis and rupture are catastrophic with significant associated morbidity and mortality. Observation of small, asymptomatic aneurysms may be reasonable in patients with multiple comorbidities. As with other vascular beds, most pseudoaneurysms require treatment.

SMAAs often appear distal to the ostial region more commonly affected by atherosclerotic occlusive disease. If infection and inflammation are present, operative exposure in the mesentery may be difficult. Treatment options of SMAAs include ligation without revascularization, which has been performed in one-third of cases historically. This relies on adequate collateral flow from the celiac artery through the inferior PDA or from the inferior mesenteric artery (IMA) through the middle colic artery. The bowel must be monitored intraoperatively for signs of ischemia with direct observation, fluorescein dye, or Doppler. More desirably, direct revascularization can be performed with primary anastomosis, interposition grafting, or aortomesenteric bypass grafting. Rarely is there enough length for direct aortic reimplantation. If the aneurysm is not mycotic, a prosthetic graft may be used. Large saccular aneurysms may be treated by aneurysmorrhaphy, taking care to avoid injury to the superior mesenteric vein, which is often adherent.[25]

Anterior transperitoneal exposure is a simple and serviceable operative approach to the visceral vessels and aorta, although it does not afford continuous exposure of the abdominal and distal thoracic aorta unless combined with a medial visceral rotation (MVR). An upper midline incision affords adequate exposure in most patients, while bilateral subcostal incisions may be advantageous in patients with previous midline incisions or large abdominal girth.

If antegrade bypass to the SMA is required, attention is first directed to exposing the supraceliac aorta. This portion of the aorta is often the last to be involved in patients with extensive atherosclerosis and is the preferred site of proximal anastomosis for a bypass graft. In some cases, it may be necessary to perform a bypass to a more distal portion of the SMA. Through the main peritoneal cavity, elevating and superiorly displacing the transverse colon allows palpation of its mesentery and identification of the middle colic artery and the SMA (**Figure 37.7**). The main vessel is exposed by incising the peritoneum directly above it at the root of the mesentery. The vessel is usually easily identified, but care must be taken to avoid injury to parallel veins and arterial branches that are often sizable. A retropancreatic tunnel is formed by blunt finger dissection to allow passage of a graft from the supraceliac aorta to the exposed portion of the SMA.

If a retrograde bypass is planned, the infrarenal aorta or left iliac artery is exposed directly by either retracting the duodenum to the right and incising the

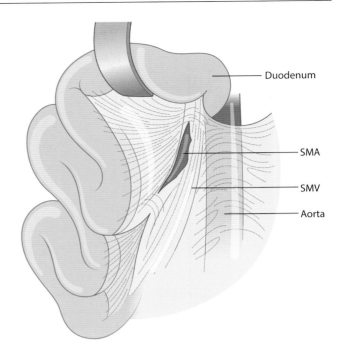

Figure 37.7 Incision at the base of the small bowel mesentery to expose the superior mesenteric artery distal to the location of vascular compromise. Reproduced from Zarins CK, Gewertz, BL eds. *Atlas of Vascular Surgery.* 2nd ed. Philadelphia, PA: Churchill Livingstone; 2005. p. 175.

retroperitoneum or medially reflecting the left colon. The vessel least involved with atherosclerosis is selected as the originating anastomotic site for a bypass graft, to be directed in a gradual curved path back to the SMA, if feasible (**Figure 37.8**). Retrograde bypass is less favored because of extensive atherosclerotic involvement of the distal aortoiliac segment and potential kinking of the graft. Specific indications for retrograde bypasses include a "hostile" upper abdomen or the presence of severe heart disease, which makes supraceliac aortic occlusion undesirable.

A most useful alternative to the one already described, a transcrural approach to the origin of the SMA is MVR. This approach is much preferred for more extensive proximal revascularizations. Incising the left lateral peritoneal reflection from the diaphragm to the pelvis allows mobilization of the descending colon (**Figure 37.9**). Next, the splenorenal and phrenocolic ligaments are carefully divided. With extension of the operator's hand under the descending colon, stomach, pancreas, and spleen, the visceral bundle is rotated anteriorly and medially. The plane of dissection can be anterior or posterior to the left kidney. This approach provides continuous exposure of the visceral aorta, as well as the proximal SMA and celiac axis (**Figure 37.10**). Rotating the patient to a lateral position with the right side down facilitates this exposure.

Endovascular therapies for SMAAs provide important alternatives to operative treatment. Embolization has been

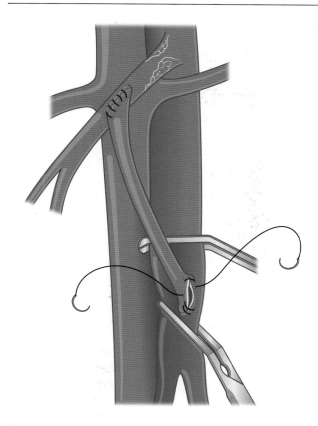

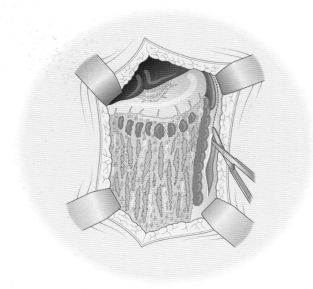

Figure 37.9 Incision of left lateral peritoneal reflection. Reproduced from Zarins CK, Gewertz, BL eds. In: *Atlas of Vascular Surgery*. 2nd ed. Philadelphia, PA: Churchill Livingstone; 2005. p. 185.

Figure 37.8 Operative reconstruction showing retrograde aortomesenteric saphenous vein bypass grafting to the superior mesenteric artery. Reproduced from Zarins CK, Gewertz BL eds. *Atlas of Vascular Surgery*. 2nd ed. Philadelphia, PA: Churchill Livingstone; 2005. p. 179.

used successfully even in patients with ruptured SMAAs.[26] Its main disadvantage is that it does not allow for the careful assessment of mesenteric ischemia as would be possible with laparotomy.

OTHER SPLANCHNIC ARTERY ANEURYSMS

Gastric artery aneurysms (GAAs) and gastroepiploic artery aneurysms (GEAAs) are rare; in combination, they account for approximately 4% of all visceral artery aneurysms.[27] GAAs occur 10 times more commonly than GEAAs.[13] Their etiology includes atherosclerosis (30%), trauma (25%), and inflammation (15%) including pancreatitis, peptic ulcer disease, and vasculitis.[27] Less common causes are mycotic aneurysms secondary to septic emboli and medial dysplasia.

More than 90% of GEAAs are ruptured at presentation; because they are intraperitoneal, the mortality rate from rupture is approximately 70%.[13,27] Other abdominal aneurysms are reported to be present in 15–40% of these patients.[27]

In patients with asymptomatic aneurysms, treatment is recommended because of the high mortality rate associated with rupture. Management of GAAs and GEAAs

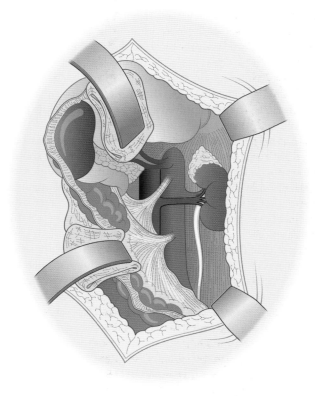

Figure 37.10 Transperitoneal medial visceral rotation. Reproduced from Zarins CK, Gewertz, BL eds. *Atlas of Vascular Surgery*. 2nd ed. Philadelphia, PA: Churchill Livingstone; 2005. p. 185.

generally consists of operative ligation with or without arterial reconstruction. If the aneurysm involves the wall of the stomach, it is resected along with a portion of the stomach wall.[13]

Aneurysms in the distribution of the jejunal, ileal, and colic arteries are rare and comprise 2% of visceral artery aneurysms.[28] These aneurysms are usually small in diameter (<1 cm) and solitary, though there is an association of such lesions with AAAs and other visceral artery aneurysms.[29] Their etiology includes inflammation, infection, trauma, atherosclerosis, medial degeneration, and iatrogenic causes. These aneurysms may also rarely be found in patients with other connective tissue disorders.[13] IMA aneurysms have been reported in association with concomitant stenosis or occlusion of the celiac trunk and SMA.[30]

Rupture of jejunal or ileal aneurysms is less common than colic aneurysms. When ruptured, these mesenteric branch vessel aneurysms can bleed into the peritoneal cavity or cause GI hemorrhage. The mortality rate for rupture is approximately 20%; therefore, all mesenteric branch vessel aneurysms should be treated.[13]

Surgical treatment varies with the location of the aneurysm. For proximal aneurysms, revascularization is ideal to preserve mesenteric flow. IMA aneurysms may be treated with either ligation, revascularization with a bypass graft, or direct reimplantation. Revascularization is required in the presence of associated celiac or SMA stenosis. Other mesenteric branch aneurysms are usually too small to undergo revascularization and therefore are treated by aneurysm resection or ligation. Intraoperative assessment of bowel viability is essential; rarely, concomitant small bowel resection or colectomy may be necessary.

Gastroduodenal artery aneurysms (GDAAs) and pancreaticoduodenal artery aneurysms (PDAAs) are uncommon and account for 1.5 and 2% of visceral artery aneurysms, respectively.[24,31] These aneurysms are most commonly associated with acute pancreatitis, which causes pseudoaneurysm formation from pancreatic inflammation or pseudocyst. Another category of pseudoaneurysms are those caused by pancreatic or biliary surgery or biliary instrumentation. Most common in this category is a pseudoaneurysm of the GDA stump after pancreaticoduodenectomy, which is a well-known cause of postoperative hemorrhage.[32]

True aneurysms of the pancreaticoduodenal arcade are less common than pseudoaneurysms. True aneurysms are thought to develop secondary to increased flow in the pancreatic arcades, such as occurs with celiac trunk occlusive disease, median arcuate ligament syndrome, or in very rare cases, congenital absence of the celiac trunk.[33]

When true PDAAs are associated with celiac occlusive disease, both aneurysm and celiac stenosis or occlusion are treated. The celiac axis must be revascularized to minimize the risk that PDAA embolization will abolish the major collateral supply to the celiac axis.[34]

Because of the strong association of GDA and PDA pseudoaneurysms with pancreatitis, most patients are symptomatic at diagnosis. These aneurysms frequently erode into the duodenum or pancreatic duct and GI hemorrhage may occur.[35] A high frequency of GDAAs and PDAAs present with rupture. As GDAAs more commonly rupture into the peritoneal cavity, mortality is greater than with PDAA rupture.[24,36]

Given the small size of feeding vessels, precise arteriographic assessment is an essential component of pretreatment evaluation. The specific objectives are to define the afferent and efferent arteries of the aneurysm, to assess whether endovascular intervention is possible, and to reveal any communication with the GI tract. Axial imaging can also reveal the presence of an underlying inflammatory process, such as pancreatitis or pseudocyst.

There is no clear correlation between GDAA and PDAA size and rupture. As a result, aggressive treatment of all true and false GDAAs and PDAAs is recommended because of the high rupture rate and high mortality associated with rupture.

Open surgical techniques include ligation, aneurysmectomy, or aneurysmorrhaphy. The disadvantages of open repair of PDAAs and GDAAs include intraparenchymal location, which makes dissection more difficult, especially in the presence of pancreatitis. Up to 70% of PDAAs have not been successfully detected during open surgery.[36] The increased application of intraoperative ultrasound (US) may address this problem.

Simple ligation of PDAAs is often difficult or impossible because of the numerous branches that supply these aneurysms. For this reason, suture ligation of all branches of a PDAA is often best achieved from within the aneurysm sac. GDAA ligation is more straightforward because of greater ease of exposure. Ligation without revascularization is used for most cases of rupture because of the difficulty of isolating the aneurysm within the pancreatic parenchyma. For PDAAs, difficulties with containing hemorrhage from a ruptured aneurysm can mandate pancreatic resection.

In circumstances where a GDAA or PDAA is associated with a pancreatic pseudocyst, the pseudocyst should be drained either internally or externally. Although rare, patients may have such extensive aneurysmal involvement that they require near total pancreatic resection including pancreaticoduodenectomy to remove all the disease.

Endovascular techniques have changed the approach to GDAAs and PDAAs.[36] Coil embolization has been the most popular option, but requires close surveillance as recanalization causing recurrent bleeding is common.[37] True PDAAs associated with celiac artery stenosis or occlusion are difficult to treat by endovascular means alone, and combined open and endovascular approaches have been reported.[34] Finally, percutaneous and open US-guided thrombin injection of GDAAs and PDAAs has been reported and may be useful in patients who are not appropriate candidates for operative intervention, such as those with acute pancreatitis.[33,38]

POSTOPERATIVE COMPLICATIONS

In a series of 55 patients with visceral artery aneurysms undergoing surgical treatment over 25 years from 1982 to 2007, there was one perioperative death (1.8% mortality) resulting from acute pancreatitis in a patient operated on for an inflammatory splenic artery aneurysm. Major complications were reported in two patients undergoing surgical treatment for SAAs in this group: a retroperitoneal hematoma requiring surgical exploration on the second postoperative day; and acute pancreatitis requiring readmission on the seventh postoperative day.[9]

A recent retrospective review including 16 patients with splanchnic or renal artery aneurysms undergoing surgical repair reported postoperative complications in 4 of 16 patients. Postoperative complications included pneumonia in four patients and one subcapsular hepatic hematoma requiring endovascular embolization. Two patients who underwent splenic artery ligation and splenectomy developed postoperative hematoma. There were also two early reoperations on the first postoperative day because of technical complications: one patient who underwent reversed saphenous vein bypass from the thoracic aorta to CHA for celiac trunk aneurysm required shortening of the saphenous vein graft which had kinked; and one patient who underwent aortohepatic prosthetic bypass for HAA had a proximal anastomotic stenosis requiring revision. There was no significant difference in postoperative complications among patients undergoing endovascular treatment (15 patients) versus open repair in this series and there were no in-hospital deaths reported in either group.[39]

CASE EXAMPLE

A 41-year-old man presented with an asymptomatic 3-cm aneurysm of a celiomesenteric trunk found on CT. A mesenteric angiogram (**Figure 37.11**) was performed and endovascular repair was considered, but it was determined that placing a stent could not be performed without jeopardizing the hepatic and splenic arteries. Therefore, an open repair was undertaken with a bilateral subcostal incision with midline cephalad extension. An extensive Kocher maneuver was performed and the head and neck of the pancreas mobilized completely to allow better exposure (**Figure 37.12**). Because the celiac artery and SMA shared a common origin, arterial reconstruction was mandatory. Each incoming and outgoing branch was controlled with atraumatic clips and the aneurysm sac was opened. A primary repair was then performed within the aneurysm by direct anastomosis of the SMA orifice to the combined orifice of the common hepatic, splenic, and celiomesenteric trunk. The posterior wall of the aneurysm was imbricated into the posterior suture line and the remainder of

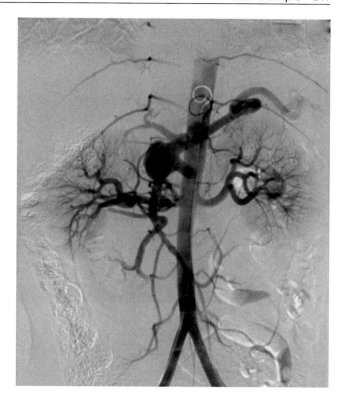

Figure 37.11 Preoperative mesenteric angiogram of a 41-year-old man (case example) showing a celiomesenteric trunk aneurysm.

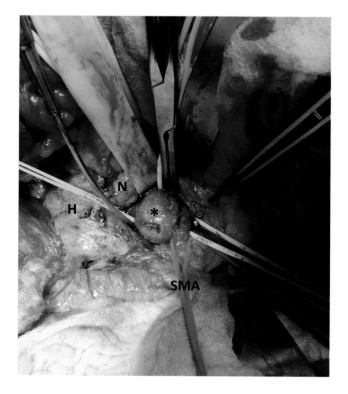

Figure 37.12 Intraoperative exposure showing the celiomesenteric trunk aneurysm sac (*), the vessel loop around the distal superior mesenteric artery, and the head (H) and neck (N) of the pancreas.

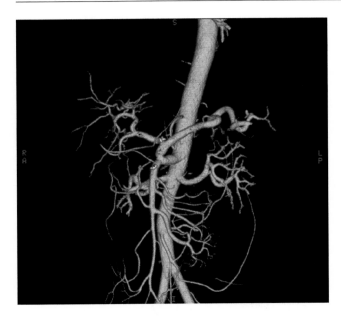

Figure 37.13 Postoperative computed tomography three-dimensional reconstruction showing no flow into the excluded aneurysm sac.

the aneurysm was effectively excluded by the primary anastomosis. The patient had an uneventful convalescence and was discharged without complications. Postoperative CTA showed all the branches to be patent with no flow within the aneurysm sac (**Figure 37.13**).

CONCLUSION

Visceral artery aneurysms are uncommon but have a significant potential for rupture resulting in high morbidity and mortality. An aggressive approach to diagnosis and treatment of these aneurysms is therefore warranted. Outcomes for patients treated electively with open surgical repair are quite good. Endovascular therapy is a viable therapeutic option and is increasingly adopted to treat patients when anatomically feasible. For patients in whom surveillance is chosen, close imaging follow-up is mandatory because of the poorly defined natural history and the high mortality associated with rupture.

REFERENCES

1. Ailawadi G, Cowles RA, Stanley JC, et al. Common celiacomesenteric trunk: aneurysmal and occlusive disease. *J Vasc Surg.* 2004;**40**:1040–1043.
2. Detroux M, Anidjar S, Nottin R. Aneurysm of a common celiomesenteric trunk. *Ann Vasc Surg.* 1998;**12**:78–82.
3. Guntani A, Yamaoka T, Kyuragi R, et al. Successful treatment of a visceral artery aneurysm with a celiacomesenteric trunk: report of a case. *Surg Today.* 2011;**41**:115–119.
4. Saltzberg SS, Maldonado TS, Lamparello PJ, et al. Is endovascular therapy the preferred treatment for all visceral artery aneurysms? *Ann Vasc Surg.* 2005;**19**:507–515.
5. Reil TD, Gevorgyan A, Jimenez JC, et al. Endovascular treatment of visceral artery aneurysms. In: Moore WS, Ahn SS, eds. *Endovascular Surgery.* 4th edn. Philadelphia, PA: Elsevier/Saunders; 2011. pp. 521–527.
6. Stanley JC, Thompson NW, Fry WJ. Splanchnic artery aneurysms. *Arch Surg.* 1970;**101**:689–697.
7. Tessier DJ, Stone WM, Fowl RJ, et al. Clinical features and management of splenic artery pseudoaneurysm: case series and cumulative review of literature. *J Vasc Surg.* 2003;**38**:969–974.
8. Tulsyan N, Kashyap VS, Greenberg RK, et al. The endovascular management of visceral artery aneurysms and pseudoaneurysms. *J Vasc Surg.* 2007;**45**:276–283.
9. Pulli R, Dorigo W, Troisi N, et al. Surgical treatment of visceral artery aneurysms: a 25-year experience. *J Vasc Surg.* 2008;**48**:334–342.
10. Sachdev-Ost U. Visceral artery aneurysms: review of current management options. *Mt Sinai J Med.* 2010;**77**:296–303.
11. Pescarus R, Montreuil B, Bendavid Y. Giant splenic artery aneurysms: case report and review of the literature. *J Vasc Surg.* 2005;**42**:344–347.
12. Martin KW, Morian JP Jr., Lee JK, et al. Demonstration of a splenic artery pseudoaneurysm by MR imaging. *J Comput Assist Tomogr.* 1985;**9**:190–192.
13. Stanley JC, Wakefield TW, Graham LM, et al. Clinical importance and management of splanchnic artery aneurysms. *J Vasc Surg.* 1986;**3**:836–840.
14. Lambert CJ Jr., Williamson JW. Splenic artery aneurysm. A rare cause of upper gastrointestinal bleeding. *Am Surg.* 1990;**56**:543–545.
15. Wagner WH, Allins AD, Treiman RL, et al. Ruptured visceral artery aneurysms. *Ann Vasc Surg.* 1997;**11**:342–347.
16. Nosher JL, Chung J, Brevetti LS, et al. Visceral and renal artery aneurysms: a pictorial essay on endovascular therapy. *Radiographics.* 2006;**26**:1687–1704.
17. Matsumoto K, Ohgami M, Shirasugi N, et al. A first case report of the successful laparoscopic repair of a splenic artery aneurysm. *Surgery.* 1997;**121**:462–464.
18. Shanley CJ, Shah NL, Messina LM. Common splanchnic artery aneurysms: splenic, hepatic, and celiac. *Ann Vasc Surg.* 1996;**10**:315–322.
19. Berceli SA. Hepatic and splenic artery aneurysms. *Semin Vasc Surg.* 2005;**18**:196–201.
20. Abbas MA, Fowl RJ, Stone WM, et al. Hepatic artery aneurysm: factors that predict complications. *J Vasc Surg.* 2003;**38**:41–45.
21. Zachary K, Geier S, Pellecchia C, et al. Jaundice secondary to hepatic artery aneurysm: radiological appearance and clinical features. *Am J Gastroenterol.* 1986;**81**:295–298.

22. Graham LM, Stanley JC, Whitehouse WM Jr., et al. Celiac artery aneurysms: historic (1745–1949) versus contemporary (1950–1984) differences in etiology and clinical importance. *J Vasc Surg* 1985;**2**:757–764.

23. Stone WM, Abbas MA, Gloviczki P, et al. Celiac arterial aneurysms: a critical reappraisal of a rare entity. *Arch Surg.* 2002;**137**:670–674.

24. Shanley CJ, Shah NL, Messina LM. Uncommon splanchnic artery aneurysms: pancreaticoduodenal, gastroduodenal, superior mesenteric, inferior mesenteric, and colic. *Ann Vasc Surg.* 1996;**10**:506–515.

25. Lorelli DR, Cambria RA, Seabrook GR, et al. Diagnosis and management of aneurysms involving the superior mesenteric artery and its branches: a report of four cases. *Vasc Endovascular Surg.* 2003;**37**:59–66.

26. Ishii A, Namimoto T, Morishita S, et al. Embolization for ruptured superior mesenteric artery aneurysms. *Br J Radiol.* 1996;**69**:296–300.

27. Rohatgi A, Cherian T. Spontaneous rupture of a left gastroepiploic artery aneurysm. *J Postgrad Med.* 2002;**48**:288–289.

28. Diettrich NA, Cacioppo JC, Ying DP. Massive gastrointestinal hemorrhage caused by rupture of a jejunal branch artery aneurysm. *J Vasc Surg.* 1988;**8**:187–189.

29. Tessier DJ, Abbas MA, Fowl RJ, et al. Management of rare mesenteric arterial branch aneurysms. *Ann Vasc Surg.* 2002;**16**:586–590.

30. Edogawa S, Shibuya T, Kurose K, et al. Inferior mesenteric artery aneurysm: case report and literature review. *Ann Vasc Dis.* 2013;**6**:98–101.

31. Iyomasa S, Matsuzaki Y, Hiei K, et al. Pancreaticoduodenal artery aneurysm: a case report and review of the literature. *J Vasc Surg.* 1995;**22**:161–166.

32. Otah E, Cushin BJ, Rozenblit GN, et al. Visceral artery pseudoaneurysms following pancreatoduodenectomy. *Arch Surg.* 2002;**137**:55–59.

33. McIntyre TP, Simone ST, Stahlfeld KR. Intraoperative thrombin occlusion of a visceral artery aneurysm. *J Vasc Surg.* 2002;**36**:393–395.

34. Bageacu S, Cuilleron M, Kaczmarek D, et al. True aneurysms of the pancreaticoduodenal artery: successful non-operative management. *Surgery.* 2006;**139**:608–616.

35. Eckhauser FE, Stanley JC, Zelenock GB. Gastroduodenal and pancreaticoduodenal artery aneurysms: a complication of pancreatitis causing spontaneous gastrointestinal hemorrhage. *Surgery.* 1980;**88**:335–344.

36. Moore E, Matthews MR, Minion DJ, et al. Surgical management of peripancreatic arterial aneurysms. *J Vasc Surg.* 2004;**40**:247–253.

37. Boudghène F, L'Herminé C, Bigot JM. Arterial complications of pancreatitis: diagnostic and therapeutic aspects in 104 cases. *J Vasc Interv Radiol.* 1993;**4**:551–558.

38. Manazer JR, Monzon JR, Dietz PA, et al. Treatment of pancreatic pseudoaneurysm with percutaneous transabdominal thrombin injection. *J Vasc Surg.* 2003;**38**:600–602.

39. Cochennec F, Riga CV, Allaire E, et al. Contemporary management of splanchnic and renal artery aneurysms: results of endovascular compared with open surgery from two European vascular centers. *Eur J Vasc Endovasc Surg.* 2011;**42**:340–346.

38

Surgical management of adult and pediatric renovascular hypertension

JAMES C. STANLEY, JONATHAN L. ELIASON, AND DAWN M. COLEMAN

CONTENTS

INTRODUCTION

Open renal revascularization for arteriosclerotic and fibrodysplastic renovascular hypertension (RVH)[1-9] in adults has been performed less often in recent years given the advances in endovascular therapy of these diseases. However, conventional open arterial reconstruction remains the mainstay of treatment for developmental pediatric RVH.[10] Proper selection of adults and children for operative intervention requires evidence of a functionally important renal artery narrowing, responsible for alterations in blood flow and activation of the renin–angiotensin system. Invariably, such individuals are on multiple antihypertensive drugs with continued difficulty in controlling their blood pressure.

ADULT RENOVASCULAR DISEASE

Open surgical treatment of arteriosclerotic renal artery stenoses entails a variety of techniques, including: (1) aortorenal endarterectomy through an axial aortotomy; (2) aortorenal endarterectomy through the transected infrarenal aorta; (3) direct renal artery endarterectomy in situ or eversion endarterectomy with subsequent aortic reimplantation of the artery; and (4) an aortorenal bypass. The chosen intervention depends on the extent of aortic and renal artery disease, and on whether a simultaneous aortic reconstruction is to be undertaken.

The usual surgical exposure when performing an endarterectomy of the renal artery is an anterior one through the base of the mesocolon and root of the mesentery, except when undertaking a direct isolated renal artery endarterectomy, in which case a medial visceral rotation is undertaken. A supraumbilical transverse abdominal incision is preferred, extended from one anterior axillary line to the other for bilateral reconstructions, and to the ipsilateral posterior axillary line when treating unilateral disease. A rolled sheet or soft bump placed under the lumbar spine enhances operative exposure. The small bowel is displaced from the abdominal cavity in a bowel bag.

The ligament of Treitz is divided and the duodenum along with the pancreas is then mobilized and retracted into the upper abdomen with the aid of a fixed retractor. The retroperitoneum over the aorta is incised and the dissection is advanced cephalad to the level of the left renal vein (LRV), which is mobilized by ligating and transecting its gonadal and adrenal branches. The inferior vena cava (IVC) is dissected sufficiently to allow access to 2 or 3 cm of the proximal right renal artery (RRA). The underlying renal arteries are skeletonized from their aortic origin to beyond their branching and the obvious plaque. Small nonparenchymal arterial branches, such as those to the adrenal gland, may be transected and ligated close to the renal artery. The aorta is dissected about its circumference for approximately 5 cm below the renal artery to above the superior mesenteric artery (SMA). This requires division of the periaortic diaphragmatic crura, which are transected perpendicular to their fibers and the aorta with electrocautery.

Systematic anticoagulation is achieved with intravenous administration of heparin (150 IU/kg) before arterial and aortic clamping. Mannitol (12.5 g in an average-sized adult) is administered intravenously at the same time to establish a diuresis. The three endarterectomy procedures differ in their performance.

Axial aortorenal endarterectomy

This is the most common method of normalizing renal blood flow in cases of aortic spillover renal artery plaque. Clamping of the proximal SMA and distal renal arteries before aortic occlusion is undertaken to prevent embolization of atheromatous debris from the aorta. The lumbar arteries are usually occluded as the operation proceeds. Arterial clamping is achieved with low-pressure (30–70 g/cm^2) microvascular Heifetz clamps. Aortic clamping is obtained proximally, just above the SMA and distally, 3–4 cm below the level of the renal arteries. Aortic occlusion above the celiac artery may be necessary when little distance exists for clamp placement between the SMA and renal arteries.

An axial aortotomy is made lateral to the SMA, extending anteriorly in a curvilinear fashion to the midline of the aorta at the level of the renal arteries and continuing for approximately 3 cm below them (**Figure 38.1**). This type of endarterectomy is particularly suited when

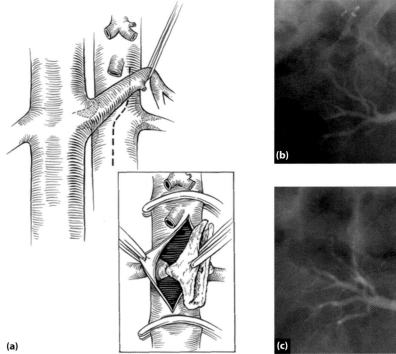
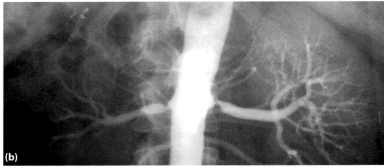
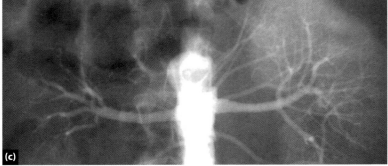

Figure 38.1 Axial aortorenal endarterectomy using a vertical aortotomy, extending from the level of the superior mesenteric artery to the anterior aorta onto the infrarenal aorta (**a**). Bilateral proximal arteriosclerotic stenoses preoperatively (**b**) and post-endarterectomy (**c**). (Reproduced with permission from Stanley JC, Messina LM, Wakefield TW, et al. Renal artery reconstruction. In: Bergan JJ, Yao JST, eds. *Techniques in Arterial Surgery*. Philadelphia, PA: W.B. Saunders; 1990. pp. 257 and 258.)

multiple (accessory) renal arteries are diseased or with bilateral arteriosclerotic stenoses limited to the proximal renal arteries. An endarterectomy plane is developed between the diseased and normal outer aortic media and this plane is extended circumferentially. The distal aortic plaque is transected approximately 1 cm below the renal artery orifices, and the proximal aortic plaque is transected immediately beneath the SMA orifice. Aortic tacking sutures may occasionally be needed to secure the residual plaque to the deeper aortic media and prevent a later aortic dissection.

Renal artery endarterectomy is accomplished by maintaining gentle traction on the aortic plaque and its extension into the renal artery, while simultaneously pushing the everted inner arterial wall away from the plaque. This is facilitated by the assistant's gentle eversion of the distal artery into the more proximal vessel. This type of endarterectomy may be easier to perform if the aortic plaque is transected into lateral halves. A well-defined renal artery end point usually occurs with distal feathering of the plaque. The aortotomy is closed with a continuous cardiovascular suture after irrigating the endarterectomized aorta and renal arteries to remove any small pieces of debris.

Once the aortotomy has been closed, circulation is restored first through the aorta to the lower extremities, then to the kidneys. This lessens the risk of renal embolization of any material loosened by the upper aortic clamp. Intraoperative duplex scanning or directional Doppler examination is undertaken to assess the adequacy of the endarterectomy. If a preocclusive intimal flap is suspected, a separate renal artery incision should be made beyond the end point of the plaque. The elevated distal plaque is then removed or tacked down and the arteriotomy is closed, usually with a vein patch to prevent narrowing of the artery. An additional dose of mannitol (12.5 g) is given just before declamping and anticoagulation is reversed with protamine sulfate administered intravenously (1.5 mg/100 IU of the previous heparin dose).

Transaortic renal artery endarterectomy

Transaortic renal artery endarterectomy for arteriosclerotic renal artery stenotic disease is often performed in patients requiring a concomitant aortic reconstruction. Vascular control is obtained in the same manner as undertaken with the axial approach, except that placement of the distal aortic clamp depends on the type and extent of aortic aneurysmal or occlusive disease being treated.

The aorta is transected approximately 1 cm below the renal arteries, and the endarterectomy is then performed through the open aorta (**Figure 38.2**). An unencumbered view of the aortic lumen and renal artery orifices is often made easier by transposing the transected aorta anterior to the LRV. The endarterectomy

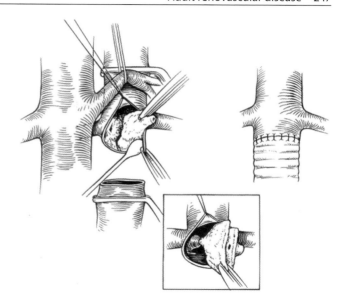

Figure 38.2 Transaortic renal artery endarterectomy through the transected aorta, undertaken in association with an aortic reconstruction for aneurysmal or occlusive disease. (Reproduced with permission from Stanley JC, Messina LM, Wakefield TW, et al. Renal artery reconstruction. In: Bergan JJ, Yao JST, eds. *Techniques in Arterial Surgery*. Philadelphia, PA: W.B. Saunders; 1990. p. 258.)

plane is extended to approximately 1 cm above the renal artery orifices, and the aortic plaque is transected transversely. The endarterectomy is facilitated by everting each renal artery while maintaining gentle traction on the plaque. Following its anastomosis to the proximal aorta, the aortic graft is then repositioned beneath the LRV. A soft-jaw clamp may then be placed on the graft, and renal blood flow is restored while the distal graft anastomosis is completed.

Direct renal artery endarterectomy

Direct renal artery endarterectomy may be undertaken for focal, unilateral renal atherosclerotic narrowing occurring independently of extensive aortic atherosclerosis. This type of endarterectomy is most useful when treating complex stenoses involving the main renal artery with early branching (**Figure 38.3**). It is not advised for treatment of bilateral disease, because it would be very time-consuming and it would markedly increase the risk of injurious renal ischemia. In such cases, an axial aortorenal endarterectomy is more appropriate. Once systemic anticoagulation and vascular control are achieved, an anterior renal arteriotomy is performed and extended proximally into the aorta and distally beyond the renal artery plaque. Following removal of the plaque, a vein or prosthetic patch graft closure of the arteriotomy is undertaken.

Occasional patients with ostial disease may be best served by reimplantation of a transected renal artery after eversion endarterectomy. This technique is well suited for

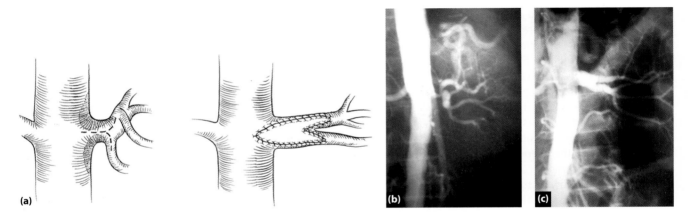

Figure 38.3 Direct renal artery endarterectomy with patch graft arterial closure (**a**), usually performed for focal renal artery arteriosclerosis of the proximal renal artery. (**b**) Complex proximal arteriosclerotic stenosis affecting early branching of the main renal artery. (**c**) Postendarterectomy with a patch closure. (Reproduced with permission from Stanley JC, Messina LM, Wakefield TW, et al. Renal artery reconstruction. In: Bergan JJ, Yao JST, eds. *Techniques in Arterial Surgery*. Philadelphia, PA: W.B. Saunders; 1990. p. 259.)

revascularization of stenotic renal arteries arising from suprarenal or pararenal aortic aneurysms. These arteries are usually transected along with a small rim of the aorta. An eversion endarterectomy is performed in a conventional manner and the endarterectomized artery is then reimplanted onto the prosthetic graft in cases of a concomitant aortic reconstruction or directly into the native aorta in other instances.

Aortorenal bypass procedures

Aortorenal bypass procedures for both arteriosclerotic and fibrodysplastic renal artery stenoses were the standard of care in many practices during the 1970s. Preference at the authors' institution was given to obtaining operative exposure of the aorta and renal artery using a transverse supraumbilical abdominal incision. In these instances, a medial visceral rotation (MVR) of the colon and foregut structures is undertaken bluntly with one's fingers in the relatively avascular plane between the splanchnic viscera and the underlying retroperitoneal structures.

The infrarenal aorta is dissected about its circumference below the origin of the renal arteries, recognizing that ligation and transection of the lumbar veins and arteries may be undertaken without consequence, if necessary. The aorta may be partially or completely occluded after systemic heparin anticoagulation is achieved. A lateral or anterolateral ovoid aortotomy is created with an aortic punch, its length being approximately twice that of the bypass graft's diameter. When completing the graft-to-aortic anastomosis, sutures should be placed so that they include the entirety of the aortic intimal and medial tissues.

Exposure of the renal artery usually requires retraction of the renal vein, which should be freed carefully from the surrounding tissues. The renal artery is dissected about its circumference from near its aortic origin to its proximal branches. The most direct route for right-sided aortorenal grafts is in a retrocaval position. However, most grafts are less likely to kink when arising from an anterolateral aortotomy and carried in a gentle curve anterior to the IVC, then posteriorly to the renal artery. Grafts to the left kidney are originated from a lateral aortotomy and positioned beneath the LRV.

The saphenous vein is the most commonly used conduit for aortorenal bypass procedures in adults (**Figure 38.4**). Whenever possible, the vein is excised with a branch included at its caudal end. This branch is incised along its lumen adjacent to the parent vein so that a common orifice is created between the main trunk and its branch. If a large branch is not present, the vein is spatulated for a few millimeters on the opposite sides. In both cases, the resultant generous circumference lessens the likelihood of anastomotic narrowing and allows for a relatively perpendicular origin of the vein graft from the aorta. The same preparation technique may be undertaken when using a branched segment of the internal iliac artery (IIA). Graft-to-aortic anastomoses are performed using a fine running cardiovascular suture. Prosthetic grafts are occasionally used if a concurrent aortoaortic, aortoiliac, or aortofemoral graft is being placed.

An end-to-end graft-to-renal artery anastomosis is facilitated by spatulation of the graft posteriorly and the renal artery anteriorly (**Figure 38.5**). This allows visualization of the artery's interior, so that inclusion of its intima with each stitch is easily accomplished. Anastomoses completed in this manner are ovoid and they are less likely to develop late strictures.

Management of stenotic disease affecting multiple main renal arteries or widely separated segmental branches may require separate implantations of the arteries into a single conduit. This is usually

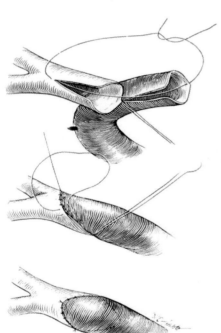

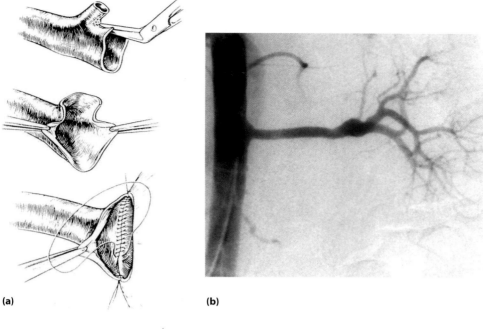

Figure 38.4 Aortorenal bypass using a reversed saphenous vein graft. (**a**) Bypass facilitated by a "branch patch" maneuver. (**b**) This creates a common orifice between the lumen of a branch and the central lumen of the saphenous vein. (Reproduced with permission from Stanley JC, Messina LM, Wakefield TW, et al. Renal artery reconstruction. In: Bergan JJ, Yao JST, eds. *Techniques in Arterial Surgery*. Philadelphia, PA: W.B. Saunders; 1990. p. 249.)

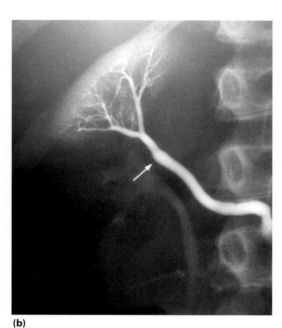

(a)   (b)

Figure 38.5 Aortorenal bypass with the vein graft-to-renal artery anastomosis following spatulation of the renal artery anteriorly and the vein posteriorly (**a**). (**b**) This creates a generous ovoid anastomosis. ((**a**) Reproduced from Ernst CB, Fry WJ, Stanley JC. Surgical treatment of renovascular hypertension: revascularization with autogenous vein. In: Stanley JC, Ernst CB, Fry WJ, eds. Renovascular Hypertension. PA: Saunders; 1984. p. 281. (**b**) Reproduced with permission from Fry WJ, Ernst CB, Stanley JC, et al. Renovascular hypertension in the pediatric patient. *Arch Surg*. 1973;**107**:692–698. p. 695.)

accomplished with a sequential end-to-side anastomosis of one artery into the side of the proximal graft, and an end-to-end anastomosis of the second artery to the distal graft (**Figure 38.6**). If a hypogastric artery with intact branches is used for the bypass, construction of multiple end-to-end, graft-to-renal artery anastomoses may be undertaken. In some patients, it may be easier to perform an anastomosis of the involved arteries in a side-to-side manner, to form a single channel, with the graft then anastomosed to this common orifice (**Figure 38.7**).

ALTERNATIVE BYPASSES

Alternative bypasses are preferable in patients with marginal cardiac function or in the presence of a hostile aorta due to coexistent aortic disease or prior aortic surgery, either of which would preclude safe aortic clamping for either an endarterectomy or origination of a renal bypass. In these cases, indirect reconstructions arising from the splenic, hepatic, SMA, or iliac arteries may be undertaken. When performing a splenorenal or hepatorenal bypass, it must be first documented by an appropriate imaging study

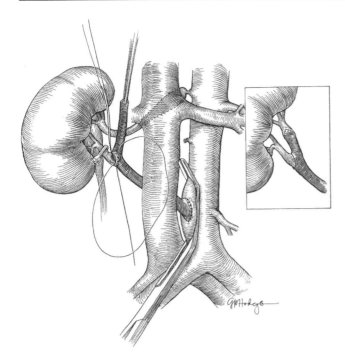

Figure 38.6 Technique of renal revascularization by sequential anastomosis of the multiple renal arteries to the graft. (Reproduced with permission from Ernst CB, Fry WJ, Stanley JC. Surgical treatment of renovascular hypertension: revascularization with autogenous vein. In: Stanley JC, Ernst CB, Fry WJ, eds. *Renovascular Hypertension*. Philadelphia, PA: Saunders; 1984. p. 283.)

that the proximal celiac artery and its branches do not harbor any narrowing that would perpetuate the hypertensive state following a reconstruction.

Splenorenal bypass

This type of bypass usually involves a direct end-to-end anastomosis of the splenic artery to the renal artery (**Figure 38.8**). Occasionally, this type of reconstruction may require placement of an interposition vein graft between the splenic and renal arteries. Mobilization of the renal artery should occur well beyond its aortic origin, to allow the distal artery to assume a gentle curve upward when anastomosed to the splenic artery, and lessen the likelihood of kinking.

The fascial plane between the mesocolon, pancreas, and Gerota capsule over the anterior surface of the kidney is relatively avascular, and allows easy elevation of the pancreas from the retroperitoneum. The splenic artery can be identified by palpation as it courses along the superior border of the pancreas, a few centimeters above and in front of the left renal artery. Some splenic arteries, especially in multiparous women, are exceedingly tortuous and may be difficult to mobilize without buckling or kinking. This is less likely to affect the proximal splenic artery. The splenic and renal arteries, or an interposition vein graft if needed, should be spatulated to create generous ovoid, end-to-end anastomoses.

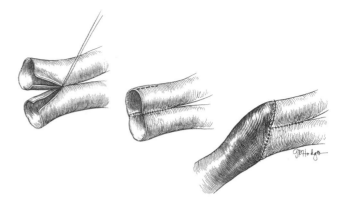

Figure 38.7 Technique of revascularization of multiple renal arteries, with sequential anastomoses of the renal vessels to the graft and side-to-side anastomoses of the affected renal arteries, followed by an anastomosis of their common orifice to the graft. (Reproduced with permission from Ernst CB, Fry WJ, Stanley JC. Surgical treatment of renovascular hypertension: revascularization with autogenous vein. In: Stanley JC, Ernst CB, Fry WJ, eds. *Renovascular Hypertension*. Philadelphia, PA: Saunders; 1984. p. 284.)

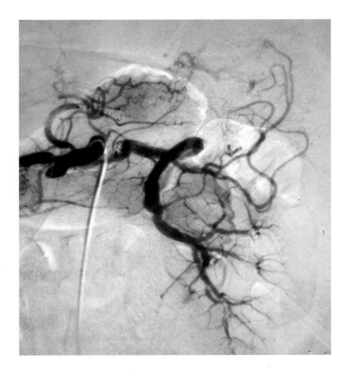

Figure 38.8 Splenorenal bypass following mobilization of the splenic artery, with an end-to-end anastomosis to the transected left renal artery. (Reproduced with permission from Stanley JC, Messina LM. Renal revascularization for recurrent pulmonary edema in patients with poorly controlled renovascular hypertension and renal insufficiency. In: Veith FJ, ed. *Current Critical Problems in Vascular Surgery*. Vol. 5. St. Louis, MO: Quality Medical Publishing; 1993. p. 311.)

Hepatorenal bypass

Hepatorenal bypass for right-sided renal artery disease usually requires interposition of an autologous saphenous vein graft, originating from the common hepatic artery (CHA) in an end-to-side manner, and anastomosed to the renal artery in an end-to-end fashion (**Figure 38.9**). The RRA is exposed through an extraperitoneal approach following an MVR of the duodenum and pancreas, as noted earlier. It is dissected from its aortic origin to the hilum to provide sufficient length for it to gently curve upward toward the hepatic vessels.

Exposure of the hepatic artery is obtained through the lesser sac following incision of the hepatoduodenal ligament. The distal CHA, gastroduodenal, and proper hepatic arteries are dissected about their circumference and encircled with vessel loops. Following systemic anticoagulation with heparin, and arterial occlusion with Heifetz clamps, an arteriotomy is made on the inferior aspect of the distal CHA.

The vein graft is anastomosed to the hepatic artery in an end-to-side manner, being spatulated as necessary to provide for a generous anastomotic circumference. The graft is then carried inferiorly in the retroperitoneum and anastomosed to the mobilized renal artery in an end-to-end fashion. Both graft and artery should be spatulated to facilitate construction of a generous anastomosis. Synthetic prostheses are not favored in these circumstances because of their proximity to the duodenum.

Iliorenal bypass

In an ileorenal bypass, either an autologous saphenous vein or a synthetic graft (**Figure 38.10**) should be considered in certain patients with a hostile aorta or upper abdomen precluding performance of conventional aortorenal, splenorenal, or hepatorenal bypasses. The graft is usually anastomosed to the anterior or anterolateral surface of the proximal common iliac artery. It is then positioned in the retroperitoneum paralleling the aorta or vena cava, with a gentle curve at the level of the kidney, where it is anastomosed to the renal artery in an end-to-end fashion. In patients with a previously placed aortofemoral graft, dissection in the region of the aortic anastomosis may lead to troublesome complications; in this setting, an iliorenal graft should originate from the limbs of the conduit rather than from the body of the graft itself.

Mesorenal bypass

Mesorenal bypass with direct implantation of the renal artery into the SMA or placement of a vein graft from the latter artery to the renal artery is an uncommon but useful alternative when other options for renal revascularization are ill-advised (**Figure 38.11**). The SMA is exposed through an extraperitoneal approach with an

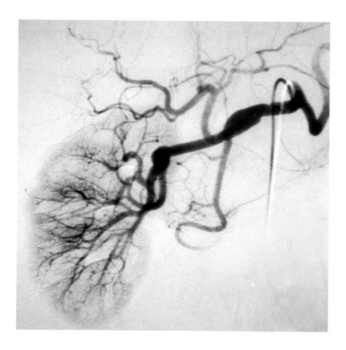

Figure 38.9 Hepatorenal bypass with a reversed saphenous vein originating from an end-to-side anastomosis to the side of the common hepatic artery and terminating in an end-to-end anastomosis to the mobilized right renal artery.

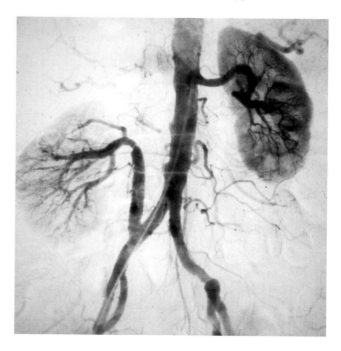

Figure 38.10 Iliorenal bypass, with the graft arising from an end-to-side anastomosis from the common iliac artery, to an end-to-end anastomosis of the graft to the renal artery. (Reproduced with permission from Stanley JC, Whitehouse WM Jr., Zelenock GB, et al. Reoperation for complications of renal artery reconstructive surgery undertaken for treatment of renovascular hypertension. *J Vasc Surg*. 1985;**2**:133–144. p. 140.)

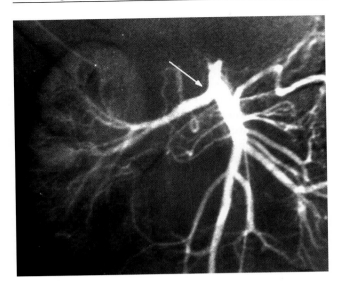

Figure 38.11 Direct renal artery end-to-side reimplantation into the superior mesenteric artery. (Reproduced from Stanley JC, Zelenock GB, Messina LM, et al. Pediatric renovascular hypertension: a thirty-year experience of operative treatment. *J Vasc Surg.* 1995;**21**:212–226. p. 219.)

extended MVR. Sufficient collateral circulation from the inferior pancreaticoduodenal and middle colic artery branches usually maintains adequate flow to the distal SMA during its occlusion.

ADULT OUTCOMES

The outcomes of carefully selected patients with renal arteriosclerotic disease undergoing open surgical treatment for their RVH result in 25% cure, 55% improvement, and 20% failure rates, with a reported mortality rate of 3%.[1–8] Renal function is improved in approximately 15%, unchanged in 75%, and worsened in 10%. The latter is often a reflection of pre-existing renal dysfunction, with chronic azotemia portending a poor response to any intervention. Acute complications, occurring <3% of the time, include thrombotic occlusions due to a distal renal artery flap or technical failures of a bypass graft associated with anastomotic narrowing. Late complications of both endarterectomy and bypass procedures are usually due to neointimal narrowing causing recurrent RVH in 5% of cases.

Open surgical therapy for fibrodysplasia-related RVH, usually involving a bypass, results in 65% cured, 30% improved, and 5% unchanged, with <1% procedure-related mortality.[9] Renal dysfunction is rare before or after operative therapy in this category of RVH. Complications include early graft occlusion in <1%, and late neointimal narrowing and recurrent RVH in fewer than 5% of these individuals. Most large clinical experiences report no operative mortality in this category of RVH.

PEDIATRIC RENOVASCULAR STENOSES

Arterial reconstructive surgery for developmental renal artery stenoses causing pediatric RVH must be individualized, considering the patient's anatomic renal artery disease, as well as concomitant aortic or splanchnic arterial disease.[10] Exposure of the renal vasculature in children is like that undertaken in adults undergoing bypass procedures.

Renal artery implantation

Implantation of the normal renal artery that has been transected beyond an existing ostial stenosis, has become an important means of treating pediatric renal revascularization (**Figure 38.12**). The divided renal artery should be spatulated anteriorly and posteriorly to create a generous anastomotic orifice. An oval lateral aortotomy is best made with an aortic punch, being a little more than twice the diameter of the renal artery being implanted. The aortorenal anastomosis is usually performed with interrupted monofilament suture. This provides for an anastomosis that will not become stenotic as the child grows. A continuous suture may be used in older adolescents with large renal arteries. Most implantations of the renal artery will be into a normal infrarenal segment of the aorta. Mobilization of the kidney medially, by incising its posterolateral attachments to retroperitoneal tissues, is an important maneuver to ensure that there is no tension on the implanted renal artery.

Small-diameter renal artery branches or accessory renal arteries beyond a stenotic segment may also be implanted into a nondiseased adjacent main or segmental

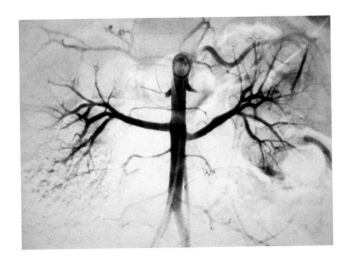

Figure 38.12 Bilateral renal artery aortic implantations. Note the ruminant proximal arteries at their aortic origins. (Reproduced with permission from Stanley JC, Zelenock GB, Messina LM, et al. Pediatric renovascular hypertension: a thirty-year experience of operative treatment. *J Vasc Surg.* 1995;**21**:212–226. p. 218.)

renal artery. This also involves spatulation of the artery to be implanted and completion of the anastomosis using fine monofilament suture.

Aortorenal bypass

Aortorenal bypass procedures using the IIA are performed when treating mid-stenoses or distal main renal artery stenoses in children (**Figure 38.13**). The excised IIA usually includes its distal branches, which are incised to create a large common orifice for the aortic anastomosis. The distal renal artery-to-IIA graft anastomoses should be completed following spatulation of both the IIA and renal artery. Anastomoses are completed with interrupted suture in very young children with small arteries. Stenoses of multiple small renal arteries may require approximation of these vessels to each other to form a large common orifice to which an aortorenal graft can be anastomosed.

Synthetic prosthetic grafts are rarely used for pediatric renal artery reconstructions because of their potential infectivity, technical difficulties in anastomosing them to small arteries, and their unpredictable long-term durability considering the many decades of life expectancy of these children. Similarly, vein grafts are not favored for aortorenal bypasses in children because of their propensity to undergo late aneurysmal dilations. When other more acceptable reconstructive procedures prove impossible and a vein is the only conduit

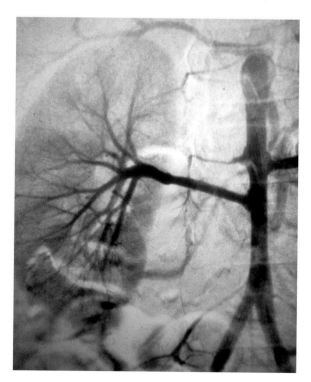

Figure 38.13 Aortorenal bypass with an internal iliac artery graft. (Reproduced with permission from Stanley JC, Zelenock GB, Messina LM, et al. Pediatric renovascular hypertension: a thirty-year experience of operative treatment. *J Vasc Surg.* 1995;**21**:219. p. 219.)

available, they should be covered with a synthetic mesh to lessen the likelihood of progressive aneurysmal dilation.

Other means of renal revascularization in children are occasionally undertaken. In certain circumstances, resections of the stenotic renal artery with primary reanastomoses, focal arterioplasties, and open operative dilations are appropriate reconstructive procedures. Splenorenal reconstructions in children, with a direct anastomosis of the renal artery to the splenic artery are not favored because of coexistent or later development of a celiac artery stenosis. Primary nephrectomy should be reserved for irreparable renovascular disease.

Many pediatric patients with renal artery stenoses have abdominal coarctations or splanchnic artery stenoses that warrant concomitant treatment at the time of their renal revascularization. Two options regarding aortic narrowing exist in these cases: patch aortoplasty or thoracoabdominal bypass. Simultaneous treatment of celiac and SMA stenoses is controversial in that most children with these lesions never experience intestinal angina.

Primary aortoplasty with an expanded polytetrafluoroethylene (PTFE) patch has become the preferred means of treating abdominal aortic coarctation or hypoplasia when technically feasible (**Figure 38.14**). Patches should be made large enough so that they are not constrictive as the child grows into adulthood. Dacron patches are no longer preferred because this material may undergo late aneurysmal deterioration over a period of years.

Primary thoracoabdominal bypass may be favored over an aortoplasty depending on the patient's age and anatomic disease affecting the renal arteries (**Figure 38.15**). Again, expanded PTFE grafts are favored over Dacron grafts because of the latter's propensity for later aneurysmal dilation. Extraperitoneal reflection of the abdominal viscera in these cases provides excellent access to the supraceliac site for the bypass origin. If a higher site is needed, a thoracotomy may be performed and the graft anastomosed to the supradiaphragmatic distal thoracic aorta. Grafts originating in the chest are easily tunneled through the posterior diaphragm, behind the left kidney to the distal aorta.

PEDIATRIC OUTCOMES

Conventional surgical revascularization for pediatric RVH that emphasizes direct renal artery implantation and single-staged concomitant aortic reconstruction offers excellent results. The hypertensive state is cured in nearly 70%, improved in 25%, and unchanged in 5%, with no operative mortality reported from most major practices treating isolated pediatric renal disease.[10] Impaired renal function before and after the operative procedure occurs in <1% of these patients. Recurrent stenoses or technical failures affect nearly 15% of these young children and will necessitate later secondary interventions. These children usually have very complex disease and optimal care demands the deft performance of carefully planned open reconstructive procedures.

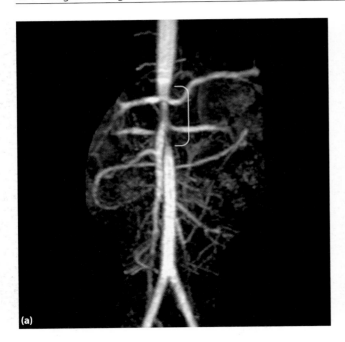
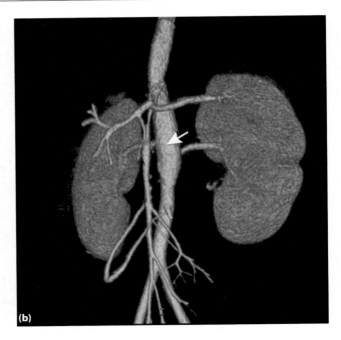

Figure 38.14 Intrarenal abdominal aortic coarctation (bracket) (**a**) associated with renal artery ostial stenoses. (**b**) Proximal abdominal patch aortoplasty (arrow) and bilateral renal artery aortic implantations. (Reproduced with permission from Stanley JC, Criado E, Eliason JL, et al. Abdominal aortic coarctation: surgical treatment of 53 patients with a thoracoabdominal bypass, patch aortoplasty, or interposition aortoaortic graft. *J Vasc Surg.* 2008;**44**:1073–1082. p. 1077.)

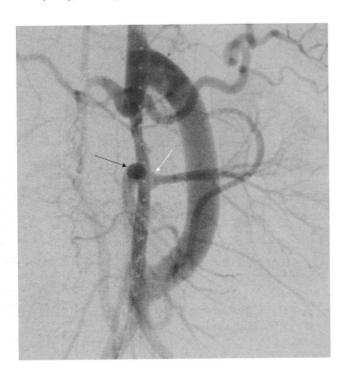

Figure 38.15 Renal artery-aortic (white arrow) and superior mesenteric artery-aortic (black arrow) implantation in conjunction with a thoracoabdominal bypass for a suprarenal abdominal aortic coarctation and severe ostial stenoses of the implanted arteries. (Reproduced with permission from Stanley JC, Criado E, Upchurch GR Jr., et al. Pediatric renovascular hypertension: 132 primary and 30 secondary operations in 97 children. *J Vasc Surg.* 2006;**44**:1219–1228. p. 1225.)

CASE EXAMPLES

Case example 1

A 55-year-old man was admitted for treatment of bilateral arteriosclerotic renal artery stenoses considered contributory to a decade of refractory hypertension despite multiple drug interventions. His serum creatinine was 1.5 mg/dL. He had a strong family history of arteriosclerotic cardiovascular disease, but preoperative studies did not reveal any evidence of carotid, coronary, or peripheral arterial disease. Given his age and evidence of bilateral ostial renal artery stenoses (**Figure 38.1b**) as his only evidence of arteriosclerosis, it was elected to undertake an aortorenal endarterectomy (**Figures 38.1a,c**) rather than bypasses to both kidneys. Endarterectomy, although more technically challenging, is considered more durable than aortorenal bypass with autogenous vein. The axial aortorenal endarterectomy was performed without complication and he continues to be normotensive on a diuretic alone 6 years postoperatively.

Case example 2

A 32-year-old woman was referred with a year's history of difficult-to-control hypertension despite treatment with an angiotensin-converting enzyme inhibitor combined with several other antihypertensive drugs. As a child, she had undergone a nephrectomy for chronic pyelonephritis and an atrophic kidney. An arteriogram of the vasculature to her remaining solitary kidney revealed medial fibrodysplasia affecting the middle and distal portions of the main renal artery with an extension into a primary branch. An aortorenal bypass was undertaken, given the concern of creating a preocclusive narrowing of the segmental artery should a percutaneous balloon angioplasty be undertaken of both the main renal artery and the involved branch. This was performed without difficulty with a segment of reversed autogenous saphenous vein, arising perpendicularly from the aorta and anastomosed in an end-to-end fashion to the distal main renal artery and involved segmental renal artery (**Figure 38.4**). She continues to be normotensive without the need for antihypertensive medications 11 years postoperatively.

REFERENCES

1. Balzer KM, Pfeiffer T, Rossbach S, et al. Prospective randomized trial of operative vs interventional treatment for renal artery ostial occlusive disease (RAOOD). *J Vasc Surg.* 2009;**49**:667–674.
2. Cherr GS, Hansen KJ, Craven TE, et al. Surgical management of atherosclerotic renovascular disease. *J Vasc Surg.* 2002;**35**:236–245.
3. Crutchley TA, Pearce JD, Craven TE, et al. Branch renal artery repair with cold perfusion protection. *J Vasc Surg.* 2007;**46**:405–412.
4. Geroulakos G, Wright JG, Tober JC, et al. Use of the splenic and hepatic artery for renal revascularization in patients with atherosclerotic renal artery disease. *Ann Vasc Surg.* 1997;**11**:85–89.
5. Grigoryants V, Henke PK, Watson NC, et al. Iliorenal bypass: indications and outcomes following 41 reconstructions. *Ann Vasc Surg.* 2007;**21**:1–9.
6. Hansen KJ, Cherr GS, Craven TE, et al. Management of ischemic nephropathy: dialysis-free survival after surgical repair. *J Vasc Surg.* 2000;**32**:472–481.
7. Khauli RB, Novick AC, Ziegelbaum M. Splenorenal bypass in the treatment of renal artery stenosis: experience with sixty-nine cases. *J Vasc Surg.* 1985;**2**:547–551.
8. Moncure AC, Brewster DC, Darling RC, et al. Use of the splenic and hepatic arteries for renal revascularization. *J Vasc Surg.* 1986;**3**:196–203.
9. Stanley JC, Fry WJ. Renovascular hypertension secondary to arterial fibrodysplasia in adults: criteria for operation and results of surgical therapy. *Arch Surg.* 1975;**110**:922–928.
10. Stanley JC, Criado E, Upchurch GR Jr., et al. Pediatric renovascular hypertension: 132 primary and 30 secondary operations in 97 children. *J Vasc Surg.* 2006;**44**:1219–1228.

39

Primary and secondary aortoenteric fistula

TIMOTHY J. NYPAVER

CONTENTS

INTRODUCTION

An aortoenteric fistula (AEF), whether primary or secondary, represents one of the most challenging and dreaded of vascular surgical complications. Primary AEFs are relatively rare and represent a direct communication between the native aorta and the overlying bowel. Secondary AEFs are related to a prior aortic reconstruction and are more common, occurring in 0.5–1.2% of all aortic reconstructions.[1-3] The patient with an AEF of either type may have significant hemodynamic compromise with active or recent gastrointestinal (GI) bleeding. In addition, increasing experience suggests that both primary and secondary AEFs can occur after endovascular abdominal aortic aneurysm (AAA) repair. While logic dictates that AEFs after endograft placement should be classified as secondary, there may be instances in which a pressurized aneurysm sac from an ongoing endoleak ruptures into an adjacent bowel segment.[4,5] Since it would have no direct communication with the endograft, it is reasonable to consider these as primary AEFs.

Important prioritizing considerations for the vascular surgeon faced with a suspected AEF include: (1) whether the patient is hemodynamically stable, or whether there is an active, life-threatening hemorrhage; (2) the overall risk to the patient for cardiopulmonary complications and their ability to undergo a difficult major operation; (3) the indication for the prior aortic reconstruction; (4) the location of the distal anastomoses (distal aorta, iliac, or femoral

arteries); and (5) based on the computed tomography (CT) findings, whether there is enough aortic neck to allow a new proximal anastomosis below the renal arteries. The hemodynamic status of the patient and whether there is active hemorrhage determine the rapidity of transit to the operating room and the algorithm for operative management (**Figure 39.1**).

SECONDARY AEF

Secondary AEFs occur because of communication between a previously placed aortic graft or endograft and the bowel, typically located at the third and fourth portions of the duodenum. The patient most often presents 2–3 years after placement of the aortic graft, with manifestations of GI bleeding. Manifestations of infection are present in up to 50% of patients and include fever and leukocytosis.[1-3] Patients often present with a "herald" bleed, which allows for timely diagnostic evaluation in any patient with previous aortic reconstruction. Massive hemorrhage, without antecedent bleeding, is unusual and accounts for <5% of presentations.[1-3] The communication between the GI tract and the graft material can either involve the anastomosis (true AEF) or the graft body or limb (prosthetic-enteric erosion).[2] The source of bleeding for the true AEF is from the aorta itself, while the prosthetic-enteric erosion typically bleeds from the edge of the bowel wall. One-fourth

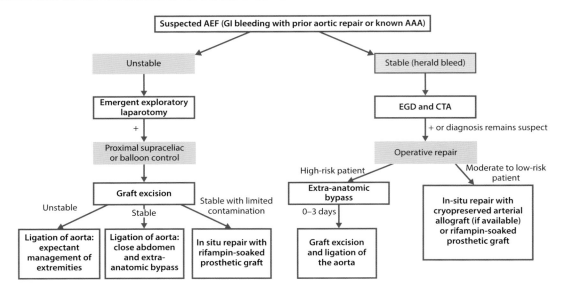

Figure 39.1 Management algorithm for the patient with suspected aortoenteric fistula. AAA: abdominal aortic aneurysm; AEF: aortoenteric fistula; CTA: computed tomography angiography; EGD: esophagogastroduodenoscopy; GI: gastrointestinal.

of patients present with manifestations of infection and sepsis alone without evidence of GI bleed.[1–3,6]

The stable patient should undergo esophagogastroduodenoscopy (EGD) with attention paid to the third and fourth portions of the duodenum, looking for ulceration. While visualization of graft material on EGD is pathognomonic, this is rarely seen and not required to make the diagnosis. CT angiography (CTA) may be of benefit by demonstrating perigraft fluid, bowel wall thickening and inflammation, periprosthetic air, or proximal anastomotic pseudoaneurysm formation, and provides important anatomic information that has an impact on the operative approach (**Figure 39.2**). While there are often indirect findings of AEF on CTA, one rarely makes a definitive diagnosis; the treating surgeon must maintain a high index of suspicion and proceed with operative repair even though the diagnosis may be in question.

In this hemodynamically stable patient, once the diagnosis is either confirmed or highly suspected, the operating surgeon must decide between two radically different approaches: (1) staged or sequential extra-anatomic bypass (clean planes) followed by aortic graft excision (infected); or (2) aortic graft excision with in-line aortic graft replacement with one of the following conduits: femoral vein (venous autograft), cryopreserved arterial allograft, or a new prosthetic graft with antimicrobial impregnation, typically with rifampin. For all in-line graft replacement options, extensive debridement of the aortic wall and any inflammatory tissue, along with omental coverage, is essential. The author prefers graft excision with in-line replacement with either cryopreserved arterial allografts or rifampin-impregnated Dacron grafts, when the former are not available. Staged extra-anatomic bypass and graft excision is reserved for patients who, because of their comorbidities, are unlikely to tolerate direct excision and in-line replacement (**Figure 39.1**). Generally, the author has not used the neoaortoiliac system (venous autograft) in the management of AEF. The patient

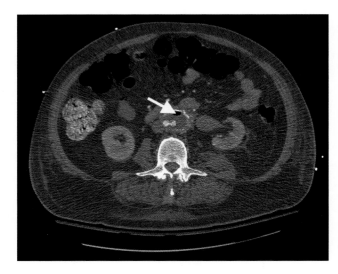

Figure 39.2 Computed tomography angiography of a patient with secondary aortoenteric fistula. There is gas accumulation within the aneurysm sac in proximity to the bifurcated graft (white arrow pointing to air within the aneurysm sac).

should receive broad-spectrum antibiotics because most cultures from AEFs yield polymicrobial organisms. The following describes the author's operative management in the setting of hemodynamic stability in a patient with good-to-moderate operative risk in whom at least 3 mm of aortic neck is present between the renal arteries and the graft.

The patient is positioned supine and prepped from the neck to the knees. The author prefers a long midline incision with control at the supraceliac aorta. This is accomplished via mobilization of the left lobe of the liver, retraction of the gastroesophageal junction to the left, and separating out the crura of the diaphragm to expose the aorta. This area is almost always free of prior adhesions. Distal control is obtained either at the level of the iliac vessels or distal graft anastomoses. This latter maneuver may require bilateral femoral artery exposure before making the abdominal incision. Any omentum encountered is preserved for later use. Finally, exposure of the graft and AEF, including a segment of aorta below the renal arteries, is undertaken. The new in-line graft should be prepared and ready for use before any exposure of the AEF. If bleeding is encountered around the AEF, supraceliac and distal clamps are quickly applied. The dissection continues expeditiously with the goal of exposing a segment of the infrarenal aorta. Proximal control is moved from the supraceliac to the infrarenal location as soon as possible to minimize visceral/renal ischemic time. Often, it is necessary to place the clamp at a between renal or suprarenal level to allow visualization of viable noninvolved aorta to accomplish an anastomosis. If suprarenal control is difficult, the supraceliac clamp is left in place while the proximal anastomosis is accomplished.

Before clamp placement, the patient is given an appropriate heparin dose and intravenous mannitol 25–50 g. If the proximal clamp is positioned suprarenal or supraceliac, the author limits the initial debridement to the proximal perirenal aorta and proceeds with the anastomosis to limit renal and mesenteric ischemia time. The opening in the bowel is encountered and covered with wet laparotomy pads with the intention of repairing this later. The anastomosis is accomplished in a typical fashion with 3-0 polypropylene suture in a circumferential fashion. The anastomosis is checked, and if hemostatic, large Fogarty clamps with soft inserts are applied to the graft. With release of the suprarenal clamp, renal perfusion is restored. Debridement of any periaortic inflammation or infection is completed, including removal of any remaining graft material. The time spent excising any grossly infected or inflammatory tissue is a critically important component of in-line replacement therapy and should not be accomplished in haste. Complete excision of the pre-existing graft is mandatory. Following this, the anastomoses are performed to each uninvolved iliac artery, preferably beyond the prior graft anastomoses (**Figure 39.3**). The duodenal defect is debrided and closed primarily. If the duodenal defect is large, a segmental resection with end-to-end anastomosis is performed.

If the infected graft extends down to the femoral arteries, groin incisions are accomplished first with exposure of the femoral arteries and graft. The native arteries are exposed proximally and distally to the site of the prior anastomosis. A two-team approach, each working on one groin, is beneficial. Access to the tunnels is maintained with an umbilical tape; laparotomy pads can be passed through the tunnels, accomplishing some minor debridement while maintaining access. Because of the significant retroperitoneal adhesions that are typically encountered, creation of a new tunnel is difficult, with a significant risk of iliac vein injury. At the time of the initial graft debridement, the author has found it helpful to divide the graft limb just above the anastomosis so that the common femoral-profunda femoris-superficial femoral artery circuit is

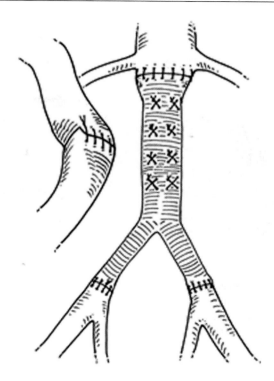

Figure 39.3 Depiction of the cryopreserved arterial allograft as an in-line repair. Note the anteriorly placed lumbar orifices that have been oversewn.

maintained, limiting distal ischemia. Once the author is ready to do the distal anastomosis of the new conduit, the arteries are clamped, any remaining graft material is completely excised, and the distal anastomosis is performed. In most instances, when doing the groin reconstruction, the author attempts to preserve retrograde flow. The author has used rotation of the sartorius muscle to provide coverage of the groin anastomoses. The skin of the groin wound is left open with the application of a vacuum-assisted closure dressing. Intra-abdominally, a segment of the omentum is mobilized on a vascular pedicle and wrapped around the newly placed prosthesis or graft (**Figure 39.4**).

PRIMARY AEF

Primary AEFs most frequently involve rupture of an infrarenal or pararenal AAA directly into the third or fourth portion of the duodenum, although other areas of the bowel may be involved. In the setting of GI bleeding and a known AAA, CTA may reveal the presence of extraluminal gas in the periaortic area in close approximation to a segment of bowel. The most common symptom is GI bleeding, with hemorrhage the most likely cause of death. The diagnosis is rarely made preoperatively and delays in diagnosis can lead to a disastrous outcome. Once suspected or diagnosed, the patient should be taken emergently to the operating room. The repair proceeds much like that of an open repair of a ruptured AAA with the following caveats: (1) temporary proximal supraceliac control

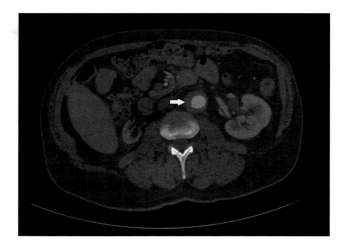

Figure 39.4 Computed tomography angiography of patient status-postexcision of infected aortic graft secondary to an aortoenteric fistula, repaired via an in-line rifampin-impregnated Dacron graft with an omental wrap. The white arrow indicates the omental wrap positioned around the prosthetic graft.

is obtained; (2) the proximal clamp is transitioned to the infrarenal aortic level as soon as possible; (3) debridement of any inflammatory tissue is performed; and (4) a two-layered closure of the bowel defect is undertaken. Throughout the operation, one attempts to minimize bowel contamination. As a primary AEF typically does not indicate long-standing infection, in-line replacement with a rifampin-impregnated Dacron graft is selected as the method of repair and revascularization. Endovascular repair can be accomplished as a bridge to definitive therapy in patients with hemodynamic instability and massive GI bleeding, or in extremely high-risk patients as a method of palliative repair.[7]

OTHER CONSIDERATIONS

Very limited to nonexistent aortic neck on CT scan

In this situation, if performed electively, the author has selectively used medial visceral rotation of the spleen and tail of the pancreas to allow for exposure of the pararenal aorta. While this is beneficial for performance of the proximal anastomosis, it carries significant risk, including splenic capsular injury, bleeding, pancreatic injury, and longer operative time and dissection, further complicating what is already a difficult operation.

The high-risk patient

If the patient's medical comorbidities make them high-risk for a prolonged operation, consideration is given to extra-anatomic bypass followed by graft excision. This approach minimizes the extent of the open abdominal portion of the

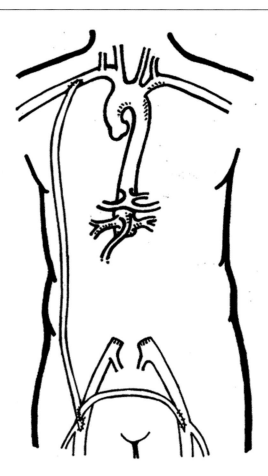

Figure 39.5 Depiction of the extra-anatomic reconstruction used in the repair of an aortoenteric fistula in which the original graft is completely intra-abdominal.

operation and reduces ischemia-reperfusion injury associated with prolonged pelvic and lower extremity clamp time. When prior aortic reconstruction is confined to the abdomen, extra-anatomic reconstruction is performed with a standard axillobifemoral bypass graft placement (**Figure 39.5**). Within 0–3 days of this operation, the patient undergoes excision of the infected graft and any inflammatory tissue, repair of the bowel defect, and closure of the aortic stump. Proximal supraceliac control and distal vessel control are necessary before dissection in the area of the AEF. Distal control is necessary because there is excellent retrograde perfusion supplied by the recently placed extra-anatomic bypass. All graft material is excised. The aortic stump is oversewn in a standard two-layered closure with 2-0 or 3-0 polypropylene suture, with a row of interrupted mattress sutures and an over-and-over stitch for the second layer. Any other foreign material (pledgeted suture) is avoided. When the original graft extends down to the femoral arteries, the extra-anatomic reconstruction by necessity becomes more elaborate. The author favors performance of bilateral axilloprofunda bypass graft placement with de novo incisions made lateral to the sartorius muscle to dissect out the mid-to-distal profunda femoral artery that serves as the site for the clean distal anastomosis and outflow (**Figure 39.6**).

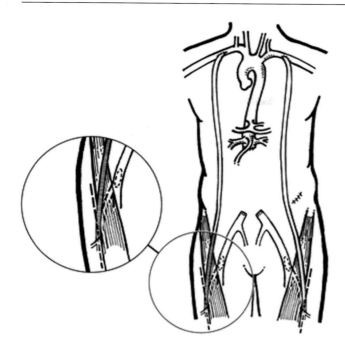

Figure 39.6 Depiction of the most common type of extra-anatomic reconstruction used in the repair of an aortoenteric fistula in which the original graft extends down to the femoral arteries. Note the lateral location of the incision used to expose the mid-to-distal profunda femoris artery.

In this high-risk patient population, endovascular therapies are also attractive alternatives. If the high-risk patient is an endovascular candidate anatomically, then consideration could be given to the application of endovascular graft placement as a definitive treatment option. However, this is to be applied to a relatively small subset of patients, as endovascular repair alone has been associated with higher rates of recurrence, sepsis, and AEF-related death.[8,9]

Hemodynamic instability

In the hemodynamically unstable patient, the decision is made to move directly to the operating room or hybrid operating room suite (**Figure 39.1**). The author has used emergent percutaneous access in instances of aortic pathology and bleeding with proximal balloon control of the hemorrhage. With ultrasound guidance, femoral access can easily be obtained, even in the setting of prior aortofemoral bypass. Once wire access is obtained to the suprarenal level, a larger-diameter sheath (>10 Fr) can be advanced into the aorta and a CODA° Balloon Catheter (Cook Medical Inc., Bloomington, IN, USA) is inflated for proximal control. This has the potential to be life-saving and allows some stabilization of the patient before operative management. If endovascular repair were an option anatomically, then the author would proceed with it as a bridge to stability. One important technique would be to avoid endografts with suprarenal fixation because this complicates subsequent open repair. If endovascular options are limited or anatomically not possible, the patient would then undergo midline incision with proximal supraceliac aortic control as described previously. Once proximal control is obtained, the operative team would proceed with infrarenal exposure and ligation of the aorta (two-layered closure). Further reconstruction of the extremities is pursued as the patient's condition allows. If there is limited contamination with minimal overall blood loss, in situ repair with an antibiotic-impregnated graft is a consideration.

Rifampin-impregnated Dacron graft

The most commonly used method for antimicrobial impregnation of prosthetic grafts is soaking the graft in an antibiotic solution of rifampin (**Figure 39.7**). Prosthetic grafts form an ionic bond with rifampin primarily through the

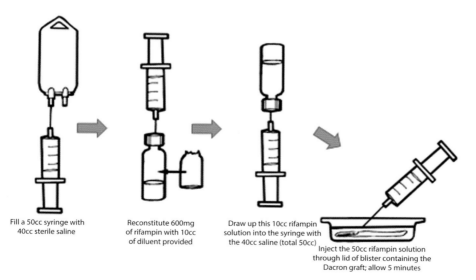

Fill a 50cc syringe with 40cc sterile saline

Reconstitute 600mg of rifampin with 10cc of diluent provided

Draw up this 10cc rifampin solution into the syringe with the 40cc saline (total 50cc)

Inject the 50cc rifampin solution through lid of blister containing the Dacron graft; allow 5 minutes

Figure 39.7 Sequence of the procedure for the preparation of a rifampin-impregnated Dacron graft to be used for in-line repair of an aortoenteric fistula.

gelatin that is used in the sealant process. The antibiotic is released locally and gradually for up to 5 days.

Cryopreserved arterial allograft

When time allows, this is the author's preferred treatment method for in-line repair of AEF. First, the graft and appropriate sizes of the aortic allograft are determined. The graft is prepared as the operation ensues because there is a defined thawing process when preparing a cryopreserved allograft. The thawing process averages approximately 30–40 minutes. Slits to enlarge the circumference of the proximal portion of the graft may have to be made to accommodate the anastomosis because of size discrepancy. Rather than using a single opening in the allograft, incisions are made into the allograft at both the 3 and 9 o'clock positions for appropriate sizing. The graft is rotated so that the lumbar orifices are positioned anteriorly; each lumbar artery is oversewn with interrupted 4-0 polypropylene suture.

CONCLUSION

The management goals of AEF, whether primary or secondary, remain the control of hemorrhage and infection, maintenance or preservation of lower extremity perfusion, and the elimination of future morbidity or recurrence related to the repair procedure. With the approaches outlined in this chapter, morbidity and mortality can be reduced (mortality <20%), and a durable, infection-resistant, limb-saving reconstruction can be accomplished.[6,9] The vascular surgeon, in addition to expeditiously arriving at the proper diagnosis, must be able to apply a variety of skills, techniques, and experience, including endovascular and complex redo abdominal open repair, to save the patient's life and maximize their long-term survival.

REFERENCES

1. Elliot JP Jr., Smith RF, Szilagyi DE. Proceedings: aortoenteric and paraprosthetic-enteric fistulas. Problems of diagnosis and management. *Arch Surg.* 1974;**108**:479–490.
2. Bunt TJ. Synthetic vascular infections. II. Graft-enteric erosions and graft-enteric fistulas. *Surgery.* 1983;**94**:1–9.
3. Hallett JW Jr., Marshall DM, Petterson TM, et al. Graft-related complications after abdominal aortic aneurysm repair: reassurance from a 36-year population-based experience. *J Vasc Surg.* 1997;**25**:277–286.
4. McPhee JT, Soybel DI, Oram RK, et al. Primary aortoenteric fistula following endovascular aortic repair due to type II endoleak. *J Vasc Surg.* 2011;**54**:1164–1166.
5. Fatima J, Duncan AA, de Grandis E, et al. Treatment strategies and outcomes in patients with infected aortic endografts. *J Vasc Surg.* 2013;**58**:371–379.
6. Kuestner LM, Reilly LM, Jicha DL, et al. Secondary aortoenteric fistula: contemporary outcome with use of extraanatomic bypass and infected graft excision. *J Vasc Surg.* 1995;**21**:184–195.
7. Marone EM, Mascia D, Kahlberg A, et al. Emergent endovascular treatment of a bleeding recurrent aortoenteric fistula as a "bridge" to definitive surgical repair. *J Vasc Surg.* 2012;**55**:1160–1163.
8. Antoniou GA, Koutsias S, Antoniou SA, et al. Outcome after endovascular stent graft repair of aortoenteric fistula: a systemic review. *J Vasc Surg.* 2009;**49**:782–789.
9. Kakkos SK, Bicknell CD, Tsolakis IA, et al. Editor's choice. Management of secondary aorto-enteric and other abdominal arterio-enteric fistulas: a review and pooled data analysis. *Eur J Vasc Endovasc Surg.* 2016;**52**:770–786.

40

Open repair of femoral and femoral anastomotic aneurysms

SEMERET T. MUNIE AND ALEXANDER D. SHEPARD

CONTENTS

INTRODUCTION

Arterial aneurysms in the lower extremities have a significant clinical importance because of their potential to cause limb-threatening ischemia from thrombosis or embolization of mural thrombus or, in rare circumstances, rupture. Intervention is preferred while aneurysms are still asymptomatic. Most true aneurysms of the lower extremities are degenerative in nature, while pseudoaneurysms are related to anastomotic, traumatic, and mycotic etiologies. Common risk factors for aneurysm formation include male sex, older age, smoking, and hypertension. In rare cases, connective tissue abnormalities (e.g., Marfan syndrome) can also lead to aneurysmal degeneration.

DEGENERATIVE FEMORAL ANEURYSMS

True femoral artery aneurysms (FAAs) are more common in the common femoral artery (CFA) (57%) than they are in the superficial femoral artery (SFA) (26%) or profunda femoris artery (PFA) (17%).[1] Aneurysms confined to the CFA are classified as type I, while those involving the origin of the PFA are type II.[2] This classification scheme is important when it comes to vascular reconstruction options.

Clinical presentation

The presentation of true FAAs can range from asymptomatic to severe lower extremity ischemia. Approximately 40% of patients are asymptomatic at the time of diagnosis, another 40% present with signs of lower extremity ischemia from embolization of mural thrombus or thrombosis, and 20% have local pain or notice a groin mass.[3]

Diagnosis

The diagnosis of a FAA is usually made on physical examination by palpation of a pulsatile groin mass. A variety of imaging modalities (ultrasonography, computed tomography (CT), or magnetic resonance imaging) can confirm the diagnosis. Catheter-based angiography has limited ability to assess the presence of an aneurysm because it only demonstrates the lumen of an artery and may miss the diagnosis in aneurysms lined with smooth mural thrombus.

Angiography, however, is helpful in evaluating the vascular anatomy of the lower extremity for operative planning.

Indications for treatment

Previous studies have shown that the diameter of the CFA increases with age, male sex, and larger body surface area. The normal size in men is approximately 10.5 mm and in women 8.5 mm.[4] In patients with asymptomatic disease, standard guidelines advise surgical repair for femoral aneurysms >2.5 cm in diameter or those containing a significant amount of mural thrombus. A recent study looking at 182 patients with degenerative FAAs raised the question that current management of isolated degenerative FAAs may be too aggressive for their natural history. This study found that acute complications rarely occurred in aneurysms <3.5 cm in diameter and recommended adjusting the current criteria.[5] On the other hand, all symptomatic FAAs should be treated regardless of size to prevent life- and limb-threatening complications (i.e., thrombosis, embolization, local compression, and rupture).

Preoperative planning

Preoperative assessment of cardiovascular risk is essential in this patient population. Imaging of the aorta, iliac, SFA, and popliteal arteries, usually with CT angiography (CTA), should also be performed to evaluate for the presence of any concurrent aneurysms. Bilateral lower extremity perfusion should also be evaluated with segmental pressure testing.

Operative repair

The surgical treatment of FAAs usually involves open repair where the aneurysmal segment is replaced with an interposition graft. Synthetic vascular grafts, such as polytetrafluoroethylene (PTFE) or Dacron are usually preferred over vein grafts because of their closer size matches and reported acceptable patency rates. General or regional (epidural) anesthesia is preferred.

A longitudinal groin incision is used to expose the aneurysm. Control of the CFA or external iliac artery (EIA) proximally, and of the SFA and PFA distally, is obtained. Most degenerative aneurysms arise just below the origins of the inferior superficial epigastric and lateral iliac circumflex branches, making control at the EIA level the norm. Efforts should be made to preserve these branches to avoid local groin wound ischemic complications. When controlling the EIA at this level, it is frequently necessary to divide a small portion of the inguinal ligament. In addition, care should be exercised in searching for (and dividing, in most cases) the crossing iliac circumflex vein, also known as "the vein of pain," to avoid later inadvertent injury. At the femoral bifurcation, one should always look for and control a posteriorly exiting branch from the CFA or the most proximal PFA. Failure to control this branch before opening the aneurysm can lead to troublesome back-bleeding. If the aneurysm is very large or ruptured, a retroperitoneal approach through a short, transverse suprainguinal incision may be necessary to obtain proximal control of the EIA. Following therapeutic

heparinization, the inflow and outflow vessels are clamped and the aneurysm is opened. Most aneurysms may be simply excised. However, it is generally not advisable to completely excise large aneurysms because they may be adherent to the common femoral/femoral veins and femoral nerve/branches. Excision of large aneurysms can also lead to more lymphatic disruption, which can induce troublesome lymphedema of the involved extremity postoperatively.

Type I aneurysms are generally reconstructed with a CFA-to-CFA interposition graft of either Dacron or PTFE (**Figure 40.1a**). Type II aneurysms can be repaired

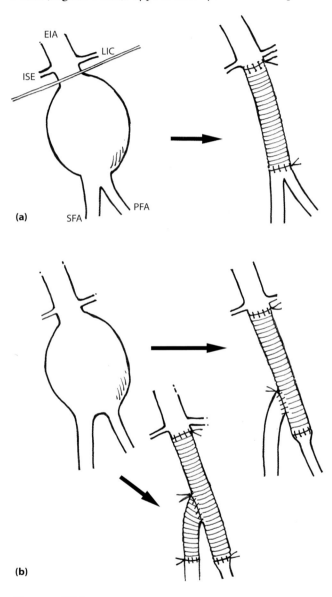

Figure 40.1 Operative repair of femoral artery aneurysms. (**a**) Type I aneurysms are confined to the common femoral artery (CFA) and can be repaired with a CFA-to-CFA interposition graft of either Dacron or polytetrafluoroethylene. (**b**) Type II aneurysms involve the origin of the profunda femoris artery (PFA) and can be repaired with an interposition graft to the PFA and reimplantation of the superficial femoral artery or vice-versa, or with a second interposition graft. EIA: external iliac artery; ISE: inferior superficial epigastric artery branch; LIC: lateral iliac circumflex branch.

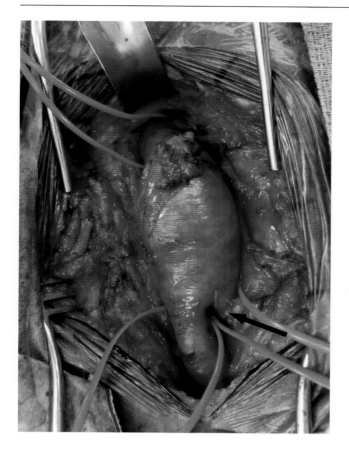

Figure 40.2 Intraoperative image of type II left femoral artery aneurysm with involvement of the profunda femoris artery (PFA) origin. Red vessel loops are around the common femoral artery proximally and the superficial femoral artery and PFA distally. The arrow points to the PFA.

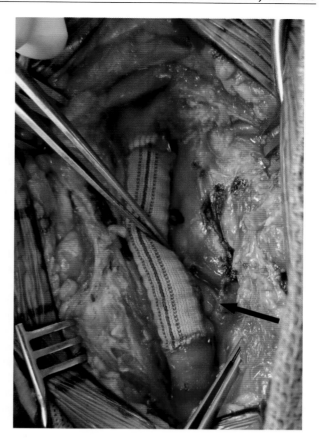

Figure 40.3 Intraoperative image of post-aneurysm excision with end-to-end Dacron graft anastomosis to the common femoral artery proximally and the superficial femoral artery distally; the profunda femoris artery is reimplanted into the side of the graft (arrow).

with an interposition graft to the PFA and reimplantation of the SFA or vice versa (**Figure 40.1b**). However, if the SFA is chronically occluded with minimal clinical symptoms before surgery, then an interposition graft to the PFA alone may be performed. Operative images of a type II left femoral aneurysm before and after repair with a Dacron interposition graft are seen in **Figures 40.2** and **40.3**.

FEMORAL ANASTOMOTIC ANEURYSMS

Anastomotic aneurysms have traditionally been described as resulting from a disrupted suture line between a graft and the host artery. In the groin, this most commonly occurs at the femoral anastomosis of an aortofemoral bypass. Careful analysis, however, suggests that degeneration of the femoral artery wall is a more important contributory factor.[6] Complications are uncommon in femoral anastomotic aneurysms <2 cm in diameter. Larger aneurysms are associated with local complications and limb ischemia. Risk factors for the development of anastomotic aneurysms include: chronic obstructive pulmonary

disease; current smoking; and postoperative groin wound infection. The incidence is higher with prosthetic than autogenous vein grafts.

Clinical presentation

Anastomotic aneurysms typically present >5 years after the original bypass surgery. The diagnosis is suggested by the complaint of a painless pulsatile mass in 60–70% of patients and symptoms of acute limb ischemia in another 20%. Less frequent presentations include a painful pulsatile mass and rupture. Patients may also present with a clinical picture suggestive of graft infection, such as groin erythema, pain, fever, chills, or night sweats.

Diagnosis

Every patient with a suspected anastomotic FAA should undergo CTA angiography of the entire graft to evaluate for the presence of infection (i.e., gas or fluid around the graft) and to rule out any synchronous aneurysms.

Indications for treatment

In a patient who presents with a history of femoral artery anastomosis, a pulsatile groin mass, and symptoms, repair is indicated. Symptoms can be pain from expansion/rupture, ischemia from thrombosis or embolization of mural clot, or venous obstruction/deep vein thrombosis from compression of the adjacent vein. Repair in asymptomatic patients depends on the size of the aneurysm (≥2.5–3 cm in diameter), the degree of associated mural thrombus, and documentation of rapid expansion.

Surgical repair

In the absence of any signs of infection, the pseudoaneurysm is ideally approached through the old groin incision, which can be extended proximally or distally as needed. Occasionally, the old incision is so poorly situated that only a portion of it can be incorporated into the new incision. In rare circumstances, it is necessary to make an entirely new incision, which should be vertically oriented to provide the most options for adequate exposure. Great care should be exercised in these situations because of the risk of healing complications from local wound ischemia. In difficult groin dissection or with very large aneurysms, proximal control can be obtained through a suprainguinal incision. Because of the reoperative nature of these cases, dense scar tissue is common and is best managed with sharp scalpel dissection, rather than scissors. These patients are at increased risk for postoperative lymphatic complications. Care must be taken to ligate any suspected lymphatic channels. It is important to avoid entry into the plane between the adventitia and media, which can often seem like an easy dissection plane. Such so-called "exarterectomy" results in a vessel wall too weak to hold stitches at the time of vascular reconstruction.

Just as with true FAAs, an attempt at control of inflow and outflow vessels should be made before opening anastomotic aneurysms. Dense scar tissue can make it challenging. Occasionally, it is easier to obtain intraluminal control with balloon occlusion catheters. Important principles to follow while performing anastomotic aneurysm repair include: good proximal and distal arterial control; excision of the aneurysm sac with debridement of the proximal and distal ends of vessels back to normal arterial wall; use of an interposition graft; anastomotic sutures placed in healthy tissue; and creation of a tension-free anastomosis. A variety of reconstruction techniques are available. Primary repair is almost never anatomically possible and even if it is, it should be avoided because such a reconstruction never addresses the root cause of the aneurysm and is therefore associated with an unacceptably high recurrence rate. The most frequent scenario involves an end-to-side anastomosis between an aortofemoral graft limb and the CFA. When the proximal CFA and SFA are occluded, an interposition graft between the graft limb and the PFA is straightforward (**Figure 40.4a**).

However, when the CFA is patent with significant retrograde flow, a decision must be made whether to preserve this vessel in the reconstruction. If so, then it may be necessary to place an interposition graft between the CFA and PFA, with a second interposition graft between the graft limb and this new graft (**Figure 40.4b**). Maintaining flow in a patent SFA is another scenario that may require reimplantation of the PFA or SFA into an interposition graft or even a second interposition graft (**Figure 40.4c**).

If graft infection is suspected preoperatively, removal of the infected graft and revascularization through non-infected tissue planes is indicated. The approach to this problem is beyond the scope of this chapter and is covered in more detail in Chapter 48. The one exception to this rule is a graft infection with *Staphylococcus epidermidis*. This low-virulence organism has been frequently cultured from uninfected-appearing anastomotic FAAs following aortofemoral bypass and has been implicated as the causative factor. Culture of this organism from surgical specimens is difficult, but when it is found, consideration should be given to lifelong suppressive antibiotics.

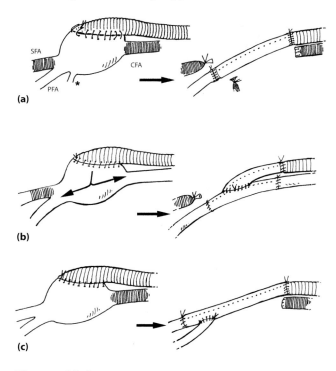

Figure 40.4 Reconstruction methods for a femoral anastomotic pseudoaneurysm. (**a**) When both the superficial femoral artery (SFA) and proximal common femoral artery (CFA) are occluded, an interposition graft between the aortofemoral graft limb and the profunda femoris artery (PFA) can be performed. (**b**) When the CFA is patent with clinically significant retrograde flow, preservation of retrograde flow requires placement of an interposition graft between the CFA and PFA, with a second interposition graft between the graft limb and this new graft. (**c**) When both the SFA and the PFA are patent, distal reconstruction can be performed to the SFA with reimplantation of the PFA or vice-versa. *: posterior branch of the CFA originating at the level of the bifurcation.

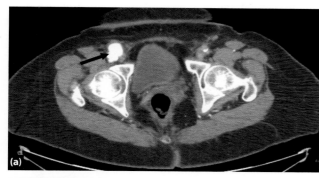

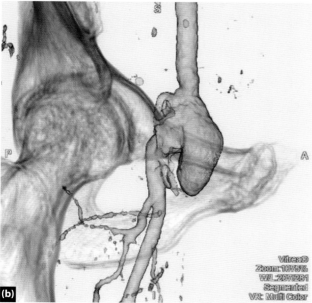

Figure 40.5 Right femoral anastomotic aneurysm (black arrow) in a 58-year-old woman 5 years following aortobifemoral bypass surgery. (**a**) Axial computed tomography (CT) image. The black arrow points to the aneurysm; note that the left femoral artery is occluded from a prior attempted revision. (**b**) Three-dimensional CT image of aneurysm documenting occlusion of the right superficial femoral artery.

Postoperative care

Postoperative complications after true femoral and anastomotic FAA repair are similar and include: hemorrhage; lymphatic leak; wound infection; graft infection; graft occlusion; major limb amputation; and recurrent anastomotic FAA. Given its redo nature, anastomotic aneurysm repair is associated with a higher incidence of local wound complications than might be expected. This finding highlights the need for meticulous operative technique.

In general, FAAs can be repaired with good success. The literature reports mortality rates <5%, which can be higher in emergency settings.[3] As with all arterial reconstructions, the key to good outcomes is thorough preoperative preparation of the patient and careful operative planning.

CASE EXAMPLE

A 58-year-old woman with multiple comorbidities, including aortobifemoral bypass surgery 5 years ago, presented to the clinic with a pulsatile swelling in her right groin. On physical examination, she was found to have a 3-cm pulsatile mass in her right groin and 1+ pedal pulses. She had no pulsatile abdominal mass. CTA showed a 3.1-cm anastomotic aneurysm at the right femoral anastomosis of her old aortobifemoral bypass (**Figure 40.5a,b**). The patient was electively taken to the operating room and underwent open repair of her anastomotic aneurysm with placement of a PTFE interposition graft from her old graft limb to her PFA. Her SFA was chronically occluded, so it was not reconstructed. Postoperatively, the patient did well and was discharged home on postoperative day 4.

REFERENCES

1. Sapienza P, Mingoli A, Feldhaus RJ, et al. Femoral artery aneurysms: long-term follow-up and results of surgical treatment. *Cardiovasc Surg.* 1996;**4**:181–184.
2. Graham LM, Zelenock GB, Whitehouse WM Jr., et al. Clinical significance of arteriosclerotic femoral artery aneurysms. *Arch Surg.* 1980;**115**:502–507.
3. Shepard AD, Jacobson GM. Anastomotic aneurysms. In: Towne JB, Hollier LH, eds. *Complications in Vascular Surgery.* 2nd ed. New York: Marcel Dekker; 2004. pp. 139–153.
4. Sandgren T, Sonesson B, Ryden-Ahlgren Å, et al. Arterial dimensions in the lower extremities of patients with abdominal aortic aneurysms: no indications of a generalized dilating diathesis. *J Vasc Surg.* 2001;**34**:1079–1084.
5. Lawrence PF, Harlander-Locke MP, Oderich GS, et al. The current management of isolated degenerative femoral artery aneurysms is too aggressive for their natural history. *J Vasc Surg.* 2014;**59**:343–349.
6. Szilagyi DE, Smith RF, Elliott JP, et al. Anastomotic aneurysms after vascular reconstruction: problems of incidence, etiology, and treatment. *Surgery.* 1975;**78**:800–816.

41

Open popliteal artery aneurysm repair

JOSEPH HERRMANN, JACOB JOHNSON, AND WILLIAM OPPAT

CONTENTS

INTRODUCTION

The normal diameter of a popliteal artery ranges from approximately 0.5 cm to 1.1 cm. The artery is considered aneurysmal if the enlargement is 1.5 times the diameter of a normal adjacent segment of the artery.[1] The minimal diameter at which the artery is considered aneurysmal is 1.2 cm. Most clinicians use a 2-cm diameter as their threshold to consider treatment.[2]

EPIDEMIOLOGY

Popliteal artery aneurysms (PAAs) are the most common peripheral artery aneurysms, accounting for 70% of peripheral aneurysms.[2] Most aneurysms occur in the proximal popliteal artery or at its midpoint.[3] Although PAAs are the most common peripheral aneurysms, they are still relatively uncommon, with an incidence of 7.4 per 100 000 men and 1 per 100 000 women. The mean age at presentation of PAA is 65 years.[4]

PAAs are often associated with other aneurysms. Fifty percent of patients with PAAs have a contralateral PAA; the prevalence of aortic aneurysms averages 40% and may be as high as 70% in patients with bilateral PAAs.[5,6] Patients treated for isolated PAAs require close continued surveillance because up to 50% of them will develop another aneurysm at a remote location over the next 10 years.[7]

CLINICAL FINDINGS

PAAs can present as an asymptomatic pulsatile mass behind the knee or may present with acute or chronic ischemia. The associated limb ischemia may be secondary to acute or chronic thrombosis of the aneurysm or secondary to distal embolization of a mural thrombus. Some patients can present with compressive symptoms if the aneurysm is large enough, such as pain or lower extremity edema, or even a deep vein thrombosis. Rarely (about 2%), patients present with PAA rupture with severe swelling and pain in the popliteal space and distal limb.[3]

PAAs are often asymptomatic for an extended period and may present with ischemic complications or, more rarely, rupture. The most feared complication is irreversible leg ischemia because of sudden aneurysm thrombosis or extensive distal embolization, with a significant risk of subsequent amputation.

DIAGNOSIS

The first tools in the diagnosis of PAAs are a high level of suspicion, a history, and a physical examination. PAAs should be suspected whenever a prominent pulsation is felt in the popliteal space. If the aneurysm is thrombosed, it will be a firm, nonpulsatile mass.[3] As previously discussed, patients with known aneurysms are more likely to have

PAAs, which could be asymptomatic, and these patients should be evaluated with a higher level of suspicion.

Physical examination can be unreliable and should be supplemented with imaging. Imaging modalities for evaluation of PAAs include duplex ultrasonography, computed tomography angiography (CTA), magnetic resonance angiography (MRA), and angiography.[2,3] Duplex ultrasonography is the most commonly used imaging modality for the diagnosis of PAAs (**Figure 41.1**). Ultrasound (US) provides information needed for treatment, such as the diameter of the aneurysm, the presence of intraluminal thrombus, vessel patency, and the velocities of flow. Duplex ultrasonography can also be used to evaluate nonvascular masses of the popliteal fossa and for mapping superficial veins to prepare for treatment of the aneurysm.[8] CTA (**Figure 41.2**) adds to the ability to provide a precise diagnosis and can identify suitable inflow and outflow target arteries for bypass to repair the aneurysm.[3] MRA provides similar information to CTA but is used less commonly because of increased cost and the time needed to obtain the images. Angiography (**Figure 41.3**) is not frequently used because of the invasive nature of the procedure, but it can be used to evaluate a PAA, precisely define runoff vessels, and identify the anatomy for potential treatment with a stent graft. In many practices, duplex US is used to screen and diagnose PAAs, while CTA or MRA is used for operative planning.

TREATMENT

The primary objective in the repair of PAAs is exclusion of the aneurysm from the circulation to prevent complications. Open surgical techniques have been the gold standard of treatment for PAAs for many years. Open surgical repair can traditionally be performed via one of two different techniques, a medial or posterior approach, each with their own advantages.[3]

MEDIAL APPROACH

The medial approach is used more frequently for small or fusiform aneurysms or for bypasses that need to extend to distal tibial or pedal vessels. The aneurysm is bypassed and ligated both proximally and distally to exclude it from the circulation. Geniculate arteries require ligation if they arise from the aneurysmal popliteal segment and have the potential to retrograde perfuse the excluded aneurysm sac.

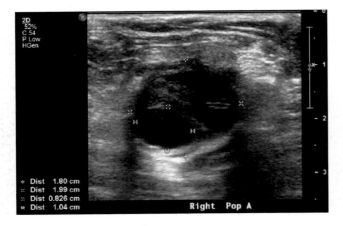

Figure 41.1 B-mode ultrasound image of partially thrombosed popliteal artery aneurysm.

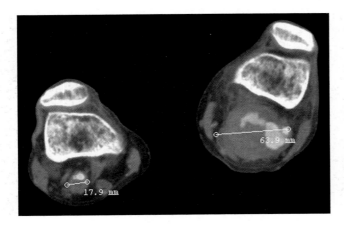

Figure 41.2 Computed tomography angiogram depicting bilateral, partially thrombosed but patent popliteal aneurysms.

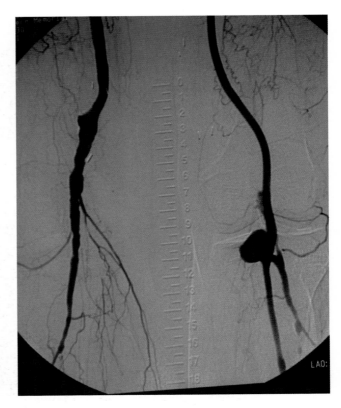

Figure 41.3 Angiogram showing a large left popliteal aneurysm. The right leg had a previous popliteal aneurysm repair with interposition bypass.

For the medial approach, the patient is positioned supine with the leg externally rotated, with a bump placed under the knee. The saphenous vein is harvested to use as a bypass conduit. The popliteal artery is then exposed above and below the knee joint; this is typically done through the same incisions used for vein harvest. Arterial exposure is typical of the femoropopliteal artery bypass, making it suitable in most elective and urgent situations (**Figure 41.4**). If it is necessary to extend the bypass to the anterior tibial or pedal arteries, or a lateral approach to the distal peroneal artery is planned, then a separate incision is required. Arterial exposure can be difficult because of arteriomegaly, venous engorgement, kinking, tortuosity, or vessel displacement.

After exposure of the target vessels, they are isolated with vessel loops. A tunnel is then typically created from the above-the-knee to the below-the-knee space between the heads of the gastrocnemius muscle. Careful attention to the anatomy of the gastrocnemius muscle is important to identify and release any possible entrapment by abnormal slips of muscle, if it exists. Tunneling can be difficult with large aneurysms, and decompression of the aneurysm sac may be required (**Figure 41.5**). The patient is then heparinized with 80–100 IU/kg of intravenous heparin.

After controlling the vessels proximally and distally, arterial bypass is performed in standard fashion with a saphenous vein bypass graft from above-the-knee to below-the-knee. The bypass anastomosis can be performed in either an end-to-end or an end-to-side fashion. If the aneurysm is occluded, the bypass is performed in standard fashion. If the aneurysm is patent, the inflow and outflow arteries to the sac also need to be ligated. This should be done as close to the aneurysm sac as possible; it is performed to exclude the sac, promote aneurysm thrombosis, and decrease the risk of continued expansion from geniculate or other collateral filling. A completion arteriography, angioscopy, or duplex ultrasonography should be considered before closure.

The medial approach is familiar to vascular surgeons because of its similarity to femoropopliteal bypass. This common exposure presents an advantage of this approach over the posterior approach. The medial approach also provides easy access to the saphenous vein and allows the procedure to be performed at a distance from the diseased vessel itself, reducing the risk of injury to adjacent structures. The main disadvantage of this approach is that the aneurysm is left intact without decompression. Up to 30% of these aneurysms do not thrombose and will continue to enlarge; they can result in pain, compression, or rupture. Some surgeons will open the aneurysm sac via the above- or below-knee incision and suture-ligate back-bleeding branches to prevent this complication.[3]

POSTERIOR APPROACH

The posterior approach is often reserved for aneurysms that displace normal anatomy, causing compressive symptoms. The patient is placed in the prone position. A lazy, S-shaped lateral incision is made starting on the medial side of the thigh, extending laterally across the flexion crease of the knee, and ending on the proximal aspect of the calf over the proximal small saphenous vein (SSV). The proximal extent of the incision is used to expose the great saphenous vein, which can be harvested to use as a bypass conduit. Alternatively, if the SSV is large enough on preoperative vein mapping, the distal incision can be extended, and the SSV can be used as the conduit.

The popliteal artery is identified proximally and exposed by separating the semimembranosus and semitendinosus muscles medially from the long head of the biceps femoris muscle laterally. The artery is dissected free circumferentially and controlled with a vessel loop. Dissection is continued distally along the artery to avoid injury of the tibial and peroneal nerves coursing laterally and posteriorly to the aneurysm. The distal popliteal artery is circumferentially controlled. The tibioperoneal trunk and proximal

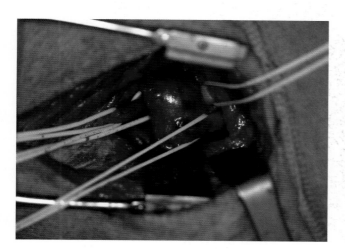

Figure 41.4 Intraoperative image demonstrating medial exposure of a popliteal artery aneurysm.

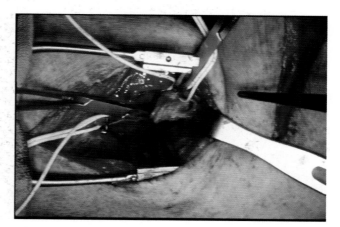

Figure 41.5 Image depicting removal of mural thrombus from a popliteal aneurysm via a medial approach.

tibial vessels might also be accessed from this approach, but the medial approach is required for bypass to the tibial vessels (**Figures 41.6** and **41.7**).

After obtaining proximal and distal control, systemic heparin is administered. The aneurysm sac is then opened longitudinally. Like open repair of an abdominal aortic aneurysm (AAA), the thrombus is removed and back-bleeding collaterals are oversewn from within. Bypass is then performed with a vein or prosthetic graft. The bypass can be performed as an interposition graft with end-to-end anastomosis or as a standard end-to-side bypass.[3]

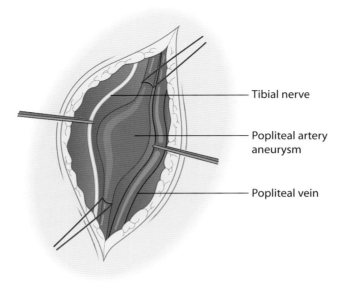

Figure 41.6 Intraoperative drawing of posterior exposure of a popliteal artery aneurysm.

- Tibial nerve
- Popliteal artery aneurysm
- Popliteal vein

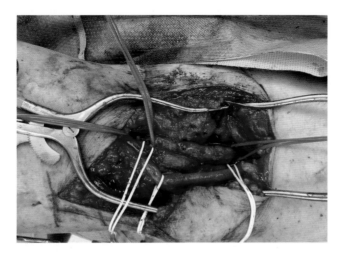

Figure 41.7 Intraoperative image demonstrating posterior exposure of a popliteal artery aneurysm (red vessel loops). The nerve has been retracted medially (bottom vessel loop). The popliteal vein is controlled with two white vessel loops.

EMERGENT SURGICAL REPAIR

Patients with PAAs who present with acute limb ischemia require immediate intervention to avoid amputation. Angiography is initially performed; surgery is performed during the same admission. If the aneurysm is occluded, but a distal outflow vessel is identified on angiography, bypass is performed as described previously. If no outflow vessel is identified, and the patient's limb is not immediately threatened, thrombolysis is started to restore flow to a potential outflow target vessel. If the limb is immediately threatened, and the patient has sensory and motor dysfunction, emergent thromboembolectomy is performed. The distal popliteal artery is exposed and controlled below the knee, exposing the area of the trifurcation. An arteriotomy is then made and a Fogarty catheter is passed into all three runoff vessels. Bypass can then be performed to the patent outflow vessel. Completion angiography is mandatory. After bypass, these patients may develop signs of reperfusion injury, like rhabdomyolysis, and they may require fasciotomy.[3]

RESULTS OF OPEN SURGICAL RECONSTRUCTION OF POPLITEAL ANEURYSMS

The outcome of open surgical repair of PAAs is affected by the scenario in which the repair is performed, that is, elective versus emergent, and the type of conduit used, that is, vein versus prosthesis. The posterior and medial approaches have been found to be equal.[9,10] As expected, the risk of graft thrombosis and amputation is higher in surgery performed for symptomatic patients. Pulli and collaborators found the risk of amputation at 30 days to be 6.5% for symptomatic patients versus 1.4% in asymptomatic patients. They also found limb salvage rates at 5 years to be 93.4% for asymptomatic patients compared to 80.4% for symptomatic patients. Those who presented with critical limb ischemia only had a 59% limb salvage rate at 5 years.[11] Huang and collaborators found similar results, with all amputations and early deaths occurring only in patients who presented with acute ischemia. They also found 1-year patency rates to be 96% in patients reconstructed with saphenous vein versus 67% for those reconstructed with prosthetic graft.[6] Based on the findings of these and other studies, PAAs should be repaired electively and with saphenous vein graft, when possible. The excellent limb salvage and patency rates are the reason why aneurysms >2 cm are treated in any patient who can tolerate open surgical repair. In patients who cannot tolerate an open surgical bypass, they should be considered for popliteal artery stenting, which is discussed in Chapter 11.

CASE EXAMPLE

A 63-year-old man with a history of hypertension and anxiety presented to the emergency department complaining of new-onset, left lower extremity rest pain. The pain was a constant, severe, aching pain in the left foot and posterior calf, and started about 2 hours before presentation. Before developing constant pain, the patient had been experiencing pain in his left lower leg, even when walking a short distance. The claudication symptoms would resolve with rest. The patient denied any provoking or relieving factors for his ongoing rest pain. He was a former smoker, but quit 15 years ago. His family history was significant for AAAs in both his father and his brother.

The patient was hemodynamically stable and afebrile. On examination, his left lower extremity was slightly cooler than the right. He had a palpable dorsalis pedis and posterior tibial artery pulses in his right lower extremity, but no palpable pedal pulses in his left lower extremity. There was a small, firm mass palpated behind his left knee with no palpable popliteal pulse. Normal movement and sensation were intact in the bilateral lower extremities. There were palpable femoral and radial pulses bilaterally.

The patient's laboratory investigations were unremarkable. Noninvasive vascular studies were obtained. The patient's ankle–brachial pressure indexes were 1.27 in the right leg and 0.39 in the left leg. An arterial duplex showed a 2.3-cm left PAA, which was thrombosed.

The patient was taken urgently to the operating room where a left lower extremity angiogram was performed. He had a thrombosed popliteal artery with reconstitution of the peroneal and posterior tibial arteries near the ankle. The popliteal artery was crossed with a Glidewire® Hydrophilic Coated Guidewire (Terumo Medical Corporation, Somerset, NJ, USA) and positioned in the posterior tibial artery. A thrombolysis catheter was placed over the guidewire and tissue plasminogen activator thrombolysis was initiated and continued for 12 hours. The patient regained a palpable posterior tibial artery pulse in his left foot with thrombolysis overnight. He was returned to the operating room the next day for a repeat angiogram that showed a patent popliteal artery with two-vessel runoff to the left foot. He then underwent an open repair of his left popliteal artery via a medial approach using a reverse saphenous vein graft.

The patient recovered well following the surgery. He was discharged home on the third postoperative day. On discharge, he was ambulating well with a strongly palpable left posterior tibial artery pulse. Before discharge, a duplex US of the abdominal aorta was obtained and was negative for AAA.

REFERENCES

1. Johnston KW, Rutherford RB, Tilson MD, et al. Suggested standards for reporting on arterial aneurysms. Subcommittee on Reporting Standards for Arterial Aneurysms, Ad Hoc Committee on Reporting Standards, Society for Vascular Surgery and North American Chapter, International Society for Cardiovascular Surgery. *J Vasc Surg.* 1991;**13**:452–458.

2. Mousa AY, Beauford RB, Henderson P, et al. Update on the diagnosis and management of popliteal aneurysm and literature review. *Vascular.* 2006;**14**:103–108.

3. Pomposelli FB, Hamdan A. Lower extremity aneurysms. In: Cronenwett JL, Johnston KW, eds. *Rutherford's Vascular Surgery.* 7th edn. Philadelphia, PA: Elsevier; 2010. pp. 2110–2111.

4. Lawrence PF, Lorenzo-Rivero S, Lyon JL. The incidence of iliac, femoral, and popliteal artery aneurysms in hospitalized patients. *J Vasc Surg.* 1995;**22**:409–415.

5. Dawson I, Sie RB, van Bockel JH. Atherosclerotic popliteal aneurysm. *Br J Surg.* 1997;**84**:293–299.

6. Huang Y, Gloviczki P, Noel AA, et al. Early complications and long-term outcome after open surgical treatment of popliteal artery aneurysms: is exclusion with saphenous vein bypass still the gold standard? *J Vasc Surg.* 2007;**45**:706–713.

7. Dawson I, van Bockel JH, Brand R, et al. Popliteal artery aneurysms. Long-term follow-up of aneurysmal disease and results of surgical treatment. *J Vasc Surg.* 1991;**13**:398–407.

8. Stone PA, Armstrong PA, Bandyk DF, et al. The value of duplex surveillance after open and endovascular popliteal aneurysm repair. *J Vasc Surg.* 2005;**41**:936–941.

9. Ravn H, Wanhainen A, Björck M. Surgical technique and long-term results after popliteal artery aneurysm repair: results from 717 legs. *J Vasc Surg.* 2007;**46**:236–243.

10. Kropman RH, van Santvoort HC, Teijink J, et al. The medial versus the posterior approach in the repair of popliteal artery aneurysms: a multicenter case-matched study. *J Vasc Surg.* 2007;**46**:24–30.

11. Pulli R, Dorigo W, Troisi N, et al. Surgical management of popliteal artery aneurysms: which factors affect outcomes? *J Vasc Surg.* 2006;**43**:481–487.

42

Open thoracic aortic aneurysm repair

ARNOUD V. KAMMAN, BO YANG, AND HIMANSHU J. PATEL

CONTENTS

INTRODUCTION

Most descending thoracic aortic aneurysms (TAAs) are due to degenerative disease that results in dilation of the aorta. The incidence of TAAs is thought to be increasing and is estimated at approximately 10 cases per 100 000 person-years.[1] Symptomatic TAAs may present with hoarseness (from left recurrent laryngeal nerve stretching), stridor (from tracheal or bronchial compression), dyspnea (from lung compression), and plethora and edema (from superior vena cava compression). Back, interscapular, or left shoulder pain may be observed in descending TAAs. However, the identification of an asymptomatic TAA is most frequently an incidental finding during evaluation of the chest for a different pathology. Simultaneous abdominal and thoracic aneurysms are seen in 20–25% of patients.[2,3] This underlines the importance of a total aortic inspection when an abdominal or thoracic aneurysm is diagnosed. Genetic predisposition, such as Marfan syndrome or bicuspid aortic valve, are phenotypes at higher risk of ascending TAA development.[1] Important risk factors for the development of descending TAAs are hypertension, smoking, and chronic obstructive pulmonary disease (COPD).

Computed tomography (CT) or magnetic resonance imaging are considered the gold standard for the proper evaluation of TAAs.[1,4] TAA treatment can be done with either thoracic endovascular aortic repair (TEVAR) or open surgical repair (OSR). Current guidelines suggest surgery for all symptomatic descending TAA patients, and for asymptomatic patients with an aneurysm diameter ≥55–60 mm (descending); rapidly expanding aneurysms (>0.5 mm/ year) should also be considered for surgery.[1,4] Lower thresholds can be maintained in patients with Marfan syndrome or a positive family history (i.e., ≥50 mm). Recent studies have described long-term data regarding TEVAR for TAA and the pathologies where OSR might provide a more durable solution in younger patients.[5,6] Although TEVAR should be strongly considered in degenerative aneurysms of the descending thoracic aorta, OSR is recommended in aneurysms resulting from chronic dissection.[1] Furthermore, it is imperative to provide the patient with a perspective of the proposed treatment options available to them and their associated risks. Finally, OSR can be the preferred treatment in younger patients, patients with connective tissue disorders, when extensive additional procedures are necessary in addition to TEVAR, or if TEVAR is not possible because of unfavorable aortic anatomy.

OPERATIVE TECHNIQUE

For an isolated descending TAA, the patient is placed in a right lateral decubitus position, with the left thorax upward. At the discretion of the surgeon, a lumbar drain is used to prevent spinal cord ischemia (SCI). The patient is generally prepped and then draped. A left posterolateral thoracotomy is performed and the left chest is entered via the fourth intercostal space (ICS) if the arch or proximal half of the TAA is to be intervened upon, or via the eighth ICS for the distal half of the TAA. The left femoral vessels are exposed with a transverse infrainguinal incision for cannulation in readiness for cardiopulmonary bypass (CPB). The descending thoracic aorta is mobilized for resection.

When a large aneurysm that contains debris is mobilized, atheromatous retrograde emboli can present to the head vessels. This suggests that the aorta should not be touched until an appropriate time of circulatory arrest. Also, the left lung should be manipulated as little as possible to avoid hemorrhage, especially when the patient is heparinized.

If there is insufficient room to cross-clamp the aorta proximally, CPB with deep hypothermic circulatory arrest (DHCA) is usually used.[7] Otherwise, left heart bypass or femoral artery-femoral vein bypass (partial CPB) techniques can be used. This does not necessitate circulatory arrest.

When CPB is performed, 2–3 units of autologous blood are withdrawn for later reinfusion. Subsequently, the patient is heparinized and a venous cannula is inserted under transesophageal echography (TEE) guidance into the right atrium with a Seldinger technique via the left common femoral vein. The left femoral artery (LFA) is isolated and an 8-mm Dacron graft is sewn in an end-to-side manner via a transverse arteriotomy to serve for arterial return.

Use of DHCA

Intercostal vessels that are not preserved are ligated and divided during this cooling process. At 18°C, systemic potassium is given to achieve cardiac arrest. CPB flow rates are reduced and a cross-clamp is set at the T5 level to maintain lower body perfusion.

After proximal incision in the descending aorta, the proximal anastomosis is constructed with a running 4-0 polypropylene suture using a Dacron graft with a single prefabricated side branch. After this, the side branch is cannulated for CPB, for flow restoration to the upper body. The proximal clamps are placed distal to the side branch after de-airing the aorta through the open distal end of the graft. Flow to the upper body and heart is now restored.

The distal thoracic aorta is mobilized and encircled, after which the distal clamp is repositioned just beyond the site of the proposed distal anastomosis. Normothermia is restored with active rewarming, and the TAA is incised fully. The graft is then tailored to an appropriate length and the distal anastomosis is created to a healthy section of the distal descending aorta.

When long segments of the aorta are replaced, the distal clamp is initially set at approximately T5 to maintain lower intercostal artery perfusion. The distal clamp is then repositioned at the distal thoracic aorta when constructing the distal anastomosis. After the proximal and distal anastomoses are constructed, the intercostal arteries are reattached, if felt necessary, by isolating a segment of the graft. Alternatively, intercostal artery patch reimplantation can occur before constructing the distal anastomosis to reduce SCI time.

Sufficient de-airing is performed, the clamps are removed, and the CPB is stopped when the patient is normothermic. During rewarming, the LFA is primarily repaired. Routine decannulation is then performed and hemostasis assured with protamine sulfate, autologous blood, and additional factors. The native aneurysm is closed over the graft to provide separation from the adjacent viscera. Chest tubes are placed and the thoracotomy and groin wounds are closed.

Partial CPB

In the setting of a partial CPB without circulatory arrest, assisted circulation can be achieved by either a left heart bypass circuit or partial CPB using the femoral artery and vein. The latter technique is preferred to be able to use pump suckers and allow blood conservation.

The aorta is clamped proximally and distally, and the aneurysm is incised in a longitudinal fashion. When possible, to preserve intercostal flow, an oblique suture line is created to include back-bleeding segmental vessels. This alleviates the need for individual vessel reimplantation. Any debris is removed and a Dacron tube graft is anastomosed proximally with polypropylene suture (**Figure 42.1**).

The distal anastomosis is then constructed to the distal aorta, again with polypropylene suture (**Figure 42.2**). The proximal clamp can then be removed and the residual aneurysm is tailored and closed over the graft.

When long segments of aorta are replaced, the distal clamp is initially set at approximately T5 to maintain lower intercostal artery perfusion. The distal clamp is then repositioned at the distal thoracic aorta when constructing the distal anastomosis. After the proximal and distal anastomoses are constructed, the intercostal arteries are reattached, if felt necessary, by isolating a segment of the graft. Alternatively, intercostal artery patch reimplantation can occur before constructing the distal anastomosis to reduce SCI time (**Figure 42.3**).

Separation from CPB is performed after routine de-airing maneuvers and the chest tubes are placed. The thoracotomy and groin wounds are closed.

Important additional intraoperative considerations should be mentioned. The vagus and left recurrent laryngeal nerves can be damaged because of entrapment or adherence of these nerves to the aneurysm (**Figure 42.4**), making dissecting and preserving these structures difficult.

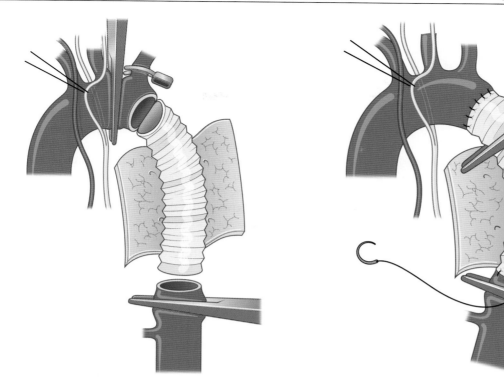

Figure 42.1 Construction of the proximal anastomosis.

Figure 42.2 Construction of the distal anastomosis.

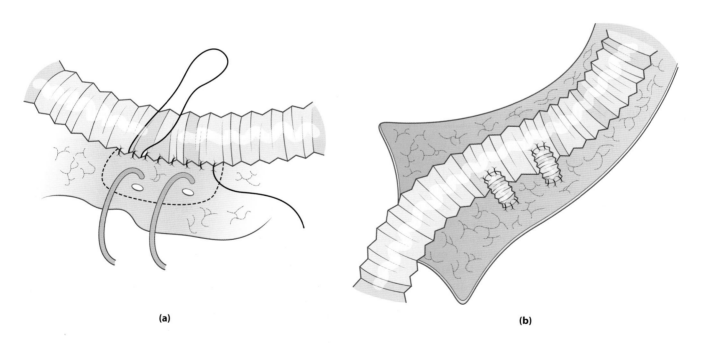

(a)

(b)

Figure 42.3 Intercostal artery patch reimplantation techniques. (**a**) Direct intercostal island implantation. (**b**) Implantation using interposition grafts.

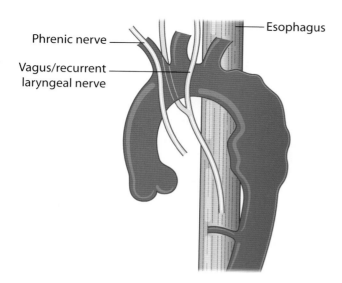

Figure 42.4 Anatomic position of the phrenic, vagus, and left recurrent laryngeal nerves.

If there is moderate or severe aortic insufficiency, prophylactic aortic valve repair or replacement may be needed before descending TAA repair. A left ventricular vent via the left superior pulmonary vein can be used for descending TAA repair with DHCA. When the right pleural space is entered during mobilization of the aorta, a chest tube should be inserted in the postoperative setting. Finally, to prevent chyle leak, it can be useful to ligate the thoracic duct at several locations in the distal thorax.

MAJOR COMPLICATIONS

Major complications can be prevented with adequate postoperative management. Respiratory failure after open repair is most commonly observed. Predictors of this complication include active smoking, COPD (even more in patients with significant reduction of forced expiratory volume in 1 second) and cardiac, renal, or bleeding complications. Pulmonary hygiene is paramount throughout postoperative care. Smoking cessation is essential in all patients; additional bronchodilator therapy for COPD patients can be prescribed to increase the chances of an acceptable outcome.

Adjuncts used to reduce the risk of SCI include the liberal use of cerebrospinal fluid drainage.[8] The authors usually maintain this for 48–72 hours postoperatively. Additional methods include the use of DHCA and intercostal artery reattachment and permissive hypertension in the postoperative phase.

Finally, renal failure is also frequently seen. This can be prevented by ensuring adequate hydration and cardiac output, minimizing infectious complications, and allowing permissive hypertension.

CASE EXAMPLES

Case example 1

A 38-year-old woman, with a medical history including tobacco use (former smoker, 4 pack years), asthma, kidney stones, and several abdominal interventions including appendectomy and two caesarean sections, presented to the authors' clinic. She had presented with chest discomfort several months prior. The workup for the thoracic pain included a CT scan. This demonstrated a 5.6-cm descending TAA extending into the distal descending aorta (**Figure 42.5**). Because she continued smoking, the operation was delayed at that time. At the time of surgery, she was asymptomatic and her physical examination revealed no abnormalities. Further investigation revealed no family history for TAA, aortic dissection, Marfan syndrome, or other connective tissue disease. The patient was encouraged to discontinue tobacco altogether. Her medical therapy included labetalol hydrochloride 100 mg three times daily and naproxen sporadically. This patient met the thresholds of repair as determined by the current guidelines. Her aneurysm of the distal arch and descending thoracic aorta had a maximum diameter of 5.8 cm. Anatomically, an endovascular intervention would have been feasible. However, for this case, an open procedure was chosen because of the young age of the patient, possible difficulty with the proximal landing zone, and the unknown long-term durability of endovascular stent grafts.

Preoperative workup included cardiac catheterization, TEE, carotid duplex scanning, pulmonary function, and ankle–brachial pressure indexes. All testing was unremarkable. She was therefore deemed fit for OSR.

The patient consented to an open procedure and subsequently underwent a successful proximal descending

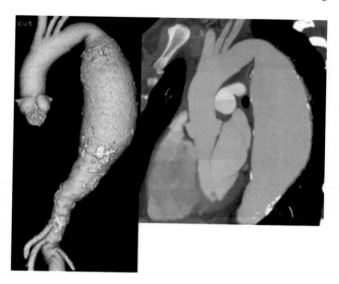

Figure 42.5 Thoracic aortic aneurysm with maximum diameter at the mid-descending thoracic aorta in a 38-year-old woman.

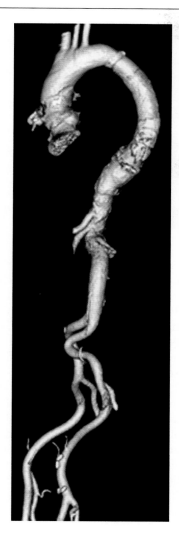

Figure 42.6 Reconstruction of the total aorta after open surgical repair with normal aortic diameters in a 38-year-old woman.

aortic aneurysm resection and repair with a 20-mm HEMASHIELD PLATINUM Woven Double Velour Vascular Graft (MAQUET Ltd., Sunderland, UK). For this procedure, the incision was made at the fourth and eighth ICS; partial CPB was used. Intraoperative findings were remarkable for a smooth intima at the proximal

anastomosis, and remarkable atherosclerotic changes at the distal anastomotic site.

She was discharged in satisfactory condition on postoperative day 6, without complications. At her 9-year follow-up visit, the repair was intact and without remarkable postoperative changes (**Figure 42.6**). She continues to be followed with CT scans to monitor the status of the aortic repair.

Case example 2

A 51-year-old man presented with a prior history of an acute type B aortic dissection complicated by visceral ischemia for which a bowel resection and an iliac-superior mesenteric artery bypass was performed. The aorta was not intervened on. During follow-up, the aortic diameter increased to thresholds of intervention for replacement of the patient's distal arch and descending thoracic aorta. The patient was asymptomatic at the time of surgery. He had an extensive medical history, including hypertension, dyslipidemia, and type B dissection. Furthermore, he had a history of substance abuse including alcohol, cocaine, and tobacco (former smoker).

Further investigation revealed no family history for TAA, aortic dissection, Marfan syndrome, or other connective tissue disease. The patient was encouraged to remain substance-free to reduce the risk of aortic complications. This patient met the thresholds of surgical repair because the diameter of the descending thoracic aorta had a maximum of 5.6 cm (**Figure 42.7**).

His medical therapy included multiple antihypertensives. Physical examination revealed no abnormalities. His preoperative workup included cardiac catheterization, which suggested normal pulmonary artery pressures, preserved cardiac output, and mild nonobstructive coronary artery disease. His ankle–brachial pressure indexes, carotid duplex scanning, and pulmonary function tests were excellent. His TEE showed normal left ventricular function, a three-cusp aortic valve with no stenosis or insufficiency, and a small persistent foramen ovale with left-to-right shunt.

The risks and benefits of remaining on medical therapy and OSR were discussed with the patient, and he consented

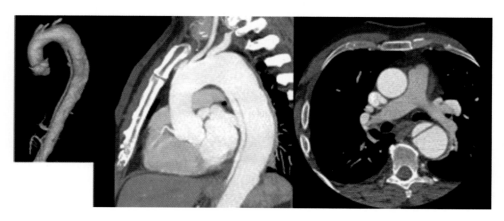

Figure 42.7 Preoperative imaging of descending thoracic aortic aneurysm measuring 5.6 cm in diameter in a 51-year-old man.

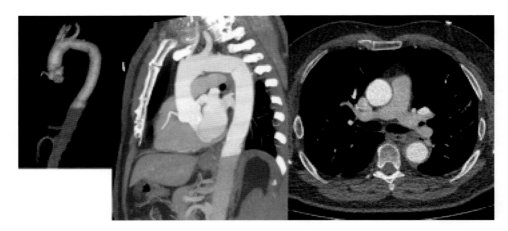

Figure 42.8 Postoperative results of open surgical repair of chronic aortic dissection in a 51-year-old man.

to undergo the open procedure to reduce his risk of aortic rupture.

He underwent a successful proximal descending aortic aneurysm resection and repair with a 28-mm Vascutek® vascular graft (Terumo Medical Corporation, Somerset, NJ, USA). For this procedure, the incision was made at the fourth and seventh ICS; CPB with DHCA was used.

His postoperative course was without complications and he was discharged in satisfactory condition on postoperative day 8. At the 3-year follow-up imaging, satisfactory repair of the chronic type B dissection could be seen (**Figure 42.8**).

REFERENCES

1. Hiratzka LF, Bakris GL, Beckman JA, et al. 2010 ACCF/AHA/AATS/ACR/ASA/SCA/SCAI/SIR/STS/ SVM guidelines for the diagnosis and management of patients with Thoracic Aortic Disease: a report of the American College of Cardiology Foundation/ American Heart Association Task Force on Practice Guidelines, American Association for Thoracic Surgery, American College of Radiology, American Stroke Association, Society of Cardiovascular Anesthesiologists, Society for Cardiovascular Angiography and Interventions, Society of Interventional Radiology, Society of Thoracic Surgeons, and Society for Vascular Medicine. *Circulation.* 2010;**121**:e266–369.

2. Chaer RA, Vasoncelos R, Marone LK, et al. Synchronous and metachronous thoracic aneurysms in patients with abdominal aortic aneurysms. *J Vasc Surg.* 2012;**56**:1261–1265.

3. Hultgren R, Larsson E, Wahlgren CM, et al. Female and elderly abdominal aortic aneurysm patients more commonly have concurrent thoracic aortic aneurysm. *Ann Vasc Surg.* 2012;**26**:918–923.

4. Erbel R, Aboyans V, Boileau C, et al. 2014 ESC Guidelines on the diagnosis and treatment of aortic diseases: document covering acute and chronic aortic diseases of the thoracic and abdominal aorta of the adult. The Task Force for the Diagnosis and Treatment of Aortic Diseases of the European Society of Cardiology (ESC). *Eur Heart J.* 2014;**35**:2873–2926.

5. Patel HJ, Williams DM, Drews JD, et al. A 20-year experience with thoracic endovascular aortic repair. *Ann Surg.* 2014;**260**:691–696.

6. Patel HJ, Williams DM, Upchurch GR Jr., et al. Long-term results from a 12-year experience with endovascular therapy for thoracic aortic disease. *Ann Thorac Surg.* 2006;**82**:2147–2153.

7. Patel HJ, Shillingford MS, Mihalik S, et al. Resection of the descending thoracic aorta: outcomes after use of hypothermic circulatory arrest. *Ann Thorac Surg.* 2006;**82**:90–95.

8. Cheung AT, Pochettino A, McGarvey ML, et al. Strategies to manage paraplegia risk after endovascular stent repair of descending thoracic aortic aneurysms. *Ann Thorac Surg.* 2005;**80**:1280–1288.

43

Common femoral and iliac artery endarterectomy

DIPANKAR MUKHERJEE, HOMAYOUN HASHEMI, ELIAS KFOURY, AND RASHAD MAJEED

CONTENTS

INTRODUCTION

Despite advances in endovascular technique, common femoral artery (CFA) endarterectomy remains an essential part of the armamentarium of the vascular surgeon because it is still the procedure of choice when indicated for CFA atherosclerotic disease.

Mukherjee and Inahara reported a 5-year patency of 94%,[1] whereas Ballotta and collaborators reported an 8-year primary patency of 96% and assisted patency of 100%.[2] In a more recent publication, Kang and collaborators, reporting their experience from the Massachusetts General Hospital (Boston, MA, USA), found that following CFA endarterectomy, there was 87% freedom from reintervention at 5 years.[3] In their opinion, all emerging endovascular options should be held to these standards to be considered acceptable.

CFA endarterectomy is a versatile operation. It can be performed as an isolated or adjunct procedure. It can be used to optimize inflow or outflow to the arterial system of the extremity, or as an isolated treatment for regional disease. A hybrid procedure involving endovascular stenting of the iliac artery with concomitant CFA endarterectomy is also a durable option. Sharafuddin and collaborators showed 75% ± 17% primary patency, or 92% ± 12% assisted patency at 40 months for the hybrid approach.[4] Piazza and collaborators from the Mayo Clinic recommend CFA endarterectomy over aortofemoral bypass irrespective of the TransAtlantic Inter-Society Consensus (TASC) classification for iliofemoral occlusive disease, with significant improvement in morbidity and length of stay.[5]

Balloon angioplasty of the CFA has not been associated with durable long-term benefits. Stenting of this vessel has not shown results comparable to endarterectomy with patch angioplasty, particularly in critical limb ischemia. Results of endovascular treatment for CFA occlusive disease as reported by interventional radiologists, cardiologists, and vascular surgeons have not matched the results of surgical intervention in the long term.[6-8] The risk of stent fracture and inaccessibility of the artery for future interventions is also a concern. In addition, the increased complexity of surgical intervention following stent thrombosis makes the endovascular option less appealing.

Iliac artery endarterectomy is performed less commonly because of the favorable outcomes of endovascular procedures, which are also relatively less invasive. However, in select cases iliac artery endarterectomy is advantageous, and can be an important adjunct procedure. One example is localized iliac artery endarterectomy for the donor iliac artery of an iliofemoral bypass.

CFA ENDARTERECTOMY

For vascular surgery purposes, the groin can be thought of as the femoral triangle. Familiarity with femoral triangle anatomy is of utmost importance for the vascular surgeon. The femoral triangle is delineated laterally by the sartorius muscle, which originates from the anterior superior iliac spine (ASIS), runs anteromedially, and inserts into the proximal medial aspect of the tibia. The proximal aspect of the sartorius muscle delineates the lateral border of the femoral triangle. The inguinal ligament forms the superior border of the femoral triangle. The inguinal ligament runs from the ASIS and inserts into the pubic tubercle. The medial border of the femoral triangle is formed by the adductor longus muscle, which originates from the superior ramus of the pubis, and inserts into the femur as it runs laterally.

Groin exposure for CFA endarterectomy starts with positioning the patient supine on the operating room table. The procedure can be done under general or epidural anesthesia, or local anesthesia with sedation.

A transverse or longitudinal incision can be used (**Figure 43.1**) to obtain exposure of the CFA, profunda femoris artery (PFA), and superficial femoral artery (SFA) at the level of the femoral triangle. The advantage of a longitudinal incision is potentially better exposure and the possibility of proximal or distal extension as needed. A transverse incision can be more cosmetically appealing, and it has been reported that it may have lower postoperative wound complications when compared to a longitudinal incision.[9] While a transverse incision may be positioned at the groin crease, often the groin crease

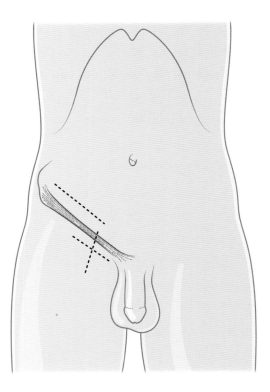

Figure 43.1 Incisions for exposure of the common femoral artery. The transverse incision should be placed just distal to the medial aspect of where the inguinal ligament is thought to be, using the anterior superior iliac spine and the pubic tubercle as landmarks for the course of the inguinal ligament. The longitudinal incision is at the midpoint of the inguinal ligament, extending from the ligament as far distally as is necessary. For external iliac artery exposure, an oblique incision below the umbilicus, lateral to the rectus muscle and directed toward the flank should be used.

might not provide adequate exposure to the proximal CFA. Therefore, a transverse incision should be placed just distal to the medial aspect of where the inguinal ligament is thought to be, using the ASIS and the pubic tubercle as landmarks for the course of the inguinal ligament. A longitudinal incision is made at the midpoint of the inguinal ligament, extending from the ligament as far distally as is necessary. Both incisions should be centered over the pulse of the femoral artery. In cases where no pulse is palpated, the surface landmarks described earlier should provide an adequate guide. Usually, a 5–10-cm-long incision is sufficient, depending on the extent of dissection and body habitus of the patient. In the authors' more recent experience, use of bedside ultrasound to locate the bifurcation of the CFA has added value when planning the incision.

After skin incision, the dissection is carried down through the subcutaneous tissues with electrocautery. The authors' preference is to tie off the lymphatic channels encountered during the exposure with suture material, because electrocautery might not be effective in sealing lymphatics and preventing lymphatic leaks postoperatively. When the femoral sheath is encountered, the authors mainly use sharp dissection with Metzenbaum scissors. The dissection is kept close to the artery to avoid injuring the adjacent structures. The CFA is dissected proximally until a healthy segment of the artery is encountered where a vascular clamp can be placed safely. Most often, the dissection is carried proximal to the inferior epigastric artery (IEA) takeoff and an angled vascular clamp is used to occlude the artery. (The authors prefer a padded vascular clamp in the case of heavily calcified vessels.) The IEA can be controlled with a small vessel loop or a 2-0 silk tie. The dissection is then carried distally to the SFA and PFA takeoff. When dissection into the distal PFA is needed, care should be taken to ligate the overlying veins. If proximal PFA control is needed, a profunda clamp or vessel loop can be used. Vessel loops may be less traumatic than vascular clamps for control. On occasion, native vessels are severely diseased and application of a clamp may be hazardous. In this situation, intravascular control of the artery with the use of balloon occlusion proximally, distally, or both, may be of value. An intravenous heparin bolus is given (80–100 IU/kg), and then dosed as needed to maintain an activated clotting time >250 seconds.

Once proximal and distal control are obtained, a No. 11 scalpel, with the blade directed upward, is used to make an arteriotomy over the anterior aspect of the CFA (**Figure 43.2a**). Care is taken not to inadvertently injure the posterior wall of the artery. The arteriotomy is then extended using Potts scissors proximally and distally until a relatively disease-free segment of the vessel is seen. The arteriotomy can be extended as necessary into the proximal, mid, or even distal PFA depending on disease burden. A FREER-Type (Modified) Elevator (Becton, Dickinson and Company, Franklin Lakes, NJ, USA) is used to develop a plane between the plaque and the media. Removal of the media may be necessary to provide a smooth flow surface after completion of the endarterectomy (**Figure 43.2b**).

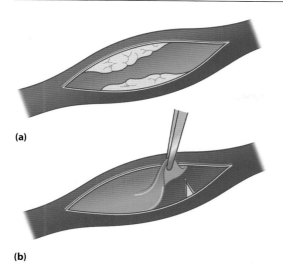

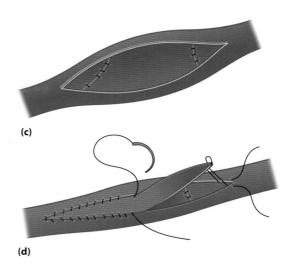

Figure 43.2 Segmental endarterectomy. (**a**) Arteriotomy is extended beyond the plaque proximally and distally to areas of minimal disease where the endarterectomy can be terminated. (**b**) The adherent circular layer of the media is carefully stripped away, leaving a smooth adventitial surface. (**c**) Endarterectomy is terminated by transverse or oblique beveling of the intima. Longitudinal 6-0 sutures are placed at the proximal and distal edges to prevent flap elevation and reduce its profile to blood flow. (**d**) Autogenous vein or prosthetic patch graft is extended proximally and distally 1–2 cm past the termination of the endarterectomy.

Care must be taken at the proximal and distal end of the plaque to ensure smooth transition and avoid a significant intimal flap, especially at the distal extent of the endarterectomy. A residual intimal flap can result in antegrade dissection and possible arterial occlusion. Fine polypropylene or polydioxanone (PDS) tacking suture can be used, if needed, to tack the plaque distally (**Figure 43.2c**). In some instances, distal external iliac artery (EIA) endarterectomy is performed through the same groin incision by carrying out an eversion endarterectomy of the distal aspect of the EIA. Partial division of the inguinal ligament can be done to assist the exposure. After the endarterectomy has been performed, and the proximal and distal end points are satisfactory, the arteriotomy is closed with autogenous vein, bovine pericardium, polytetrafluoroethylene (PTFE), or Dacron patch with a fine polypropylene running suture (**Figure 43.2d**). The vessel should be flushed before restoring flow. Flow should be restored to the PFA before the SFA to avoid direct distal embolization. After hemostasis is satisfactory, the wound is closed in multiple layers to obliterate potential dead space that may accumulate into a lymphocele or a hematoma.

ILIAC ARTERY ENDARTERECTOMY

In contemporary vascular surgery, iliac artery endarterectomy has become an uncommonly performed procedure with the advent of endovascular interventions for focal iliac artery stenoses or occlusion (TASC type A and B lesions). The iliac artery can be exposed either transperitoneally or retroperitoneally. The authors' preference is a retroperitoneal approach. A retroperitoneal approach involves an oblique incision extending

approximately 10 cm in length and located anywhere from just below the umbilicus to 2 cm cephalad to the inguinal ligament, depending on the level of occlusion in the iliac system. For exposure of the common iliac artery, the incision should be at the level of the umbilicus. For external iliac artery exposure, the incision can be placed more caudad (**Figure 43.1**). The external oblique muscle is encountered and is divided in the direction of its fibers. The internal oblique and transversalis muscles are then opened, with care taken not to inadvertently enter the peritoneum. Should inadvertent peritoneal entry occur, the peritoneal opening can be closed with an absorbable suture. While closing the peritoneal tear, care should be taken to approximate gently, because excess tension can create additional peritoneal tears. After the transversalis muscle is opened and the preperitoneal space is entered, the peritoneum is swept bluntly lateral to medial. Special attention should be given to the spermatic cord in men at the inferomedial aspect of the exposure. In women, the round ligament can be divided if necessary. The IEA may also be encountered inferomedially. This should be protected, but can also be divided if necessary.

At this stage, the authors place a self-retaining retractor in the incision to facilitate exposure. The ureter should be identified. After exposure, the iliac artery is dissected sharply using Metzenbaum scissors. The CIA and EIA can both be exposed in their entirety through this incision. Note that the iliac veins may be adherent to the adjacent artery secondary to the chronic inflammatory response from atherosclerosis. Proximally, care should be taken to minimize unnecessary dissection, which can cause autonomic sexual dysfunction in male patients if pelvic splanchnic nerves are transected. The EIA can be controlled with either atraumatic vascular clamps or vessel loops. The CIA needs to be controlled with atraumatic vascular clamps. A longitudinal arteriotomy is made over the anterior wall of the artery. The arteriotomy is then extended proximally and distally with Potts scissors until the nondiseased portion of the artery is encountered. A FREER-Type (Modified) Elevator (Becton, Dickinson and Company) is used to dissect away the atherosclerotic plaque from the remainder of the media and adventitia, being careful to remain in the correct endarterectomy plane to avoid inadvertent thinning of the blood vessel. The endarterectomy plaque is then feathered out gently proximally and distally. The distal end point should be carefully assessed for an intimal flap, and if need be, a fine polypropylene or PDS tacking suture can be used. As explained earlier, a patch angioplasty can be performed if the disease is isolated to the iliac artery and there is no plan for a bypass as part of the procedure.

COMPLICATIONS

Complications of CFA endarterectomy reported in the literature range from 0% in small series to up to 17%.[10-12] Commonly reported short-term complications include infection, hematoma, and nerve damage. Long-term complications include aneurysmal dilation of the repair, and failure or occlusion of the endarterectomy. In one series by Mukherjee and Inahara, the only complication reported was aneurysmal dilation in 1 out of 29 patients who underwent the procedure.[1] In a recent study that used the National Surgical Quality Improvement Program®, 1843 CFA endarterectomies were identified between 2005 and 2010. The procedure had 3.4% mortality with approximately 8% wound complication, which was accounted for by superficial (5.9%) and deep infection (2%), along with 0.8% wound dehiscence.[12] Other complications include systemic complications, which are relatively infrequent. These include myocardial infarction (0.6%), pneumonia (1.6%), cardiac arrest (0.9%), and urinary tract infection (1.6%). Risk factors for higher complications with surgical intervention are morbid obesity, steroid dependence, and end-of-life disease. In these situations, endovascular intervention for short-term benefit would be a reasonable option.

At the authors' institution, early ambulation of patients and deep venous thrombosis prophylaxis are recommended. Foley catheter placement preoperatively is not necessary. Most of the authors' patients are discharged on the first postoperative day.

Complications of iliac endarterectomy or iliofemoral bypass are like those for CFA endarterectomy. Infection risk may be less. In one series, it was as low as 1%.[13] This is in stark contrast to femorofemoral bypass, which can have a higher rate of wound infection, given the need for bilateral groin exposure. This has been reported to be 6–8%.[14] Sexual dysfunction is less common than in aortobifemoral bypass, and has been reported to be as low as 0%. Long-term patency of iliofemoral bypass is excellent.

Primary patency of 76% at 5 years, and secondary patency of up to 100% have been reported.[3]

APPLICATIONS OF COMMON FEMORAL ENDARTERECTOMY

The most common application of CFA endarterectomy is in a patient with isolated CFA disease presenting with claudication (**Figure 43.3**).

With increasing severity of occlusive disease, CFA endarterectomy can be used adjunctively with other revascularization procedures, as shown in this example. **Figure 43.4** shows a patient with right lower extremity critical limb ischemia who underwent CFA, PFA, and SFA endarterectomy, with aortobifemoral bypass. **Figure 43.5** shows a patient with bilateral critical limb ischemia, requiring left-sided CFA and PFA endarterectomy to optimize inflow for a femoropopliteal bypass (**Figure 43.5b,c**). Revascularization for the right lower extremity was obtained by means of a left-right femorofemoral bypass along with a right CFA endarterectomy (**Figure 43.5a**).

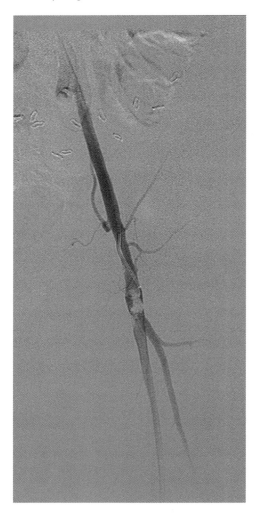

Figure 43.3 Patient presenting with disabling claudication, with disease isolated to the common femoral artery.

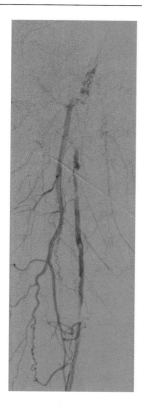

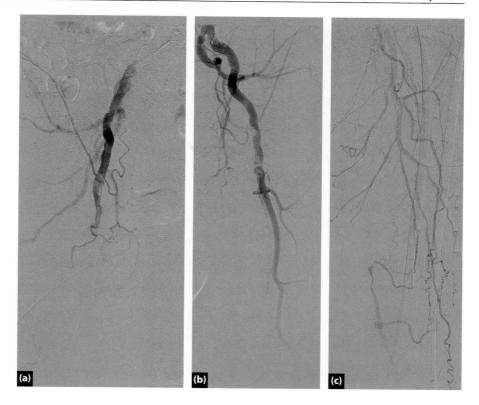

Figure 43.4 Common femoral, profunda femoris, and proximal superficial femoral artery endarterectomy with patch angioplasty combined with an aortobifemoral bypass in a patient with critical limb ischemia.

Figure 43.5 Patient with bilateral critical limb ischemia. This patient required left common femoral artery (CFA) endarterectomy and femoropopliteal bypass for left-sided critical limb ischemia, and right CFA endarterectomy with left-right femorofemoral bypass for right-sided critical limb ischemia. (**a**) Right common iliac artery (CIA) angiogram with severely limited flow to the CFA. (**b**) Left CIA angiogram with multiple lesions limiting flow to the CFA. (**c**) Left femoral angiogram showing severely limited inflow and extensive collateralization.

APPLICATIONS OF ILIAC ENDARTERECTOMY

Iliac artery endarterectomy is currently mainly used as an adjunct to iliofemoral bypass where there is complete occlusion of either the CIA, EIA, or both. The surgical options are: (1) aortounifemoral bypass; (2) femorofemoral bypass; or (3) iliofemoral bypass using iliac endarterectomy. Each procedure has its own advantages and disadvantages. Aortounifemoral bypass uses the aorta as the source of inflow and has the best patency rate.[15] However, this procedure is rather extensive and often requires a long hospital stay with significant morbidity. Femorofemoral bypass is an extra-anatomic bypass that can be performed under local anesthesia with less morbidity. However, the patency of this bypass is significantly inferior to in-line bypass.[16,17] Femorofemoral bypass grafting involves the contralateral femoral artery; in cases of infection, the contralateral limb can be put at risk.

When iliofemoral bypass is performed, the inflow can be the endarterectomized CIA or EIA.

In the case of a completely occluded CIA and patent EIA (**Figure 43.6a**), the CIA is transected approximately

3–4 cm from its origin and an eversion endarterectomy is performed in standard fashion. Following completion of the endarterectomy, proximal control can be obtained by applying a vascular clamp to the CIA or inserting a Fogarty balloon into the aorta. The conduit used is usually an 8-mm Dacron or PTFE graft, which is anastomosed in an end-to-end fashion. The distal anastomosis can be performed end-to-side to the disease-free segment of the EIA. If both CIA and EIA are occluded (**Figure 43.6b**), then CIA endarterectomy is performed, with distal anastomosis to the CFA, by passing the graft under the inguinal ligament. If the CFA requires endarterectomy, it can be performed as explained earlier. An example of a lesion for which this repair was performed is shown in **Figure 43.7**.

If the entire length of the EIA is occluded (**Figure 43.6c**), it can be transected 3–4 cm from its origin, eversion endarterectomy is performed, and an end-to-end anastomosis to the endarterectomized EIA is carried out. The graft is then tunneled under the inguinal ligament and anastomosed end-to-side to the CFA. Another alternative is to perform the proximal anastomosis to the distal CIA in an end-to-side fashion (**Figure 43.8**).

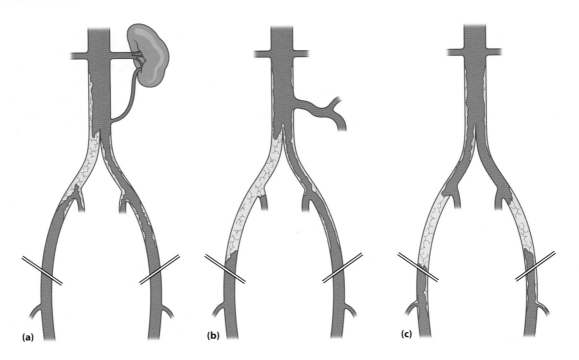

Figure 43.6 Common patterns of common iliac artery (CIA) and external iliac artery (EIA) occlusion. (**a**) Occluded common iliac artery (CIA) with patent external iliac artery (EIA). (**b**) Occluded CIA and EIA. (**c**) Occluded EIA.

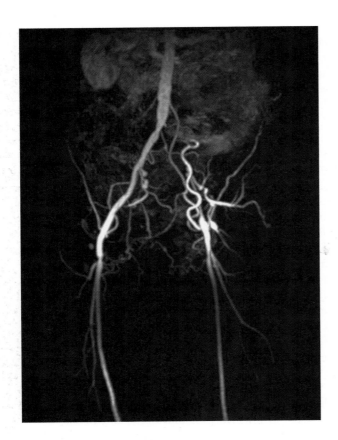

Figure 43.7 Common iliac artery (CIA)/external iliac artery (EIA) occlusion requiring CIA endarterectomy with CIA-CFA bypass.

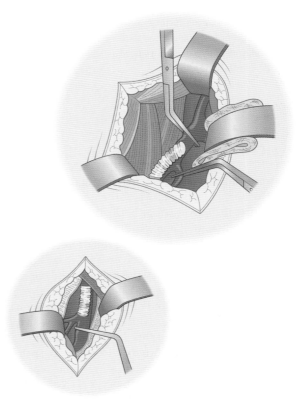

Figure 43.8 With the entire external iliac artery occluded, one option is end-to-side anastomosis to the distal common iliac artery and distal anastomosis to the common femoral artery.

If only the EIA is occluded, the saphenous vein can be used as a conduit, especially if there is concern for possible infection. However, use of the saphenous vein in this location may result in size mismatch. In this location, there is also tendency for vein kinking and compression compared to a prosthetic graft. Using this retroperitoneal approach, the donor vessel is usually the ipsilateral CIA. In rare situations, the donor vessel can be the contralateral iliac artery with the bypass graft tunneled through the retropubic space superior to the bladder. Careful hemostasis and layered wound closure are once again of paramount importance.

REFERENCES

1. Mukherjee D, Inahara T. Endarterectomy as the procedure of choice for atherosclerotic occlusive lesions of the common femoral artery. *Am J Surg.* 1989;157:498–500.
2. Ballotta E, Gruppo M, Mazzalai F, et al. Common femoral artery endarterectomy for occlusive disease: an 8-year single-center prospective study. *Surgery.* 2010;147:268–274.
3. Kang JL, Patel VI, Conrad MF, et al. Common femoral artery occlusive disease: contemporary results following surgical endarterectomy. *J Vasc Surg.* 2008;48:872–877.
4. Sharafuddin MJ, Kresowik TF, Hoballah JJ, et al. Combined direct repair and inline inflow stenting in the management of aortoiliac disease extending into the common femoral artery. *Vasc Endovascular Surg.* 2011;45:274–282.
5. Piazza M, Ricotta JJ 2nd, Bower TC, et al. Iliac artery stenting combined with open femoral endarterectomy is as effective as open surgical reconstruction for severe iliac and common femoral occlusive disease. *J Vasc Surg.* 2011;54:402–411.
6. Paris CL, White CJ, Collins TJ, et al. Catheter-based therapy of common femoral artery atherosclerotic disease. *Vasc Med.* 2011;16:109–112.
7. Davies RS, Adair W, Bolia A, et al. Endovascular treatment of the common femoral artery for limb ischemia. *Vasc Endovascular Surg.* 2013;47:639–644.
8. Bonvini RF, Rastan A, Sixt S, et al. Angioplasty and provisional stent treatment of common femoral artery lesions. *J Vasc Interv Radiol.* 2013;24:175–183.
9. Beirne C, Martin F, Hynes N, et al. Five years' experience of transverse groin incision for femoral artery access in arterial reconstructive surgery: parallel observational longitudinal group comparison study. *Vascular.* 2008;16:207–212.
10. Derksen WJ, Verhoeven BA, van de Mortel RH, et al. Risk factors for surgical-site infection following common femoral artery endarterectomy. *Vasc Endovascular Surg.* 2009;43:69–75.
11. Nguyen BN, Amdur RL, Abugideiri M, et al. Postoperative complications after common femoral endarterectomy. *J Vasc Surg.* 2015;61:1489–1494.e1.
12. Siracuse JJ, Gill HL, Schneider DB, et al. Assessing the perioperative safety of common femoral endarterectomy in the endovascular era. *Vasc Endovascular Surg.* 2014;48:27–33.
13. Harrington ME, Harrington EB, Haimov M, et al. Iliofemoral versus femorofemoral bypass: the case for an individualized approach. *J Vasc Surg.* 1992;16:841–852.
14. Goldstone J, Moore WS. Infection in vascular prostheses. Clinical manifestations and surgical management. *Am J Surg.* 1974;128:225–233.
15. de Vries SO, Hunink MG. Results of aortic bifurcation grafts for aortoiliac occlusive disease: a meta-analysis. *J Vasc Surg.* 1997;26:558–569.
16. Schneider JR, Besso SR, Walsh DB, et al. Femorofemoral versus aortobifemoral bypass: outcome and hemodynamic results. *J Vasc Surg.* 1994;19:43–55.
17. Criado E, Burnham SJ, Tinsley EA Jr., et al. Femorofemoral bypass graft: analysis of patency and factors influencing long-term outcome. *J Vasc Surg.* 1993;18:495–504.

44

Aortobifemoral bypass graft

MACIEJ UZIEBLO

CONTENTS

INTRODUCTION

The development of minimally invasive endovascular techniques has revolutionized the surgical approach to arterial occlusive disease, so much so that extensive endovascular reconstructions are being taken out of the hospital setting into the outpatient environment. In this setting, "endovascular first" has become the mantra in modern vascular surgery, and open reconstructions have taken on the stigma of a plan B or failure.

In many cases, suprainguinal arterial reconstructions lend themselves well to durable endovascular interventions. Excellent patency of stents used to treat iliac artery occlusive disease has been achieved. Hybrid techniques, including common femoral artery (CFA) endarterectomy and the use of aortoiliac endografts, have been used successfully to treat complex aortoiliac occlusive disease, thus reducing the situations in which aortobifemoral bypass is used as the first-line operative treatment. Thus, the days of an "easy" aortobifemoral bypass are in the past. There are clear situations, however, where an endovascular method will not bring satisfactory results. In the author's view, they include: extensive CFA occlusion; small-caliber iliac vessels with heavy calcifications; associated renovascular disease; and juxtarenal aortic occlusion. (**Figures 44.1** and **44.2** exemplify these complex scenarios.)

For clinical situations where either approach may be applicable, such as distal aortic and iliac disease, the age of the patient and their medical fitness for surgery may settle

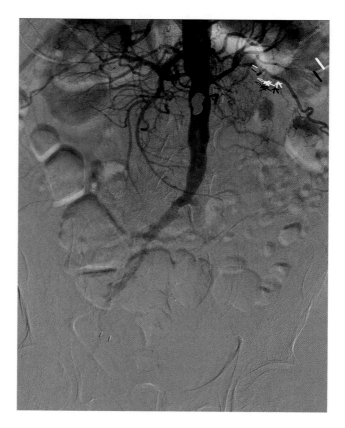

Figure 44.1 Aortic disease suited to open intervention.

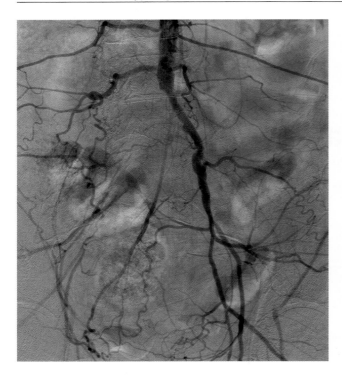

Figure 44.2 Aortic occlusion with collaterals not amenable to endovascular intervention.

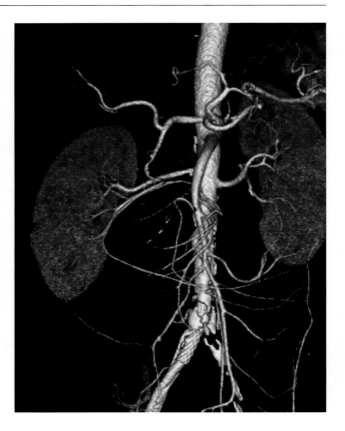

Figure 44.3 Aortic disease amenable to open or endovascular reconstruction.

the choice (**Figure 44.3**). Younger patients are more likely to experience restenosis of any reconstruction. An endovascular option first, including endograft relining of the aorta and iliac arteries, does not negate a future open approach, which may be preferable to redo aortic surgery or groin redissection.

PREOPERATIVE EVALUATION

Preoperative evaluation is crucial and should include high-quality computed tomography (CT) angiography to define the anatomy of the aorta, and iliac and femoral artery segments. Attention should focus on vessel size and location, the extent of areas of stenosis and occlusion, the degree of vessel wall calcification, the presence of renal or mesenteric artery occlusive disease, and any associated aneurysmal disease or vascular anomaly, such as a retroaortic left renal vein or caval duplication. Any other intra-abdominal pathology should be sought. Three-dimensional and maximum intensity projections are part of most CT machines. They guide proximal clamp placement with respect to the calcium load present in the vessels that could cause dissection during clamping or embolization and distal reconstruction. Occasionally, severe calcification and severe iliac disease limit the accuracy of CT evaluation regarding the flow lumen patency of the vessel because of the differential rate of phase-contrast flow in the iliac arteries. Also, severe proximal occlusive disease may render CT evaluation of distal extremity runoff as nondiagnostic. In this case, transbrachial angiography is helpful. The author

uses the left brachial approach to minimize the risk of traversing the cervical vessels and stroke. The brachial artery is superficial just above the elbow crease and can be easily controlled or repaired at that level. The author uses the 5-Fr Glidesheath Slender® transradial introducer sheath (Terumo Medical Corporation, Somerset, NJ, USA) because of its small outside diameter and lesser risk of complications with the brachial artery. The sheath allows using any 5-Fr catheter, but the author's standard way is to place a long pigtail catheter over a soft guidewire and direct the wire into the descending aorta after partially unfolding the pigtail over the ostium of the left subclavian artery. Standard anterior–posterior (AP) and lateral views are obtained to evaluate mesenteric patency, the amount of calcium, and any collateral mesenteric flow. Iliac imaging is improved with contralateral 20–30-degree obliquity with femoral evaluation at 20-degree ipsilateral obliquity. Lower extremity runoff is performed with digital subtraction arteriography acquisition, with selective iliac cannulation for dedicated views of the legs. This allows precise anatomic evaluation, and repeated magnified and oblique views of any regions of interest, while minimizing contrast. For patients with renal insufficiency, dilute 50:50 contrast is used in preference to CO_2, which limits the evaluation of areas with heavy calcification. A 15-minute pressure hold over the brachial artery is sufficient for hemostasis with the arm fixed on an armboard for 4 hours after. The patient is allowed normal arm use in 24 hours.

PATIENT PREPARATION

For open reconstructions, the author places the patient supine. Warming devices are placed under the patient; they are not used on the legs because of concern for warm ischemia during clamping. An arterial line is placed for hemodynamic monitoring and activated clotting time samples; a urinary catheter and naso/orogastric drainage tubes are implemented. Surgery is performed in three stages: distal dissection; proximal dissection; and arterial reconstruction. Dissection is started in the groin to avoid prolonged open abdomen time. Many aortic reconstructions are done in patients with a history of prior interventions and complex femoral anatomy, and the additional work of outflow preparation may be well anticipated. Starting with abdominal exposure should be considered only if suspected abdominal disease, for example, cirrhosis or a tumor were to be assessed before proceeding and were not satisfactorily explained by preoperative CT.

DISTAL DISSECTION

Incision is made one-third of the way toward the pubis; one-third of the incision is placed above the inguinal ligament. Vertical incisions work best because often there is more extensive reconstruction to be done and hence the need for extensive CFA and possibly profunda femoris artery (PFA) exposure. The inguinal ligament is dissected first by deepening the incision. Electrocautery is used preferentially for precise, bloodless dissection. Ultrasonic dissectors may offer an advantage in lymphatic leak, but do not afford the precision of cautery as a dissecting tool. Digital retraction is used in the initial dissection to allow easy tissue manipulation because retractors distort the tissue. Ultimately, retractors are placed once the anterior femoral sheath is encountered. Because often there is no pulse in the artery, it may be located as it exits from under the ligament medial to the sartorius muscle. Effort should be made to avoid excessive false tunneling in search of the artery, which brings the risk of a postoperative lymphocele. The author does not believe that approaching the artery laterally mitigates the lymphatic leak risk, and makes it harder to perform the anastomosis. Dissection should include the PFA and the superficial femoral artery (SFA) with preservation of any large preformed collaterals. The PFA is often the distal outflow target; thus, it should be dissected to its branching point. Sufficient PFA length is obtained after division of the crossing vein. If preoperative CT, angiogram, and clinical intraoperative assessment show the CFA and its branches to be widely patent, it should be used as the distal target, although this is not a frequent scenario. Making a retrograde subinguinal passage completes the femoral dissection. The inguinal ligament is dissected, elevated with a Richardson retractor and the crossing veins are ligated, with the remainder of tunneling done on the anterior surface of the artery with one's index finger.

PROXIMAL DISSECTION

Midline laparotomy is performed from under the rib cage to above the pubis. The position of the nasogastric tube within the stomach is verified. Routine exploration is made and the small bowel is eviscerated to the right over a towel. Digital traction is applied from the right while the assistant uses a DeBakey pickup to place tension on the tissues overlying the aorta to be dissected. Cautery is encouraged to keep the field dry and control the lymphatics. Large channels are clipped or ligated. The author does not find ultrasound dissectors helpful. The aorta is exposed along its length from the left renal vein to the iliac bifurcation. Digital dissection is done anteriorly on the iliac arteries to complete the tunnels, with one index finger from above and one from the groin incision. Keeping the dissection in the plane of the artery ensures subureteral placement. After the tunnels are completed, a long aortic clamp is passed along the surgeon's finger by the assistant from below; it is guided into the abdomen and used to pass an umbilical tape to mark the tunnel. Next, lateral aortic dissection is completed to allow the tissues on the side to be retracted. At this point, the bowel is returned to the abdomen and packed under the abdominal wall with towel corners. Towel-corner packing allows "lip-like" retractor function of the towels to maximize mechanical retraction, which is placed ideally after anterior aortic dissection, lysis of the ligament of Treitz, and inguinal tunnel completion to avoid multiple retractor adjustments. The author recommends using the Codman Bookwalter Wishbook Adjustable Frame, because of the multiple degrees of freedom of its arms and tiltable blades.

Additional dissection is made now, including assessment for clamp placement based on the level of aortic occlusion and calcium at the proposed clamp site. Aortic occlusion to the level of the renal arteries and calcification mandate suprarenal dissection and renal artery dissection, to allow vessel loop placement for renal occlusion and protect from emboli during clamping. The left renal vein should be ligated in this situation, which is easier than its mobilization and affords a better view with less risk of injury. Tying the vein with a 2-0 silk suture over a right angle works well. The author does not reconstruct the vein after ligation. In rare events of extensive calcification, a supraceliac clamp may be needed, but this eventuality should be anticipated from reviewing the preoperative imaging. During preparation of the proximal clamp site with lateral aortic retraction, to diminish bleeding from the aorta, small lumbar vessels can be clipped. It is generally easier to do this in the case of occlusive disease rather than with a relatively less mobile aneurysm.

RECONSTRUCTION

Heparin is given per kg of weight. The graft is selected and cut to size. The author prefers GORE-TEX® vascular grafts (W. L. Gore & Associates, Flagstaff, AZ, USA) for occlusive disease, sized 16 × 8 mm for men and 14 × 7 mm for women. The proximal end of the graft should be folded on itself over 5 mm to make a double wall collar, which diminishes needle hole bleeding when using a polypropylene suture. The author uses a long SH 36-inch polypropylene suture for a sturdy needle to handle any calcified tissue, especially when sewing the posterior wall. A long polypropylene suture is also easy to follow.

The aorta is clamped distally, first above the level of the occlusion with a long aortic clamp or it can be oversewn with a 2-0 polypropylene suture. The suture is passed around the aorta catching a small amount of adventitia posteriorly, away from the vena cava, and it is tied anteriorly. Alternately, if a clamp is used distally and the aorta is opened, its distal end can be closed with a heavy polypropylene suture over the clamp, which is then removed to free up space in the operative field. A totally occluded aorta does not need distal clamping. A portion of it may be resected and oversewn to make room for the graft.

Subsequently, proximal clamping is ideally applied in an AP direction, which allows the divided aorta to rise up to make sewing easier. In cases of a nonaneurysmal, nondegenerated aortic wall, or one that contains calcification, endarterectomy of the carotid cuff can be performed to the level of the clamp for easy handling. Glover or Satinsky clamps can be used with the posterior tine of the clamp passed behind the posterior wall protected with a red rubber catheter. For a total aortic occlusion, the author applies the proximal clamp temporarily above the renal arteries and controls those vessels with loops to prevent emboli. After endarterectomy of the aortic core, the clamp is replaced below the renal arteries in an AP position.

Proximal anastomosis is performed, posterior wall first, with the parachute technique. Flushing is done through the graft and hemostasis is checked. Heparinized saline is used to flush the graft and the aortic clamp is moved to the graft body. Next, the limbs are tunneled to the groins with the previously placed umbilical tapes to guide a large, curved aortic clamp from the bottom, which is used to grasp the graft limbs in the abdomen and bring them to the groin incisions (**Figure 44.4**).

Distal anastomoses are completed depending on disease extent in the CFA and PFA. If the PFA is well developed and there is total CFA occlusion, no proximal endarterectomy is performed (**Figure 44.5**). Small vessels or an extensively long endarterectomy call for placement of a bovine pericardium patch, then sewing the graft onto the patch, rather than using the distal anastomotic hood as the patch. Using an endarterectomized SFA as patch closure is a time-honored technique, but a bovine pericardium patch is very simple to apply, especially when dealing with a PFA endarterectomy. Occasionally, one encounters posterior CFA plaque with a spillover stenosis into the origin of the PFA. An eversion PFA endarterectomy, if the distal end of the plaque is palpable within 1 cm of the orifice, is feasible and allows the anastomosis to be placed comfortably onto the CFA. Using a GORE-TEX® CV-6 suture (W. L. Gore & Associates) with a small needle prevents bleeding from the distal reconstruction.

Closure is performed in a routine fashion with a running polydioxanone suture for the abdomen after closing the retroperitoneum. A large bovine pericardium patch can be used to cover the aortic reconstruction if the retroperitoneum is attenuated (**Figure 44.6**). The groin is closed in layers with a running suture. For heavier individuals, vacuum-assisted skin closure is employed. The author uses interrupted nylon sutures for the final skin layer.

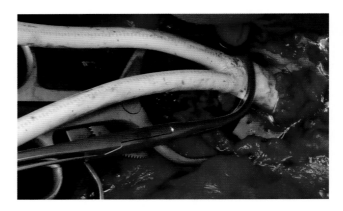

Figure 44.4 Completed proximal end-to-end anastomosis.

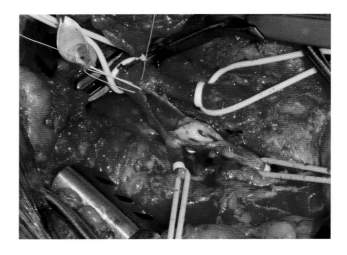

Figure 44.5 Profunda femoris artery endarterectomy with plaque tacking in preparation for direct anastomosis.

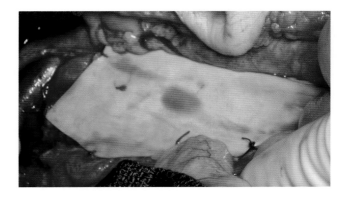

Figure 44.6 Graft coverage with bovine pericardium.

SPECIAL CONSIDERATIONS

End-to-side or end-to-end reconstruction

Sufficient soft-quality proximal aorta should exist for an end-to-side configuration (**Figure 44.7**) to be viable, which is not common with today's patient selection and availability of novel endovascular techniques. End-to-end anastomosis is easier to perform and has, in the author's opinion, better lay and flow characteristics. It is also easier to cover on completion. A large renal artery with a distal takeoff, or a large inferior mesenteric artery may constitute an indication for end-to-side bypass in very rare patients with good proximal aortic patency. Bilateral external iliac artery occlusion as indication for an end-to-side configuration is questionable. Patients the author has encountered seem to have significant diffuse, including hypogastric, disease; thus, a well-placed distal anastomosis on a large PFA may satisfy the pelvic perfusion requirement, rather than relying on prograde flow through stenosed vessels.

Mesenteric or renal disease

Asymptomatic mesenteric, non-preocclusive stenosis should not be corrected at the time of surgery because endovascular options exist. Preocclusive stenosis must be evaluated on an individual basis. Symptomatic mesenteric disease is addressed with bypass to the superior mesenteric artery (SMA) with a 6-mm side graft presewn onto

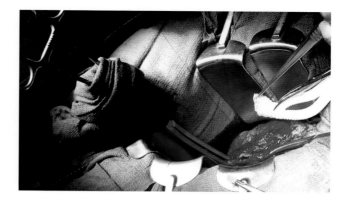

Figure 44.7 Proximal end-to-side anastomosis.

the main body of the graft, after completion of the aortofemoral portion of the procedure. GORE-TEX® vascular grafts (W. L. Gore & Associates) with prefabricated mesenteric side branches are not available. Mesenteric ischemia is mostly addressed with SMA reconstruction alone, which is a relatively easy and elegant procedure, without the need for additional dissection of the hepatic artery for celiac reconstruction.

Preemptive renal reconstruction is also controversial and may be considered for a nonatrophic kidney with hypertension and severe stenosis. Grafting of the renal artery with a presewn side branch is easiest. Renal artery stenting is preferable, to be performed after an open aortobifemoral bypass to avoid possible injury to the stents during aortic clamping.

45

Renal artery aneurysms

JAMES C. STANLEY, DAWN M. COLEMAN, AND JONATHAN L. ELIASON

CONTENTS

INTRODUCTION

Symptomatic renal artery aneurysms and those coexisting with functionally important renal artery stenoses warrant operative treatment.[1–3] Asymptomatic aneurysms >2 cm in diameter, especially in hypertensive patients, justify treatment by experienced interventionists; aneurysms <2 cm in diameter provide a relative indication for elective treatment, but only when a high degree of suspicion exists that they are the cause of refractory renovascular hypertension (HTN). Because of the potential for catastrophic rupture during pregnancy, therapy is recommended for all aneurysms in women of childbearing age who might conceive in the future.

SURGICAL EXPOSURE

The renal arteries are approached through an anterior abdominal incision. A transverse supraumbilical incision is favored at the authors' institution. When treating unilateral disease, the incision is carried from the contralateral anterior axillary line to the ipsilateral posterior axillary line. The rectus abdominis muscles are transected and the abdominal oblique muscles are divided in the direction of their fibers. A rolled sheet or soft bump placed under the lumbar spine enhances operative exposure. When bilateral renal reconstructive procedures are undertaken, the incision is extended into both flanks. Transverse abdominal incisions facilitate the handling of instruments in a direction perpendicular to the longitudinal axis of the body; this technical advantage has caused this type of incision to be preferred over midline vertical incisions.

The right renal artery (RRA) and vein are exposed by medial reflection of the colon and duodenum to the left. This exposure is accomplished by incising the lateral parietes from the hepatic flexure to the cecum, and separating the mesocolon from the retroperitoneal structures, usually by blunt finger dissection. The duodenum and the pancreas overlying the right kidney are carefully displaced to the left as the dissection progresses. This method provides excellent visualization of the renal vessels, as well as the aorta and vena cava (**Figure 45.1**). Before renal artery dissection is begun, the renal vein from its caval junction to the renal pelvis is dissected from the surrounding tissues, with ligation and transection of its adrenal and ureteric tributaries. The vein may then be retracted during dissection of the underlying distal renal artery.

Although an aneurysm may be easily palpable in the hilum of the kidney, it is unwise to approach the aneurysm directly. If one dissects the more proximal renal artery first before proceeding distally, troublesome injury to small arterial and venous branches is lessened. The aneurysm is dissected circumferentially about its dome and the exiting renal artery branches are encircled with elastic vessel loops as they are encountered.

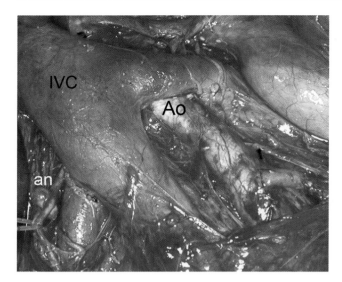

Figure 45.1 Exposure of the right kidney's vasculature following performance of a transverse supraumbilical incision and a medial visceral rotation. The renal artery with a small saccular aneurysm at its bifurcation (an) is clearly visible within the operative field, as are the inferior vena cava (IVC) and aorta (Ao).

Aneurysms involving the proximal main RRA are exposed by lateral retraction of the vena cava after it is skeletonized by ligation and transection of its entering lumbar venous branches. This provides unimpeded access to the involved renal artery from its aortic origin to the hilum of the kidney.

Exposure of the left renal artery (LRA) follows a retroperitoneal dissection similar to that performed on the right, with reflection of the viscera, including the left colon, medially. The tail and body of the pancreas are retracted to expose the superior pole of the kidney. Only rarely does a low-lying or large spleen obscure the operative field. This retroperitoneal approach ensures much better visualization of the renal vessels than does exposure through the mesocolon at the root of the mesentery. Treating aneurysms of the proximal and middle portions of the LRA requires extensive mobilization and retraction of the overlying renal vein.

It is fortuitous that larger aneurysms invariably stretch and displace the overlying veins. This redundancy makes the dissection and retraction of the renal vein branches much easier, with less risk of their being inadvertently torn when reconstructing the affected artery. Dorsal renal artery aneurysms are occasionally approached from behind by mobilizing the kidney and rotating it medially to expose the vessels posteriorly. Such a posterior approach is somewhat cumbersome, but it carries the advantage that the renal veins are not overlying the involved artery.

Once exposure of the renal artery and aneurysm has been accomplished, and before clamping the renal artery, systemic anticoagulation is achieved with the administration of intravenous heparin 150 IU/kg. Microvascular Heifetz clamps, developing tensions ranging from 30 to 70 g/cm^2, are preferred over conventional vascular clamps for occluding arteries in juxtaposition to the aneurysm. Clamps should be placed behind the artery to be occluded, so that the blades, rather than their handles, are positioned toward the operating surgeon. This lessens the likelihood of entanglement of suture material in the clamp during the reconstruction.

Ischemic renal injury following clamping may occur unless a stenotic renal artery exists proximal to the aneurysm and demonstrable collateral arteries circumvent the aneurysm. The latter may provide some degree of continuous blood flow to the kidney parenchyma following clamp application. In the absence of protective collaterals, the kidney should be cooled. Some have advocated mobilizing the kidney and surrounding it with ice slush. It is the preference at the authors' institution to clamp the proximal renal artery, quickly unroof the aneurysm, and flush each of the exiting arterial branches with cold (4°C) balanced electrolyte solution, followed by their immediate clamping. Some surgeons, usually those with practices involving renal transplantation, prefer to undertake ex vivo reconstruction of the renal arteries when multiple aneurysms involve the segmental vessels. Laparoscopic aneurysmectomy and renal artery reconstructive surgery have been advocated by several contemporary surgeons, but have not gained wide clinical application.[4,5]

SPECIFIC OPERATIVE INTERVENTIONS

Aneurysmectomy and primary or patch graft closure

This is the most appropriate means of treating most renal artery aneurysms (**Figure 45.2**). Solitary aneurysms involving the main renal artery and segmental branch bifurcations, may be excised and the vessel closed primarily in a simple manner (**Figures 45.3 and 45.4**).

The aneurysm in these cases is resected, leaving a 1–2-mm rim of aneurysmal tissue at the base of the affected artery. Closure of the arterial defect with a simple continuous suture is then performed, using fine cardiovascular suture incorporating the rim of aneurysmal tissue. If such a closure is likely to cause luminal narrowing, then a patch graft closure is warranted. Autogenous saphenous vein is preferred over synthetic materials when closing small vessels. Initial sutures should be placed in the distal apex of the arteriotomy when reconstructing segmental arteries, to facilitate visualization of the vessel margins and lessen the likelihood of luminal compromise during the closure.

Aneurysmectomy and reimplantation

This may be appropriate when the aneurysm is so intimately involved with the segmental branches that its excision necessitates a formal arterial reconstruction.

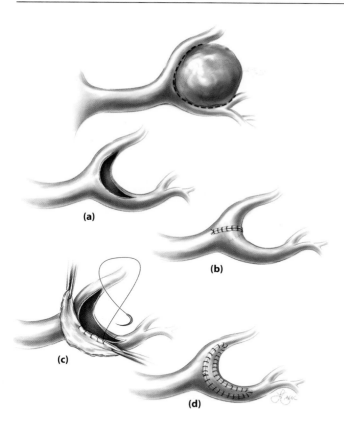

Figure 45.2 Excision of a large saccular renal artery aneurysm at the primary branching of the main renal artery. (**a**) Arterial defect. (**b**) The arterial defect may be closed directly in a transverse manner (Heineke–Mikulicz fashion). (**c,d**) Alternatively, it may be closed with a patch of autogenous vein. (Reproduced from Coleman DM, Stanley JC. Renal artery aneurysms. *J Vasc Surg*. 2015;**62**:779–785.)

In most instances, reimplantation of the segmental artery into the parent vessel (**Figure 45.4**) is preferred over an aortorenal bypass. Limited spatulation in the longitudinal axis of the affected renal artery allows for the creation of a more generous anastomosis. Interrupted suture when reimplanting particularly small-caliber arteries lessens anastomotic narrowings that might result from a purse-string effect associated with a continuous suture closure.

Multiple segmental artery involvement may on occasion require initial approximation by lateral anastomosis of these small branches before reimplantation. The technique of suturing together segmental vessels that have been spatulated, to create a common orifice before implantation, is useful. Although such techniques may be successfully performed in situ, in certain instances they are best performed as ex vivo repairs, particularly if an in situ reconstruction is expected to cause prolonged renal ischemia.

Closed aneurysmorrhaphy

Closed aneurysmorrhaphy of small renal artery aneurysms (2–3 mm in diameter) may be accomplished by plicating the aneurysm with a fine running monofilament suture (**Figure 45.4**). Such aneurysms, while not necessarily requiring operation themselves, are often encountered during treatment of other larger and more clinically relevant aneurysms.

Aneurysmectomy and aortorenal bypass

This is appropriate when treating aneurysms affecting the main proximal or mid-renal artery, and distal aneurysms

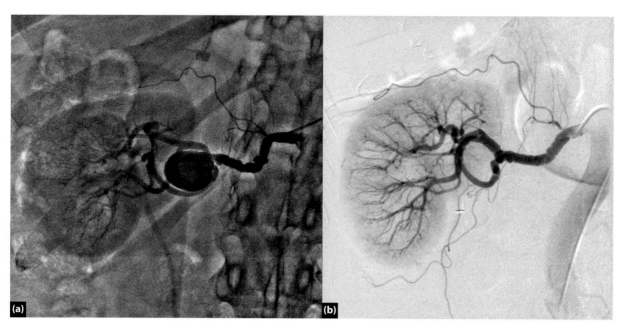

Figure 45.3   Aneurysmectomy and primary closure. (**a**) Large aneurysm affecting the main renal artery branching. (**b**) Following the aneurysmectomy, the arterial defect was closed primarily.

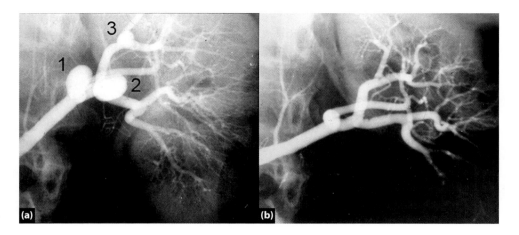

Figure 45.4 (**a**) Preoperative and (**b**) postoperative arteriogram of three renal artery aneurysms. Each aneurysm was treated differently: (1) the proximal aneurysm was excised with the arterial defect closed primarily in a transverse manner; (2) the middle aneurysm was excised and the normal segmental artery beyond the aneurysm was reimplanted onto the main renal artery; and (3) the small distal aneurysm at the bifurcation of a second-order renal artery was obliterated by a closed aneurysmorrhaphy with a fine cardiovascular suture. (Reproduced from Stanley JC. Renal artery aneurysms and dissections. In: Veith FJ, ed. *Current Critical Problems in Vascular Surgery*. St. Louis, MO; Quality Medical Publishers, 1991. p. 311.)

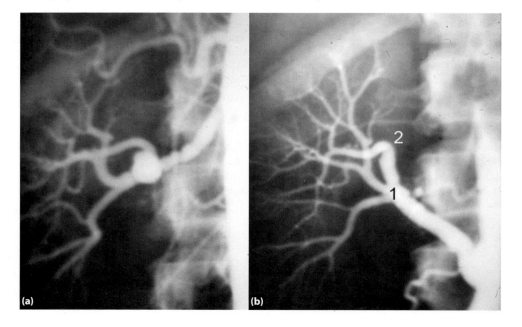

Figure 45.5 Aneurysmectomy and aortorenal bypass. (**a**) Aneurysm involving branching of the main renal artery affected by arterial dysplasia. (**b**) Treatment included an aneurysmectomy followed by autogenous saphenous vein aortorenal bypass, with an end-to-side implantation of one exiting branch (1) and end-to-end anastomosis of the other exiting branch (2).

occurring with concomitant arteriosclerotic or fibrodysplastic stenoses (**Figure 45.5**). In adults, a conventional aortorenal bypass graft procedure using a saphenous vein is preferred over a prosthetic graft because of the precise manner in which anastomoses to small arteries may be fashioned. In children requiring an aortorenal bypass, a segment of the internal iliac artery is the preferred conduit.

After the graft-to-aortic anastomosis has been completed, attention is directed to performing the distal renal anastomosis. The proximal renal artery and branches

arising from the aneurysm are occluded with microvascular clamps and the aneurysm is resected. The most direct route for an aortorenal vein graft to the right kidney is in the retrocaval position, but an antecaval position may lessen the likelihood of anastomotic kinking.

The graft-to-renal artery anastomosis is performed in an end-to-end manner. This anastomosis is facilitated by spatulation of the renal artery on its anterior aspect, and spatulation of the vein graft on its posterior aspect. This method allows visualization of the interior of the renal artery as each stitch is placed. The anastomosis initially involves placing two fine sutures through the apex of the spatulated vessels and the tongue of the opposite vessel. These sutures are tied and used as stay stitches. The anastomosis is usually completed with a continuous suture, although interrupted sutures are placed when reconstructing very small arteries or those in young children. These spatulated anastomoses are ovoid with increased suture line circumferences that, with healing, are less likely to develop late narrowings.

SURGICAL OUTCOMES

Perioperative mortality following open renal aneurysmectomy has not occurred in most high-volume centers. Nevertheless, early complications can occur including acute thrombosis of the reconstructed renal artery or one of its branches in 1–2% of cases.[6–8] Segmental arterial occlusions usually cause a limited infarction of a small segment of the kidney. This is usually of little consequence if preformed collateral vessels circumventing the aneurysm are nonexistent. However, if they are present, the patient may develop renovascular HTN. A similar clinical scenario occurs with late stenoses of the reconstructed arteries that may affect 2% of cases. Improvement in blood pressure (BP) has been observed in >50% of patients undergoing surgical treatment of their renal artery aneurysms without known coexisting stenotic disease.[6] Whether the latter is a benefit of the surgical procedure or simply better postoperative medical management of the patient's HTN is unknown. Most large series document excellent postoperative renal artery patency rates well above 90% at 10 years.[6]

CASE EXAMPLE

A 58-year-old woman was referred for treatment of a 2.2-cm RRA aneurysm affecting the main renal artery bifurcation (**Figure 45.3a**). She had been hypertensive for two decades and was on an angiotensin-converting enzyme inhibitor, beta-blocker, and a diuretic. She had persistently elevated BP when admitted. She underwent an aneurysmectomy with a primary arterioplastic closure of the renal artery without placement of a patch (**Figures 45.2b** and **45.3b**). The medial fibrodysplasia that affected her RRA may have contributed to her preoperative hypertensive state and this vessel was dilated in a retrograde fashion at the time of her aneurysmectomy. She was normotensive at the time of discharge and was not receiving any antihypertensive drugs.

REFERENCES

1. Chandra A, O'Connell JB, Quinones-Baldrich WJ, et al. Aneurysmectomy with arterial reconstruction of renal artery aneurysms in the endovascular era: a safe, effective treatment for both aneurysm and associated hypertension. *Ann Vasc Surg.* 2010; **24**:503–510.
2. Coleman DM, Stanley JC. Renal artery aneurysms. *J Vasc Surg.* 2015;**62**:779–785.
3. English WP, Pearce JD, Craven TE, et al. Surgical management of renal artery aneurysms. *J Vasc Surg.* 2004;**40**:53–60.
4. Gallagher KA, Phelan MW, Stern T, et al. Repair of complex renal artery aneurysms by laparoscopic nephrectomy with ex vivo repair and autotransplantation. *J Vasc Surg.* 2008;**48**:1408–1413.
5. Giulianotti PC, Bianco FM, Addeo P, et al. Robot-assisted laparoscopic repair of renal artery aneurysms. *J Vasc Surg.* 2010;**51**:842–849.
6. Henke PK, Cardneau JD, Welling TH 3rd, et al. Renal artery aneurysms: a 35-year clinical experience with 252 aneurysms in 168 patients. *Ann Surg.* 2001;**234**:454–462.
7. Klausner JQ, Lawrence PF, Harlander-Locke MP, et al. The contemporary management of renal artery aneurysms. *J Vasc Surg.* 2015;**61**:978–984.
8. Robinson WP 3rd, Bafford R, Belkin M, et al. Favorable outcomes with in situ techniques for surgical repair of complex renal artery aneurysms. *J Vasc Surg.* 2011;**53**:684–691.

46

Extra-anatomic reconstruction for aortoiliac occlusive disease

SCOTT M. SILVER AND FARAH MOHAMMAD

CONTENTS

INTRODUCTION

Operative selection for the treatment of aortoiliac disease must consider multiple factors. Aortobifemoral bypass offers excellent long-term patency, but is not appropriate for many patients given the physiologic demands, morbidity, and mortality associated with a laparotomy and clamping of the aorta. A femorofemoral bypass graft is an extra-anatomic bypass popularized by Vetto's comprehensive series published in 1962.[1] In conjunction with stent angioplasty of the iliac inflow vessel, a femorofemoral bypass offers high-risk patients an alternative to aortobifemoral bypass. It has also become a useful adjunct to endovascular treatment of abdominal aortic aneurysms during primary unibody stent graft placement and as treatment for stent graft limb occlusion. Axillary bifemoral bypass can be used when iliac inflow is inadequate bilaterally and cannot be corrected with stent angioplasty.

FEMOROFEMORAL BYPASS

There are several factors to consider in selecting an appropriate patient for a femorofemoral bypass graft. Unlike most vascular operations, cardiac status is less of a concern. This bypass is well tolerated even by high-risk cardiac patients because of the short operative time required and the superficial arterial anatomy. It is helpful to carefully examine the condition of the patient's groin. Morbid obesity, multiple arterial accesses, and previous operations can increase the complexity and length of the operation, as well as predict the occurrence of postoperative complications. Inflow is via the aorta and one iliac artery, hence occlusive disease in the inflow artery must be carefully evaluated and treated. Arteriography with pressure gradients is ideal.

Use of physical examination to determine inflow is sometimes necessary in a "bailout" or salvage situation. An easily palpable femoral pulse is usually adequate to support a femorofemoral bypass. Computed tomography angiography and duplex ultrasound (US) can be used in conjunction with physical examination to evaluate the adequacy of inflow. The axillary artery can also serve as an inflow source if one iliac artery cannot be adequately reconstructed. In this circumstance, an axillary bifemoral bypass graft can be used to revascularize both lower extremities. The common femoral (CFA), superficial femoral (SFA), or profunda femoris (PFA) arteries can be used as a distal target for an outflow vessel. The operator should be prepared to expose these vessels and perform an endarterectomy to complete the bypass.

A femorofemoral bypass graft can be performed under general, regional, or local anesthesia. Careful evaluation of the factors mentioned earlier helps to determine which anesthetic is most appropriate. The authors' own practice has favored general anesthesia if cooperation, experience, and expertise in vascular anesthesia are available.

In the operating room, the patient is placed supine with their arms extended on arm boards. A table-mounted mechanical retraction system (e.g., a Thompson retractor, Thompson Surgical Instruments, Traverse City, MI, USA) should be available for cephalad retraction of the inguinal ligament(s). Sterile towels and adhesive antimicrobial drapes are used with standard surgical preparation. Preoperative antibiotics are given.

It is best to avoid imprecise dissection of the groin because devitalized fat, transected lymph nodes, and interrupted lymphatic channels add to the risk of groin wound complications. However, a pulseless CFA is expected and easily identified with careful attention to the available anatomy. A line between the anterior superior iliac spine (ASIS) and pubic tubercle is drawn identifying the underlying inguinal ligament. A vertical incision is started at this line 2.5 cm lateral to the pubic tubercle and extending distally for 8–10 cm. Electrocautery is used to deepen the incision through the subcutaneous fat and Scarpa's fascia until the inguinal ligament is identified. It is helpful to mobilize the inguinal ligament to locate a pulseless CFA. This can be done by retracting the inguinal ligament superiorly, and the fascia lata overlying the femoral triangle inferiorly, and incising obliquely along the inferior border of the inguinal ligament. The femoral triangle contents can then be palpated medially and laterally. The CFA should be palpated and visualized to assure the distal dissection continues directly overlying the artery. Exposure is facilitated with two sharp Weitlaner retractors. If external iliac artery (EIA) control is required, a Thompson retractor is placed under the mobilized inguinal ligament. Adipose tissue is incised with electrocautery and lymph nodes can be mobilized medially or laterally to avoid transection. Large lymphatic vessels should be ligated between sutures. The CFA, PFA, and SFA are dissected circumferentially and encircled with vessel loops. Care should be taken to identify and ligate the lateral circumflex femoral vein that overlies the proximal segment of the PFA because it can cause troublesome bleeding.

Once the vessels have been adequately exposed for bypass and possible endarterectomy, a tunnel is created. The tunneler can meet significant resistance at the midline and care should be taken to avoid subfascial passage. Preperitoneal space tunneling can be helpful in the case of previous surgery and excessive scarring. C-shaped and S-shaped bypass grafts are described and have similar patency. A C-shape generally allows for a more limited dissection (**Figure 46.1**). The S-shape is used if the inflow EIA requires endarterectomy. In this configuration, the hood of the graft is elongated and becomes the patch of the endarterectomized artery. A tunnel is created from the right to left groin incision between the anterior surface of the abdominal wall fascia and adipose layer. Care should be taken to tunnel the graft so it does not meet the femoral vessels at an acute angle. If the graft approaches the femoral vessels at a right angle, it can kink when the patient is upright causing thrombosis (**Figure 46.2a,b**). Dacron or expanded polytetrafluoroethylene (PTFE) grafts can be used and generally are 6–8 mm in diameter. Oversizing the graft should be avoided because a larger-diameter graft can result in diminished flow velocity through the graft and increase the risk of thrombosis. Externally

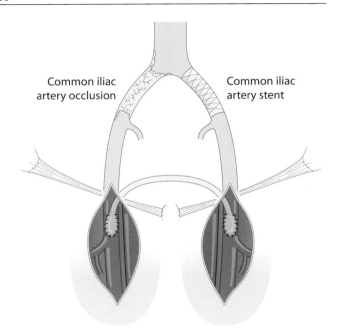

Figure 46.1 Typical femorofemoral bypass reconstruction with a C-shaped suprapubic tunnel. Inflow has been optimized with left common iliac stenting.

ring-supported grafts are preferred to diminish the risk of graft compression in the suprapubic tunnel.

The surgeon should have multiple options for vascular control of the femoral vessels because calcified atherosclerotic plaque is frequently encountered. A right angle vascular (e.g., renal) clamp on the EIA and vessel loops on the PFA and SFA is efficient when the vessels are soft. If the EIA cannot be occluded with a renal clamp, a 5-Fr sheath, three-way stopcock, and No. 5 Fogarty catheter can be used for proximal balloon occlusion. Plaque frequently extends into the origin of the PFA. A "baby" renal clamp can replace the vessel loop to gain a centimeter of proximal PFA to complete the endarterectomy. In planning the location of the anastomoses, care should be exercised to ensure that the graft does not make an acute bend immediately adjacent to the anastomosis (**Figure 46.3a–c**). The inflow anastomosis is created first, after the graft has been passed through the suprapubic tunnel to minimize unanticipated angulation. An arteriotomy is made with a fresh No. 11 blade and extended with Potts scissors. Endarterectomy is performed as needed. Extensive endarterectomy with an arteriotomy that extends to the inguinal ligament may necessitate patch closure of the artery first before a graft-to-artery anastomosis is constructed. This avoids the angulation problems sometimes associated with a long graft hood used to patch the artery. The graft is spatulated and an end-to-side anastomosis is created. If an expanded PTFE graft is chosen, a 5-0 expanded PTFE suture should be used to decrease suture line bleeding. Avoiding a hematoma is paramount. Any groin wound complication puts the graft at risk for infection. The distal anastomosis is constructed in similar fashion to the proximal anastomosis, though endarterectomy of the artery proximal to

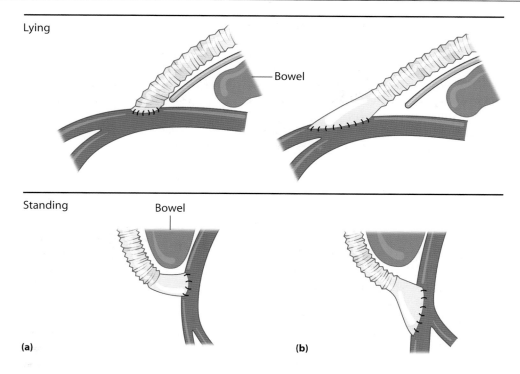

Figure 46.2 Femorofemoral graft showing avoidance of acute angulation at the inguinal ligament. (a) Kinking of the graft at the anastomosis when placed too close to the inguinal ligament. (b) Anastomosis placed further distal on the femoral artery to avoid kinking.

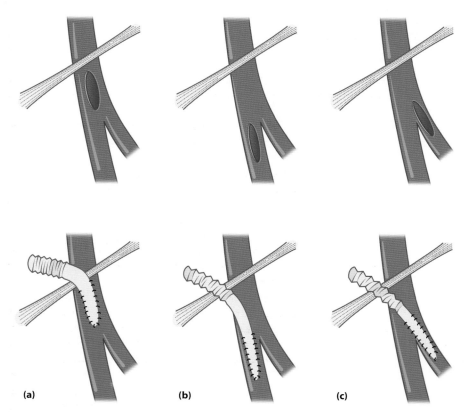

Figure 46.3 Construction of femorofemoral bypass anastomoses. (a) Arteriotomy on the proximal common femoral artery can lead to angulation. (b) More distal femoral arteriotomy, usually over bifurcations or onto either the superficial femoral artery or profunda femoris artery (PFA) can avoid this angulation. (c) Oblique arteriotomy onto the proximal PFA lessens the angle of curvature of the graft.

the anastomosis is usually unnecessary. On completion of both anastomoses, thrombin-soaked sterile compressed sponge is applied and protamine is given to reverse heparin anticoagulation after checking pedal Doppler flow. The incisions are closed with three layers of absorbable polyglycolic acid suture in the subcutaneous fat and vertical mattress nylons to approximate the skin edges.

AXILLARY BIFEMORAL BYPASS

Using the axillary artery for inflow proximal subclavian artery (SCA) stenosis should be ruled out. Upper extremity segmental pressures, CT angiography, and arterial duplex have largely replaced conventional angiography. The right axillary artery is usually chosen because the right SCA is more reliably disease-free than the left. The right arm is placed 90 degrees to the patient. The preparation is extended to include the arm, shoulder, thorax, abdomen, and both groins. A 10-cm incision is made 1.5 cm inferior to the lateral two-thirds of the clavicle. The dissection is continued through the subcutaneous fat, muscular aponeurosis, pectoralis major muscle, and clavipectoral fascia.

The pectoralis minor muscle is incised laterally to provide wide exposure of the axillary vein and artery. The axillary vein is encountered inferior to the artery; careful dissection with branch ligation is required to expose the artery. Exposure of the first portion of the axillary artery is undertaken with recognition of dissection hazards. First, the surgeon should have knowledge of the nerve anatomy in this dissection. (This is beyond the scope of this chapter.) Second, the axillary artery is a notoriously delicate artery and gentle technique in exposing, handling, and clamping this artery is mandatory. Bleeding in this location is difficult to control and further injury to the artery can be expected when attempting to hastily repair an injury. Once the first portion of the axillary artery is exposed, a 4-cm segment is mobilized to allow proximal and distal control. Distally, the femoral arteries are exposed as for a femorofemoral bypass.

A subpectoral tunnel is then created with blunt digital dissection parallel to the axillary artery and inferiorly into the subcutaneous tissue of the axilla. This tunnel is continued in a gentle arc along the anterior axillary line and curved just medial to the ASIS into the right groin. Creation of this tunnel is aided by a counterincision at the midpoint between the inferior costal margin and the iliac crest. An externally supported expanded PTFE graft is tunneled retrograde to the infraclavicular incision from the ipsilateral groin incision. The authors favor a prereconstructed 8-mm expanded PTFE graft with a cross-femoral limb already attached (**Figure 46.4**). After tunneling the cross-femoral limb to the left groin incision, the graft is positioned in the axillary tunnel to avoid kinking and angulation at any of the three anastomotic sites. Proximally, the graft should have enough length to run parallel to the axillary artery for 4 cm with some redundancy to prevent graft avulsion from the axillary

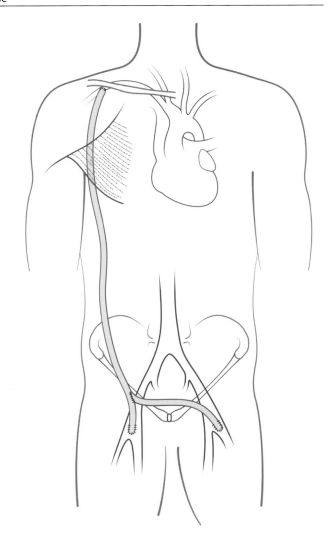

Figure 46.4 Axillobifemoral graft configuration.

artery with extreme arm abduction. Anastomosis to the relatively fixed first portion of the axillary artery also reduces the risk of this complication. After heparin anticoagulation, the axillary artery is occluded proximally and distally and an arteriotomy is made on the antero-inferior surface of the artery (10:30 on the clock face) to avoid graft angulation. An end-to-side anastomosis is constructed with 5-0 expanded PTFE suture to limit needle hole bleeding (**Figure 46.5**). Femoral anastomoses are constructed as described in the femorofemoral bypass section of this chapter, taking care to avoid graft angulation. Following a check of distal flow in the right wrist and both feet, anticoagulation is reversed with protamine sulfate and the incisions are meticulously closed.

POSTOPERATIVE MANAGEMENT

In the postoperative period, most complications specific to this operation are related to the groin incision. Careful daily inspection, groin hygiene, and occlusive dressings

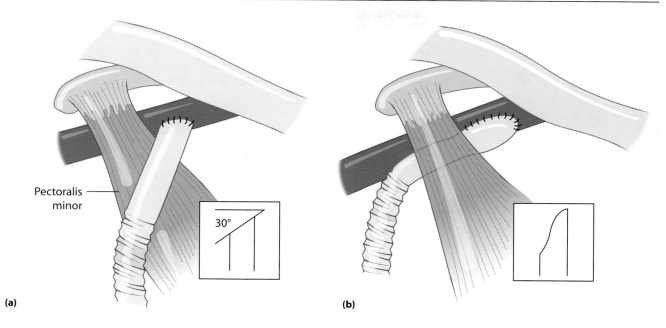

Pectoralis
minor

30°

(a)   **(b)**

Figure 46.5 Axillary anastomosis construction technique. (**a**) Classic construction with graft cut at a 30-degree bevel and tunneled between the pectoralis muscles. (**b**) Modified technique favored by the authors with a more traditional, acutely angled graft bevel tunneled behind the pectoralis minor.

are required. Medical management should include aspirin 81 mg daily and statin therapy. Routine surveillance with duplex US and ankle–brachial pressure indexes are performed at 1, 3, and 6 months and thereafter annually. Progressive disease of the distal anastomoses and outflow vessels is the most common cause of graft thrombosis. Anastomotic peak systolic velocities (PSV) >300 cm/s should be evaluated with angiography and appropriate intervention. A mid-graft PSV <60 cm/s is also predictive of thrombosis. With surveillance, 5-year patency rates for femorofemoral bypass of 50–60% can be achieved. Axillary bifemoral bypass patency rates are more variable (35–80%), because of variable patient selection.

CASE EXAMPLE

An older woman was a high-risk candidate for an aortobifemoral bypass graft because of known coronary artery disease and chronic obstructive pulmonary disease. Severe, short-distance, bilateral buttock and thigh claudication limited her ability to live independently. Arteriography demonstrated severe aortoiliac disease with an occluded right common iliac artery (CIA) and a patent left iliac system with high-grade stenoses of the proximal CIA and distal EIA (**Figure 46.6**). The patient was deemed a candidate for femorofemoral bypass following stenting of her left iliac system to optimize arterial inflow (**Figure 46.7**). **Figure 46.1** illustrates the final reconstruction.

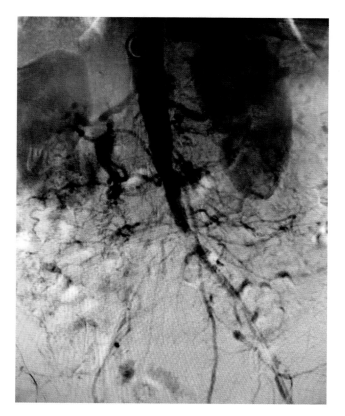

Figure 46.6 Preoperative arteriography demonstrating aortoiliac disease in a patient deemed to be a candidate for femorofemoral bypass after treatment of disease in the left iliac (inflow) artery.

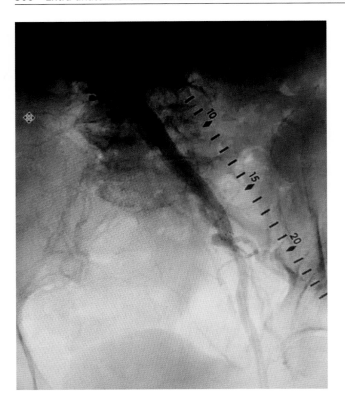

Figure 46.7 Arterial inflow via the left common and external iliac arteries was optimized with stent angioplasty.

REFERENCE

1. Vetto RM. The treatment of unilateral iliac artery obstruction with a transabdominal, subcutaneous, femorofemoral graft. *Surgery.* 1962;**52**:342–345.

SUGGESTED READING

Angle N, Dorafshar AH, Farooq MM, et al. The evolution of the axillofemoral bypass over two decades. *Ann Vasc Surg.* 2002;**16**:742–745.

Darling RC 3rd, Leather RP, Chang BB, et al. Is the iliac artery a suitable inflow conduit for iliofemoral occlusive disease: an analysis of 514 aortoiliac reconstructions. *J Vasc Surg.* 1993;**17**:15–19.

Rutherford RB. Axillobifemoral bypass: current indications, techniques, and results. In: Veith FJ, ed. *Current Critical Problems in Vascular Surgery.* St. Louis, MO: Quality Medical Publishing; 1996. pp. 201–205.

Schneider JR, McDaniel MD, Walsh DB, et al. Axillofemoral bypass: outcome and hemodynamic results in high-risk patients. *J Vasc Surg.* 1992;**15**:952–963.

47

Thoracofemoral bypass graft for aortoiliac occlusive disease

I. PIPINOS AND HERNAN HERNANDEZ

CONTENTS

INTRODUCTION

Thoracofemoral bypass for aortoiliac occlusive disease is a challenging procedure best-suited for the subset of patients with aortoiliac disease who have either a complication (usually occlusion) after previous aortobifemoral bypass or a hostile abdomen from a history of prior abdominal procedures or other abdominal pathology.

INDICATIONS AND PREOPERATIVE PLANNING

The presenting symptoms in these patients with severe aortoiliac occlusive disease include lifestyle-limiting chronic functional (claudication) or critical (rest pain or tissue loss) limb ischemia. Diagnosis can usually be made with a detailed history and physical examination and confirmed with noninvasive vascular studies. This procedure is ideal for good-risk patients with preserved lung function and a healthy thoracic aorta who need improved arterial flow to the lower extremities while avoiding entering the abdomen. Usually, these patients have a history of multiple abdominal operations, intra-abdominal scarring, failed prior infrarenal aortic reconstruction, infected aortic prosthesis, or other retroperitoneal disease. For patients who can tolerate a thoracofemoral bypass, this approach can be superior to the alternative solution of an extra-anatomic, axillofemoral bypass because of its superior cumulative 5-year patency rates of 81 versus 63%, with axillofemoral bypass usually reserved for higher-risk patients with limb-threatening acute or chronic ischemia.[1,2]

Preoperative evaluation includes basic risk stratification and comorbidity optimization, cardiac stress test, echocardiogram, and pulmonary function testing. Evaluation of the descending thoracic aorta is performed with computed tomography angiography (CTA) of the chest, abdomen, and pelvis with bilateral lower extremity runoff, to ensure that the thoracic aorta is healthy and there are adequate infrainguinal, disease-free arterial segments that will serve as good recipient sites for the distal anastomoses. Contraindications include aneurysm or occlusive disease of the descending thoracic aorta or the inability to tolerate one-lung ventilation. Relative contraindications include severe obstructive pulmonary disease or prior left thoracotomy with residual dense adhesions.[3] Before operating, there should be a discussion involving the patient, anesthesiologist, and surgeons to fully address the operative plan and the risks and benefits involved.

PROCEDURE DESCRIPTION

Positioning

The patient is transferred to the operating table with a vacuum beanbag extending from the shoulders to the proximal thigh. After induction of general anesthesia and placement of a double-lumen endotracheal tube, the patient's left hemithorax is elevated to an angle of 45–65 degrees with the table, while maintaining the pelvis as flat as possible; this facilitates the thoracotomy while allowing adequate exposure for the groin dissection. The left arm is supported in an arm cradle, helping to extend the lower thorax and avoid a brachial plexus injury. A roll is positioned under the right axilla and the air is evacuated from the beanbag. Pillow rests are placed under the knees and between the legs to prevent hyperextension; the patient's legs are secured to the table with a safety strap. Should a full thoracotomy become necessary, a generous operative field should be fully prepared, making sure to include the left scapula and thoracic spine (**Figure 47.1**).

Groin incisions and retroperitoneal access

The procedure begins in the groins to reduce the length of time that the chest cavity is open, thereby minimizing the associated heat loss. Standard incisions for the exposure of the femoral vessels are used in both groins and the femoral vessels are dissected free bilaterally. The left groin incision is then extended approximately 10 cm cephalad above the inguinal ligament. At the cephalad aspect of the left groin incision, the retroperitoneum is accessed and this access point facilitates the creation of the tunnel connecting the left groin to the left thorax (**Figures 47.2–47.4**). Specifically, a 10-cm incision is made through the aponeurosis of the external and internal oblique muscles on

the left, extending parallel to the inguinal ligament and approximately 2 cm cephalad to its caudal border. The internal oblique muscles are divided bluntly in the direction of their fibers, and the transverse abdominal muscle and transverse fascia are opened in the lateral aspect of the incision (**Figure 47.2**). The retroperitoneal space is then

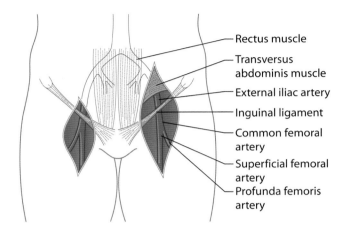

Rectus muscle

Transversus abdominis muscle

External iliac artery

Inguinal ligament

Common femoral artery

Superficial femoral artery

Profunda femoris artery

Figure 47.2 Standard groin exposures with left incision extending 10 cm above the inguinal ligament and an additional 10-cm incision through the aponeurosis of the external and internal oblique muscles on the left, extending parallel to the inguinal ligament and approximately 2 cm cephalad to its caudal border. The internal oblique muscles are divided bluntly in the direction of their fibers, and the transverse abdominal muscle and transverse fascia are opened in the lateral aspect of the incision. This incision is used for the creation of the retroperitoneal tunnel to the left chest. When a bifurcated graft is used, this incision is also used to route the right limb of the graft from its retroperitoneal location to a preperitoneal channel and into the right groin.

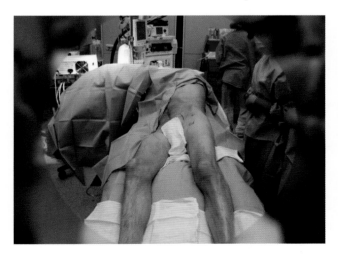

Figure 47.1 Patient positioned in a right side down thoracoabdominal position with the left arm in a supportive arm cradle and hips as flat as possible to facilitate exposure of both groins.

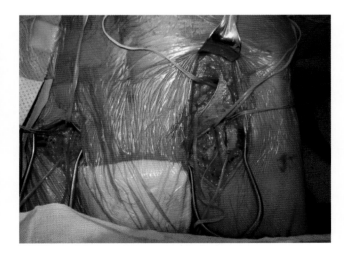

Figure 47.3 Completed groin dissections with controlled femoral vessels and left retroperitoneal incision.

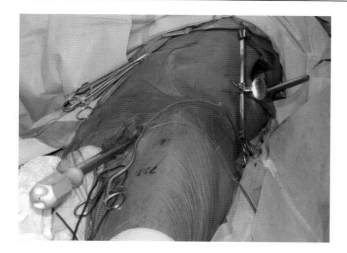

Figure 47.4 An olive-tipped femoropopliteal tunneler is passed from the left retroperitoneal incision, through the previously created retroperitoneal tunnel and into the left chest.

entered medial to the anterior superior iliac crest; this is the caudal end of the graft tunnel.

Thoracic aorta exposure

Thoracic dissection begins by tilting the operating table to the patient's right side to facilitate exposure and then performing a limited (mini) left posterolateral thoracotomy through the eighth intercostal space (ICS) to reach the descending thoracic aorta. The specific choice of ICS is based on the patient's body habitus and final positioning. The skin incision is extended laterally beyond the margins of the latissimus dorsi muscle, carefully so that the muscle itself is not incised. The authors then create superior and inferior skin flaps to help retract the muscle, thus avoiding incising the muscle and any subsequent associated postoperative pain. The intercostal muscles are then incised along the superior border of the inferior rib of the chosen ICS and the pleural cavity is entered with care so that injuring or incising the lung parenchyma itself are avoided. A rib spreader is inserted and opened cautiously to prevent rib fractures. If necessary, additional exposure may be obtained by excising the cephalad rib or transecting it at the posterior margin of the incision. Once the authors have entered the thoracic cavity, the left lung is deflated and retracted away into the upper thorax. Two "figure-of-eight" sutures are placed in the center of the diaphragm using a 0 silk suture and these are brought through the inferior and anterior chest wall and secured to retract the diaphragm to allow adequate exposure of the distal descending thoracic aorta. The inferior pulmonary ligament is taken down to the level of the inferior pulmonary vein, and the lung is retracted further superiorly. The pleura around the distal descending thoracic aorta is incised, and approximately a 6-cm segment of aorta immediately above the diaphragm is exposed. Next, the

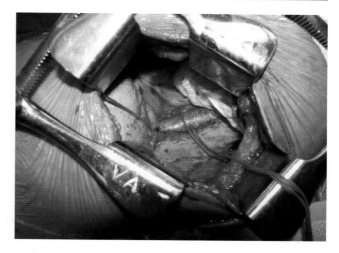

Figure 47.5 A rib spreader through the eighth intercostal space showing control of the descending thoracic aorta with umbilical tapes proximal and distal to the planned aortotomy site to facilitate subsequent clamping and proximal anastomosis. Notice the diaphragm retracted anteriorly and inferiorly with silk suture that is placed through its dome and brought out at the inferior and anterior chest wall. The deflated left lung is retracted superiorly to facilitate exposure and dissection of the descending thoracic aorta.

authors choose the proximal anastomosis site by gently palpating the aorta and finding a spot that is relatively free of atherosclerotic disease. It is helpful to completely dissect the aorta circumferentially, both proximally and distally, and control this by placing umbilical tapes so that they can be used later as a "handle" to stabilize the aorta and help position the clamp (**Figure 47.5**). The authors take special care in these steps to preserve all the intercostal arteries, because the anterior spinal artery originates from one of the intercostal arteries between the 8th and 12th thoracic vertebrae. The site of the aortotomy is carefully situated so that it is high enough above the crus of the diaphragm to avoid lateral kinking of the proximal graft after tunneling.

Tunneling

The authors then create a retroperitoneal tunnel to facilitate passing the graft limbs from the thorax to the groins. A 2-cm incision is made in the posteromedial aspect of the left diaphragm over the ribs through the open thoracic incision. The location of the aortotomy and the exit site through the diaphragm must be aligned carefully so that they correctly position the thoracic segment of the graft in a way that avoids lateral kinking of the graft. The authors place the left hand through the left retroperitoneal incision and the right hand through the left thoracic cavity. The left hand enters through the left retroperitoneal incision and dissects slowly the left retroperitoneal plane, aiming cephalad and slightly medial, over the external iliac vessels and the psoas major muscle, posterior to the left kidney and posteromedial to the spleen to meet the right hand, which is also following this route starting from the left thorax. A long tunneler is then guided through the tunnel and used to pass an umbilical tape that ultimately facilitates passing the graft itself (**Figure 47.4**). When a standard bifurcated prosthetic graft is used for the bypass, the shaft and two limbs of the graft are tunneled through the retroperitoneal channel and brought through the left retroperitoneal incision. Then, a preperitoneal tunnel is created that allows the right limb of the graft to reach the right groin incision. Again, simultaneous blunt finger dissection is used to create this second tunnel between the left suprainguinal, retroperitoneal space and the right groin that courses immediately posterior to the rectus muscles and both anterior and cephalad to the bladder in the preperitoneal space. If creation of the second tunnel is very difficult, this may be helped by dividing the caudal border of the inguinal ligament on the right. The second option is to first use a straight graft (usually 8 or 10 mm in diameter) to create the thoracic aorta-to-left groin bypass and then use a second graft (usually 6 or 8 mm in diameter) to do a standard cross-femoral bypass connecting the left femoral hood of the first graft to the right femoral vessels. In this case, the femoral crossover tunnel is created in a standard subcutaneous plane.

Anastomoses and choice of grafts

It is the authors' preference to perform the anastomosis to the thoracic aorta using a partially occluding, side-biting clamp. This maintains antegrade blood flow through the aorta, potentially limiting the magnitude of the ischemia to the lower torso, visceral vessels, and anterior spinal artery (**Figure 47.6**). The authors' preferred clamp for this location is a side-biting Cobra aortic clamp because of its excellent control. If a partially occluding, side-biting

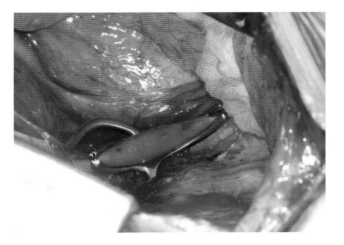

Figure 47.6 A partially occluding aortic clamp is preferred because it helps maintain antegrade blood flow through the aorta during the proximal anastomosis, potentially limiting the magnitude of ischemia to the lower torso, visceral vessels, and anterior spinal artery.

clamp cannot be used, then the aorta may be clamped with an upper vertical and lower-angled clamp; the lower-angled clamp is useful to control intercostal bleeding. After systemic heparinization (100 IU/kg), the jaws of the partially occluding clamp should be directed caudally to prevent it from accidentally becoming dislodged; the aorta caudal to the clamp should be interrogated with continuous wave Doppler to confirm that antegrade flow is preserved. These steps are unnecessary if straight clamps are used. An appropriately sized graft is chosen to match the size of the aorta and femoral vessels. When a bifurcated graft is used, a 16 × 8 or 14 × 7-mm graft is appropriate. When a vertical limb from the thoracic aorta to the left groin with a left-to-right femorofemoral crossover is used, then the authors use 8- or 10-mm grafts for the vertical limb and a 6- or 8-mm graft for the crossover graft. Both Dacron and polytetrafluoroethylene grafts are suitable alternatives. The aortotomy is created and the body of the graft is spatulated appropriately. When a bifurcated graft is used, the authors leave the body of the graft for as long as possible to make sure that there is sufficient length to reach the right groin without excess stretch and tension. If the graft is not long enough to comfortably reach the right groin, excess graft from the left limb can be used to construct a composite right limb (graft-graft composite). A tension-free aortic anastomosis is created in a continuous fashion with 2-0 polypropylene monofilament vascular suture. After completing the proximal anastomosis, an atraumatic vascular clamp is positioned on the body of the graft itself to check for leaks.

Tunneling the graft from the left chest to the left groin is safely performed with the previously placed tunneler (**Figure 47.6**). The opening must be enlarged sufficiently through the diaphragm so that the graft is not constricted as it passes through. It is imperative to maintain the correct orientation and tension on the limbs during this step to prevent them from twisting or kinking. The distal anastomosis of the left limb is constructed first. When a bifurcated graft is used, then the right limb is smoothly brought around from the left retroperitoneum to the preperitoneal space behind the rectus and anterior to the bladder (retropubic space). The right femoral anastomosis is then completed (**Figure 47.7**). If this is a "redo" operation, this may require anastomosis to the previously undissected profunda femoris arteries (PFAs) or anastomoses to the limbs of the older graft. The specific anastomosis configuration is chosen based on the distribution of the occlusive disease. Good flow in the PFAs must be established because the superficial femoral and external iliac arteries are frequently diseased in a patient scenario like this one. This may require extending the anastomosis further distally into the PFA and performing a common femoral/PFA endarterectomy. If it is necessary to perform an extensive profundaplasty, the authors usually do a patch angioplasty and then hood the anastomosis of the prosthetic graft onto the patch.

Heparin can be slowly decreased or it can be reversed with protamine sulfate. The thoracic and femoral incisions are closed in layers using standard techniques. A large chest

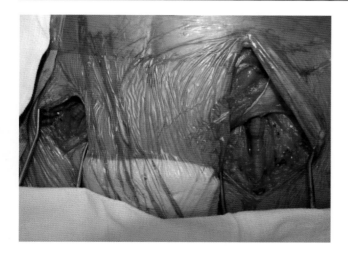

Figure 47.7 Completed distal anastomoses of a 16 × 8-mm thoracobifemoral textile graft with the right limb passing through the preperitoneal tunnel behind the rectus and anterior to the bladder (retropubic space).

tube (36 Fr) is placed through a separate incision caudal to the thoracotomy and positioned with the tip in the apex of the thoracic cavity. The lung is then reinflated under direct vision. The ribs are approximated using interrupted absorbable suture in a figure-of-eight configuration. The chest wall muscles are closed with running absorbable suture. If skin flaps were created for adequate exposure, the authors suggest leaving closed suction drains in the subcutaneous space.

POSSIBLE COMPLICATIONS

Major complications include reoperation for bleeding, respiratory failure, myocardial infarction or cardiac failure, renal failure, and paraplegia.

CASE EXAMPLE

A 56-year-old man initially presented with complaints of bilateral buttock and thigh pain after as little as 3 meters of walking and increasing rest pain. His ankle–brachial pressure indexes were 0.1 bilaterally; CTA with bilateral runoff demonstrated infrarenal aortic occlusion with reconstitution of the common iliac arteries just before their bifurcation. The patient had a history of multiple abdominal operations and retroperitoneal lymphadenectomy for testicular cancer. After discussion with the patient and his family, it was felt that aortobifemoral bypass would be too risky secondary to scarring; it was decided to proceed with thoracofemoral bypass to avoid the hostile abdomen. The patient tolerated the procedure well; at his 12-month follow-up, he could ambulate well and reported no signs of claudication.

REFERENCES

1. Schneider JR. Extra-anatomic bypass. In: Cronenwett JL, Johnston KW, eds. *Rutherford's Vascular Surgery*. 7th edn. Philadelphia, PA: Saunders/Elsevier; 2010. pp. 1137–1153.
2. Martin D, Katz SG. Axillofemoral bypass for aortoiliac occlusive disease. *Am J Surg*. 2000;**180**:100–103.
3. Fulton JJ, Keagy BA. Redo aortobifemoral and thoracobifemoral bypass for aortoiliac occlusive disease. In: Zelenock GB, ed. *Mastery of Vascular and Endovascular Surgery*. Philadelphia, PA: Lippincott Williams & Wilkins; 2006. pp. 375–384.

SUGGESTED READING

Barrett SG, Bergamini TM, Richardson JD. Descending thoracic aortobifemoral bypass: an alternative approach for difficult aortic revascularization. *Am Surg*. 1999;**65**:232–235.

Branchereau A, Magnan PE, Moracchini P. Use of descending thoracic aorta for lower limb revascularisation. *Eur J Vasc Surg*. 1992;**6**:255–262.

Criado E, Johnson G Jr., Burnham SJ, et al. Descending thoracic aorta-to-iliofemoral artery bypass as an alternative to aortoiliac reconstruction. *J Vasc Surg*. 1992;**15**:550–557.

Fukui S, Paraskevas N, Soury P, et al. Totally videoendoscopic descending thoracic aorta-to-femoral artery bypass. *J Vasc Surg*. 2010;**51**:1560–1563.

Kalman PG. Thoracofemoral bypass: a useful addition to a vascular surgeon's armamentarium. *Perspect Vasc Surg Endovasc Ther*. 2004;**16**:59–64.

Köksal C, Sarikaya S, Zengin M. Thoracofemoral bypass for treatment of juxtarenal aortic occlusion. *Asian Cardiovasc Thorac Ann*. 2002;**10**:141–144.

Kolvenbach R, Da Silva L, Schwierz E, et al. Descending aorta-to-femoral artery bypass: preliminary experience with a thoracoscopic technique. *Surg Laparosc Endosc Percutan Tech*. 2000;**10**:76–81.

Lee HK, Kim KI, Lee WY, et al. Descending thoracic aorta to bilateral femoral artery bypass in a hostile abdomen. *Korean J Thorac Cardiovasc Surg*. 2012;**45**:257–259.

McCarthy WJ, Mesh CL, McMillan WD, et al. Descending thoracic aorta-to-femoral artery bypass: ten years' experience with a durable procedure. *J Vasc Surg*. 1993;**17**:336–347.

Passman MA, Farber MA, Criado E, et al. Descending thoracic aorta to iliofemoral artery bypass grafting: a role for primary revascularization for aortoiliac occlusive disease? *J Vasc Surg*. 1999;**29**:249–258.

Sapienza P, Mingoli A, Feldhaus RJ, et al. Descending thoracic aorta-to-femoral artery bypass grafts. *Am J Surg*. 1997;**174**:662–666.

48

Aortic graft infections

SHERAZUDDIN QURESHI AND MITCHELL R. WEAVER

CONTENTS

INTRODUCTION

The use of prosthetic grafts as conduits for the treatment of aortic aneurysmal or occlusive disease is a cornerstone of vascular surgery. Its success is based not only on the technicalities of graft implantation, but also in maintaining graft sterility in vivo. Unfortunately, this is not always achieved. These infections pose a significant morbidity and mortality risk for the patient, are a considerable challenge to the surgeon charged with the patient's care, and generate significant socioeconomic costs.

PRESENTATION AND DIAGNOSIS

Diagnosing patients with aortic graft infection (AGI) requires a high index of suspicion in the face of often nonspecific symptomatology. Patient presentations range from generalized malaise and subtle systemic signs all the way to overt sepsis. The studies of collaborating laboratories are nonspecific, but may include leukocytosis with or without a left-shifted differential count and elevated inflammatory markers, such as erythrocyte sedimentation rate and C-reactive protein. Multiple sets of blood cultures should be obtained, but these may not yield positive results even with obvious infection. Nevertheless, every effort should be undertaken to identify the offending organism. Common pathogens include *Staphylococcus aureus* and *S. epidermidis*, the latter with a penchant for foreign bodies given its biofilm-producing property.[1] Imaging studies usually begin with a high-quality computed tomography angiography (CTA), which can confirm the diagnosis, evaluate the extent of the infection, and direct operative planning for definitive treatment. Typical findings include perigraft enhancement, adjacent soft tissue stranding, pockets of gas (**Figure 48.1**), pseudoaneurysm formation, and even frank rupture. In the face of a subtler clinical picture or uncertain findings, a short-term follow-up CTA or a tagged white blood cell scan may further clarify the presence of AGI.[2]

MANAGEMENT PRINCIPLES

Initially, appropriate antibiotic therapy should be administered and the patient should be physiologically optimized. Goals of treatment include infection eradication, hemorrhage prevention, and maintenance of organ and limb perfusion. Infection eradication typically requires excision of all prosthetic graft material, along with

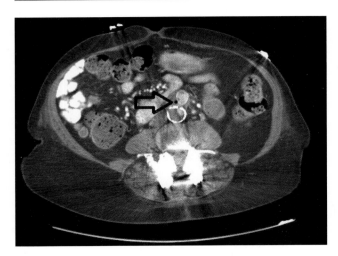

Figure 48.1 Computed tomography angiogram demonstrating an air pocket (arrow) adjacent to the proximal end-to-side anastomosis of an aortofemoral bypass with a Dacron graft.

aggressive debridement of surrounding infected and devitalized tissue. In certain cases, graft preservation has been successful when antibiotic therapy has been coupled with multiple washouts and eventual soft tissue coverage. This approach is typically limited to early, nonvirulent, peripherally located graft infections *not* involving an anastomosis, and is typically not feasible for intracavitary AGI. Options for arterial reconstruction can be divided into either extra-anatomic bypass (e.g., axillobifemoral bypass) with aortic ligation, or in situ arterial reconstructions with one of several conduits (femoral vein, cryopreserved allograft, or antibiotic-impregnated prosthetic graft). An individualized approach to AGI is best because each treatment option has its own benefits and limitations.

GENERAL OPERATIVE PRINCIPLES

General anesthesia is standard for these operations. Blood products should be available to replace blood loss and correct coagulopathy. Prolonged operative times are the norm; thus, ergonomic patient positioning with appropriate padding is paramount to avoid unintended neurapraxia and pressure-related complications. Warming devices should be used to avoid hypothermia. Both a transperitoneal midline approach and a left flank retroperitoneal approach can be used depending on the operative plan (see Chapter 32).

A supine position allows for the most flexibility when dealing with AGI. The aorta from the diaphragmatic hiatus and as far distally as the external iliac arteries (EIAs) can be exposed through a midline celiotomy incision. While the pararenal aorta can be controlled through a standard inframesocolic approach, more proximal supraceliac control requires partial mobilization of the left lobe of the liver and subsequent division of the gastrohepatic ligament. The supine position also allows for the chest and lower extremities to be prepped into the operative field

should an axillobifemoral bypass be planned or to harvest a lower extremity vein. A disadvantage of this approach is the scarring encountered from the initial aortic graft implantation or from previous abdominal surgeries, which makes the identification of tissue planes and subsequent dissection difficult.

A left flank retroperitoneal approach has some significant advantages. First, it avoids a hostile abdomen and provides a direct approach to the aorta without impediment from the peritoneal contents. Second, depending on the interspace chosen for the incision, exposure of the descending thoracic aorta is possible. Disadvantages include the potential difficulty in controlling the distal right iliac artery system, and the right femoral artery. This position is not conducive to harvesting lower extremity veins; exposure and tunneling for right axillofemoral bypass is impossible from this position.

The conduct of the operation first involves obtaining exposure for vascular control of the noninfected artery proximal and distal to the infected graft. One must be cognizant of the risk to adjacent organs during dissection including the ureters, bowel, and major veins. Placement of ureteral stents, to aid in their intraoperative identification, should be considered preoperatively. Should an enteric fistula be present, one must be prepared to repair or resect the bowel. Depending on the level of aortic control, individual visceral branches off the aorta may need to be isolated and controlled. Should the surrounding infection require sufficient debridement to interrupt in-line flow to the renal or visceral branches, cold perfusion techniques should be available.

Aortic cross-clamping requires close and constant communication with the anesthesia care team to adjust hemodynamic fluctuations. Once the patient is anticoagulated and aortic control is established, the goal should be to remove all prosthetic material from the field. Aggressive and thorough debridement of the area is mandatory. Not only is the graft itself sent for culture, but multiple samples of any obvious purulence encountered, as well as the involved tissue, should be submitted. The microbiology laboratory should be asked to sonicate graft material and allow for prolonged culture times to identify any slow-growing bacteria within a protective biofilm. Once debridement is completed, attention is focused on in situ revascularization or ligation of the aorta.

After completing the aortic reconstruction, an attempt is made to provide soft tissue coverage of the graft, typically with the greater omentum. The greater omentum is carefully freed of its attachments to the transverse colon and lengthened. The omentum can then be divided, creating a tail of omentum to cover the graft. The left side of the omentum with the blood supply based on the left gastro-epiploic artery is typically used (**Figure 48.2**). A fenestration is created at an avascular site within the transverse mesocolon through which the omental flap is passed to cover the graft (**Figures 48.3–48.5**). Consultation with plastic surgery colleagues is useful when more complex flaps are required for coverage.

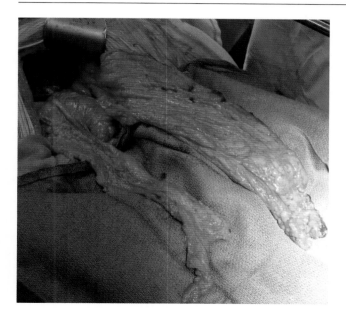

Figure 48.2 Intraoperative image demonstrating the greater omentum after being freed of its attachments to the transverse colon and divided to create a tail of omentum to cover the graft.

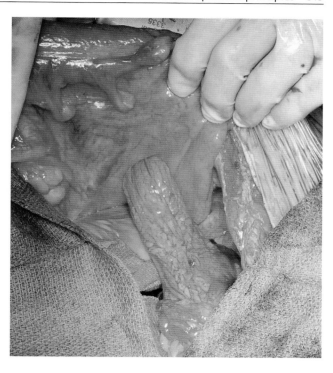

Figure 48.4 Intraoperative image demonstrating a tongue of omentum passed through the mesocolic fenestration.

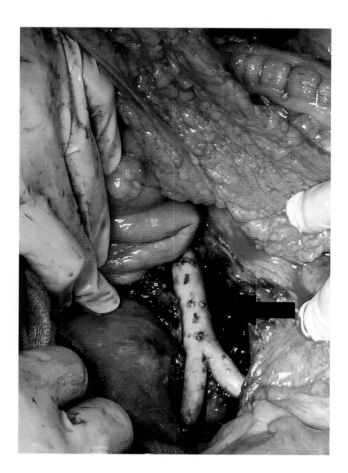

Figure 48.3 Intraoperative image demonstrating a cryopreserved allograft (arrow).

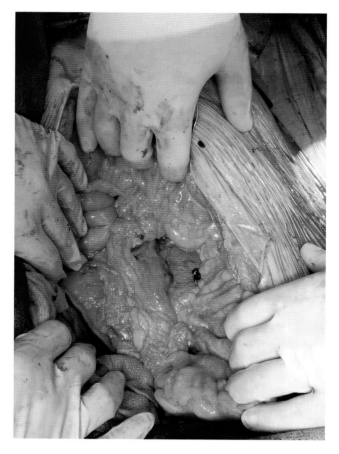

Figure 48.5 Intraoperative image demonstrating complete coverage of a cryopreserved allograft with an omental flap.

ARTERIAL RECONSTRUCTION

Extra-anatomic bypass with aortic ligation

Axillobifemoral bypass with aortic ligation has long been recognized as the standard therapy for AGI involving the infrarenal aorta. The benefits of this approach include the ability to stage what are typically long and difficult operations in compromised patients by performing the arterial reconstruction at one setting and the graft excision at a second, later setting. Another benefit is that the new graft is placed in clean tissue planes. In cases with severe contamination and virulent organisms, this may be the best option. The major disadvantages for this approach include poor graft patency and the risk of aortic stump blowout.[3] In addition, because emergent cases require addressing the aortic graft before arterial reconstruction, this approach may lead to prolonged and intolerable limb ischemia times. If there is inadequate, healthy infrarenal aorta to allow for oversewing the aortic stump, this method may not be an option.

When the common femoral arteries (CFAs) are not involved with the infection, typically an axillobifemoral bypass may be performed in the usual fashion (see Chapter 46). If the CFAs are involved, bilateral axillary to either superficial femoral artery (SFA) or, more commonly, deep femoral artery (DFA) bypass is required. The distal DFA can be approached along the lateral aspect of the sartorius muscle, thus remaining in clean tissue planes and avoiding a contaminated groin incision. Later, when excising the graft from the CFA, an attempt should be made to preserve flow at the femoral bifurcation.

During the abdominal procedure, care should be taken not to extend the midline incision too far distally and risk exposure/contamination of the cross-femoral limb. Ligation of the aorta is performed with either a stapling device or polypropylene suture in two-layered running fashion. Fascial pledgets may be helpful to reinforce the closure. If available, the omentum can be sutured in place to bolster the aortic stump.

Historical operative mortality for this approach is as high as 27% and higher than more recently reported series of in situ reconstructions. A risk of infecting the new extra-anatomic graft exists and approaches 15% in one series. Regarding aortic stump disruption, mortality can exceed 75%. The risk of this occurrence is reported to be as high as 25%. Lastly, limb loss rates have been reported as high as 15%. Overall, patient survival rates at 1 year of ≥70% have been achieved with this approach.[3–5]

IN SITU AORTIC RECONSTRUCTION

Neoaortoiliac system (NAIS) with femoral vein

Creation of a NAIS with the femoral vein is one choice of conduit that may be used for arterial reconstruction in the face of AGI. This method involves harvesting the femoral vein from the origin of the deep femoral vein (DFV) to the popliteal vein. Preoperative duplex vein mapping is performed to ensure that the vein is patent and of adequate size, typically >6–7 mm in diameter. Care is taken to preserve the saphenous vein, and especially the DFV, to provide adequate venous drainage for the leg. A longitudinal incision is made along the lateral aspect of the sartorius muscle, which is retracted medially. The vein is mobilized from its confluence with the DFV distally to the above-knee popliteal vein, including dividing the adductor magnus tendon, if necessary, to enter the adductor canal to obtain additional length. During dissection, care is taken to preserve collateral branches of the SFA and popliteal artery. Once exposed, the vein is typically left in place until the required length of vein is determined. When harvested, the vein is divided flush with the DFV, taking care not to leave a stump that may be a nidus for thrombus formation. Depending on the size match, the femoral vein can either be reversed or more typically left in its native orientation following valve lysis. Valves are typically lysed by everting the vein and excising them. The vein is then distended and any identified branches are oversewn with fine polypropylene suture. Since a bifurcated reconstruction is typically required, both veins can be harvested and then anastomosed to each other in a side-to-side fashion proximally to create a bifurcated vein graft. Postoperative venous thromboembolic prophylaxis is maintained both mechanically (intermittent pneumatic compression) and pharmacologically (subcutaneous heparin).

NAIS, using autogenous tissue to decrease the risk of reinfection, may allow for a short-duration antibiotic regimen. Overall, recent series reported late mortality to compare favorably with the other methods of reconstruction.[5,6] Disadvantages of NAIS include the added operative time. If available, a second surgical team to harvest the femoral veins can help ameliorate this. Another disadvantage is the size mismatch between the infrarenal aorta, particularly when the initial operation was for aneurysmal disease, and the proximal end of the graft even when a bifurcated vein graft is created. In cases of an unstable patient from hemorrhage or sepsis, an alternative conduit should be considered. NAIS is subject to the same issues affecting lower extremity vein bypasses, namely vein graft stenosis from intimal hyperplasia and aneurysmal degeneration. Finally, postoperative venous complications, including disruption of venous drainage with subsequent leg swelling, deep vein thrombosis, and compartment syndrome with need for fasciotomy have been reported.[6]

Cryopreserved allografts

Cryopreserved allografts are an alternative conduit for in situ aortic replacement (**Figure 48.3**). This approach avoids placement of a prosthetic graft in an infected field, as well as the time and morbidity associated with femoral vein harvest. Current cryopreservation techniques have improved the integrity of these grafts leading to fewer long-term complications than have been reported in the past. The downside to their use includes cost, and the lead time necessary for their acquisition. Thus, cryopreserved allografts may not be an option in an urgent or emergent situation. Specific handling and storage techniques are also required for the allograft. Once thawed, it is sewn in place in the standard fashion with the one caveat that the lumbar branches are placed facing up, to allow for ease of repair if there is any bleeding once the allograft is pressurized.

A recent study detailed the results of a multi-institutional database of 220 patients who underwent the use of cryopreserved aortoiliac allografts for aortic reconstruction in the USA in the setting of infection, including enteric fistula, with a mean follow-up of 30 months. Survival was 75% at 1 year and 51% at 5 years. Primary graft patency was 97% at 5 years. At 5 years, freedom from graft-related complications was 80%, freedom from graft explant 88%, and freedom from limb loss 97%.[7]

Antibiotic-treated grafts

A third option for in-line aortic reconstruction for AGI is the use of an antibiotic-treated prosthetic graft. Currently available Dacron grafts pretreated with gelatin can be easily impregnated with an antibiotic when soaked in rifampin. Typically, 600 mg of rifampin is reconstituted in 50 mL of solution in which the graft is soaked for 5–30 minutes, after which excess is allowed to drain off before implantation. Therefore, any chosen graft size may be quickly prepared in the operating room.

Advantages of using antibiotic-treated prosthetic grafts include having a readily available, appropriately sized graft. As with other in-line arterial reconstructions, it avoids aortic stump blowout complications and has superior graft patency compared to extra-anatomic bypass. Like other in situ reconstructions, limb loss is rare and 5-year survival is around 50%.[5,8] Disadvantages of antibiotic-treated grafts are largely related to the risk of reinfection, ranging from 4 to 22%.[1,8] Obviously, antibiotic treatment with rifampin is of no value for nonsusceptible organisms. Reinfection is encountered more frequently with virulent organisms, particularly methicillin-resistant *S. aureus* and may be largely unavoidable. Radical debridement of the affected retroperitoneal tissue and use of an omental wrap are important adjuncts to reduce reinfection rates.

POSTOPERATIVE CARE

The postoperative complications of procedures to treat AGI are like the complications following any infrarenal aortic reconstruction with the additional burden of problems related to infection and sepsis. When femoral artery anastomoses are involved, open groin wounds frequently result and are best managed with negative-pressure wound therapy. The duration of postoperative antibiotic coverage is controversial and depends on several factors, including the offending pathogen, the type of reconstruction, and the patient's immune status. Most patients require a minimum of 6 weeks of intravenous antibiotics. Some need longer courses; occasionally, lifelong oral suppressive antibiotics are used.

CONCLUSIONS

The diagnosis and treatment of AGI remains a major challenge even for the most experienced vascular surgeon. A variety of reconstructive options are available, but all depend on the administration of culture-specific antibiotics, aggressive debridement of all infected tissue, and maintenance of vital organ and limb perfusion.

CASE EXAMPLE

A 71-year-old man with a history of aorta-to-bilateral EIA reconstruction for treatment of an aortic aneurysm presented with recurrent episodes of fevers, chills, and bacteremia despite treatment with antibiotics. A CT scan of the abdomen revealed air and perigraft inflammation. The patient was treated in a staged fashion. First, an axillobifemoral bypass was performed. After closure and

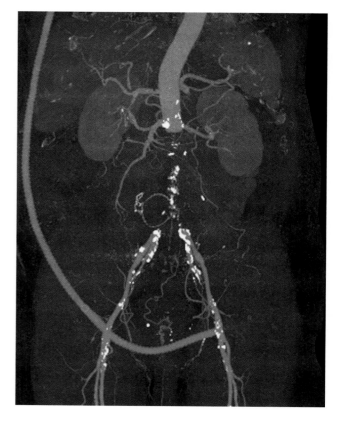

Figure 48.6 Three-dimensional reconstruction of computed tomography imaging obtained 2 years postoperatively for the patient described in the case example; it demonstrates axillobifemoral bypass and ligation of infrarenal aorta.

exclusion of the incisions, but during the same operation, the right limb of the aortic graft was excised and the right EIA was repaired with a vein patch. Four days later, the patient returned to the operating room and, through a left retroperitoneal exposure, the remainder of the graft was excised, the infrarenal aorta was ligated, and the left EIA was repaired with a vein patch. A graft enteric fistula was identified; this required resection of the small bowel and primary anastomosis. The patient was treated with antibiotics postoperatively and had an uneventful postoperative recovery (**Figure 48.6**).

REFERENCES

1. Hodgkiss-Harlow KD, Bandyk DF. Antibiotic therapy of aortic graft infection: treatment and prevention recommendations. *Semin Vasc Surg.* 2011;**24**:191–198.
2. Lawrence PF. Conservative treatment of aortic graft infection. *Semin Vasc Surg.* 2011;**24**:199–204.
3. Berger P, Moll FL. Aortic graft infections: is there still a role for axillobifemoral reconstruction? *Semin Vasc Surg.* 2011;**24**:205–210.
4. Charlton-Ouw KM, Sandhu HK, Huang G, et al. Reinfection after resection and revascularization of infected infrarenal abdominal aortic grafts. *J Vasc Surg.* 2014;**59**:684–692.
5. Kilic A, Arnaoutakis DJ, Reifsnyder T, et al. Management of infected vascular grafts. *Vasc Med.* 2016;**21**:53–60.
6. Dorweiler B, Neufang A, Chaban R, et. al. Use and durability of femoral vein for autologous reconstruction with infection of the aortoiliofemoral axis. *J Vasc Surg.* 2014;**59**:675–683.
7. Harlander-Locke MP, Harmon LK, Lawrence PF, et al. The use of cryopreserved aortoiliac allograft for aortic reconstruction in the United States. *J Vasc Surg.* 2014;**59**:669–674.
8. Lew W, Moore W. Antibiotic-impregnated grafts for aortic reconstruction. *Semin Vasc Surg.* 2011;**24**:211–219.

49

Infrainguinal bypass graft for lower extremity arterial occlusive disease

FRANK M. DAVIS AND PETER K. HENKE

CONTENTS

INTRODUCTION

It is estimated that 8–12 million Americans are affected by peripheral arterial disease (PAD) and this prevalence will continue to rise.[1] Infrainguinal bypass remains one of the most common open vascular operations to treat patients with PAD. In the current era, endovascular interventions are increasingly successful as stand-alone procedures. However, a significant number of patients require open bypass for lower extremity occlusive disease because of the atherosclerotic burden or endovascular therapy failure.

The two primary indications for infrainguinal bypass remain critical limb ischemia (CLI) and lifestyle-limiting claudication. For patients with CLI, defined as rest pain, tissue loss, or ankle pressure <40 mmHg, only 5% will achieve limb survival at 1 year without revascularization.[2] For patients with claudication, the natural history is

progressive decline in ambulatory distance before the onset of pain. Despite intensive medical management, 20–30% develop increased disability.[3] Interventions for claudication are done to improve function in the setting of significant ongoing disability.

PREOPERATIVE PLANNING

Preoperative planning is crucial for infrainguinal bypass procedures. Detailed anatomic characterization of the extent of arterial disease must be obtained before arterial reconstruction. Generally, arteriography is the gold standard for most patients with CLI. However, advances in computed tomographic angiography (CTA) have led to an increasing number of patients undergoing CTA, especially those with absent femoral pulses. Ultimately, preoperative imaging should identify major anatomic lesions, the inflow site, and the potential outflow vessel.

Proximal anastomotic site

The common femoral artery (CFA) is typically the inflow vessel of choice, although distal locations such as the superficial femoral (SFA), profunda femoris, or popliteal artery may be used with equivalent patencies. Intraoperatively, if there is uncertainty about the suitability of the inflow site, direct arterial pressures can be compared to a radial arterial pressure. A resting pressure gradient >10 mmHg is significant and a more proximal location for the site of bypass inflow should be investigated. In addition, consideration of CFA endarterectomy is prudent.

Distal anastomotic site

The general principle with infrainguinal reconstruction is that the distal target vessel should bypass all significant atherosclerotic disease to the most proximal limb artery that has at least one runoff artery to the foot. Therefore, the below-knee popliteal artery is the most commonly used target. Improper distal target selection can decrease long-term graft patency. Although most claudicants require only femoropopliteal bypass, a high proportion of CLI patients require tibial or pedal bypasses. Arteries distal to the outflow target should be free of hemodynamically significant disease.

CONDUIT SELECTION

The choice of conduit is a critical aspect of infrainguinal bypass procedures and consists of a variety of autogenous or prosthetic options. Autogenous options include: ipsilateral and contralateral great saphenous vein (GSV); in situ GSV; upper extremity vein; and, occasionally, superficial femoral vein. Prosthetic options include: Dacron; heparin-bonded Dacron; polytetrafluoroethylene (PTFE) with or without distal cuff; and expanded PTFE.

Autogenous grafts

Overall, autogenous conduits provide the best patency for infrainguinal arterial reconstruction.[4,5] The preferred autogenous conduit is the GSV. Reversed and in situ configurations of the GSV are equally effective; however, some proponents of in situ GSV bypass have suggested that it provides better size matching.[6] Assessment of vein quality, with duplex imaging, is conducted to evaluate vessel diameter, compressibility, and wall thickness. For optimal patency, the vein should be at least 3 mm in diameter, although compressible veins between 2 and 3 mm in diameter can be used. Studies have shown that 5-year

patency of appropriately chosen GSV conduit for above-knee bypass is >70%,[4,7] while the 3-year patency for below-knee bypasses with GSV is 50–70%.[8]

When the GSV is not available, a variety of veins or combination of veins can be used. The cephalic or basilic veins can provide an adequate conduit but are demanding to harvest.[9,10] Short segments of veins can be connected with venovenostomies to create a conduit of sufficient length for the intended bypass. When performing spliced vein bypasses, the ends of each vein are spatulated to aid in the creation of a wide anastomosis free of stenosis.

Prosthetic grafts

Prosthetic grafts are non-autogenous options for patients who do not have a suitable vein conduit. In comparison to reversed GSV grafts, PTFE grafts have the same patency for above-knee popliteal bypasses during the first 2–3 years; however, thereafter vein grafts have superior long-term patency.[4,5,11] Prosthetic bypasses to the below-knee popliteal artery have uniformly poor patency (54% 3-year patency of PTFE versus 61% 3-year patency for GSV).[8] In an effort to improve the long-term patency of prosthetic grafts, expanded PTFE grafts covalently bonded to heparin or heparin-bonded Dacron grafts were created.[12,13] An additional way to improve the patency of below-knee prosthetic bypasses involves the use of a Miller vein cuff or Taylor vein patch (**Figure 49.1**). Randomized trials have shown that the addition of vein cuffs significantly improves the patency of prosthetic grafts for

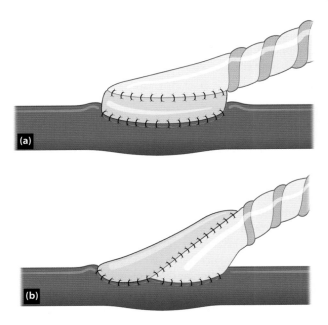

Figure 49.1 Improving the patency of below-knee prosthetic bypasses. (**a**) Autogenous vein cuff (Miller vein cuff). (**b**) Autogenous vein patch (Taylor vein patch). Either patch can be applied to a prosthetic graft to improve the patency of infrageniculate polytetrafluoroethylene bypass grafts.

infrageniculate bypasses (52% patency at 2 years for PTFE with vein cuff versus 29% for PTFE without cuff), with the addition of warfarin.[14]

OPERATIVE TECHNIQUE

Vein harvest and preparation

When harvesting the GSV for bypass conduit, the vessel can be found in the medial aspect of the femoral triangle. Preoperative duplex vein mapping is helpful in following the course of the vessel. Incision with a No. 10 blade is made directly over the vein to prevent skin flaps. Once the main vein is identified, excision is continued distally directly over the vein. Circumferential dissection is facilitated with silicone elastomer loops to avoid direct grasping of the vein. During the dissection, all side branches are carefully ligated using 3-0 silk suture. When tying the side branches, it is preferable to leave a short stump compared to placing a ligation close to the main trunk to prevent vessel stenosis.

Once an appropriate length of vein is identified, a small clamp is placed flush with the common femoral vein and the vessel is ligated proximally and distally. The stump is oversewn in two layers with monofilament suture. The proximal aspect is clamped with a bulldog clamp and heparinized blood with papaverine is flushed under

gentle pressure from the distal end to identify tears or untied branches. Missed or small avulsed side branches are repaired with longitudinally oriented 6-0 polypropylene suture. Overdistension of the vein should be avoided to prevent shearing of the endothelium. For in situ GSV bypasses, the technique varies slightly and is described later in the chapter.

Femoral to above-knee popliteal bypass

The CFA is most frequently used as the inflow vessel for infrainguinal bypasses. A vertical incision is made directly over the femoral pulse (**Figure 49.2a**). If a femoral pulse cannot be palpated, the CFA can be identified in the medial third between the pubic tubercle and the anterior superior iliac spine. The incision is deepened with electrocautery to the level of the deep fascia (**Figure 49.2b**), which is incised exposing the femoral sheath with the aid of self-retaining retractors (**Figure 49.2c**). Adequate time should be spent ligating all lymphatics to reduce the risk of a lymphocele. On entering the femoral sheath, the CFA is dissected proximally to the inguinal ligament. Distally, the CFA divides into the SFA and the profunda femoris artery. Exposure of these vessels is best accomplished by dissecting distally on the anterior surface of the parent trunk. The lateral femoral circumflex vein crosses anterior to the profunda femoris artery at the level of bifurcation (**Figure 49.2d**).

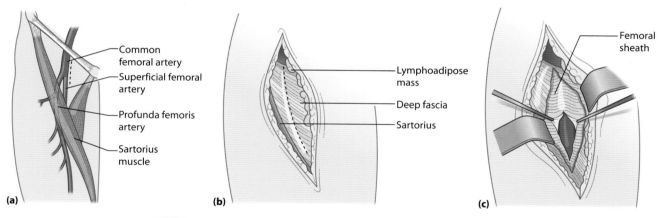

(a) (b) (c)

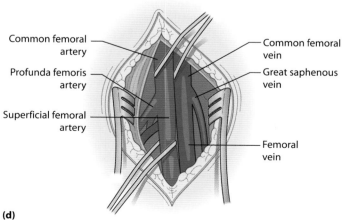

(d)

Figure 49.2 Femoral to above-knee popliteal bypass. (**a**) The femoral triangle is bordered by the inguinal ligament, and the sartorius and adductor magnus muscles. The dashed line represents the proposed incision to adequately expose the common femoral (CFA), superficial femoral (SFA), and profunda femoris arteries. (**b**) The incision is carried down through the skin and subcutaneous fat to the fascia lata. Special attention should be paid to ligating the lymphatic tissue. (**c**) The deep fascia is incised exposing the femoral sheath that is opened along its axis. (**d**) The CFA and SFA are mobilized and controlled with silicone elastomer vessel loops. The profunda femoris artery arises laterally off the common femoral trunk. Its origin is crossed by the lateral femoral circumflex vein.

Following identification of all vessels, silicone elastomer vessel loops are placed around each vessel to establish vessel control.

For the distal target, the above-knee popliteal artery is approached through a medial incision with the leg externally rotated and the knee flexed 30 degrees (**Figure 49.3a**). The incision is made along the anterior border of the sartorius muscle in the distal third of the thigh. The subcutaneous tissue and fascia are divided with electrocautery and the sartorius muscle is retracted posterolaterally (**Figure 49.3b**). The vastus medialis muscle is retracted anteriorly exposing the fascia, which is divided entering the popliteal fossa. Additional exposure of the popliteal artery can be obtained by dividing the tendon of the adductor magnus muscle (**Figure 49.3c**). The popliteal artery is analyzed for a healthy segment with palpation. After adequate length of the popliteal artery is exposed, vessel loops are placed proximally and distally.

Following exposure of the proximal and distal targets, the conduit tunnel is created. The tunneler device is passed from the femoral incision to the popliteal fossa behind the sartorius muscle. The chosen conduit is marked for orientation to prevent twists, and then attached to the tunneler and pulled into position, with proper positioning of the conduit checked. Before arterial occlusion, heparin (100 IU/kg) is given. The proximal anastomosis is performed first after the application of clamps or vessel loops. A No. 11 blade is used to make an arteriotomy on the anterior CFA wall and is extended with Potts scissors. The graft is anastomosed to the inflow vessel in an end-to-side fashion with a running 5-0 polypropylene suture. The heel of the graft is sutured first, and the graft is sutured to a point halfway toward the toe. A second suture is then placed in the toe of the graft and continued toward the first stitch. After flushing, the clamps are released and hemostasis is evaluated. Single 6-0 polypropylene repair sutures are used if bleeding is encountered through the anastomosis. Hemostatic agent can be applied to the anastomosis and a soft bulldog clamp is placed on the graft until the distal anastomosis is complete.

Regarding the distal anastomosis, care should be taken to identify a site of distal arteriotomy that is free of

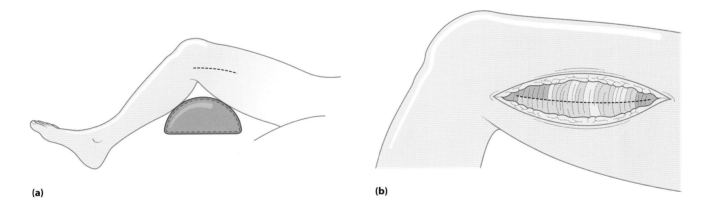

(a)

(b)

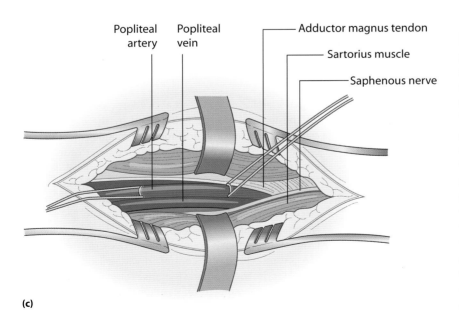

Popliteal artery | Popliteal vein | Adductor magnus tendon | Sartorius muscle | Saphenous nerve

(c)

Figure 49.3 Femoral to above-knee popliteal bypass (distal target). (**a**) The above-knee popliteal artery is approached with an incision along the distal third of the thigh, anterior to the sartorius muscle. The knee should be flexed to 30 degrees to aid in exposure. (**b**) The incision is continued through the subcutaneous fat where the deep fascia is incised and the sartorius muscle is retracted posteriorly. (**c**) The above-knee popliteal artery is seen exiting the adductor canal. The adductor magnus tendon is seen covering the proximal portion of the popliteal artery and it may be divided to provide better exposure. Once the popliteal artery is freed of venous plexus it can be mobilized with silicone elastomer vessel loops.

excessive calcification. The above-knee popliteal artery is controlled with vessel loops or small vascular clamps. A longitudinal arteriotomy approximately 1.5 times the graft diameter is created. The orientation of the graft is checked and the bulldog clamp is released to ensure pulsatile bleeding. An end-to-side anastomosis is created with 6-0 running polypropylene suture, using a similar technique to the proximal anastomosis.

For in situ vein grafts, the proximal GSV is exposed in the groin as described previously and the distal GSV is mobilized in the region of the suspected anastomosis. Following division of the saphenofemoral junction, the first venous valves are divided under direct visualization with Potts scissors. The proximal anastomosis is then performed in an end-to-side fashion. A variety of valvulotomes are then inserted distal-to-proximal to lyse the valves. The quality of the vein and the success of lysis are analyzed; flow should be pulsatile before completion of the distal anastomosis. After completion of the distal anastomosis, the entire in situ graft is evaluated with Doppler interrogation and manual compression of the bypass distal to the probe. Continuous outflow indicates the presence of an arteriovenous fistula, which must be ligated before completion.

Femoral to below-knee popliteal bypass

Exposure of the infrageniculate popliteal artery is achieved through a medial incision 1–2 cm posterior to the medial edge of the tibia with the leg externally rotated and the knee flexed 30 degrees (**Figure 49.4a**). The incision is extended a third of the way down the calf, with care taken to avoid injuring the GSV. The subcutaneous tissue is divided with electrocautery and the crural fascia is incised 1 cm posterior to the tibia extending to the semitendinosus tendon (**Figure 49.4b**). More proximal exposure can be obtained by dividing the tendons of the semitendinosus, gracilis, and sartorius muscles. The medial head of the gastrocnemius muscle is retracted posteriorly, exposing the popliteal fossa. The popliteal vein is often the first structure encountered, and bridging veins must be divided with 3-0 silk suture (**Figure 49.4c**). The origin of the soleus muscle is taken down from the soleal line. The anterior tibial vein crossing the popliteal artery bifurcation is exposed and is suture-ligated with 3-0 cardiovascular silk toward the popliteal vein; a silver clip is applied distally and the anterior tibial vein is divided in the middle. One can see the origin of the anterior tibial artery (ATA) and tibioperoneal trunk from the distal popliteal artery. The arteriotomy

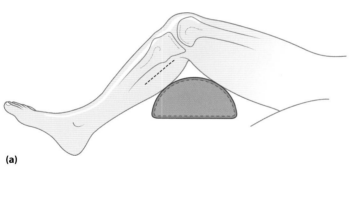
(a)

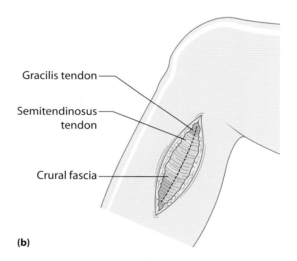
(b)

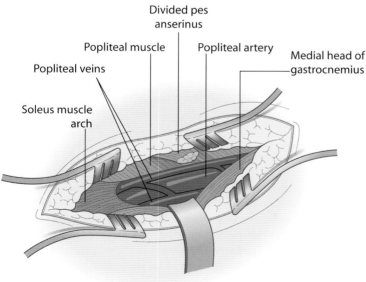
(c)

Figure 49.4 Femoral to below-knee popliteal bypass. (**a**) For medial exposure of the below-knee popliteal artery, an incision is made approximately 2 cm behind the posteromedial surface of the tibia. (**b**) The incision is continued through the subcutaneous tissue to the crural fascia, which is incised below the semitendinosus tendon. (**c**) The popliteal fossa below the knee is exposed by retracting the medial head of the gastrocnemius muscle. The popliteal artery is surrounded by paired popliteal veins that are dissected off and ligated.

incision is made in the distal popliteal artery in preparation for distal anastomosis. Proximal and distal arterial control is obtained with vessel loops. The tunneling device is passed from the popliteal fossa between the heads of the gastrocnemius muscle and posterior to the knee between the femoral condyles. It is then passed in the subsartorial space to the groin incision. The graft is passed through the tunnel maintaining proper orientation. Anastomoses proceed in the same manner as for the femoral to above-knee popliteal bypass. Proximal and distal control can be obtained with vessel loops or small vascular clamps.

Although we do not use a tourniquet for distal arterial control, some authorities advocate tourniquets for all bypasses to infrageniculate arteries. An appropriate sized tourniquet is placed around the distal thigh prior to exsanginating the leg with an Esmarch dressing.

Purported advantages include less dissection and manipulation of the target artery. Tourniquet control, however, can be problematic with heavily calcified arteries.

Anterior tibial artery bypass

With the patient supine, the leg internally rotated, and the knee flexed to 30 degrees, a vertical incision is made in the anterolateral leg midway between the tibia and fibula (**Figure 49.5a**). The incision is continued along the lateral border of the tibialis anterior muscle. A plane is developed between the tibialis anterior and extensor digitorum longus muscles allowing access to the neurovascular bundle lying on the interosseous membrane (**Figure 49.5b**). The ATA is isolated from the neurovascular bundle with attention to the deep peroneal nerve (**Figure 49.5c**).

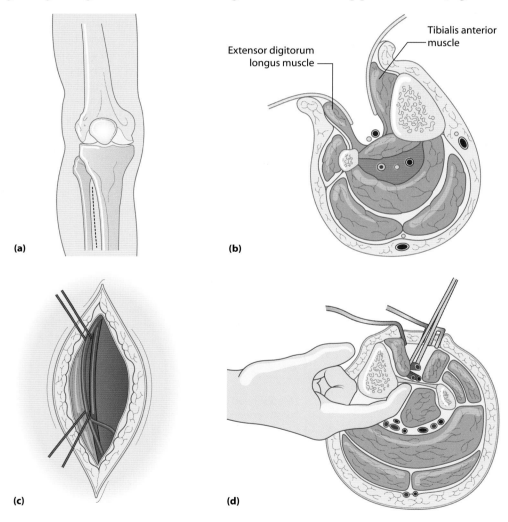

(a) (b) (c) (d)

Figure 49.5 Above-knee to anterior tibial artery (ATA) bypass. (**a**) For exposure of the ATA, an anterolateral incision is made between the tibia and fibula. Small medial incisions are also made above and below the knee for tunneling. (**b,c**) The incision is carried through the deep fascia and a plane is developed between the tibialis anterior and extensor digitorum longus muscles. The ATA lies above the interosseous membrane and can be mobilized. (**d**) A tunnel is created for passage of a vascular conduit from the medial leg through the interosseous membrane to the anterior compartment. The tunneler is introduced through the interosseous membrane under direct visualization into the anterior compartment 2 cm proximal to the level of anastomosis. A long, curved vascular clamp is then passed through the defect in the interosseous membrane and the graft is pulled from the popliteal space to the anterior compartment for anastomosis.

Tunneling of the bypass from the above-knee inflow site to the ATA is typically performed anatomically to protect the graft from wound breakdown. A medial calf exposure of the below-knee popliteal artery is conducted as described previously. From the popliteal fossa to the ATA, the tunneler is introduced through the interosseous membrane under direct visualization into the anterior compartment 2 cm proximal to the level of anastomosis (**Figure 49.5d**). The graft is pulled from the popliteal space to the anterior compartment for anastomosis. An end-to-side anastomosis is created with 6-0 polypropylene running suture.

Posterior tibial artery bypass

The posterior tibial artery can be exposed at either its proximal or distal portion. For proximal exposure, an extension of the below-knee popliteal artery is employed as a 10-cm incision is created 2 cm posterior to the medial edge of the tibia (**Figure 49.6a**). Dissection is carried through the crural fascia to the medial head of the gastrocnemius muscle, which is retracted posteriorly (**Figure 49.6b**). The soleus is then encountered; its muscle fibers, originating from the tibia, are divided to expose the underlying vessels. A complex network of venous branches overlying the posterior tibial artery are carefully divided (**Figure 49.6c**).

For distal exposure of the posterior tibial artery, the patient is placed in the supine position and the leg is externally rotated with the knee flexed at 60 degrees. A vertical incision is made at the distal tibia around the medial malleolus onto the foot. Division of the flexor retinaculum exposes the neurovascular bundle lying between flexor digitorum longus and flexor hallucis longus. The posterior tibial artery lies anterior to the tibial nerve. Grafts to the posterior tibial artery are tunneled anatomically through the popliteal fossa.

Peroneal (fibular) artery bypass

A vertical incision is made 2 cm behind the posterior border of the tibia in the middle third of the calf and extended from 10 cm. Dissection is carried through the crural fascia and the tibial attachment of the soleus is divided (**Figure 49.6b**). Posterior retraction of the soleus reveals the flexor digitorum longus; the dissection is continued into the deep posterior fascial compartment. The posterior tibial artery is often seen and should be retracted to avoid injury (**Figure 49.6c**). Deep in the incision, the peroneal vessels are located on the anterior surface of the flexor hallucis longus. Following exposure of the peroneal (fibular) artery and adequate vessel control, grafts are tunneled anatomically to the peroneal artery for distal anastomosis.

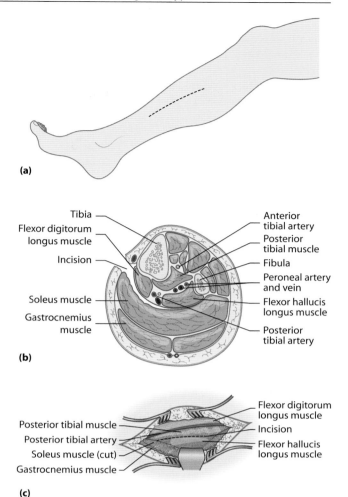

Figure 49.6 Above-knee to posterior tibial/peroneal artery bypass. (**a**) The posterior tibial and peroneal arteries are approached through an incision along the medial calf. (**b**) The posterior tibial artery is encountered between the flexor digitorum longus and soleus muscles whose muscle fibers originating from the tibia must be divided. (**c**) Once the posterior tibial artery is cleared of surrounding veins it can be controlled with silicone elastomer vessel loops. The peroneal artery is encountered deeper in the wound on the anterior surface of the flexor hallucis longus muscle. The dotted line represents the site of incision through the flexor digitorum longus muscle that must be made to expose the peroneal artery.

INTRAOPERATIVE ASSESSMENT OF INFRAINGUINAL BYPASS AND WOUND CLOSURE

Intraoperatively, a duplex Doppler provides qualitative assessment of infrainguinal bypasses by analyzing changes in velocity or spectral broadening to detect conduit defects. If there are concerns, a completion angiogram is performed with contrast injection into the hood of the proximal anastomosis.

Once the bypass has been determined successful and hemostasis is achieved with reversal of heparin, the fascia is reapproximated using absorbable suture, taking care not to close the deep fascia. Subcutaneous tissue is closed in layers, obliterating anatomic dead space. The skin is closed subcuticularly; in patients with significant edema or diabetes, the skin should be closed with running nylon suture.

COMPLICATIONS

The major early postoperative complications of infrainguinal bypass are multiple. The PREVENT III (Project or Ex-Vivo vein graft Engineering via Transfection III) study, with 1400 infrainguinal grafts in patients with CLI, reported wound complications (4.8%), graft occlusion (5.2%), amputations (1.8%), and death (2.7%).[15] Regarding early thrombosis (<30 days), the most common causes are poor conduit, kinking/twisting of the graft, or inadequate inflow/outflow. If early graft thrombosis is identified, patients should be taken to the operating room for thrombectomy and arteriography of the entire graft.

Late complications include persistent lymphedema, aneurysm, stenosis, and infection. Postoperative surveillance includes regular visits with physical examinations and duplex ultrasound. Measurement of peak systolic velocity (PSV) should be performed at 1, 3, 6, and 12 months after surgery and then every 12 months thereafter. Abnormal findings, such as a change in the ankle–brachial pressure index >0.2, increased PSV (>300 cm/s or velocity ratio >3.5), or very low velocity (<40 cm/s) warrants further investigation with angiogram.

CASE EXAMPLES

Case 1

A 61-year-old man presented with a 1-month history of tissue loss of right lower extremity. He underwent a diagnostic angiogram that revealed a distal SFA and popliteal artery occlusion at the adductor hiatus (**Figure 49.7**). There were numerous collaterals about the knee joint. The posterior tibial, peroneal, and ATA all reconstituted in the mid-calf, while only the posterior tibial artery extended onto the foot. Vein mapping showed adequate conduit of the ipsilateral GSV. A right SFA-to-posterior tibial bypass was performed with an ipsilateral reverse GSV graft resulting in symptomatic resolution.

Case 2

A 53-year-old woman presented with a 6-month history of right lower extremity rest pain. One year prior she had undergone angioplasty and stenting of her SFA for claudication and presented for a second opinion of her worsening symptoms. CTA demonstrated proximal occlusion of the SFA stent with reconstitution of the below-knee popliteal artery (**Figure 49.8**). Preoperative vein mapping demonstrated inadequate superficial vein for conduit in the upper or lower extremities. Given the absence of an autogenous conduit, a right femoral-to-below-knee popliteal bypass was performed with a 7-mm PTFE graft and a Taylor vein patch.

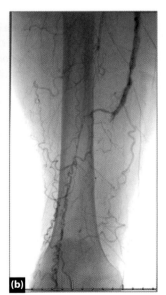 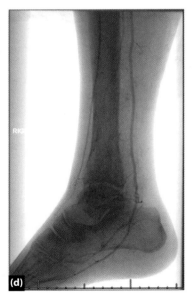

Figure 49.7 Diagnostic angiogram of 61-year-old man (case example 1). (**a**) A right lower extremity arteriogram revealed widely patent common femoral, proximal and mid-superficial femoral, and profunda femoris arteries without aneurysm. (**b**) The distal SFA appears somewhat irregular without focal stenosis and occluded at the adductor hiatus. (**c**) There are numerous collaterals about the knee joint. The popliteal artery and tibioperoneal trunk are occluded as are all three tibial vessels. The posterior tibial, peroneal, and anterior tibial arteries all reconstitute in the mid-calf. (**d**) The dorsalis pedis artery occludes at the ankle, but the posterior tibial artery extends onto the foot with a distal target for bypass confirmed.

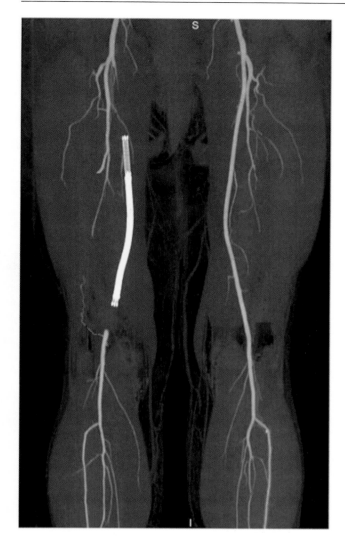

Figure 49.8 Computed tomography angiography of 53-year-old woman (case example 2). Patent common and external iliac arteries with proximal occlusion of the superficial femoral artery can be seen. There is distal reconstitution of the below-knee popliteal artery with patent three-vessel runoff to the ankle.

REFERENCES

1. Hirsch AT, Hartman L, Town R, et al. National health care costs of peripheral arterial disease in the Medicare population. *Vasc Med.* 2008;**13**:209–215.

2. Wolfe JH, Wyatt MG. Critical and subcritical ischaemia. *Eur J Vasc Endovasc Surg.* 1997;**13**:578–582.

3. Norgren L, Hiatt WR, Dormandy JA, et al. Intersociety consensus for the management of peripheral arterial disease (TASC II). *J Vasc Surg.* 2007;**45**:S5–67.

4. Klinkert P, Schepers A, Burger DH, et al. Vein versus polytetrafluoroethylene in above-knee femoropopliteal bypass grafting: five-year results of a randomized controlled trial. *J Vasc Surg.* 2003;**37**:149–155.

5. Pereira CE, Albers M, Romiti M, et al. Meta-analysis of femoropopliteal bypass grafts for lower extremity arterial insufficiency. *J Vasc Surg.* 2006;**44**:510–517.

6. Harris PL, Veith FJ, Shanik GD, et al. Prospective randomized comparison of in situ and reversed infrapopliteal vein grafts. *Br J Surg.* 1993;**80**:173–176.

7. Johnson WC, Lee KK. A comparative evaluation of polytetrafluoroethylene, umbilical vein, and saphenous vein bypass grafts for femoral-popliteal above-knee revascularization: a prospective randomized Department of Veterans Affairs cooperative study. *J Vasc Surg.* 2000;**32**:268–277.

8. Veith FJ, Gupta SK, Ascer E, et al. Six-year prospective multicenter randomized comparison of autologous saphenous vein and expanded polytetrafluoroethylene grafts in infrainguinal arterial reconstructions. *J Vasc Surg.* 1986;**3**:104–114.

9. LoGerfo FW, Paniszyn CW, Menzoian J. A new arm vein graft for distal bypass. *J Vasc Surg.* 1987;**5**:889–891.

10. Hölzenbein TJ, Pomposelli FB Jr., Miller A, et al. The upper arm basilic-cephalic loop for distal bypass grafting: technical considerations and follow-up. *J Vasc Surg.* 1995;**21**:586–592.

11. Mills JL Sr. P values may lack power: the choice of conduit for above-knee femoropopliteal bypass graft. *J Vasc Surg.* 2000;**32**:402–405.

12. Devine C, Hons B, McCollum C. Heparin-bonded Dacron or polytetrafluoroethylene for femoropopliteal bypass grafting: a multicenter trial. *J Vasc Surg.* 2001;**33**:533–539.

13. Devine C, McCollum C. Heparin-bonded Dacron or polytetrafluorethylene for femoropopliteal bypass: five-year results of a prospective randomized multicenter clinical trial. *J Vasc Surg.* 2004;**40**:924–931.

14. Stonebridge PA, Prescott RJ, Ruckley CV. Randomized trial comparing infrainguinal polytetrafluoroethylene bypass grafting with and without vein interposition cuff at the distal anastomosis. The Joint Vascular Research Group. *J Vasc Surg.* 1997;**26**:543–550.

15. Conte MS, Bandyk DF, Clowes AW, et al. Results of Prevent III: a multicenter, randomized trial of edifoligide for the prevention of vein graft failure in lower extremity bypass surgery. *J Vasc Surg.* 2006;**43**:742–751.

50

Open surgical management of visceral artery occlusive disease

JAE S. CHO

CONTENTS

INTRODUCTION

Open revascularization for chronic mesenteric ischemia (CMI) consists of bypass grafting, endarterectomy, or reimplantation. Bypass grafting, the most common method, can be constructed with either an antegrade or a retrograde configuration. Each has its advantages and disadvantages. The salient advantages of an antegrade configuration are that the supraceliac aorta provides the best inflow source, because it is usually free of atherosclerosis, and it has a higher patency rate compared with a retrograde configuration. The disadvantages are that some vascular surgeons may not be familiar with this anatomic region and there is a higher potential for hemodynamic disturbances with clamping and unclamping of the supraceliac aorta. This latter problem can be reduced by partial aortic occlusion using a side-biting clamp. A retrograde configuration is favored by some vascular surgeons because of their familiarity with this exposure and it involves a lower risk for hemodynamic disturbances. Disadvantages of a retrograde bypass include: a potential for graft kinking and occlusion; graft contact with the bowel; and compromised inflow from a diseased infrarenal aorta. The ultimate choice for bypass configuration is based on surgeon comfort, an adequate inflow source, and minimal disease at the anastomotic inflow site.

Mesenteric endarterectomy is useful when the disease is limited to the proximal segments of the target vessels or when concomitant aortic reconstruction is required. In this setting, transaortic endarterectomy with a "trapdoor" incision is most effective. Isolated reimplantation is rarely used except in the case of the inferior mesenteric artery during aortic reconstruction.

OPERATIVE TECHNIQUE

Antegrade supraceliac aortomesenteric bypass graft

A transperitoneal midline incision is made from the xiphoid process to the umbilicus. A bilateral subcostal incision with midline extension to the xiphoid process (transplant incision) may also be used, especially in patients with a large body habitus or in those with a wide costal angle. A self-retaining retractor such as an Integra® Omni-Tract® retractor (Integra LifeSciences Corporation, Plainsboro, NJ, USA) facilitates exposure. The table is placed in a slight reverse Trendelenburg position with superolateral retraction of the costal margins. The left triangular ligament of the liver is divided and the left lateral segment retracted to the patient's right. The gastrohepatic ligament is incised to enter the lesser sac. Using a nasogastric tube/echocardiography probe, the esophagus is identified and protected by retracting it to the patient's left. The esophagophrenic ligament is preserved to protect the anterior and posterior vagus nerve fibers. Attention is paid near the lesser curvature of the stomach to avoid injuries to the vagus nerves and a replaced left hepatic artery, if present.

The median arcuate ligament and interdigitating fibers of the crura are divided longitudinally to expose the aorta, which lies just posteriorly. A sufficient length of the supraceliac aorta is dissected and isolated along the anterior two-thirds of its circumference so that a side-biting clamp can be accommodated. The celiac ganglion that surrounds the celiac axis at its origin is divided. Dissection is continued caudally to the proximal few centimeters of the celiac axis (CA) (**Figure 50.1**). The inferior phrenic artery may be found in about 50% of cases and should be controlled. The left gastric artery is divided to facilitate end-to-end anastomosis to the CA. When an end-to-side anastomosis is chosen, the common or proper hepatic artery is chosen.

The superior mesenteric artery (SMA) can be exposed in its proximal segment or at the root of the mesentery, depending on the extent of disease and the patient's body habitus. When the disease is confined to the orifice of the SMA in a cachectic individual with a short distance between the CA and SMA, the latter vessel can be exposed by continuing dissection of the aorta caudally, aided by caudal retraction of the pancreas. The superior border of the pancreas is mobilized and retracted anteroinferiorly. The origin of the SMA is exposed posterior to the neck of the pancreas and the splenic vein. Care should be taken to avoid injuries to adjacent vascular structures, such as the inferior pancreaticoduodenal artery.

Exposure of the SMA at the base of the mesentery is the most frequently used approach, because this segment of the artery is more reliably disease-free and suitable as a target vessel. The transverse colon is reflected superiorly and the duodenum to the patient's right. The SMA can be easily palpated at the root of the mesentery just to the left of the reflected duodenum. If the artery is not easily localized, the ligament of Treitz is divided to mobilize the fourth portion of the duodenum and the artery can be isolated just cephalad to the duodenum. Alternatively, the middle colic artery can be traced retrograde to the SMA. In patients with CMI who have suffered weight loss, this can be done without much difficulty. About 2.5–3 cm of the vessel should be dissected circumferentially, along with jejunal branches that arise at this level.

A retropancreatic tunnel is prepared using gentle bimanual finger dissection from the supraceliac aorta and the root of the mesentery. It is safest to route the tunnel along the left side of the aorta to avoid any injury to adjacent structures. This maneuver should be performed with caution because the tunnel courses adjacent to the superior mesenteric vein and beneath the splenic vein. An umbilical tape or a silastic tubing is placed in the tunnel.

Following systemic heparinization (100 IU/kg), a bifurcated prosthetic graft is selected. The author prefers to

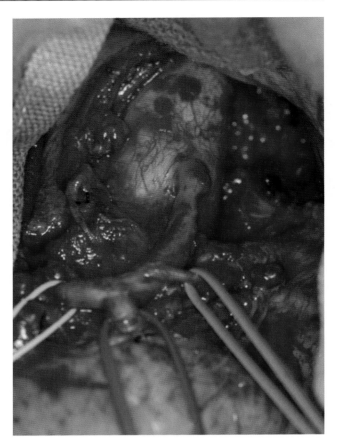

Figure 50.1 The supraceliac aorta, celiac axis, and its branches are dissected free. The blue loop encircles the left gastric artery, the red the splenic artery, and the yellow the common hepatic artery.

use a 12 × 7-mm Dacron graft. However, 12 × 6-mm or 14 × 7-mm grafts are good alternatives. Mannitol may be given (0.5 g/kg IV), especially when complete occlusion of the aorta is required. Partial occlusion of the aorta is preferred over complete occlusion, because the former prevents back-bleeding through the lumbar arteries, which may be significant. A side-biting clamp, such as a Lemole-Strong aortic clamp (Becton, Dickinson and Company, Franklin Lakes, NJ, USA), is an excellent choice in this location. When partial occlusion is not feasible, complete occlusion is obtained with a standard technique. A side-biting clamp is applied and a longitudinal aortotomy is made. The graft is placed with the main body as short as possible. Additionally, the heel of the anastomosis should be within 1 cm of the graft bifurcation and the SMA limb should be posterior/posterolateral to the CA limb to avoid kinking of the SMA limb as it enters the retropancreatic tunnel (**Figure 50.2**).

The main body of the graft is sewn end-to-side to the aorta with a 4-0 polypropylene suture. After anastomotic hemostasis is assured, the CA is divided at its origin and the proximal stump is oversewn. The anterior limb of the bifurcated graft is anastomosed end-to-end to the CA with a running 5-0 polypropylene suture. After appropriate

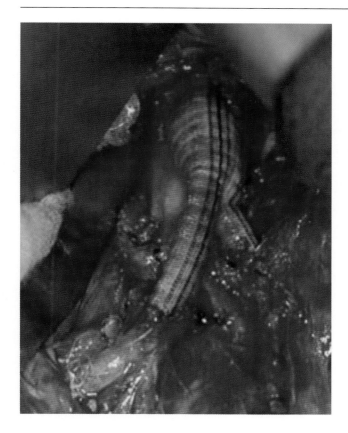

Figure 50.2 Completed antegrade aortoceliac/superior mesenteric artery (SMA) bypass. Note the posterior orientation of the SMA limb to avoid kinking as it enters the retropancreatic tunnel.

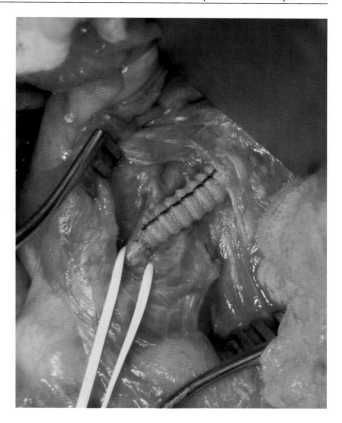

Figure 50.3 The superior mesenteric artery (SMA) limb is sewn end-to-side to the SMA.

back-bleeding and forward-bleeding, the suture line is secured and flow is restored to the CA. The SMA limb is then brought into approximation with the SMA through the retropancreatic tunnel. Control of the SMA and its branches is obtained and a longitudinal arteriotomy is made. The graft is fashioned to fit and sewn end-to-side with a running 6-0 polypropylene suture. After appropriate back-bleeding and forward-bleeding, flow is restored to the SMA (**Figure 50.3**).

When an isolated bypass to the CA is planned (such as in median arcuate ligament syndrome), a flanged 8-mm limb may be used to bypass to the CA (**Figure 50.4**). In case of gross contamination with enteric contents, an autogenous (saphenous or femoral vein) conduit or allograft should be used.

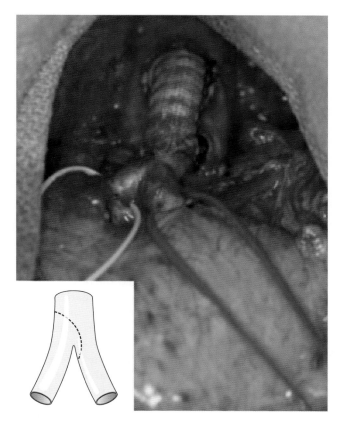

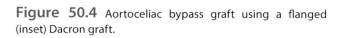

Figure 50.4 Aortoceliac bypass graft using a flanged (inset) Dacron graft.

Retrograde aortomesenteric bypass graft

The inflow source for this operation is usually the distal infrarenal aorta, common iliac, or external iliac artery, depending on the quality of the inflow vessel (atherosclerotic burden) and graft configuration. The chosen inflow vessel is isolated and dissected free with standard technique after incising the retroperitoneum. The SMA is dissected and prepared as noted earlier. The inflow anastomosis is performed first in an end-to-side fashion. The SMA anastomosis is performed in antegrade fashion, end-to-side. It is imperative to allow a gentle curve for the graft as it traverses from the inflow vessel to the target vessel to avoid kinking when the bowel is returned to its normal anatomic position within the abdomen. The graft is covered with the retroperitoneum to protect it from the bowel. Alternatively, the graft may be covered with omentum.

Trapdoor transaortic visceral endarterectomy

The patient is placed in a modified left thoracotomy position. The left hemithorax, shoulder, and arm are positioned at 70 degrees to the table while the left hip is rotated posteriorly as far as possible (usually 30 degrees off the table). Both groins should be accessible, as is the case with any aortic operation. An oblique incision is made from the 9th or 10th intercostal space (ICS) across the abdominal muscles to the umbilicus, with the distal extent to the pubis along the midline as needed. The incision may be extended more proximally as needed along the intercostal space. A self-retracting retractor is invaluable.

Exposure can be provided via the retroperitoneal or transperitoneal route, depending on the need to evaluate the viability of the intestines. The viscera are mobilized medially with the left kidney left in situ. When the atherosclerotic burden of the aorta extends beyond the origins of the renal arteries, the left kidney should be mobilized anteriorly along with the viscera. The left crus of the diaphragm is divided to expose the paravisceral aorta. Sufficient lengths of the branch vessels are isolated and dissected free. The left renal vein (LRV) is dissected and retracted caudally (**Figure 50.5a**). When more extensive endarterectomy of the pararenal aorta is needed, or when concomitant aortic resection is planned for aneurysmal disease, the left kidney is better reflected anteriorly along with the rest of the viscera.

After control is obtained of the aorta and its branches, a trapdoor aortotomy is made around the orifices of the CA and SMA (**Figure 50.5b**). The plane of endarterectomy is then developed around the visceral vessel orifices and extraction endarterectomy of these vessels is carried out. The aortotomy is closed primarily with a 4-0 polypropylene suture. On occasion, it may become necessary to extend the endarterectomy of the visceral arteries when plaque extends beyond their orifices. In such a setting, a separate arteriotomy is made in the proximal segment of

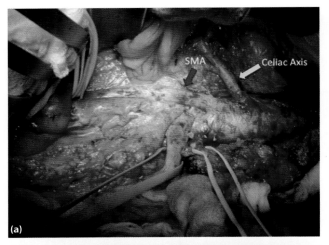

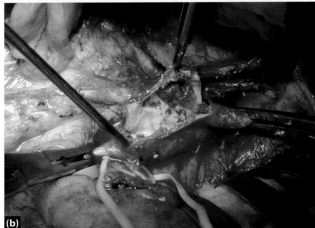

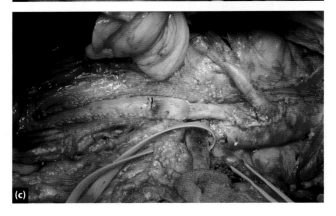

Figure 50.5 Trapdoor transaortic visceral endarterectomy. (**a**) Retroperitoneal exposure of the entire abdominal aorta, celiac axis, superior mesenteric artery (SMA), and left renal artery (yellow loop). The left kidney is left in situ; the left renal vein is encircled with a thick blue loop. (**b**) A trapdoor aortotomy is made exposing the plaque and acute thrombus at the orifice of the celiac axis. (**c**) The trapdoor aortotomy is primarily closed. A long SMA endarterectomy with patch angioplasty is also shown.

the visceral artery (usually the SMA), an endarterectomy is performed, and the artery is closed with a patch angioplasty (**Figure 50.5c**).

Thoracovisceral bypass graft

In the setting of a hostile abdomen, or in the case of inadequate inflow (such as a diseased supraceliac aorta or severe infrarenal aortoiliac occlusive disease that precludes retrograde bypass or warrants concomitant aortic reconstruction), thoracovisceral bypass grafting can be performed. The patient is positioned as described for trapdoor transaortic visceral endarterectomy. An oblique incision is made through the seventh ICS across the abdominal muscles to the umbilicus. The diaphragm is divided circumferentially. The viscera are mobilized medially as described earlier. A side-biting clamp is applied to the descending thoracic aorta and a bifurcated graft is then used to reconstruct the visceral vessels with the technique described earlier (**Figure 50.6a,b**). Once hemostasis of the proximal anastomosis is assured, the patient is systemically heparinized and the distal reconstruction completed.

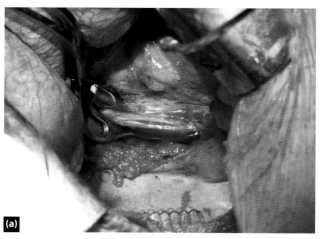

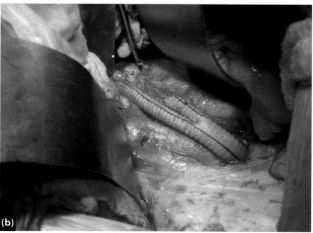

Figure 50.6 Thoracovisceral bypass graft. (**a**) A Lemole-Strong clamp (Becton, Dickinson and Company, Franklin Lakes, NJ, USA) is applied to the descending thoracic aorta for partial occlusion. (**b**) Descending thoracic aortoceliac/SMA bypass is performed.

Transabdominal medial visceral rotation (MVR)

Access to the paravisceral aorta may also be gained by MVR through a full-length midline incision. After the small bowel is reflected to the right, the left lateral peritoneal reflection is incised to reflect the left colon medially. Dissection is continued cephalad and the spleen is mobilized. If the left kidney is to be left in situ, a plane of dissection is developed anterior to the left kidney between the pancreas and the Gerota's fascia. Dissection should be kept in the correct plane to avoid bleeding and injury to the pancreas, kidney, and adrenal gland. The stomach, pancreas, spleen, and descending colon are mobilized to the right, leaving the left kidney and associated structures in situ. The left crus of the diaphragm and the triangular ligament are divided. The anterior and posterior trunks of the vagus nerve are preserved. The autonomic ganglia over the SMA and CA are freed to expose the vessels. The LRV that is crossing the aorta is mobilized to its confluence with the inferior vena cava (IVC). By retracting the LRV caudally, the origins of the renal arteries can be exposed, if needed. The left renal artery can easily be dissected to the hilum. The proximal 2–3 cm of the right renal artery can be exposed with caution by retracting the IVC to the right. The entire abdominal aorta can be mobilized by incising the loose areolar tissue along its left lateral aspect of the aorta and reflecting the entire viscera to the right. The aortic bifurcation and the iliac arteries can be exposed, if necessary (**Figure 50.7**). Visceral reconstruction, endarterectomy, or bypass grafting can be performed as described earlier.

Closure

Meticulous closure of the abdominal wall is critical to avoid leak of ascites that frequently develops after mesenteric revascularization because the bowel may weep fluid in the early postoperative period.

POSTOPERATIVE COMPLICATIONS

Visceral reperfusion syndrome that frequently occurs after mesenteric revascularization causes both local and remote organ injury, manifested by multisystem organ dysfunction. Acute respiratory distress syndrome, elevation of serum hepatic transaminase, thrombocytopenia, coagulopathy resistant to vitamin K supplementation, renal dysfunction, and prolonged postoperative ileus are commonly observed. Prolonged ventilator support and parenteral alimentation may be necessary.

Once the patient recovers, vessel patency should be interrogated with radiologic imaging, preferably computed tomography arteriography to ascertain adequacy of the reconstruction and to serve as a reference against which future studies may be compared, before the patient is discharged.

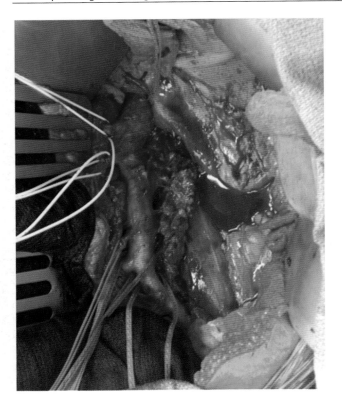

Figure 50.7 Transabdominal left medial visceral rotation, with the left kidney retracted anteriorly to expose the entire abdominal aorta and its branches (except the right renal artery) from hiatus to bifurcation. Upper white vessel loop around celiac; middle white vessel loop (somewhat loose) around superior mesenteric artery (SMA), lower white vessel loop around left renal artery; red vessel loop around inferior mesenteric artery. The three umbilical tapes are around the distal aorta just above bifurcation and both common iliac arteries. Note that the exposure is not much different from that of retroperitoneal route shown in **Figure 50.5** except that only the origin of the SMA can be exposed when the left kidney is reflected anteriorly.

CONCLUSION

Significant advances have been made over the past 30 years in the management of CMI. The operation must be individualized to fit the patient's anatomy and risk factors. Not every patient requires complete revascularization, whether it be all mesenteric vessels or concomitant mesenteric and aortic reconstruction, unless it is necessary (i.e., aortic occlusion, symptomatic aortoiliac occlusive disease, or large aortic aneurysm). Unlike in the past, hybrid procedures may obviate the need for aortic reconstruction while minimizing postoperative morbidity.

SUGGESTED READING

Stoney RJ, Effeney DJ. *Wylie's Atlas of Vascular Surgery: Thoracoabdominal Aorta and Its Branches.* Philadelphia, PA: J.B. Lippincott Company; 1992.

Foley MI, Moneta GL, Abou-Zamzam AM Jr., et al. Revascularization of the superior mesenteric artery alone for treatment of intestinal ischemia. *J Vasc Surg.* 2000;**32**:37–47.

Stoney RJ, Wylie EJ. Recognition and surgical management of visceral ischemic syndromes. *Ann Surg.* 1966;**164**:714–722.

Reilly LM, Ramos TK, Murray SP, et al. Optimal exposure of the proximal abdominal aorta: a critical appraisal of transabdominal medial visceral rotation. *J Vasc Surg.* 1994;**19**:375–389.

Harward TR, Brooks DL, Flynn TC, et al. Multiple organ dysfunction after mesenteric artery revascularization. *J Vasc Surg.* 1993;**18**:459–467.

Jimenez JG, Huber TS, Ozaki CK, et al. Durability of antegrade synthetic aortomesenteric bypass for chronic mesenteric ischemia. *J Vasc Surg.* 2002;**35**: 1078–1084.

Cho JS, Carr JA, Jacobsen G, et al. Long-term outcome following mesenteric artery reconstruction: a 37-year experience. *J Vasc. Surg* 2002;**35**;453–60

51

Truncal vascular trauma

DANON GARRIDO, JOSEPH RABIN, AND SHAHAB TOUR SAVADKOHI

CONTENTS

INTRODUCTION

Penetrating traumatic injury to the heart, great vessels, and major abdominal vasculature is a challenge for the surgeon. Patients often present hemodynamically unstable with life-threatening injuries that require emergent intervention. The variability of these injuries leads to additional uncertainty for surgeons in how to best manage these patients. On arrival to the trauma unit, all patients should be assessed in accordance with the Advanced Trauma Life Support (ATLS) guidelines. The airway must be secured quickly and systematically, adequate breathing and ventilation stabilized, life-threatening hemorrhage located and controlled, large-bore intravenous access obtained for resuscitation, vital signs measured, and obvious neurologic deficits identified as the patient is exposed. A Focused Abdominal Sonogram for Trauma (FAST) examination is often performed early to help identify potential sources of active bleeding. This standard primary survey in the context of the underlying mechanism of injury helps identify life-threatening injuries and enables rapid treatment and hemorrhage control to be efficiently initiated. In general, patients who present with hemodynamic instability and shock following a penetrating injury require emergent surgical intervention.

DAMAGE CONTROL SURGERY FOR NONCOMPRESSIBLE TORSO HEMORRHAGE (NCTH)

Damage control surgery describes a staged or delayed approach to the definitive repair of injuries to limit or reverse physiologic deterioration and subsequent consequences on patients who are exsanguinating. The most important resuscitative maneuver available for patients with NCTH and severe shock is thoracic aortic occlusion. The effects of aortic clamping performed through a left anterolateral thoracotomy (resuscitative thoracotomy) are basically to slow distal hemorrhage and improve cerebral

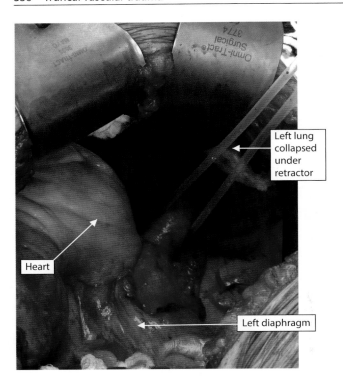

Figure 51.1 Left thoracotomy for control of descending thoracic aorta.

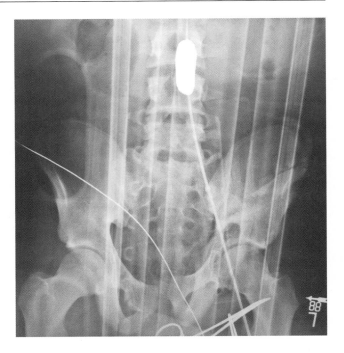

Figure 51.2 Resuscitative endovascular balloon occlusion of aorta for severe pelvic and abdominal hemorrhage through left femoral access. The balloon is inflated between the third and fourth lumbar vertebral bodies.

and myocardial perfusion (**Figure 51.1**). In addition, lung parenchymal bleeding can be compressed, air leaks from bronchial injuries controlled, and the pericardium opened to release any tamponade. This maneuver can be applied to patients with tense hemoperitoneum to control inflow to the abdomen.

RESUSCITATIVE BALLOON OCCLUSION OF THE AORTA

The physiologic effects of resuscitative thoracotomy with aortic clamping can also be accomplished with a compliant endovascular balloon, resuscitative balloon occlusion of the aorta (REBOA) without the physiologic burden of a thoracotomy (**Figure 51.2**). Technically, access can be gained on the femoral or axillary artery under ultrasound guidance or direct cutdown. A 150–180-cm, 0.35-inch guidewire is advanced and exchanged for a 180-cm stiff wire (Amplatz Stiff Wire, Cook Medical Inc., Bloomington, IN, USA). The 5-Fr sheath is exchanged for a 12-Fr sheath and a 32mm Coda® Balloon Catheter (Cook Medical Inc.) is inflated in the supraceliac aorta. Exactly how long the balloon can be occlusive without causing irreversible vital organ or neurologic damage is unknown. The authors' recommendation is to maintain balloon occlusion for the time needed to stabilize the patient or obtain the desired operative exposure, as long as these efforts are performed expeditiously.

TEMPORARY FLOW STABILIZATION

A different way of maintaining physiologic homeostasis is the restoration of blood flow across a significant vascular disruption with a temporary vascular shunt. These devices allow the patient to undergo either repair of concomitant injuries (e.g., orthopedic fixation), a damage control procedure, or transport to a higher-level facility to undergo definitive repair of the injured vessels. Inserting a vascular shunt, although seemingly straightforward, has the potential to cause injury if not done properly. The steps for shunt placement are well-outlined in Chapter 52 (*Extremity Vascular Trauma*).

PENETRATING INTRATHORACIC INJURY

Emergent thoracic exploration is indicated for patients in shock following a penetrating thoracic injury, for those with chest tube output >1000–1500 cc immediately after insertion, continued chest tube output or ongoing bleeding >200–300 cc per hour, massive air leak, or evidence of cardiac tamponade.[1,2] High chest tube output is indicative of continued bleeding that requires surgical control, while a large air leak is concerning for a major tracheobronchial injury, which is fully evaluated with the addition of bronchoscopy. Up to one-third of patients undergoing surgical exploration for traumatic hemorrhage also require a pulmonary resection because of associated parenchymal injury.[3]

Approaches

Managing patients with severe chest trauma requires an understanding of thoracic surgical approaches that can be effectively employed in unstable, actively bleeding patients. The first issue is to determine the most appropriate incision to use; the second is to determine what procedure to perform. Each surgical exposure has advantages and disadvantages. Whichever approach is used, it should be versatile enough to address potential injuries in adjacent locations including the neck and abdomen. Standard options include the following.[4,5]

ANTEROLATERAL THORACOTOMY

This is the most common approach for the unstable patient undergoing an emergent resuscitative procedure. It provides rapid access to the thorax with good exposure to the hilum and avoids the time-consuming positioning associated with the traditional posterolateral thoracotomy. It is also versatile enough to allow for a concomitant exploratory laparotomy. Limited exposure of the heart, entire lung, and posterior mediastinum, especially the esophagus, are its drawbacks. The incision is made in the inframammary crease with division of the pectoralis muscles followed by the intercostal muscles within the desired (usually fourth) intercostal space (ICS). The internal mammary artery and vein are in close proximity medially and should be preserved if possible.

CLAMSHELL THORACOTOMY

A clamshell thoracotomy is performed by extending an anterolateral thoracotomy across the midline into an anterolateral thoracotomy on the contralateral side. It provides excellent exposure of the anterior mediastinum, and both lungs and pleural cavities. In cutting across the sternum, a Lebsche knife, sternal saw, or Gigli saw may be used followed by ligation of the internal mammary vessels bilaterally.

POSTEROLATERAL THORACOTOMY

This incision provides the best exposure of the thorax, but requires time-consuming lateral positioning. It should only be used if the patient is hemodynamically stable and the injury is confined to the ipsilateral hemithorax. Single-lung isolation is often desired and obtained through placement of either a double-lumen endobronchial tube or bronchial blocker by anesthesia. The thorax is usually entered in the fifth ICS.

STERNOTOMY

This incision provides excellent exposure to the anterior mediastinum and rapid access to the heart and great vessels. The standard incision is carried down from the suprasternal notch to the xiphoid process. The sternal midline is identified and divided with a sternal saw; a retractor is placed after controlling sternal edge bleeding.

PENETRATING CARDIAC INJURY

Patients present following civilian gunshot wounds, stab wounds, and rarely following shotgun wounds (e.g., hunting trauma, gang-related violence), impalements, or rib fractures. A direct hit from a high-velocity military rifle is usually immediately fatal. Hemodynamic status may range from stable to hypotensive to frank cardiac arrest. If the injury caused a large pericardial defect, the patient may exsanguinate into the left pleural cavity with a massive hemothorax. Patients with an essentially intact pericardium may develop cardiac tamponade. Tamponade may prevent a massive hemothorax and paradoxically produce a brief protective interval. However, if not quickly corrected, tamponade will cause cardiac failure and death. Cardiac injury must be ruled out in any patient with a penetrating injury to the "box" region, defined as the area inferior to the clavicles, superior to the costal margin, and medial to the midclavicular line. Injuries outside the "box" may also cause cardiac damage. Patients need rapid transport to a trauma center, prompt assessment, and resuscitation based on the ATLS guidelines, and a FAST examination to detect a pericardial collection. Stable patients can undergo a structured workup, while unstable patients should go directly to the operating room. Those in cardiac arrest require immediate intervention and may benefit from a salvage emergency thoracotomy.

The left anterolateral thoracotomy is the incision of choice for patients in extremis. If necessary, this incision can be extended across the sternum into a clamshell thoracotomy that provides complete exposure of the mediastinum, pericardium, and bilateral thoracic cavities. A sternotomy provides excellent mediastinal exposure and can be easily performed. Atrial injuries can be controlled with a vascular clamp and repaired with 4-0 polypropylene suture, while the right ventricle can be digitally controlled and repaired with a horizontal mattress suture. The sutures may be buttressed with pledgets if necessary.[6]

Injuries adjacent to the coronary arteries can be quite challenging because the repair may narrow or occlude the native artery. Repair sutures should be placed under the coronary vessel, in a horizontal mattress fashion, and tied. Actual coronary artery injuries are not usually difficult to locate due to their superficial location. Distal coronary artery injury and injuries to the diagonal or obtuse marginal branches rarely cause global dysfunction; they can usually be ligated without development of significant cardiac failure. However, a proximal coronary artery injury, especially the left anterior descending artery, which is associated with severe cardiogenic shock, may require emergent bypass. Mild cardiac dysfunction associated with coronary injury may be managed with an intra-aortic balloon pump to provide afterload reduction and improved cardiac output in the hope of avoiding an emergent coronary artery bypass.[6,7] Most valvular injuries are discovered while evaluating a new murmur heard following the initial repair. Rarely, a septal defect is created and in such cases elective repair is often possible.

PENETRATING GREAT VESSEL INJURY

Penetrating injuries to the great vessels are found in approximately 5% of thoracic gunshot wounds and 2% of thoracic stab wounds.[8] Many patients arrive to definitive care in hemorrhagic shock requiring rapid treatment and emergent surgery for hemorrhage control. Some patients arrive with stable hemodynamics and often remain stable throughout their workup. Stable patients can undergo imaging studies, such as computed tomography angiography (CTA), to help define the injury and plan an optimal operative strategy for repair. Unstable patients can undergo a sternotomy with supraclavicular or neck extension enabling rapid control of proximal great vessels bilaterally, although many favor a left anterolateral thoracotomy to control the proximal left subclavian artery (SCA). The internal mammary artery should always be inspected to rule out injury as a cause of hemorrhagic shock.[9]

The role of endovascular repair of great vessel injuries continues to evolve. This minimally invasive option eliminates the need for an extensive open surgical procedure along with its associated risks. Access can be obtained via the femoral or brachial arteries. Factors against using an endovascular approach include: inadequate proximal or distal landing zones; hemodynamic instability; other injuries in the same region requiring exploration; and vascular occlusion or transection preventing guidewire traversal of the traumatic lesion. A final consideration is the use of an endovascular proximal artery occlusion balloon in conjunction with open surgery. This approach allows rapid proximal hemorrhage control with minimal dissection to facilitate a standard open repair.

Brachiocephalic artery (BCA) injury

The standard approach for a BCA injury is via a sternotomy. In the setting of penetrating injury, there is often concomitant injury to the brachiocephalic vein; ligation and division of this vein helps control hemorrhage and enhances exposure. A few select patients with only limited BCA injury can be managed with primary repair using 4-0 polypropylene suture (**Figure 51.3**). However, most patients should be managed with the "bypass exclusion technique." This involves sewing a 10-mm Dacron graft to the ascending aorta using a partially occluding aortic clamp for the proximal anastomosis. Distally, the graft is sewn to the BCA beyond the point of injury after the artery has been divided between two clamps. Ideally, the distal BCA clamp should not interfere with the bifurcation of the carotid and SCAs so that collateral perfusion is preserved between the SCA and carotid artery while proximal inflow is clamped. Once the distal anastomosis is completed, the proximal BCA is oversewn. A similar approach is used for the management of proximal left carotid artery injuries that cannot be primarily repaired.[10]

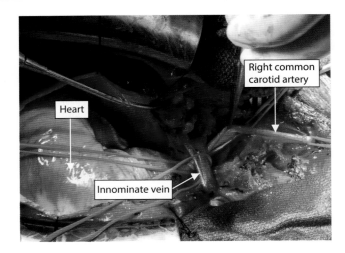

Figure 51.3 Stab wound to posteromedial wall of brachiocephalic artery (BCA). The patient's head is to the right. The forceps are pulling the edges of the lacerated artery wall apart. The red vessel loop to the left is cinched down around the proximal BCA for proximal control. On the right, distal control of the right common carotid artery is provided by a red vessel loop, while in the background the right subclavian artery is controlled by a red vessel loop.

SCA injury

Most SCA injuries require repair with either an interposition graft or an endovascular stent graft.[11] The challenge to open repair is obtaining adequate exposure. The standard approach to a right SCA injury is via sternotomy with a supraclavicular or cervical extension. For a left SCA, many authorities advocate proximal control via a left anterolateral thoracotomy through the third or fourth ICS and a supraclavicular incision as necessary. Others (including the authors' group) find that a sternotomy with a distal supraclavicular extension provides adequate exposure.[9] Because of the challenging location, initial hemorrhage control can be either via direct digital compression or insertion of a Foley balloon catheter through the injury tract to tamponade the bleeding. The injury itself is managed directly with either primary repair, patch angioplasty, or interposition grafting. Options for an interposition graft include prosthetic graft or autologous vein, which is preferred in the setting of a contaminated wound. A final option for unstable patients who would not tolerate a vascular reconstruction is to follow damage control principles and place a temporary shunt. Patients can be further resuscitated in the intensive care unit and returned to the operating room for definitive repair after their physiology has been optimized.

PULMONARY AND VENOUS INJURY

The superior and inferior vena cava (IVC), and pulmonary artery and veins, often cause a significant amount of hemorrhage despite being low-pressure systems. Repair can be challenging because of the weaker structural integrity of their walls. Control can be obtained with partially occluding intestinal Allis or Babcock clamps and the injury repaired by running a 4-0 polypropylene suture under the clamps. Opening the pericardium to obtain more proximal control can also be helpful. While the vena cava and main pulmonary artery must be repaired, a pulmonary vein or lobar pulmonary artery can be ligated with subsequent pulmonary lobar resection. In cases involving a significant hilar injury, a pneumonectomy may be required followed by aggressive support for subsequent right heart failure. Such support includes aggressive use of inotropic and afterload-reducing agents with occasional need for extracorporeal membrane oxygenation. The azygos vein can also be a source of large-volume hemorrhage that can be quickly life-threatening. It is best managed with rapid suture ligation.

INTRA-ABDOMINAL VASCULAR INJURY

Blunt abdominal vascular trauma is produced by local tissue compression or acceleration/deceleration resulting in significant shear forces that can disrupt the normal integrity of the layers of the blood vessel wall (intima, media, and adventitia). Intra-abdominal hemorrhage from a vascular injury is often associated with a retroperitoneal hematoma. Such hematomas are categorized according to their location: zone 1 is the midline retroperitoneum (aorta, IVC); zone 2 the upper lateral retroperitoneum (the renal vessels); and zone 3 the pelvic retroperitoneum (the iliac vessels and pelvic bone fracture) (**Figure 51.4**). In general, retroperitoneal hematomas following penetrating injury are routinely explored, while only zone 1 injuries from blunt trauma are explored (**Figure 51.5**). Recently, however, this practice has been questioned in light of successful observation of stable, nonexpanding zone 2 hematomas away from the renal hila, and in cases of stable retrohepatic hematomas that once opened can easily lead to exsanguination. While early adoption of REBOA may be useful in select cases to initially control hemorrhage, the operative approach to these life-threatening injuries is to rapidly control and stop bleeding through a midline laparotomy. The approach and appropriate techniques for managing such challenging injuries depend on the location of the injury.

In cases involving the superior aspect of zone 1, an injury to the aorta or one its main branches, including the celiac axis, superior mesenteric artery (SMA), or proximal renal arteries is of primary concern. The ideal approach is to perform a left-sided medial visceral rotation (MVR; e.g., Mattox maneuver), which exposes the entire abdominal aorta and its major branches from the hiatus to the bifurcation. If there is active hemorrhage that requires more rapid proximal control, supraceliac control can be obtained by opening the lesser omentum between the inferior edge of the liver and distal esophagus. The esophagus and stomach are retracted to the left, while the liver is retracted to the right. The right crus of the diaphragm is divided, bluntly if necessary, and the aorta exposed and clamped. An aortic compressor or other form of manual compression can also provide temporary aortic control at this proximal location.

The inferior aspect of zone 1 is concerning for injuries to the infrarenal aorta or IVC. In such a case, a standard inframesocolic approach, retracting the transverse colon superiorly and the small bowel to the right side, provides exposure of the retroperitoneum over these vessels, which is then opened. On identifying the left renal vein, the underlying infrarenal aorta can be rapidly dissected free and clamped for proximal control. For zone 1 injuries with predominantly right-sided hematomas or after exploration has ruled out an aortic injury, trauma to the IVC is of concern. Access to these injuries is obtained by performing a right-sided MVR (Cattell–Braasch maneuver). The right-sided parietal peritoneum is divided along the white line of Toldt from the cecum to the hepatic flexure. The cecum/right colon is then retracted medially and superiorly providing exposure to the IVC, iliac vessels, and right renal vasculature. If more proximal control is required,

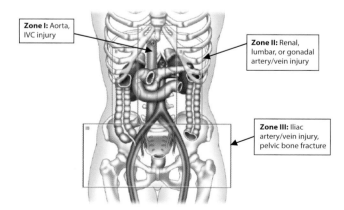

Figure 51.4 Retroperitoneal hematoma zones.

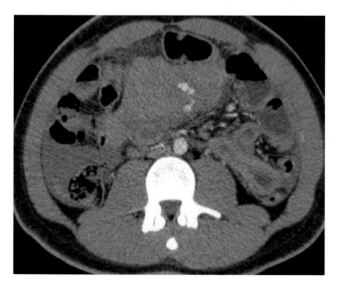

Figure 51.5 Zone 1 hematoma from visceral blunt injury.

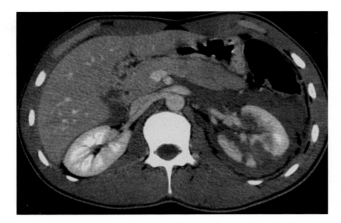

Figure 51.6 Superior mesenteric artery (SMA) interposition graft with greater saphenous vein performed to repair an SMA dissection/occlusion after a motor vehicle accident with blunt abdominal trauma. (The patient's head is to the right, their feet to the left.)

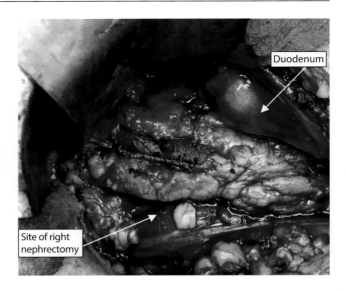

Figure 51.7 Left renal trauma with a zone 2 hematoma.

a Kocher maneuver can be performed, which also provides good pancreatic exposure.

After adequate exposure has been achieved, specific injuries are identified and managed. Injuries to the aorta can often be repaired primarily with 3-0 or 4-0 polypropylene suture. Injuries to the celiac axis or its branches should either be repaired primarily, if technically feasible, or in most cases simply ligated. Proximal SMA injuries are managed with either a shunt for cases requiring a rapid damage control procedure or more definitively with an interposition graft (**Figure 51.6**). Another option for proximal injuries involves ligating the vessel proximal to the injury and then reconstructing it with a graft from the distal aorta. In cases of IVC injuries, obtaining control proximally and distally to the injury can be accomplished with sponge sticks or with intestinal Allis or Babcock clamps to align the edges of the injury. The defect is then repaired, either directly or under the clamps, with a running 4-0 or 5-0 polypropylene suture. In cases of exsanguinating hemorrhage, the infrarenal IVC can be ligated.

Zone 2 injuries are concerning for renal and renal vascular injuries. While small injuries can be repaired primarily, more complex injuries associated with active bleeding and other intra-abdominal trauma are most prudently managed with a nephrectomy as long as a contralateral kidney can be identified (**Figure 51.7**).

Zone 3 injuries often involve the iliac vasculature. As proximal and distal control is obtained, direct pressure on the site of injury should be applied to control hemorrhage. Exposure is obtained with an MVR, and if uncertain as to which side to mobilize, a right-sided approach (Cattell–Braasch maneuver) is used since it provides excellent exposure of both proximal iliac vessels, the entire right iliac system, the IVC, and the distal aorta. After obtaining proximal and distal control, the iliac arteries are managed with either primary repair for

a simple isolated injury, an interposition graft if more significant and minimal contamination exists, an extra-anatomic femorofemoral bypass in situations with significant contamination, or a shunt if the patient requires a damage control procedure. Iliac venous injuries are often difficult to control and should only be repaired with a simple suture closure if it can be easily accomplished; otherwise, ligation should be undertaken. Zone 3 hematomas, from pelvic fracture, are often managed with external fixation of pelvic bones and endovascular coil embolization of internal iliac branches.

Operative management of bleeding from the portal-retrohepatic area (sometimes referred to as zone 4) is fraught with difficulty. Control of bleeding from the retrohepatic vena cava is especially challenging and is associated with high mortality. Contained hematomas should be left undisturbed, and expanding lesions should be packed when first encountered. Complete mobilization of the liver by division of the suspensory ligaments, including the right triangular, coronary, and falciform ligaments, provides some mobility to access the retrohepatic portion of the IVC. However, attempts to mobilize the liver in this region usually result in increased bleeding from the retrohepatic injury, as torque on the liver and IVC may increase the size of the laceration. Much has been written in the literature regarding the use of intracaval shunts (large-caliber chest tubes inserted through the right atrial appendage into the infrarenal IVC and secured with Rummel tourniquets above and below the injury site) to control and treat these injuries. While theoretically appealing, the authors have found that practically speaking this maneuver is almost always associated with mortality and have therefore abandoned its use.

For portal vein injuries, local proximal and distal control is obtained with the assistance of direct compression (sponge sticks), while dissecting the vein free from the hepatic artery and bile duct. Once the injury is visualized, it can be gently grasped with Allis clamps and mobilized to allow suture repair. Injuries to the proximal portal vein or distal superior mesenteric vein (SMV) may require division of the pancreas for successful control and repair. Temporary shunts should be considered for portal and SMV injuries in the subset of unstable patients whose injury anatomy is such that a shunt can be inserted without causing further damage. In this situation, the authors use a very short segment of an Argyle™ shunt (28-Fr for the portal vein; Medtronic, Minneapolis, MN, USA), which is carefully inserted through the defect and held in place proximally and distally with vessel loop tourniquets.

POSTOPERATIVE CARE AND COMPLICATIONS

Given the significant physiologic responses often seen after severe truncal trauma, postoperative care must be organized with a coherent team effort. Early mortality is usually due to ongoing hemorrhage from either unrecognized injury or inadequate control of the known injury site; hemodynamic monitoring for bleeding and other complications is the key to postoperative management. Complications of REBOA can be divided between access site injury and ischemia/reperfusion-induced organ damage. Lower extremity pulses and compartments should be monitored frequently for the first 24 hours along with serum lactate, creatine phosphokinase levels, and liver function tests. Abdominal compartment syndrome is another complication of torso trauma that needs to be monitored frequently and treated promptly with surgical decompression. Delayed mortality of patients with truncal trauma is usually because of uncontrolled sepsis from hollow organ injuries. Source control with effective surgical repair, surgical drainage, and supportive antibiotics are important post-trauma management steps that can improve overall mortality and morbidity.

CASE EXAMPLE

A 31-year-old man was brought to the trauma bay after sustaining several stab wounds to his abdomen and right flank during a gang street fight. He arrived with a patent airway; lungs were clear to auscultation and he had a systolic blood pressure of 80 mmHg. He partially responded to resuscitative crystalloid fluid and blood product transfusion. His primary survey revealed several wounds in his abdominal wall. A rapid trauma, whole-body CTA showed a grade II splenic laceration and right kidney hilar blush with perihilar hematoma. Bedside REBOA was performed to reduce hemorrhage and the patient was taken to the operating room for an exploratory laparotomy. Cattel–Braasch and Kocher maneuvers were performed to expose the right renal hilum and to explore a right-sided

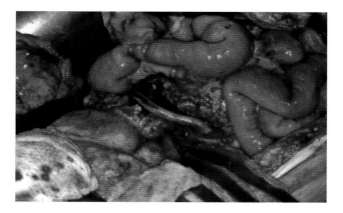

Figure 51.8 Lateral repair of inferior vena cava injury following right nephrectomy in a 31-year-old man (case example). (The patient's head is to the left, their feet to the right.)

zone 1 and 2 retroperitoneal hematoma. Massive bleeding was encountered from both the IVC and renal vessels. Proximal and distal control of the IVC injury was accomplished with sponge sticks. A right nephrectomy was rapidly performed to control renal hilar bleeding and to create better exposure of the IVC injury. The IVC venotomy was extended to explore the posterior wall, where a second laceration was encountered and repaired. The anterior venotomy was then closed with a running 4-0 polypropylene suture (**Figure 51.8**). No other zone 1 lesion was identified. The splenic injury had no active bleeding and no intervention was performed. At the end of the operation, the patient was hemodynamically stable and the REBOA catheter was removed.

REFERENCES

1. Meredith JW, Hoth JJ. Thoracic trauma: when and how to intervene. *Surg Clin North Am.* 2007;**87**:95–118.
2. Demetriades D, Velmahos GC. Penetrating injuries of the chest: indications for operation. *Scand J Surg.* 2002;**91**:41–45.
3. Huh J, Wall MW Jr., Estrera AL, et al. Surgical management of traumatic pulmonary injury. *Am J Surg.* 2003;**186**:620–624.
4. DuBose JA, O'Connor JV, Scalea TM. Lung, trachea, and esophagus. In: Moore EE, Feliciano DV, Mattox KL, eds. *Trauma.* 7th ed. New York: McGraw Hill; 2013. pp. 468–484.
5. Rabin J. The lungs. In: Scalea TM, ed. *The Shock Trauma Manual of Operative Techniques.* New York: Springer Science; 2015. pp. 157–172.
6. Kang N, Hsee L, Rizoli S, et al. Penetrating cardiac injury: overcoming the limits set by Nature. *Injury.* 2009;**40**:919–927.
7. Wall MJ Jr., Mattox KL, Chen CD, et al. Acute management of complex cardiac injuries. *J Trauma.* 1997;**42**:905–912.

8. Søreide K. Epidemiology of major trauma. *Br J Surg.* 2009;**96**:697–698.

9. O'Connor JV, Scalea TM. Penetrating thoracic great vessel injury: impact of admission hemodynamics and preoperative imaging. *J Trauma.* 2010; **68**:834–837.

10. Mattox KL, Wall MJ Jr., Lemaire S. Thoracic great vessel injury. In: Feliciano DV, Mattox KL, Moore EE, eds. *Trauma.* 6th ed. New York: McGraw Hill; 2008. pp. 589–603.

11. Carrick MM, Morrison CA, Pham HQ, et al. Modern management of traumatic subclavian artery injuries: a single institution's experience in the evolution of endovascular repair. *Am J Surg.* 2010;**199**:28–34.

52

Extremity vascular trauma

DANON GARRIDO, SHAHAB TOUR SAVADKOHI, AND RAJABRATA SARKAR

CONTENTS

INTRODUCTION

Unlike occlusive disease, extremity vascular trauma occurs mostly in young healthy individuals. As a result, collateral circulation is usually undeveloped and injury to an axial vessel may result in significant ischemia and limb loss. Signs and symptoms of arterial injury have been classically defined as either hard or soft. Hard signs include: obvious pulsatile bleeding; absent distal pulse; expanding hematoma; and arterial thrill or bruit over or close to the site of suspected arterial injury. Soft signs include: a history of significant hemorrhage; diminished distal pulse compared to the contralateral side; distal neurologic abnormalities; and proximity of a vessel to the wound or bone fragments. In the presence of hard signs, it is appropriate to proceed directly to the operating room without further workup. Performance of Doppler-derived ankle–brachial pressure indexes (ABPIs) is the easiest way to screen for vascular injuries. For lower extremities, if the ABPI is ≥1.0 and there is no pulse deficit, then the risk of vascular injury is defined as low. For all practical purposes, in

any instance in which the ABPI for an extremity is <1.0, there is a significant risk for arterial injury and additional imaging should be obtained.[1] Several orthopedic injuries are associated with a high risk of injury to an associated vessel. In this setting, the index of suspicion for vascular injury should be high (**Table 52.1**).

Table 52.1 Vascular injuries associated with orthopedic injuries

Orthopedic injury	Vascular injury
Supracondylar humerus fracture	Brachial artery with associated ischemic contracture
Elbow dislocation	Brachial artery
Distal femoral fracture	Superficial femoral artery fracture Popliteal artery
Posterior dislocation of the knee	Popliteal artery
Tibial plateau fracture	Popliteal artery Tibioperoneal trunk

IMAGING MODALITIES IN THE EVALUATION OF EXTREMITY VASCULAR TRAUMA

Color-flow duplex, computed tomography (CT), and angiography are the primary modalities used in the evaluation of extremity injury when suspicion exists. Color-flow duplex is inexpensive and the examination can be performed at the bedside without the need for contrast CT angiography (CTA). It provides rapid and detailed information on extremity blood vessels and surrounding anatomic components and has a high sensitivity (93%) and specificity (95%) in the evaluation of extremity trauma.[2] Angiography is the gold standard in the evaluation of suspected vascular trauma. It should be selectively used on patients with soft signs and an abnormal ABPI in lower extremity traumatic injuries. It is particularly useful in the setting of suspected junctional zone vascular injuries of the subclavian (SCA) and iliac arteries. In these cases, angiography provides a rapid diagnosis along with a direct pathway to definitive endovascular intervention.[3]

TREATMENT OPTIONS

Treatment is dependent on the severity of the injury, the status of the affected extremity, and the overall status of the patient. Nonocclusive arterial injuries, including pseudoaneurysms, intimal flaps, stenosis/spasm, and arteriovenous fistulas may be managed nonoperatively if the disruption is not flow-limiting. Anticoagulant or antiplatelet therapy should be considered in contained flap or dissection-type injuries, and prompt angiography with endovascular or open intervention should be performed if ischemic symptoms develop. For those requiring operative intervention for ischemia or hemorrhage, one must also consider the "salvageability" of the extremity and the stability of the patient before undertaking definitive

vascular repair. In cases of a mangled extremity, primary amputation may be the best option.

ASSESSMENT OF THE MANGLED EXTREMITY AND PRIMARY AMPUTATION

A mangled extremity is defined as an extremity with a complex injury that involves the soft tissue, bone, nerve, and vasculature. There are several methods available to calculate the degree of injury and associated outcome after attempted reconstruction. In the authors' practice, the Mangled Extremity Severity Score (MESS) is used (**Table 52.2**). A MESS score of <4 predicts salvage with 100% accuracy and a score of ≥7 predicts amputation with 100% accuracy. In severe cases, a primary amputation may lead to a superior functional outcome and avoids the misdirection of care when other life-threatening injuries should take priority. The decision to amputate is usually dictated by the degree of soft tissue injury, Gustilo open fracture classification, and the resources available to accomplish and maintain a complex extremity reconstruction (such as an intensive care unit (ICU)), and the presence of other life-threatening injuries.[3]

DAMAGE CONTROL AND TEMPORIZING MEASURES

Patients too unstable for definitive vascular repair include those presenting with nonresponsive hemodynamic instability, coagulopathy, acidosis, hypothermia, higher-priority life-threatening injuries, unstable orthopedic fractures, and large contaminated wounds where there is insufficient tissue to provide immediate graft coverage. In these patients, damage control maneuvers should be undertaken.

Table 52.2 Mangled Extremity Scoring System (MESS)

Injury type	Characteristics	MESS score
Skeletal/soft-tissue injury	Low-energy (stab wound, simple fracture, pistol gunshot wound)	1
	Medium-energy (open or multiple fractures, dislocation)	2
	High-energy (high-speed MVA or rifle GSW)	3
	Very-high-energy (high-speed trauma + gross contamination)	4
Limb ischemia	A pulsatile limb without signs of ischemia	0
	Pulse reduced or absent but perfusion normal	1[a]
	Pulseless, paresthesias, diminished capillary refill	2[a]
	Cool, paralyzed, insensate, numb	3[a]
Shock	Systolic blood pressure always >90 mmHg	0
	Hypotensive transiently	1
	Persistent hypotension	2
Age, years	<30	0
	>30–50	1
	>50	2

[a] Multiply by 2 if injury >6 hours. GSW: gunshot wound; MVA: motor vehicle accident.

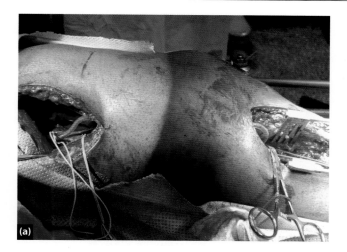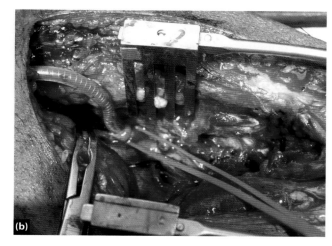

Figure 52.1 An intraluminal (Sundt™, Integra LifeSciences Corporation, Plainsboro, NJ. USA) shunt was placed between the above-knee and below-knee popliteal arteries in a patient with popliteal artery injury. (**a**) Intraluminal shunt in the below-knee popliteal artery. (**b**) The shunt is held in place with a vessel loop tourniquet.

Temporary intravascular shunts allow for rapid restoration of distal limb perfusion when immediate vascular reconstruction is not possible. When an arterial injury is identified, thrombectomy, regional heparin, and temporary shunt placement provide distal reperfusion while orthopedic lengthening and fixation is secured and autogenous vein harvest occurs. This not only allows for expedited perfusion to the extremity, but buys time to develop a more thoughtful fixation, along with an easier platform for definitive arterial or venous reconstruction (**Figure 52.1a,b**).

Inserting a vascular shunt, although seemingly straightforward, has the potential to cause injury if tissues are not respected. The vessel should be dissected proximally and distally to allow the application of vascular clamps. Edges should be debrided to obtain a clean, healthy vascular edge. Thromboembolectomy with an appropriately sized Fogarty balloon catheter proximally and distally should be performed. Forward- and back-bleeding should be confirmed, and both ends should be flushed with heparinized saline. An appropriately sized and contoured shunt should then be selected and inserted distally first and allowed to back-bleed.

Then, the proximal end of the shunt should be inserted and secured with a heavy tie, and antegrade flow should be reestablished. Doppler confirmation of flow should be performed before proceeding. The shunt should be covered with either soft tissue or an occlusive

negative-pressure dressing. Consider fasciotomy and document shunt placement time.

DEFINITIVE MANAGEMENT: GENERAL PRINCIPLES

The rate of ischemic complications increases with longer ischemia times, and all efforts should be made to reestablish perfusion to the limb within 3 hours of the limb injury. Once the decision is made to reconstruct, the affected extremity and the contralateral limb must be prepped in the operating room should autogenous conduit harvest be needed. In the case of an affected upper extremity, one lower extremity should be available for great saphenous vein (GSV) harvest. If no significant venous injury is identified, the ipsilateral GSV can be harvested to limit morbidity of the incision on the affected side. However, when the injured vein is part of the deep venous system, as many veins as possible in the affected extremity must be preserved, and the contralateral GSV should be harvested for conduit. A variety of prosthetic conduits are available, with polytetrafluoroethylene (PTFE) being the most commonly used. All prosthetic grafts perform with similar patency rates, which are inferior to autogenous grafts for arterial or venous reconstructions, especially in infrapopliteal vessels. They also have higher rate of graft infections in contaminated wounds (**Table 52.3**).

Table 52.3 General principles and adjuncts of open vascular repair

Type of repair	Indication	Examples
Vessel ligation	Damage control situations. Perfused organ should be removed	Subclavian, brachial, radial, and ulnar arteries
Lateral repair	<50% loss in vessel diameter	Repair of common femoral artery with a patch
Direct anastomosis	No tension after debridement of nonviable vessel wall	Repair of brachial artery after sharp transection
Bypass	Inability to perform a direct repair or a primary anastomosis without undue tension	Not suitable in hemodynamically unstable patients. Conduit considerations

In general, long bone fractures should be brought to length with either permanent or temporary fixation before definitive vascular repair. A prosthetic conduit is an acceptable option in upper and lower extremity junctional zone injuries. Repair of venous injury should be considered in all cases because venous repair may improve limb outcomes. This consideration is particularly relevant with axillary, subclavian, common femoral, and external iliac injuries. When other life-threatening injuries do not require high prioritization, venous repair should surely be pursued.

Proximal and distal control can be secured either via separate incisions or by extending the original wound along the affected arterial segment. Proximal control at junctional areas can be obtained via endovascular balloon occlusion from a remote access site. Barring contraindications to anticoagulation, systemic heparinization should be initiated at this point. The injured segment is dissected and nonviable adjacent tissue debrided away. An embolectomy catheter should be passed proximally and distally to remove any associated thrombus, and the segment then flushed with heparinized saline. At this point, the use of a shunt is considered. After both ends of the vessel are dissected and cleaned, surgical judgement dictates the type of repair that can accomplish restoration of flow. Doppler examination or completion angiography should be used to confirm reestablishment of flow to the distal beds.

SPECIFIC INJURIES: LOWER EXTREMITIES

Open management of iliofemoral injuries

Standard exposure of the femoral vessels can be obtained in most situations. When local hemorrhage is too extensive to allow direct exposure despite local pressure, more proximal and distal exposure may be necessary. Intraluminal balloon control from the contralateral groin can be very helpful in this situation. Sometimes, proximal control is best achieved with a retroperitoneal approach to the iliac vessels. The femoral incision can be extended to run parallel to the lateral border of the rectus, or a second incision can be made centered on this site. Reconstructing the femoral bifurcation is usually not necessary for limb salvage if in-line flow is restored to either the superficial femoral (preferable) or profunda femoris vein (PFV). Either the femoral vein or the PFV, but not both, can be ligated with little risk of trouble, but the common femoral vein should be reconstructed if possible to avoid postoperative limb morbidity (e.g., swelling, compartment syndrome, postthrombotic state).

Open management of the popliteal artery

Injuries to the popliteal vessels can be quite challenging.[4] Popliteal artery exposure is usually gained through

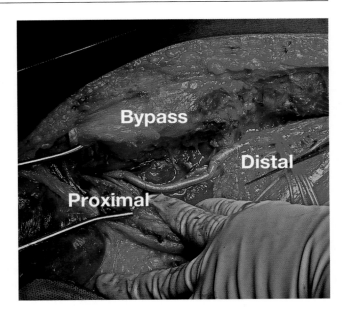

Figure 52.2 Gunshot wound to the popliteal artery was repaired with an interposition (contralateral saphenous vein) bypass graft.

standard medial distal thigh and proximal calf incisions. In severe popliteal artery injuries or those directly behind the knee, above- and below-knee incisions can be connected by cutting through all medial tendon attachments to the knee; this gives excellent exposure to the popliteal fossa (**Figure 52.2**). When dealing with concomitant popliteal venous injuries, the authors make every effort to repair the vein because of the documented improvement in limb salvage. In these situations, the vein is repaired first, followed by the artery. A temporary shunt allows restoration of arterial flow earlier in this situation and usually requires some form of partial anticoagulation. Exsanguinating the leg with an Esmarch bandage before completion of the venous anastomoses reduces the risk of retained venous clot. The risk of compartment syndrome with these injuries is high and the authors have a low threshold for proceeding with fasciotomy. In situations with prolonged preoperative ischemia, the authors usually perform fasciotomies first, before any attempt at revascularization. Unstable orthopedic injuries must be dealt with before vascular reconstruction, and someone from the vascular team must be present if orthopedic intervention is planned after vascular repair to ensure that the reconstruction is not compromised.

Open management of tibial arteries

When managing tibial vascular injuries, one must control bleeding, reduce any fractures, warm and resuscitate the patient, and examine the foot with continuous-wave Doppler. In most cases, after these maneuvers, an arterial signal will be present in the foot indicating viability and obviating the need for additional maneuvers. If there is no Doppler signal after these steps, one must consider that there may be injury to more than one tibial vessel or to the tibial peroneal trunk. The options in this scenario are: (1) attempt to restore flow with a small-caliber, temporary vascular shunt; (2) perform vascular reconstruction with a below-knee popliteal-to-tibial bypass or interposition graft using the saphenous vein; or (3) accept ligation and continue expectant management. One should be mindful that in some cases primary amputation should be performed when ischemic damage has been present for >6 hours, there is severe orthopedic injury to the foot or ankle with associated injuries, or when the severity of the mangled extremity is such that a safe attempt at limb salvage is precluded. In general, patency of at least two tibial vessels is considered optimal.

SPECIFIC INJURIES: UPPER EXTREMITIES

Management of SCA and axillary arteries

Exposure of the proximal portion of the right SCA can be accomplished with a median sternotomy. The left SCA originates and courses in a posterior location from the aortic arch. Optimal and expeditious exposure is granted through a high (third or fourth intercostal space) left anterolateral thoracotomy. Further exposure requires a clavicular extension of the incision, with or without resection of the clavicular head. A supraclavicular incision is made parallel to the clavicle, and a horizontal, infraclavicular incision is made at the middle third of the clavicle and extended laterally when exposure of the total length of the artery is desired. If the medial clavicle is resected, the resected bone should not be replaced to avoid bulky callus formation. Prosthetic conduits are typically used for reconstruction of these vessels with excellent long-term patency and low risk of infection. Venous injuries should be reconstructed rather than ligated to avoid long-term disability.[5]

Management of the brachial artery

Brachial artery injuries should be reconstructed primarily or with autogenous veins (GSV or ipsilateral basilic vein, assuming there is no concomitant ipsilateral deep venous injury). Prosthetic conduits should be avoided because of poor patency. Care must be exercised to avoid injury to the brachial vein and median nerve during exposure and reconstruction.[6]

Management of radial and ulnar arteries

An S-shaped incision over the antecubital fossa allows access to the distal brachial artery and the proximal radial and ulnar arteries. Identifying the brachial artery and tracing it distally may aid in identifying these forearm arteries. The radial artery follows the medial border of the brachioradialis muscle, and the medial groove of this muscle can be used as a landmark to make an incision in the mid-forearm. The ulnar artery dives deep to the pronator teres muscle slightly beyond the bifurcation and remains deep to the flexor muscles of the proximal forearm before emerging into a more superficial course at the midpoint of the forearm. Injury to only one artery (radial or ulnar) can be managed with simple ligation if the palmar arch is complete. Otherwise, these injuries should be repaired with an autogenous vein graft.

ENDOVASCULAR MANAGEMENT

Endovascular tools for temporary and definitive repair are extremely useful, particularly in central junctional zones. Endovascular techniques allow for the avoidance of emergent operative dissection adjacent to critical structures, such as the brachial plexus or major veins. Furthermore, the use of covered stents is becoming recognized as a feasible alternative in definitive management in both penetrating and blunt trauma. For lower extremity injuries, endoluminal access is usually gained via a contralateral femoral access point, but antegrade access is sometimes extremely valuable; 180-cm wires and 60–100-cm catheters are normally used if the femoral artery is accessed. The wire is advanced far enough to support the sliding of a catheter and subsequently a long sheath past the injury site. A covered stent (e.g., iCast™ Balloon Expandable Covered Stent, Atrium Medical Corporation, Hudson, NH, USA; Fluency, BARD Peripheral Vascular, Inc., Tempe, AZ, USA; GORE® VIABAHN® Endoprosthesis, W. L. Gore & Associates, Flagstaff, AZ, USA) is then pushed into the proper location and the sheath is retracted before deployment. Less aggressive oversizing (<20%) based on CTA measurements is recommended for extremity arteries because these vessels are prone to dissection and disruption from overstretching. For upper extremity arteries, endoluminal access is generally achieved via femoral access, but retrograde access through radial or brachial vessels is extremely valuable; 260-cm wires and 90–100-cm catheters are normally used in the setting of femoral access. More aggressive oversizing (>20%) based on CTA measurements is recommended since these vessels (as opposed to the lower extremity arteries) are very compliant and the risk of endoleak is high (**Table 52.4**).

POSTOPERATIVE CARE

The immediate postoperative care setting for these patients is the ICU to facilitate close monitoring for other injuries or derangements. The reconstructed extremity should be protected, warmed, and positioned to avoid the formation of pressure ulcers. Specific plans for dressing and external fixators should be followed. Neurovascular checks should be continued during the postoperative course.

Immediate complications are related to ischemia/reperfusion injury and prophylactic measures should be instituted in conjunction with the anesthesia team.

Table 52.4 Open versus endovascular techniques

Objective	Open techniques	Endovascular techniques
Temporary control of flow	Arterial clamping, sponge stick control of venous bleeding	Balloon control (REBOA) for lower extremities. Occlusive sheath control
Permanent occlusion of flow	Surgical ligation	Amplatz vascular plug, coil occlusion, stent graft plugs
Mass control of bleeding	Open surgical packing	Mass embolization with coil or sterile compressed sponge/thrombin
Control of bleeding and restoration of flow	Open bypass, patch repair, primary anastomosis, shunts	Stent graft repair, covered stent coverage, or closed cell stenting/coiling

Note: REBOA: Resuscitative Endovascular Balloon Occlusion of the Aorta.

These complications are a product of electrolyte efflux and washout of free radicals into the systemic circulation after flow has been established. Myoglobinuria should be watched for and aggressively treated to prevent acute kidney injury. If fasciotomies were not performed at the time of repair, the patient should be followed very closely for the development of compartment syndrome with a low threshold for performance of fasciotomies.[7] The authors have found the use of negative-pressure wound therapy very helpful in the management of fasciotomies. Limb elevation is important to reduce swelling and maximize the chances for early closure of fasciotomies. Antithrombotic therapy should consist of aspirin and a prophylactic dose of subcutaneous low-molecular-weight heparin at a minimum. For patients who undergo venous reconstruction, the authors sometimes consider full-dose anticoagulation. In this situation, sequential compression sleeves (if tolerated) are also helpful to maximize venous flow through the reconstructed venous segment. Graft thrombosis can occur, with technical failure and development of a hypercoagulable state as the most common causes. Postoperative Doppler interrogation is of utmost importance in screening for this complication; however, in young patients with healthy arteries, one should expect palpable distal pulse to be present as soon as hemodynamic stability is reached, usually within 12 hours of surgery. If graft thrombosis is detected, all attempts to restore flow should be made, given that the patient is otherwise stable.

CASE EXAMPLE

A 67-year-old woman presented to the emergency department after sustaining a penetrating injury to her left groin. Airway was patent, lungs were clear to auscultation, heart rate 110 bpm, and blood pressure 100/70 mmHg. Pulsatile bleeding was seen when pressure was released from the left groin. She was taken emergently to the operating room for exploration. The contralateral right groin was accessed percutaneously and endovascular balloon occlusion control was obtained of the external iliac artery (EIA) just proximal to the injury. Exploration of the wound was carried out with minor back-bleeding. Her injuries consisted of distal EIA and common femoral artery, femoral bifurcation, and femoral vein disruption. The femoral

artery and its bifurcation was recreated using a 6-mm PTFE graft, which was constructed in the back table in a Y fashion (end-to-side graft-to-graft anastomosis). A distal iliac-to-SFA and profunda femoris artery bypass was then performed (**Figures 52.3** and **52.4**). The patient had a palpable dorsalis pedis and posterior tibial pulse at the end of the case.

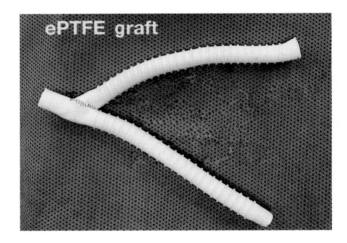

Figure 52.3 Back table reconstruction of bifurcated expanded polytetrafluoroethylene graft.

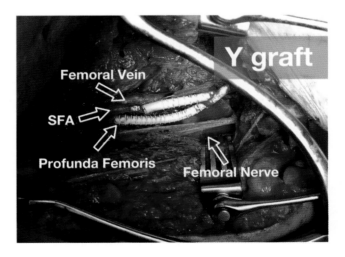

Figure 52.4 Interposition graft reconstruction of femoral bifurcation.

REFERENCES

1. Conrad MF, Patton JH Jr., Parikshak M, et al. Evaluation of vascular injury in penetrating trauma: angiographers stay home. *Am Surg.* 2002;**68**:269–274.

2. Busquéts AR, Acosta JA, Colón E, et al. Helical computed tomography angiography for the diagnosis of traumatic arterial injuries of the extremities. *J Trauma.* 2004;**56**:625–628.

3. de Mestral C, Sharma S, Haas B, et al. A contemporary analysis of the management of the mangled lower extremity. *J Trauma Acute Care Surg.* 2013;**74**:597–603.

4. Dua A, Desai SS, Shah JO, et al. Outcome predictors of limb salvage in traumatic popliteal artery injury. *Ann Vasc Surg.* 2014;**28**:108–114.

5. Franz RW, Skytta CK, Shah KJ, et al. A five-year review of management of upper-extremity arterial injuries at an urban level I trauma center. *Ann Vasc Surg.* 2012;**26**:655–664.

6. Ergunes K, Yilik L, Ozsoyler I, et al. Traumatic brachial artery injuries. *Tex Heart Inst J.* 2006;**33**:31–34.

7. Donaldson J, Haddad B, Kahn WS. The pathophysiology, diagnosis, and current management of acute compartment syndrome. *Open Orthop J.* 2014;**8**:185–193.

53

Management of penetrating extracranial carotid and vertebral artery trauma

TAEHWAN YOO AND MOUNIR HAURANI

CONTENTS

INTRODUCTION

Penetrating neck trauma represents 1% of all traumatic injuries in the USA, making up 3–6% of all mortalities largely from great vessel injury.[1] Advances in imaging and endovascular techniques are supplanting traditional surgical therapy and continue to change how these injuries are managed. However, surgical exploration and vascular repair remain critical skills because of the high morbidity and mortality associated with major arterial vascular injury.

EXTRACRANIAL PENETRATING CAROTID INJURY

The initial decision to operate is based on the presence of hard signs of vascular trauma (**Table 53.1**). Patients who present with a penetrating neck injury and hard signs should undergo emergent exploration. Additional indications include evidence of damage to aerodigestive

Table 53.1 The signs of cervical penetrating vascular injury

Signs/indications	Description
Hard signs (surgical exploration warranted)	1. Pulsatile bleeding 2. Palpable thrill 3. Audible bruit 4. Expanding hematoma
Soft signs (further diagnostic imaging warranted)	1. History indicative of moderate hemorrhage 2. Diminished pulse 3. Small, stable hematoma

Additional indications (surgical exploration warranted)	1. Evidence of cerebral ischemia
	  a. Hemiparesis/neurologic deficit
	  b. Altered mental status
	2. Evidence of tracheobronchial/esophageal disruption
	  a. Crepitus
	  b. Air bubbling from penetrating injury
	  c. Respiratory distress

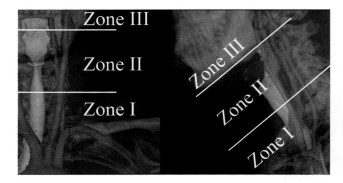

Figure 53.1 Zones of injury. Zone I: below the cricoid cartilage and above the clavicles at the thoracic inlet. Zone II: between the cricoid cartilage and the angle of the mandible. Zone III: above the angle of the mandible.

structures resulting in crepitus, respiratory distress, or air bubbles being present from the wound, or a neurologic deficit suggesting cerebral ischemia (**Table 53.1**). Given the often-unknown location of vessel injury, the operating surgeon must be able to gain vascular control in multiple cavities of the body. Generally, the decision to enter the chest or the neck is made based on the zone of the injury (**Figure 53.1**).

Zone I injuries are challenging to control because access to the proximal common carotid artery (CCA) is impeded by the clavicle and sternum. Zone III injuries above the angle of the mandible are difficult to control because of the entry of the internal carotid artery (ICA) into the skull base. Zone II injuries are readily accessible via cervical incision for proximal and distal control.

In patients who are hemodynamically stable without evidence of hard signs, the level of injury traditionally dictated management. For zone I or III injuries, angiography was the gold standard. Angiography provides a thorough evaluation of the extracranial vessels from their intrathoracic origin to their intracranial termination. However, it requires significant expertise to perform. Zone II injuries with platysma muscle violation were traditionally managed with mandatory diagnostic neck exploration. However, this approach resulted in historically high rates of negative findings ranging from 30 to 89%.[2]

Cervical computed tomography angiography (CTA) is becoming the initial modality of choice for the evaluation of all stable patients because of scanning speed, widespread availability, and technical ease. The sensitivity of CTA for detecting vascular injury approaches 100%, making it a suitable replacement for angiography with the added benefit of identifying aerodigestive tract injuries.[3] Therefore, the authors advocate initial CTA evaluation in all stable patients, sparing them from potentially morbid and unnecessary procedures (**Figure 53.2**).

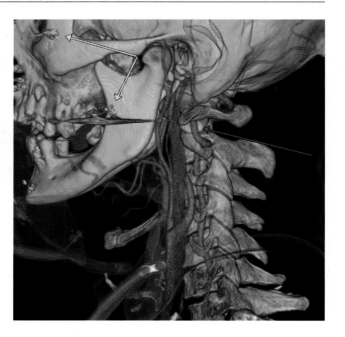

Figure 53.2 Diagnostic computed tomography angiography (CTA). CTA reconstruction of a patient who was shot in the neck. The blue arrow marks the bullet entry site. Yellow arrows mark bullet fragments. In this case, CTA effectively ruled out vascular injury.

SPECIAL OPERATIVE CONSIDERATIONS IN OPEN NECK EXPLORATION AND VASCULAR REPAIR

Before the operation, the authors advise prepping the bilateral lower extremities into the field for access to the great saphenous veins, which can be used for vein patching or interposition grafting as necessary. The authors also advise widely prepping from the angle of the mandible superiorly to the chest below the xiphoid in case further exposure is necessary.

Controlling carotid bleeding often requires direct manual pressure over the site, necessitating the compressing hand be prepped into the field. In areas where direct manual pressure cannot be adequately applied, balloon catheter tamponade by inserting a Foley catheter into the wound tract or bleeding cavity can create extrinsic compression on the vessel, allowing temporary control while further exposure is gained.

An oblique incision is made along the anterior border of the sternocleidomastoid muscle (SCM). The platysma muscle is divided along the medial border to allow adequate exposure for evaluation of proximal and distal injuries (**Figure 53.3a–c**). The SCM is retracted laterally and the internal jugular vein is followed along its anterior border to the facial vein. Division of the facial vein allows complete access to the carotid sheath and bifurcation. The incision can be continued proximally along the SCM down to the sternal notch.

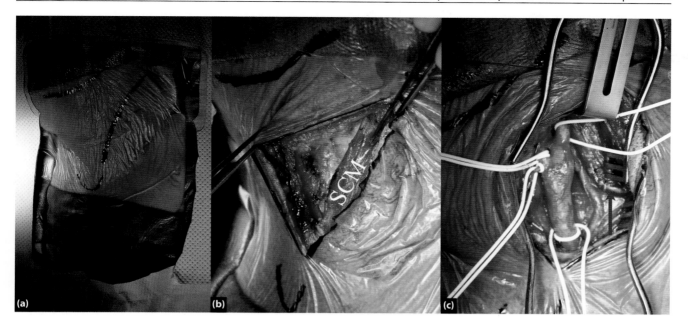

Figure 53.3 Cervical surgical exploration for carotid injury. Incision should be made along the anterior border of the sternoclei-domastoid muscle (SCM). (**a**) The sternal notch and the angle of the jaw are marked out. (**b**) The SCM is dissected along its anterior border and retracted laterally along with the internal jugular vein (IJV). (**c**) The common, external, and internal carotid arteries can be quickly explored and controlled. The blue arrow shows the ligated facial vein that needs to be divided to fully mobilize the IJV.

Once the injury is identified, proximal and distal control is obtained. The digastric muscle can be divided to gain further distal access. High distal injuries in zone III are particularly challenging to control because of the entry of the ICA into the petrous bone. A No. 2–3-Fr Fogarty balloon catheter can be carefully inflated for temporary distal control until the ICA is ligated or better exposed to facilitate repair. Mandibular or zygomatic arch osteotomy can be performed to improve exposure. Placement of a temporary shunt in settings where the patient is hemodynamically unstable, may allow for resuscitation and rewarming before complex repairs of the injured vessel are attempted.

Obtaining proximal control of low, zone I common carotid injuries is challenging given their location posterior to the sternoclavicular joint bilaterally. A partial or full median sternotomy can be performed to control the proximal arch vessels (**Figure 53.4**). Alternatively, for left-sided injuries, the proximal subclavian artery (SCA) and CCAs can be reached with an anterolateral thoracotomy through the fourth intercostal space (ICS). If more proximal control is needed on the right, the manubrium can be split and divided into the second ICS, providing access to the origin of the brachiocephalic artery and aortic arch (**Figure 53.4**). Side-biting clamps can be used to control a noncalcified aortic arch proximal to the brachiocephalic origin.

Once control is obtained, the degree of injury and patient status dictate whether to repair or ligate. Every reasonable attempt to revascularize the carotid artery should be made given the significant mortality and morbidity that

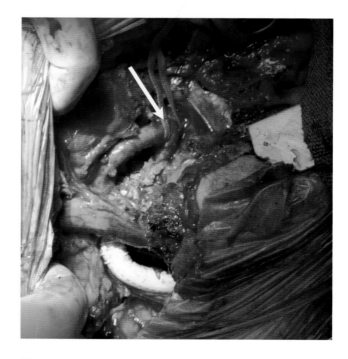

Figure 53.4 Proximal control of the arch vessels for zone I injuries. The patient's head is to the left, with a Finochietto retractor (rib spreader) to the right holding the divided manubrium apart, which is further mobilized laterally by dividing the second intercostal space. The umbilical tapes and white arrow are showing the brachiocephalic artery, with the brachiocephalic (blue arrow) vein crossing over the artery. Distally, the subclavian artery needed to be reconstructed with a short interposition prosthetic graft.

accompanies carotid ligation.[4–6] However, in case of hemo-dynamic instability or extensive and difficult-to-repair injuries, carotid ligation should be considered. If there is no back-bleeding from the distal carotid in patients presenting with profound neurologic deficit, revascularization is contraindicated because of the risk of distal embolization with restoration of blood flow.[7] Typically, a distal stump pressure of >70 mmHg indicates that the distal carotid can be ligated safely.[8]

The devitalized arterial wall should be debrided to healthy clean edges for an adequate repair. Injuries involving >50% of the wall circumference, or inability to achieve a tension-free repair, necessitate saphenous vein interposition bypass. If a vein is unavailable, prosthetic grafts have been placed successfully with equivalent patency as autogenous repair.[6] However, the likelihood of postoperative infection is greater with prosthetic grafts in the emergent setting in a contaminated surgical field due to penetrating injury.

ENDOVASCULAR APPROACH TO CAROTID ARTERY INJURIES

If a zone I or III injury is recognized, endovascular access is the preferred method of intervention because of the anatomic challenges presented by the thoracic inlet and skull base. A four-vessel cervical and cerebral angiogram is used to assess location and extent of injury, dissection, pseudoaneurysm, and collateral cerebral circulation.

Endovascular repair is determined based on injury type. Complete or nearly complete transection, usually with the presence of a large pseudoaneurysm, may not be amenable to stenting. In these injuries, balloon occlusion of the ICA can be used to quickly obtain control and prevent exsanguination, though there is increased risk of neurologic morbidity. However, control of hemorrhage through ICA occlusion may allow for adequate resuscitation with improvement in cerebral perfusion pressure through collateral blood flow. Otherwise, penetrating carotid injuries can be managed with endovascular stent grafting with pseudoaneurysm coiling and exclusion (**Figure 53.5a,b**).

Complications

Carotid ligation is particularly morbid, with a stroke rate of 30%,[9] and procedural mortality rate of 45%,[5] albeit this method is used more commonly on already comatose patients for whom the prognosis is generally poor. Open repair in patients without neurologic deficit has a 1% risk of permanent deficit.[4] Patients with neurologic deficit have a 50% chance of improvement with revascularization.[4] In addition, cranial nerve injury, wound/graft infection, and postoperative bleeding can all occur.

Carotid stenting has an overall primary patency of 80% at 2 years, with procedural mortality of <1% and a stroke

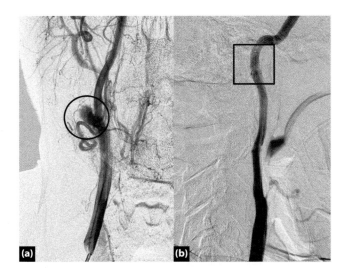

Figure 53.5 Stent repair of carotid artery pseudoaneurysm. (**a**) Patient with unstable neck fractures and carotid artery pseudoaneurysm (circled). Given his concurrent neck injury, the injury was treated with a stent graft. (**b**) Notice the embolic protection device in place (squared).

risk of 3.5%.[10] Long-term outcomes data is lacking. Other complications associated with endovascular therapy are a <1% incidence of femoral artery pseudoaneurysm[11] and a 6.6% rate of contrast-induced nephropathy in trauma patients.[12]

Follow-up

Standard follow-up with annual carotid duplex imaging following repair can be used. The authors recommend antiplatelet therapy after any open repair. Though data is sparse, lifelong antiplatelet therapy is recommended in patients with carotid or SCA stents.[13]

EXTRACRANIAL PENETRATING VERTEBRAL ARTERY INJURY (VAI)

Penetrating VAIs are particularly rare and are most often discovered incidentally on four-vessel angiography after penetrating injury.[14] The vertebral artery is divided into four distinct anatomic segments: V1; V2; V3; and V4 (**Figure 53.6**). Because of the difficulty in exposing these areas for open repair, all injuries should be addressed by endovascular techniques if possible. The robust collateral circulation of the vertebrobasilar system makes ligation of the vertebral artery significantly less likely to result in ischemic insult compared to carotid ligation. Therefore, the goal of vertebral artery intervention is hemorrhage control and prevention of posterior circulation embolic stroke with ligation or embolization, rather than revascularization (**Figure 53.6**).

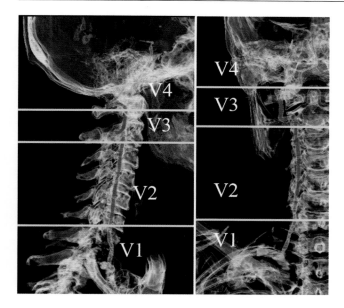

Figure 53.6 Segments of the vertebral artery (V1–V4). The V1 segment is accessible via a cervical incision either just superior to the clavicle or through an extended incision parallel to the anterior border of the sternocleidomastoid muscle. The V1 segment begins from its origin off the subclavian artery to the C6 transverse process. The V2 segment runs from the C2 to the C6 transverse process. Once the artery enters the C6 transverse process, and until it exits again at C2, it is relatively protected, but also difficult to access surgically. The V3 segment is the extracranial segment between the C2 transverse process and the vertebral canal of the skull base. The V4, or intracranial segment, continues until it joins with the contralateral vertebral artery to form the basilar artery at the lower border of the pons.

Operative consideration in open neck exploration involving the vertebral artery

When endovascular therapy is unavailable, an open surgical approach is warranted based on the location of the injury. Exposure of the extracranial vertebral artery is encompassed by standard neck exploration. An oblique incision is made along the anterior SCM from below the mastoid to the sternoclavicular junction. If more proximal control is needed for ligation of the vertebral artery at its origin on the SCA, the incision can be extended laterally, parallel to, and approximately 1–2 cm above the clavicle.

For V1 injuries, transection of the clavicular head of the SCM and anterior scalene muscle (ASM) may be necessary. Care should be taken to avoid injury to the phrenic nerve that lies on the ASM. Branches of the thyrocervical trunk are divided to gain access to the vertebral artery and the subclavian vertebral junction. Proximal control may require median sternotomy to expose the SCA. A small Fogarty catheter is a useful adjunct to obtain temporary control. The vertebral artery is then clipped above and below the injury.

V2 injuries can be difficult to ligate because of their interosseous location. A standard incision is made along the anterior border of the SCM. The carotid sheath is retracted laterally. The middle thyroid vein is divided to allow access to the prevertebral space. Bone wax can be pushed firmly into the bleeding interspace between the transverse processes for control. Further direct exposure of the interosseous vertebral artery is not necessary because the space between the transverse processes can be palpated. Metal clip appliers can be guided along a probing index finger to the vertebral artery segments above and below the injured vessel under the longus colli muscle. Metal clips are placed above and below the site of injury within the same interspace, or one interspace above and below if necessary. The cervical nerve roots exit the spinal cord posterior to the vertebral artery. To avoid inadvertent nerve root injury during clipping, the clips should be applied from an anterior approach, just below the transverse process.[15]

Endovascular approach to VAIs

Endovascular intervention is not restricted by a challenging anatomy, making it the preferred approach. Outcomes in penetrating VAIs are sparse because of the overall low incidence. Thus, endovascular management strategies are based on the literature about blunt vertebral trauma. Pseudoaneurysms or arteriovenous fistula formation warrant intervention with coil embolization because of the high risk of posterior circulation embolic stroke. Patients with vertebral dissection without any other sequelae can be managed with antiplatelet or anticoagulation therapy, with many of these resolving over time.[16]

Complications

Vertebrobasilar insufficiency after ligation has been reported in 1.8–3.1% of patients, and is denoted by specific neurologic symptoms, including altered mental status, dysphagia, dysarthria, diplopia, and nystagmus.[17] Literature about blunt trauma VAI studies has shown the risk of posterior circulation stroke ranging from 5 to 24%,[6,18] with neurologic symptoms usually starting 4–5 days after initial trauma.[18] Other complications are associated with femoral artery access and contrast-induced nephropathy.[11,12]

Follow-up

Patients with VAIs should remain on either anticoagulation or antiplatelet therapy. Heparin therapy was found to decrease neurologic events from 20–35% to 0–14% with further studies showing no significant difference in patients receiving antiplatelet therapy (either clopidogrel or aspirin) compared to anticoagulation.[6,18,19] The degree of injury, from partial dissection to complete transection, does not predict posterior circulation stroke.[17,18] Current recommendations based on expert opinion are to treat all asymptomatic patients, regardless of VAI severity, with antiplatelet therapy or anticoagulation. All symptomatic patients without contraindications should receive anticoagulation therapy. All VAIs should be treated with antithrombotic therapy for 3–6 months or resolution on radiographic imaging.

CASE EXAMPLES

Case example 1

This patient presented with a large stab wound to zone II of his neck. There was clear violation of the platysma muscle and partial transection of the SCM (**Figure 53.7a**; the arrow demonstrates the defect). Given that there were no hard signs, or vascular or airway injury, CTA was used to evaluate the vascular structures. Three-dimensional reconstruction (**Figure 53.7b**) and conventional axial imaging ruled out any vascular injury. CT imaging also demonstrated

that there was subcutaneous air more central than anticipated (**Figure 53.7c**, arrow) and further evaluation of the trachea and esophagus should be performed.

Case example 2

This patient presented with a large defect in his neck, face, and oropharynx secondary to a gunshot wound. He was hemodynamically unstable and comatose, with a large circumferential defect of the carotid artery. On surgical exploration, the distal ICA was found to have brisk back-bleeding and was ligated, given the extent of vessel damage. Once stabilized, angiography was performed. **Figure 53.8a** shows filling of the right vertebral artery (RVA) and a ligated right CCA (arrow). Selective angiography of the left carotid artery (**Figure 53.8b**) shows brisk filling of the right hemisphere. The arrow in **Figure 53.8c** shows retrograde filling of the right external carotid artery via muscular branches of the RVA. The bullet (circled) as well as multiple surgical clips can be seen at the level of the ligated artery. **Figure 53.8d** demonstrates further right hemispheric filling via left vertebral artery injection.

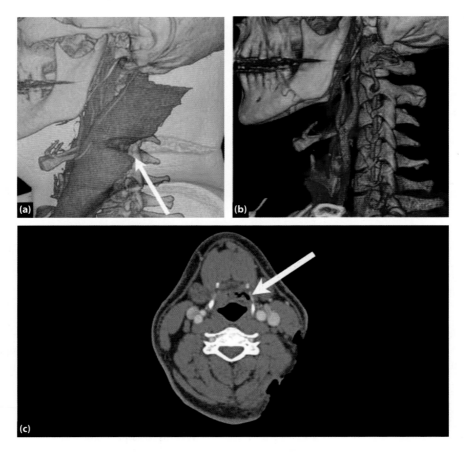

Figure 53.7 Computed Tomography angiography (CTA) after zone II injury. (**a**) CTA reconstruction shows platysma violation and partial transection of the sternocleidomastoid muscle. (**b**) Three-dimensional reconstruction demonstrates no vascular injury, sparing the patient a negative neck exploration. (**c**) Imaging also demonstrated the presence of air (arrow) centrally, mandating further evaluation of the trachea and esophagus.

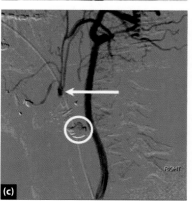
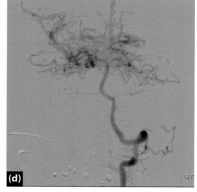

Figure 53.8 Head and neck angiogram after right carotid ligation. (**a**) Post-carotid ligation angiography shows filling of the right vertebral artery and ligated right common carotid artery (arrow). (**b**) Selective left carotid angiography shows brisk filling of the right cerebral hemisphere. (**c**) Retrograde filling of the right external carotid artery via the muscular branches of the right vertebral artery. The bullet (circle) and multiple surgical clips can be seen at ligated carotid artery site. (**d**) Left vertebral artery angiography demonstrates further collateral flow to the right cerebral hemisphere.

REFERENCES

1. Brywczynski JJ, Barrett TW, Lyon JA, et al. Management of penetrating neck injury in the emergency department: a structured literature review. *Emerg Med J.* 2008;**25**:711–715.

2. Múnera F, Soto JA, Palacio DM, et al. Penetrating neck injuries: helical CT angiography for initial evaluation. *Radiology.* 2002;**224**:366–372.

3. Demetriades D, Asensio JA, Velmahos G, et al. Complex problems in penetrating neck trauma. *Surg Clin North Am.* 1996;**76**:661–683.

4. Liekweg WG Jr., Greenfield LJ. Management of penetrating carotid arterial injury. *Ann Surg.* 1978;**188**:587–592.

5. du Toit DF, van Schalkwyk GD, Wadee SA, et al. Neurologic outcome after penetrating extracranial artery trauma. *J Vasc Surg.* 2003;**38**:257–262.

6. O'Brien PJ, Cox MW. A modern approach to cervical vascular trauma. *Perspect Vasc Surg Endovasc Ther.* 2011;**23**:90–97.

7. Thal ER, Snyder WH 3rd, Hays RJ, et al. Management of carotid artery injuries. *Surgery.* 1974;**76**:955–962.

8. Ehrnefeld WK, Stoney RJ, Wylie EJ. Relation of carotid stump pressure to safety of carotid artery ligation. *Surgery.* 1983;**93**:299–305.

9. Lawrence KB, Shefts LM, McDaniel JR. Wounds of common carotid arteries: report of 17 cases from World War II. *Am J Surg.* 1948;**76**:29–37.

10. DuBose J, Recinos G, Teixeira PG, et al. Endovascular stenting for the treatment of traumatic internal carotid injuries: expanding experience. *J Trauma.* 2008;**65**:1561–1566.

11. Stone PA, Campbell JE, AbuRahma AF. Femoral pseudoaneurysms after percutaneous access. *J Vasc Surg.* 2014;**60**:1359–1366.

12. Matsushima K, Peng M, Schaefer EW, et al. Posttraumatic contrast-induced acute kidney injury: minimal consequences or significant threat? *J Trauma.* 2011;**70**:415–419.

13. Bhatt DL, Kapadia SR, Bajzer CT, et al. Dual antiplatelet therapy with clopidogrel and aspirin after carotid artery stenting. *J Invasive Cardiol.* 2001; **13**:767–771.

14. Reid JD, Weigelt JA. Forty-three cases of vertebral artery trauma. *J Trauma.* 1988;**28**:1007–1012.

15. Hatzitheofilou C, Demetriades D, Melissas J, et al. Surgical approaches to vertebral artery injuries. *Br J Surg.* 1988;**75**:234–237.

16. Franz RW, Goodwin RB, Beery PR 2nd, et al. Postdischarge outcomes of blunt cerebrovascular injuries. *Vasc Endovascular Surg.* 2010;**44**:198–211.

17. Thomas GI, Anderson KN, Hain RF, et al. The significance of anomalous vertebral-basilar artery communications in operations on the heart and great vessels: an illustrative case with review of the literature. *Surgery.* 1959;**46**:747–757.

18. Biffl WL, Moore EE, Elliott JP, et al. The devastating potential of blunt vertebral arterial injuries. *Ann Surg.* 2000;**231**:672–681.

19. Alterman DM, Heidel RE, Daley BJ, et al. Contemporary outcomes in vertebral artery injury. *J Vasc Surg.* 2013;**57**:741–746.

54

Blunt thoracic aortic injury

ADRIANA LASER, SHAHAB TOURSAVADKOHI, AND ROBERT CRAWFORD

CONTENTS

INTRODUCTION

Blunt thoracic aortic injury (BTAI) is a spectrum of lesions in the aortic wall ranging from an abnormality seen only on modern imaging to a life-threatening surgical emergency. BTAI is the second leading cause of death among blunt trauma patients after head injury. It is estimated that only 13–15% of BTAI patients make it to the hospital alive.[1] Specific factors correlated with BTAI from motor vehicle crash are: velocity changes of at least 20 mph; side impact; and intrusion into the vehicle. The etiology of BTAI is a deceleration injury from a point of anatomic tethering (aortopulmonary ligament). A computed tomography (CT) scan of a BTAI requiring treatment is shown in **Figure 54.1a–c**. BTAI is graded as: grade I, an

intimal tear (minimal aortic injury); grade II, an intramural hematoma; grade III, a pseudoaneurysm; and grade IV, a rupture or transection.[2] Recently, a more simplified scheme has been proposed (**Figure 54.2**).[3] The natural history depends on severity, or grade, of injury.

BACKGROUND

BTAI was historically treated in the 1960s–1980s with immediate open repair. The 1990s brought the delayed management concept: medically controlling blood pressure (BP) and heart rate (beta-blockade) while addressing other life-threatening injuries first. Thoracic endovascular aortic repair (TEVAR) was first reported as

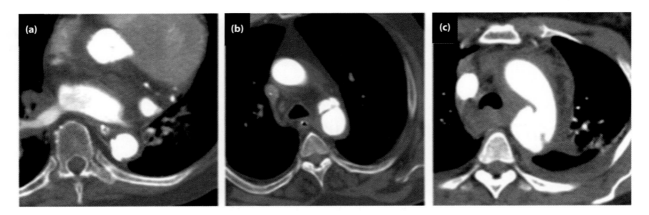

Figure 54.1 Computed tomography of blunt thoracic aortic injury: low; moderate; and high-risk traumatic aortic pseudoaneurysms. (**a**) Small pseudoaneurysm with trace periaortic hematoma, managed with surveillance imaging. (**b**) Moderately sized pseudoaneurysm with minimal periaortic hematoma, managed with delayed endovascular repair during the patient's index admission. (**c**) Large lesion with extensive mediastinal hematoma and left hemothorax, managed with emergency endovascular repair (courtesy of Harris DG, Rabin J, Bhardwaj A, et al. Non-operative management of traumatic aortic pseudoaneurysms. *Ann Vasc Surg.* 2016;**35**:75–81).

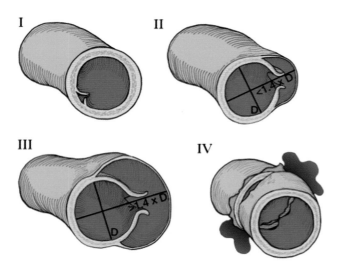

Figure 54.2 Proposed grades of blunt traumatic aortic injury. **I**: intimal. **II**: small pseudoaneurysm <50% circumference and injury diameter <1.4 × normal diameter. **III**: large pseudoaneurysm >50% circumference or injury diameter >1.4 normal diameter. **IV**: frank rupture (courtesy of Rabin J, Harris DG, Drucker C, et al. The evolution of management strategies for blunt aortic injury. *Curr Surg Rep.* 2016;**4**:3).

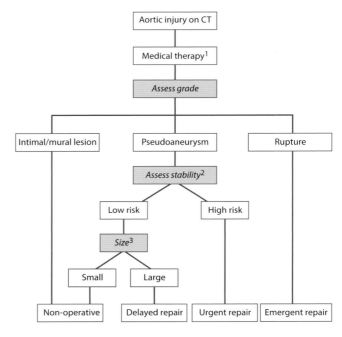

Figure 54.3 Suggested management algorithm for blunt thoracic aortic injury (courtesy of Harris DG, Rabin J, Starnes BW, et al. Evolution of lesion-specific management of blunt thoracic aortic injury. *J Vasc Surg.* 2016;**64**:500–505).

a treatment for BTAI in 1997. A covered stent graft uses radial force to remain in position, along with proximal barbs, hooks, or struts. Specific concerns in the younger trauma population are more acute angles of curvature, smaller aortic diameters, smaller access vessels, and longer life expectancy (possible aortic diameter growth) potentially causing "bird beaking," endoleaks, or graft migration, fracture, and collapse. Challenges to stent grafting the thoracic aorta as compared to the abdominal aorta include: increased hemodynamic forces and

variability over the cardiac cycle; greater elasticity and movement of the aortic wall; and a curvature to deal with. Because our understanding of the natural history of BTAI has changed, management has evolved from immediate "clamp and sew" open repair of all operative candidates to a selective approach with often delayed repair (largely endovascular). The authors' management algorithm is outlined in **Figure 54.3**.[4]

INDICATIONS FOR TREATMENT

Definitive indications include grade IV injuries and all grade III injuries with active extravasation and other high-risk features; treatment for lesser injuries is under debate. The authors' approach has been medical management for most grade I and II injuries, with urgent or emergent intervention for grade III and IV injuries. Patients without secondary signs of injury (pseudocoarctation, mediastinal hematoma, or large left hemothorax) are generally safe to wait for delayed repair. A novel BTAI score was recently developed to predict early rupture in high-grade injuries more accurately than with clinical assessment. This score is based on the size of the pseudoaneurysm-to-aortic diameter ratio (>1.4), the presence of a descending thoracic aortic hematoma (>10 mm), and lactate (>4 mmol/L). There is a high risk for rupture when two or more of these three risk factors are present suggesting the need for immediate repair in these cases (**Figure 54.4**).[5]

GENERAL PROCEDURAL GUIDELINES FOR TEVAR

Imaging

CT angiography (CTA) is the imaging modality of choice for diagnostic and operative planning, with a greater sensitivity than catheter angiography. It is important to image

Risk Score Criteria:

Lactate >4 mM
Mediastinal hematoma >10 mm
Lesion/normal aortic ratio >1.4

High risk for aortic rupture when any 2 factors are present.

Figure 54.4 Risk score criteria for predicting aortic injury rupture (courtesy of Harris DG, Rabin J, Kufera JA, et al. A new aortic injury score predicts early rupture more accurately than clinical assessment. *J Vasc Surg.* 2015;**61**:332–338).

from the neck through to the mid-thighs to evaluate access vessels and vertebral artery anatomy.

Blood pressure

Perioperative BP should be maintained at a mean arterial pressure of 50–60 mmHg and a systolic BP of 110–130 mmHg. Beta-blockers are typically the agents used.

Heparinization

Other injuries are assessed to ensure feasibility of heparinization and patient positioning. Need for general anesthesia and spinal drainage is assessed based on the patient's clinical status and anatomic considerations. Routine performance of the procedure without heparinization has been described and can be performed with minimal additional morbidity.

Three-dimensional (3-D) imaging

3-D imaging programs offer enhanced preoperative planning abilities to measure and size grafts. Aortic diameters at the proximal and distal landing zones are measured, as is the length of required coverage. Aortic arch angulation, location of the left subclavian artery (SCA), vertebral artery, and left common carotid origins, and the presence of anatomic variations are also evaluated.

Access vessels

Access vessels are assessed for diameter extent and disease. This helps make the decision regarding cutdown versus percutaneous access, and whether a conduit is needed. The iliac and femoral vessels need to be a minimum of 6 mm to accommodate a 16–25-Fr delivery sheath. The devices used primarily in the USA are listed in **Table 54.1**.

Table 54.1 Thoracic endovascular aortic repair stent grafts currently on the market in the USA

Product	Aortic diameter	Access	Proximal end	Material
GORE®TAG® Thoracic Endoprosthesis, Conformable GORE®TAG® Thoracic Endoprosthesis[a]	16–42 mm	18–24-Fr outer diameter sheaths	Partially uncovered stent	Expanded PTFE graft, nitinol stent
Valiant™ Captivia™ Thoracic Stent Graft[b]	22–46 mm	22–25-Fr outer diameter; sheathless	Uncovered stent	Polyester graft, nitinol stent
Zenith Alpha™ Thoracic Endovascular Graft[c]	15–42 mm	16–20-Fr inner diameter sheaths	Uncovered stent	Dacron graft, stainless steel stent

[a] W. L. Gore & Associates, Flagstaff, AZ, USA.
[b] Medtronic, Minneapolis, MN, USA.
[c] Cook Medical Inc., Bloomington, IN, USA. PTFE: polytetrafluoroethylene.

Stent graft

Stent graft type is chosen based on patient anatomy; sizing is based on CT measurements with ≤10% oversizing compared to TEVAR for degenerative aneurysms. Shortened landing zones (<2 cm) and sharp angulation are factors associated with early graft failure.

Graft predeployment and deployment

Predeployment aortography should be performed with device and stiff wire in place. Techniques for deployment are specific to each device. In general, familiarity with a device is key to technical success.

Goal of TEVAR

The goal of TEVAR is injury coverage, usually with the shortest-length device suitable for the lesion. Other than preservation of a left internal mammary artery graft or a dominant left vertebral artery (LVA), coverage of the left SCA can be performed safely. In a small minority of cases, revascularization for left arm symptoms needs to be performed, typically later. A carotid-SCA bypass or SCA-to-carotid transposition should be performed if the left SCA is covered in elective situations.

Postdeployment imaging

Postdeployment angiography should be performed to evaluate great vessel and iliac artery patency, stent graft patency, injury coverage, seal, and possible endoleaks. Ballooning is almost never required and should be avoided.

Follow-up

Follow-up is with CT scans at 1, 6, and 12 months. Without concerning findings, annual surveillance is resumed.

GENERAL PROCEDURAL GUIDELINES FOR OPEN REPAIR

Although TEVAR is the procedure of choice for BTAI, open repair has a role depending on the availability of urgent TEVAR at some facilities. If pursuing open repair, single-lung ventilation is usually required and the most appropriate exposure is obtained through a fourth intercostal space posterolateral thoracotomy incision. The site of injury is left undisturbed and the aorta is preferentially clamped distal to the left SCA, although control between the left carotid and left SCA is sometimes necessary. Following distal control in the mid-descending thoracic aorta, an interposition Dacron graft is sewn in place with

3-0 or 4-0 polypropylene suture. Techniques to maintain distal perfusion via left heart bypass or total cardiopulmonary bypass are associated with better outcomes and lower rates of spinal cord ischemia (SCI).

MANAGEMENT CONTROVERSIES

Open versus endovascular therapy

The advantages of TEVAR in the older thoracic aneurysm patient with multiple comorbidities have been well documented. But what about TEVAR for BTAI in the young trauma patient, with a longer life expectancy and no comorbidities? Recent meta-analyses have demonstrated decreased short-term mortality, SCI, and stroke with TEVAR compared to open repair. The first prospective trial of TEVAR versus open repair for BTAI was carried out by the American Association for the Surgery of Trauma. It demonstrated superior results for TEVAR, with decreased in-hospital mortality (23.5 versus 7.2%) and decreased blood transfusion requirements.[6] Looking only at patients without critical extrathoracic injuries, TEVAR resulted in a 13-fold mortality reduction. The benefits of TEVAR include decreased anticoagulation intensity, and avoidance of thoracotomy, single-lung ventilation, and left heart bypass. The Society for Vascular Surgery (SVS) clinical practice guidelines recommend TEVAR over open repair for grade II–IV injuries[2] and this has been the authors' practice for nearly a decade.

Minimal aortic injuries

Minimal aortic injuries are intimal flaps with no or minimal periaortic hematoma.[4] Early evidence showed most type I injuries heal spontaneously. Nonoperative management of minimal injury patients rarely results in aortic rupture or the need for salvage repair. The authors recommend CT follow-up of grade I and II injuries, with repair considered only for progressing lesions.

Timing

Delayed operative repair with interval medical management has been shown to be a safe option for many stable BTAI patients.[4] This strategy allows management of other life-threatening injuries (intra-abdominal or intracerebral hemorrhage) first. Another reason for delayed repair is to reduce the risks associated with intraoperative heparinization, though recent reports have shown that patients undergoing TEVAR for BTAI without heparinization have a very low complication rate (iliac thrombus).[7] However, delayed surgical repair is still preferred in many situations, especially in older patients and patients with coronary artery disease, pulmonary injury, and nonoperative solid organ injuries. In fact, a recent study addressing the issue of timing showed that early treatment of BTAI in patients with concurrent BTAI and traumatic brain injury (TBI) worsens TBI, and that TEVAR can be safely delayed (days to weeks).[7]

A recent review of almost 200 patients with traumatic thoracic aortic pseudoaneurysms managed nonoperatively because of prohibitive risks (severe comorbidities or concurrent injuries) demonstrated low aortic risk. (Inpatient aortic-related mortality was 2% and late interventions were required in 4%.)[8] Patients who are hemodynamically stable at 4 hours postinjury are generally thought of as safe for delayed repair (low risk of developing aortic rupture).[9] The authors feel that delayed treatment is preferable for the many reasons outlined previously, and that recognition of high-risk features (listed earlier) can help delineate the injuries that need emergent treatment.

Left SCA revascularization

Although the SVS guidelines recommend routine revascularization of the left SCA after coverage with elective TEVAR,[2] there is no supportive level I evidence. Revascularization is important with patent left internal mammary grafts, left-sided arteriovenous dialysis fistulas, left hand dominance, LVA off the aortic arch, and supra-aortic pathology (carotid or vertebral artery stenoses). The authors do not recommend routine left SCA revascularization after TEVAR for BTAI with left SCA coverage, except in the situations listed previously, and do not hesitate to cover the left SCA if necessary (approximately 40% of the time in the authors' experience).

Routine spinal drainage

Guidelines from the SVS recommend against routine cerebrospinal drainage for TEVAR in the setting of BTAI.[2] The risk of SCI is lower with TEVAR for BTAI compared to TEVAR for other pathologies. Specific risk factors for SCI with TEVAR are: aortic coverage length; intraoperative hypotension; renal insufficiency; atherosclerosis or prior coverage of the left SCA; patency of internal iliac or vertebral arteries; and history of prior abdominal aortic aneurysm repair. Because most of these factors are not present with BTAI and because most lesions are covered with one 10-cm stent graft, the authors do not recommend routine spinal drainage. High-risk individuals can be monitored with motor and sensory evoked potentials and drained selectively.

COMPLICATIONS

Complications of TEVAR for BTAI include a 1% risk of stroke compared to 3–5% for all TEVARs.[10] There is an approximate risk of 1% for SCI, but this increases with certain risk factors (**Table 54.2**). Endoleaks, bird beaking, and

Table 54.2 Complications of thoracic endovascular aortic repair for blunt thoracic aortic injury

Complication	Description
Stroke	Increases with left subclavian artery (SCA) coverage
Spinal cord ischemia	Increases with risk factors: prior infrarenal aortic surgery; renal failure; hypotension; occluded hypogastric or lumbar arteries
Endoleak	Types I–IV
"Bird beaking"	Graft encroaches into the aortic arch leading to endograft collapse or migration
Excessive aortic coverage	Left SCA, left common carotid, or celiac artery coverage
Retrograde type A aortic dissection	Rare, risk increased with proximal ballooning
Access	Iliac artery rupture, femoral artery dissection, distal embolization

accidental excessive aortic coverage are also low but not insignificant risks. Mortality at 30 days is 6% after TEVAR for BTAI compared with 14% for open repair of BTAI; mortality is largely influenced by associated injuries.[10]

CONCLUSIONS

Management of BTAI has undergone a transformation over the last several decades from universally early, open repair to selective, expectant, nonoperative medical treatment for grade I and II injuries, urgent versus delayed repair for grade III injuries, and immediate treatment for grade IV injuries. TEVAR for BTAI is recommended over open repair whenever anatomically feasible.

REFERENCES

1. Parmley LF, Mattingly TW, Manion WC, et al. Nonpenetrating traumatic injury of the aorta. *Circulation*. 1958;**17**:1086–1101.
2. Lee WA, Matsumura JS, Mitchell RS, et al. Endovascular repair of traumatic thoracic aortic injury: clinical practice guidelines of the Society for Vascular Surgery. *J Vasc Surg*. 2011;**53**:187–192.
3. Rabin J, Harris DG, Drucker C, et al. The evolution of management strategies for blunt aortic injury. *Curr Surg Rep*. 2016;**4**:3.
4. Harris DG, Rabin J, Starnes BW, et al. Evolution of lesion-specific management of blunt thoracic aortic injury. *J Vasc Surg*. 2016;**64**:500–505.
5. Harris DG, Rabin J, Kufera JA, et al. A new aortic injury score predicts early rupture more accurately than clinical assessment. *J Vasc Surg*. 2015;**61**:332–338.

6. Demetriades D, Velmahos GC, Scalea TM, et al. Operative repair or endovascular stent graft in blunt traumatic thoracic aortic injuries: results of an American Association for the Surgery of Trauma Multicenter Study. *J Trauma*. 2008;**64**:561–770.

7. Rabin J, Harris DG, Crews GA, et al. Early aortic repair worsens concurrent traumatic brain injury. *Ann Thorac Surg*. 2014;**98**:46–51.

8. Harris DG, Rabin J, Bhardwaj A, et al. Nonoperative management of traumatic aortic pseudoaneurysms. *Ann Vasc Surg*. 2016;**35**:75–81.

9. Fortuna GR Jr., Perlick A, DuBose JJ, et al. Injury grade is a predictor of aortic-related death among patients with blunt thoracic aortic injury. *J Vasc Surg*. 2016;**63**:1225–1231.

10. Cheng D, Martin J, Shennib H, et al. Endovascular aortic repair versus open surgical repair for descending thoracic aortic disease: a systematic review and meta-analysis of comparative studies. *J Am Coll Cardiol*. 2010;**55**:986–1001.

55

Dialysis access

P.C. BALRAJ, ARIELLE HODARI-GUPTA, AND G. HADDAD

CONTENTS

INTRODUCTION

More than 300,000 individuals in the USA rely on vascular access to receive hemodialysis treatment. The number of patients with end-stage renal disease (ESRD) in the USA continues to increase on a yearly basis. Current Kidney Disease Outcomes Quality Initiative guidelines stipulate that all patients should be referred for the creation of autogenous access when they reach stage 4 chronic kidney disease (glomerular filtration rate <30 mL/min/1.73 m^2).[1] This allows sufficient time for fistula creation and maturation before starting hemodialysis.

ACCESS TYPE

An ideal access permits a flow rate that is adequate for hemodialysis (600 mL/min), can be used for extended periods, and has a low complication rate (e.g., infection, stenosis, thrombosis, aneurysm, and limb ischemia). Studies have demonstrated consistently that native fistula accesses have the best 4–5-year patency rates and require the fewest interventions compared with other access types.[2–4]

A native arteriovenous fistula (AVF) is the preferred access. A radial–cephalic direct wrist access fistula (Brescia–Cimino fistula) (**Figure 55.1**), with a 2-year patency of 55–89%, is the goal standard against which all other fistulas are measured. Other autogenous options include: (1) radial branch–cephalic direct access (snuffbox fistula) (2) ulnar–basilic forearm transposition; (3) brachial–cephalic upper arm direct access (antecubital vein to brachial artery); and (4) brachial–basilic upper arm transposition (basilic vein transposition). Prosthetic options for arteriovenous access are constructed by interposing a prosthetic graft between an artery and a vein, typically with expanded polytetrafluoroethylene (PTFE) grafts 4–8 mm in diameter. The arteriovenous graft can be constructed in a straight or looped fashion.

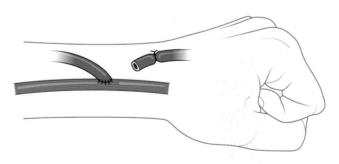

Figure 55.1 Autogenous radial-cephalic arteriovenous fistula (Brescia-Cimino Fistula).

PREOPERATIVE EVALUATION

In these patients, who often have multiple active comorbidities, preoperative evaluation requires a thorough history, and physical and medical optimization. Specific historical findings to review include prior vascular access procedures, such as venous catheters, presence of pacemaker wires, arm swelling, and symptoms of arterial insufficiency. Physical examination should include a pulse examination, Allen's test, and bilateral upper extremity blood pressure (BP) to evaluate the arterial system, edema, and the presence of collateral veins on the upper arm and chest wall, which may suggest central venous occlusive disease. Routine preoperative venous and arterial duplex imaging are performed, which have been shown to increase both the construction and maturation rate of upper extremity autogenous AVFs.[5] Arterial requirements include the absence of a pressure differential of 20 mmHg between arms and, in the distal forearm, a patent palmar arch and arterial luminal diameter of at least 2.0 mm. Any abnormality on physical examination or noninvasive studies can be further evaluated with arteriography if the limb is still to be considered for use in vascular access. For a successful AVF, venous requirements include: a diameter ≥2.5 mm; absence of obstruction; straight segment for cannulation (within 1 cm from the surface); and continuity with proximal central vein. Again, abnormalities on physical examination or noninvasive studies require further evaluation with phlebogram.

ANESTHESIA

The procedure can be done with multiple forms of anesthesia and depends on the patient's comorbid conditions, the anesthesiologist, and the surgeon. A regional nerve block is the anesthesia of choice for the authors' institution. This is done in the preoperative area by a dedicated block team while the preceding case is underway. This helps to maximize efficiency and shorten turnover time.

RADIAL–CEPHALIC FISTULA

Exposure for a radio–cephalic fistula begins with a longitudinal incision at the wrist that is deepened through the subcutaneous tissue. The cephalic vein is identified and isolated from the surrounding structures. The fascia is entered and the radial artery is isolated with the radial veins in a bundle and surrounded with a vessel loop. The vein and artery are inspected to ensure that they are of adequate size to proceed. After the patient is anticoagulated with heparin, the cephalic vein is divided and the distal end is ligated. With vascular control of the radial artery, a longitudinal arteriotomy is created. The cephalic vein end is slightly beveled and brought over to the artery. An end of cephalic vein-to-side of radial artery anastomosis is then performed with fine running (7-0) polypropylene suture. Before completing the anastomosis, the vein and the artery are allowed to bleed; the anastomosis is then completed. Next, it is important to assess the fistula by palpating a thrill at the anastomosis. The incision is closed with 3-0 absorbable suture for the subcutaneous tissue and staples for the skin.

BRACHIAL–CEPHALIC FISTULA

A brachial–cephalic fistula is created by anastomosing the cephalic vein to the brachial artery in the antecubital fossa or just above the elbow (transposition). For the former, a transverse incision is made in the antecubital fossa and is deepened through the subcutaneous tissue. The cephalic vein is identified, isolated from the surrounding structures, and surrounded with vessel loops. Next, attention is paid to the brachial artery. The fascia is entered, the bicipital aponeurosis is partially divided, and the brachial artery is isolated and surrounded with vessel loops. At this point, heparin (3000 IU) is given intravenously, and after allowing it to circulate, the cephalic vein is divided and the distal end is ligated. The cephalic vein is then beveled and brought over to the brachial artery; after obtaining control and creating an arteriotomy, an end-to-side anastomosis is created. It is created more easily than a brachial–basilic fistula because it requires less dissection. Because of the lateral and relatively superficial location of the cephalic vein, a brachial–cephalic fistula is easy to cannulate. It also provides a long length of straight vein and has the potential for higher blood flow than a radial–cephalic fistula.

BASILIC VEIN TRANSPOSITION

In one-stage procedures, the basilic vein is usually mobilized through a single-arm incision along the course of the basilic vein (**Figure 55.2**); if necessary, the incision is extended transversely to the antecubital fossa. The medial antebrachial cutaneous nerve is carefully protected. The basilic vein is disconnected and dilated with heparinized

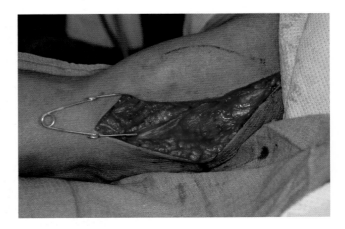

Figure 55.2 Basilic vein mobilized through a single incision along the medial aspect of the arm in preparation for a one-stage transposition procedure.

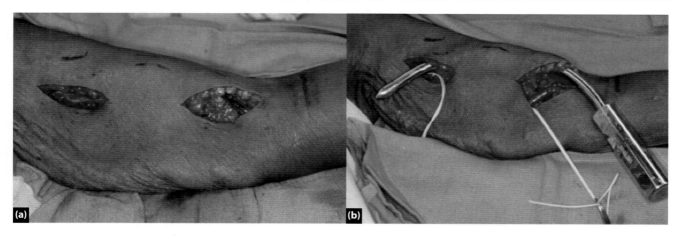

Figure 55.3 Basilic vein transposition. **(a)** Second stage of a two-stage procedure with mobilization of the basilic vein through two longitudinal small "skip" incisions along the course of the basilic vein, one over the distal part of the basilic vein near its anastomosis and one at the level of the proximal part. **(b)** The basilic vein is divided and tunneled with a tunneler over the anterolateral aspect of the arm.

solution and then transposed inside an anterolateral subcutaneous tunnel; following patient heparinization (3000 IU unfractionated heparin, given intravenously), the basilic vein is anastomosed to the brachial artery, or proximal radial or ulnar arteries, with fine running (7-0) polypropylene suture.

In two-stage procedures, the basilic vein is mobilized through a transverse antecubital fossa incision followed by creation of the fistula. Following a period of 4–6 weeks necessary for maturation, the second stage involves mobilization of the basilic vein through two longitudinal "skip" incisions (**Figure 55.3**), one over the distal part of the basilic vein near its anastomosis and one at the level of the proximal arm to allow full mobilization of the basilic vein up to its confluence with the brachial vein; the basilic vein is then mobilized by dividing all tributaries. Subsequently, a superficial anterolateral arm tunnel is created between the two incisions with a tunneler, taking care not to make the tunnel too deep; the patient is given 3000 IU unfractionated heparin intravenously; the anterior surface of the arterialized fistula is marked with a marker pen and the proximal part of the fistula near the anastomosis is controlled with a bulldog clamp, followed by fistula transection. The vein is retracted off the proximal incision, dilated with the heparinized solution, and placed inside the tunnel using the top marks, taking care not to twist the fistula. Then, the two ends of the fistula are reanastomosed with 7-0 polypropylene suture.

ARTERIOVENOUS GRAFT

A longitudinal skin incision is made above the antecubital fossa and is deepened through the subcutaneous tissue. The fascia is entered and the brachial artery is identified, isolated, and surrounded with vessel loops. A second incision is made in the proximal upper arm near the axilla.

The proximal brachial vein/axillary vein is then identified and isolated with vessel loops. A tunnel is created in a lateral fashion between the two incisions and the graft is introduced through the tunnel. After heparinization, proximal and distal control is obtained. A longitudinal arteriotomy is performed and the graft is beveled and sutured to the artery in an end-to-side fashion with fine running (6-0) polypropylene suture. The graft is injected with heparinized saline and a bulldog clamp is placed on the arterial end of the graft. Control is then obtained on the vein. A longitudinal venotomy is performed; then, the graft is beveled and sutured to the vein in an end-to-side fashion with continuous fine (6-0) polypropylene suture. Before completing the anastomosis, the vein and the graft are allowed to back-bleed, and the anastomosis is completed.

For a loop graft, a single longitudinal incision is made in the axilla and deepened through to the subcutaneous tissue; then, the fascia is entered. The neurovascular bundle is identified. The deep brachial/axillary vein and axillary artery are identified and dissected out. A tunnel is created with a counterincision in the arm, using the appropriate device for each type of graft. Arterial and venous anastomoses are created in a standard fashion.

POSTOPERATIVE CARE: MONITORING AND SURVEILLANCE

The patient should be seen postoperatively for evaluation of the surgical wound. Isometric exercise has been shown to increase the diameter of forearm veins; thus, exercise should be recommended. The exercises can increase handgrip strength (e.g., squeezing a rubber ball) and may increase blood flow, thereby enhancing vein maturation.[6]

Monitoring and surveillance of dialysis access can lead to fistula preservation. Increased placement of native

AVFs and detection of dysfunctional access before thrombosis occurs improve quality of life and overall outcome. Possible complications include infection, stenosis, thrombosis, aneurysm, and limb ischemia. The following are all indicators for further evaluation: patient history (pain during hemodialysis and prolonged bleeding time after hemodialysis); abnormal findings on clinical examination (graft occlusion or weak thrill, ipsilateral arm edema suggestive of a central venous stenosis, or aneurysms/pseudoaneurysms); high venous pressures (>300 mmHg); suboptimal blood flow (<400 mL/min); and recirculation while the patient is receiving hemodialysis.

A thorough physical examination should be performed. First, inspection can be used to assess for the presence of aneurysms. Next, the patient should lift their arm; a fistula that does at least partially collapse is likely to have an inflow stenosis.[7] Downstream stenosis also produces an overall dilation of the vein, giving it "aneurysmal" proportions. For graft evaluation, one can determine the direction of flow in a loop configuration and avoid inadvertent recirculation by erroneous needle insertion. A strong pulse is often misinterpreted as evidence of good flow, rather than the opposite. A pulse suggests lower flows.[8]

In a newly thrombosed graft, the arterial pulse is often transmitted into the proximal end of the graft, leading to erroneous cannulation, which could be avoided easily by simply using a stethoscope to confirm absence of flow. When auscultating with a stethoscope, a bruit over an access system that is only systolic is always abnormal; it should be continuous. An intensification of the bruit suggests a stricture or stenosis. Palpable thrill at the arterial, middle, and venous segments of the graft predicts flows >450 mL/min.[8] A hemodynamically significant stenosis is the substrate for thrombosis by reducing flow, increasing turbulence, and increasing platelet activation and residence time against the vessel wall. When a test indicates the likely presence of a stenosis, angiography should be used to definitively establish the presence and degree of stenosis.

Indications for intervention include a failing or failed graft or fistula based on abnormal results of access monitoring or surveillance.[9-11] Interventions include angiogram, angioplasty with or without stenting, and thrombectomy/thrombolysis of a failing/failed or nonmaturing arteriovenous graft or AVF. Stenting is performed very selectively in cases of suboptimal angioplasty, dissection, or if extravasation occurs.[12] Thrombectomy can be performed with the "crossing sheath technique,"[13] and a variety of catheters that extract or macerate the clot (e.g., Fogarty® Arterial Embolectomy Catheter, Edwards Lifesciences, Irvine, CA, USA; AngioJet™ Peripheral Thrombectomy System, Boston Scientific Corporation, Marlborough, MA, USA). Lytics can also be used, either alone or in combination with the mechanical devices described here. Finally, for those whose options for an upper extremity vascular access are precluded by a central venous stenosis or occlusion, the Hemodialysis Reliable Outflow (HeRO)® graft (Merit Medical Systems, Inc, South Jordan, UT, USA) is a reasonable alternative to a lower extremity access or tunneled dialysis catheter.

HERO® GRAFT

The HeRO® graft (**Figure 55.4**) has two components: a graft component with titanium connector; and a venous outflow component. The graft component has a 6-mm inner diameter, 7.4-mm outer diameter, and is 53 cm long, inclusive of the connector. It consists of an expanded PTFE hemodialysis graft with PTFE beading to provide kink resistance near the proprietary titanium connector. The titanium connector attaches the arterial graft component to the venous outflow component; it has radiopaque silicone with braided nitinol reinforcement, a 5-mm inner diameter, and is 40-cm long. The graft component can be cannulated with a standard technique. The key features are: no venous anastomosis; kink and crush resistance; removable and replaceable outflow; and radiopaque band (at the distal tip).

Patients who are considered for HeRO® graft placement usually have undergone multiple tunneled dialysis catheter and upper extremity access procedures. It is very important to evaluate their entire venous and arterial anatomy to identify the reason for the failure. Evaluation would include a complete physical examination, noninvasive vascular testing, and venography. If central venous stenosis or occlusion is the reason for failure, the HeRO® graft would be a good option. The U.S. Food & Drug Administration has approved the HeRO® graft for catheter-dependent patients with central venous stenosis or occlusions. Few relative contraindications include inflow artery diameter <3 mm, systolic BP <100 mmHg, active infection, or ejection fraction <20%.

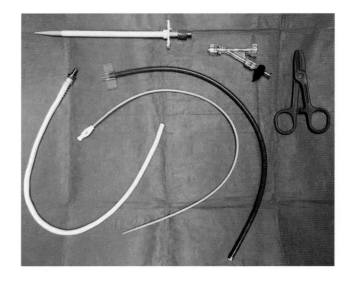

Figure 55.4 Hemodialysis Reliable Outflow (HeRO)® graft (Merit Medical Systems, Inc, South Jordan, UT, USA).

CASE EXAMPLE

A 66-year-old man who had significant comorbidities including hypertension, diabetes mellitus, ESRD on hemodialysis, inflammatory bowel disease needing colectomy with ostomy, and reversal of ostomy, presented to the authors' vascular access center after failing multiple hemodialysis access attempts. He was evaluated and found to have exhausted his options on the left arm; he had a failing right arm arteriovenous graft. He was an obese patient who was minimally ambulatory. It was decided that he was at high risk for infected graft if a thigh graft was attempted. He underwent a right arm graftogram (**Figure 55.5**) that showed central venous occlusion of the right subclavian vein and right internal jugular vein (IJV). However, his superior vena cava (SVC) was patent through collaterals. The nature of his problems and the risk of not having hemodialysis was discussed and he was counselled about the HeRO® graft. The risk/benefits were explained and he was prepped for surgery the next day.

Technique

The procedure can be done with the patient under general or regional anesthesia, depending on the comfort zone of the surgeon. The patient can be either a catheter-dependent patient or someone with a failing/failed fistula or graft because of central occlusion. If the patient already has a tunneled catheter, the outflow portion of the case becomes very simple. The patient is brought to the operating room and placed in a supine position with the upper extremity extended to 90 degrees on an armboard with the head turned to the opposite side. The operating room should have both open and endovascular capabilities. The entire arm, including the ipsilateral neck and chest wall, is prepped and draped in a sterile fashion. The authors recommend prepping the catheter with chlorhexidine gluconate solution. The authors prefer to give vancomycin and gentamicin for perioperative antibiotic prophylaxis because they would use the catheter to access the central veins. The existing catheter is wired with the tip placed into the inferior vena cava. The catheter is then released from the subcutaneous tissue, retracted, and a central cavogram is performed to identify any stenosis that may preclude passage of the venous outflow component. If stenotic, then the GLIDEWIRE® Hydrophilic Coated Guidewire (Terumo Medical Corporation, Somerset, NJ, USA) is exchanged for a stiff wire and balloon angioplasty is performed; the authors prefer to carry the angioplasty up to the exit site of the catheter. Then, the short peel-away sheath is placed, the dilator is removed, and the sheath is plugged with the white/translucent plug provided in the kit. Next, the venous outflow device is introduced with the tip at the SVC-atrial junction. The dilator, wire, and peel-away sheath are removed, followed by clamping the outflow device with the green clamp provided in the kit.

The arterial portion is like any arteriovenous access procedure. Either the brachial or axillary artery is chosen for inflow. Once exposed, a deltopectoral incision is made. The graft component is placed in a tunnel created between those incisions. The outflow device is tunneled, cut to length, and the titanium connector is attached to the outflow component making sure the distal tip is in the SVC-atrial junction (**Figure 55.6**). Heparin is given and arterial anastomosis is performed in the usual fashion.

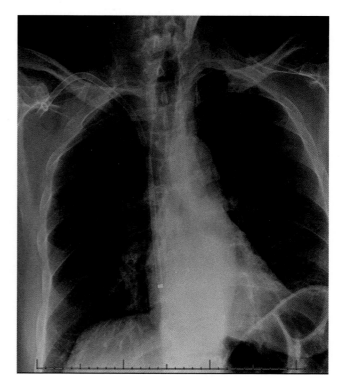

Figure 55.6 Postoperative X-ray showing the outflow component tip in the superior vena cava-atrial junction.

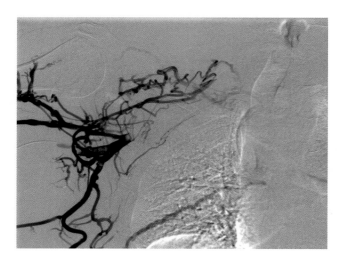

Figure 55.5 Venogram showing right subclavian and internal jugular vein occlusion with collateralization in a 66-year-old man (case example).

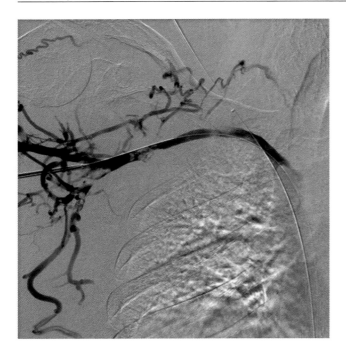

Figure 55.7 Venogram showing wire access to the superior vena cava with ultrasound-guided puncture of collateral vein.

A thrill should be palpated in the graft. The graft should be ready to be used in 2–4 weeks.

If the patient does not have an existing catheter, using ultrasound guidance, the IJV or a collateral is cannulated with a micropuncture needle; under fluoroscopy, the wire is placed into the central veins (**Figure 55.7**). This might be the rate-limiting step of the entire procedure. The authors perform their own venipuncture; however, if you are time-limited, it is prudent to get your interventional radiology colleagues to perform central venous cannulation the day before the surgery and have a catheter placed. The above steps are followed in the operating room the next day.

Occasionally, in a catheter-dependent patient with no other alternative sites, the catheter is removed over the wire and the HeRO® outflow device is placed. In such cases, the authors create a "hybrid" graft component by anastomosing a prosthetic graft designed to allow early cannulation, such as the Vectra® Vascular Access graft (BARD Peripheral Vascular, Inc., Tempe, AZ, USA), FLIXENE™ (Atrium Medical Corporation, Hudson, NH, USA), or GORE® ACUSEAL Vascular Graft (W. L. Gore & Associates, Flagstaff, AZ, USA). The graft can be cannulated immediately, thereby eliminating the need for placement of a tunneled catheter.

REFERENCES

1. National Kidney Foundation. Clinical practice guidelines for vascular access. *Am J Kidney Dis.* 2006;**48**:S176–247.
2. Pisoni RL, Young EW, Dykstra DM, et al. Vascular access use in Europe and the United States: results from the DOPPS. *Kidney Int.* 2002;**61**:305–316.
3. Mehta S. Statistical summary of clinical results of vascular access procedures for hemodialysis. In: Sommer BG, Henry ML, eds. *Vascular Access for Hemodialysis II.* 2nd edn. Chicago, IL: W. L. Gore & Associates and Precept Press; 1991. pp. 145–157.
4. Kaufman JL. The decline of the autogenous hemodialysis access site. *Semin Dial.* 1995;**8**:59–61.
5. Kakkos SK, Haddad GK, Stephanou A, et al. Routine preoperative venous and arterial mapping increases both, construction and maturation rate of upper arm autogenous arteriovenous fistulae. *Vasc Endovascular Surg.* 2011;**45**:135–141.
6. Leaf DA, MacRae HS, Grant E, et al. Isometric exercise increases the size of forearm veins in patients with chronic renal failure. *Am J Med Sci.* 2003;**325**:115–119.
7. Beathard GA. Physical examination of AV grafts. *Semin Dial.* 1992;**5**:74.
8. Trerotola SO, Scheel PJ Jr., Powe NR, et al. Screening for dialysis access graft malfunction: comparison of physical examination with US. *J Vasc Interv Radiol.* 1996;**7**:15–20.
9. Kakkos SK, Haddad GK, Haddad J, et al. Percutaneous rheolytic thrombectomy for autogenous fistulae and prosthetic arteriovenous grafts: outcome after aggressive surveillance and endovascular management. *J Endovasc Ther.* 2008;**15**:91–102.
10. Kakkos SK, Andrzejewski T, Haddad JA, et al. Equivalent secondary patency rates of upper extremity Vectra Vascular Access Grafts and transposed brachial–basilic fistulas with aggressive access surveillance and endovascular treatment. *J Vasc Surg.* 2008;**47**:407–414.
11. Beathard GA, Welch BR, Maidment HJ. Mechanical thrombolysis for the treatment of thrombosed hemodialysis access grafts. *Radiology.* 1996;**200**:711–716.
12. Kakkos SK, Haddad R, Haddad GK, et al. Results of aggressive graft surveillance and endovascular treatment on secondary patency rates of Vectra Vascular Access Grafts. *J Vasc Surg.* 2007;**45**:974–980.
13. Vogel PM, Parise C. Comparison of SMART stent placement for arteriovenous graft salvage versus successful graft PTA. *J Vasc Interv Radiol.* 2005;**16**:1619–1626.

56

Vascular thoracic outlet syndrome

J. KARAM AND R. THOMPSON

CONTENTS

INTRODUCTION

Upper extremity deep vein thrombosis (DVT) accounts for 4–10% of all DVT. It is usually associated with indwelling catheters, pacemaker leads, known hypercoagulable disorders, and malignancies.[1]

Effort-induced axillary-subclavian vein thrombosis, also known as Paget–Schroetter syndrome, is an underrecognized cause of upper extremity DVT. This condition is considered the venous manifestation of thoracic outlet syndrome (TOS), where the underlying cause is the compression of and repetitive injury to the subclavian vein (SCV), between the first rib and clavicle.[2]

VENOUS THORACIC OUTLET SYNDROME (VTOS)

Patients with VTOS typically present with spontaneous, sudden-onset swelling in the entire affected limb, with symptoms of pain, heaviness, and cyanosis. They are typically young (15–45 years) and otherwise healthy, physically active individuals. They typically report a history of frequent intense exercise, repetitive overhead activity, or heavy lifting.[3,4]

On physical examination, patients with VTOS usually exhibit a markedly swollen upper extremity. Multiple subcutaneous collateral veins may be visible in the affected arm, shoulder, and anterior chest (**Figure 56.1**).

Although attractive from a theoretical standpoint, Duplex imaging of the SCV is limited by the clavicle. The thrombosis might be apparent on Duplex if the clot extends into the axillary vein or the distal SCV below the clavicle. Venous obstruction and collateral flow can also affect hemodynamic parameters and waveform analyses.

Contrast-enhanced upper extremity computed tomography or magnetic resonance venography are often used as a first step in imaging evaluation. This allows the presence, location, and extent of the thrombosis to be accurately assessed. However, in patients with acute presentation (<6 weeks from the onset of symptoms), the authors prefer direct, catheter-based contrast venography as the first step in imaging evaluation, because it can provide accurate diagnostic information and immediate therapeutic intervention in cases where thrombolysis and possible balloon angioplasty are options.

In patients with acute-to-subacute presentation of VTOS, the authors focus their initial approach on restoring a patent SCV. This is critical for evaluating residual stenosis and positional venous compression and is most rapidly achieved by pharmacomechanical thrombolysis. Balloon angioplasty to diameters of 10–12 mm can give good radiographic results; however, the benefit is usually incomplete and short-lived unless the source of extrinsic compression has been addressed. Placement of stents in the SCV should not be performed as part of the initial treatment, because mechanical deformation and stent fractures are predictable outcomes that can cause more harm than benefit.

After thrombolysis, patients are maintained on systemic anticoagulation to prevent early recurrent thrombosis. In general, the authors do not believe that long-term

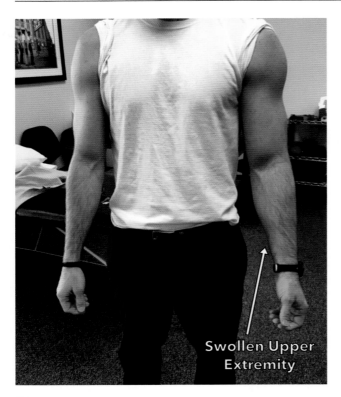

Figure 56.1 Left upper extremity swelling (arrow) in young athlete with venous thoracic outlet syndrome.

anticoagulation as a stand-alone treatment for VTOS is sufficient, whereas surgical treatment offers optimal outcomes. The goal of surgical intervention is complete thoracic outlet decompression and definitive treatment of residual subclavian stenosis or occlusion. Surgical treatment is typically conducted within 4–6 weeks of thrombolysis.

SURGICAL TECHNIQUES

Surgical management of VTOS can be performed with several different strategies and approaches. The transaxillary approach to VTOS was promoted in the early 1990s, as exemplified by Freischlag,[5] who provided detailed descriptions and outcomes of this technique.

The infraclavicular approach to VTOS was developed and described by Molina and colleagues.[6] In this protocol, all patients suspected to have VTOS undergo venography and initial thrombolysis. Patients with long-segment occlusions of the axillary vein and SCV are excluded from surgical management and receive lifelong anticoagulation. All other patients undergo surgery through an infraclavicular approach, with the first rib resected along with portions of the anterior scalene and subclavius muscles. The SCV is exposed along its length underneath the clavicle and vein patch angioplasty with saphenous vein is performed in all patients. The incision is extended medially to a partial median sternotomy if needed, for completion of a long-patch angioplasty or a SCV bypass graft. In this

protocol, a venogram is performed the day after the operation and a stent is placed in the treated SCV.

At the authors' medical center, the paraclavicular approach for VTOS has long been favored, which allows for complete decompression of the thoracic outlet and possible reconstruction of the SCV, if needed, in the same operation. Compared to the transaxillary and infraclavicular approaches, the paraclavicular approach provides the following advantages: (1) direct surgical treatment for all patients with VTOS by complete thoracic outlet decompression; (2) the potential to treat the SCV by thorough external venolysis, when appropriate; and (3) the potential to reconstruct the SCV, when necessary, with either vein patch angioplasty or bypass grafting, with no need for a sternotomy or postoperative stent placement.

Paraclavicular thoracic outlet decompression for VTOS involves several additional considerations to the standard, previously described supraclavicular exploration for neurogenic TOS (NTOS). Positioning is like NTOS (semi-Fowler's) on a fluoroscopic table. A 4-Fr micropuncture sheath is placed in the basilic vein for the initial venogram, to confirm the level of disease and to serve as a baseline for comparison at the end of the procedure.

Following the standard supraclavicular decompression, the authors focus on two critical aspects of surgery for VTOS: complete medial resection of the first rib and external venolysis of the SCV.

To completely resect the anteromedial portion of the first rib, a second transverse skin incision is made 1 cm below the head of the clavicle and immediately over the medial first rib. Flaps are created at the level of the pectoralis major fascia. The tissue plane between the lower and middle portions of the pectoralis major muscle is spread in a muscle-sparing manner until the cartilaginous portion of the first rib is encountered. The rib is exposed and dissected free of surrounding tissue attachments with electrocautery. The clavicle is elevated with protection of the SCV, and all intercostal muscle attachments to the rib are divided along with the tendon of the subclavius muscle on its upper surface. The anteromedial aspect of the first rib is transected at the level of the sternum with a bone rongeur and the whole first rib is removed as a single specimen. The cut edge of the bone is remodeled to a smooth surface and sealed with bone wax. The remaining subclavius muscle and its tendon are resected to provide additional exposure to the SCV.

External venolysis of the SCV

The axillary vein is then identified and exposed from the infraclavicular incision where it emerges from underneath the clavicle. When necessary, the pectoralis minor muscle may be divided at its insertion on the coracoid process, to allow more distal exposure of the axillary vein. The authors then turn their attention to the proximal SCV by tracing it up to the supraclavicular space. From the supraclavicular exposure, the SCV,

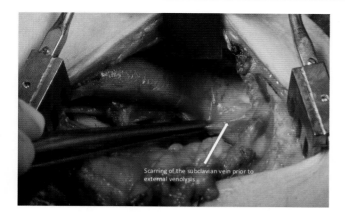

Figure 56.2 Typical appearance of scarred subclavian vein before external venolysis.

the lower aspect of the internal jugular vein, and the upper aspect of the brachiocephalic vein are all exposed. Circumferential external venolysis is performed by excising the thick fibrous tissue that typically encases the SCV. Once venolysis is complete, a venogram is performed to assess the lumen of the SCV and determine the need for further reconstruction (**Figure 56.2**).

SCV reconstruction

The patient is systemically anticoagulated with intravenous heparin and continuous infusion of dextran. The decision on patch angioplasty or bypass grafting is made using the venogram, visualization of the vein, and digital palpation. The authors routinely use adequately sized, cryopreserved femoral vein grafts for patch angioplasty or bypasses, although bovine pericardium may also be used for patch angioplasty. In some cases, where a particularly long bypass graft is constructed, a temporary (12-week) adjunctive radiocephalic fistula may also be constructed at the wrist to improve venous flow. The authors believe it allows for preferential high venous outflow through the bypass graft and not the multiple collaterals (**Figures 56.3–56.5**).

POSTOPERATIVE CARE

A multidisciplinary team comprised of surgeons, physical therapists, pain specialists, and trained nurse practitioners is responsible for the postoperative management of patients with VTOS. Our protocol for VTOS includes keeping the patient on 48 hours of low-molecular-weight dextran, then gradually starting systemic anticoagulation with intravenous heparin, followed by oral anticoagulation on discharge and for 12 weeks.

Closed suction drains are removed 6–7 days after surgery. The authors do not use postoperative ultrasound surveillance, but they recommend venography if arm swelling occurs during follow-up.

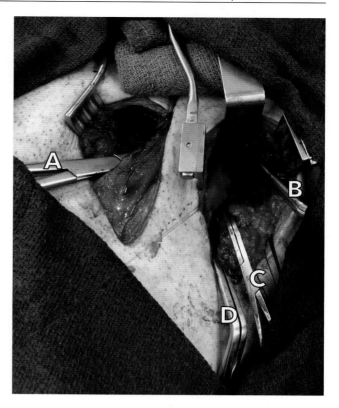

Figure 56.3 Clamp placement for venous reconstruction in the paraclavicular approach. (A) Brachiocephalic vein clamp. (B) Internal jugular vein clamp. (C) Clamp on large collateral veins. (D) Distal subclavian vein clamp.

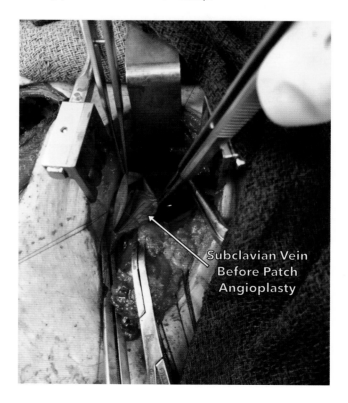

Figure 56.4 Preparation of the subclavian vein before patch angioplasty (arrow).

ARTERIAL THORACIC OUTLET SYNDROME (ATOS)

ATOS is the least frequent form of TOS. It represents 1–3% of all TOS. The authors reserve the definition of ATOS for patients who have fixed arterial lesions (stenosis, occlusion, or aneurysmal dilation) of the subclavian artery (SCA) as it passes over the first rib. This is usually due to compression by an osseous abnormality (cervical rib or other bony anomaly); however, in some cases, it may be due to a tight ligamentous band (**Figure 56.5**).[7] In the authors' series of ATOS patients, 75% had cervical ribs, whereas anomalous first ribs and tight fascial bands accounted for the rest of structural anomalies causing compression of the SCA.

There are two clinical manifestations of ATOS: one related to the injury to the SCA; the second related to distal manifestations of arterial ischemia caused by embolic or thrombotic occlusions. The treatment for ATOS focuses on relieving arterial compression and removing the source of the emboli, to restore normal circulation to the arm.

At the authors' center, patients presenting with acute arm ischemia from ATOS are treated first with thrombolysis or surgical thrombectomy, depending on the level of occlusion and the type of presentation. After distal circulation is restored, the patients are prepared for ATOS repair within a few days of the initial procedure.

The authors' approach is like that used for NTOS, in that they focus on complete decompression of the thoracic outlet with anterior and middle scalenectomy and removal of the first rib and cervical rib, if present (**Figure 56.6**).

The decision to repair the SCA with a bypass graft versus patch angioplasty depends on the extent of the aneurysm or embolizing lesion along its course. The authors have typically used a paraclavicular approach as previously

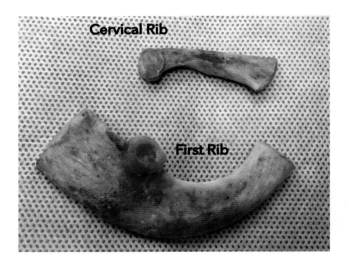

Figure 56.5 First rib with cervical rib, typically connected by a joint.

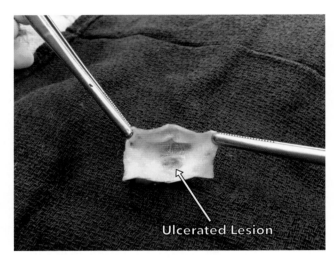

Figure 56.7 Ulcerated lesion inside a subclavian aneurysm (arrow). This is typically the cause of distal embolization.

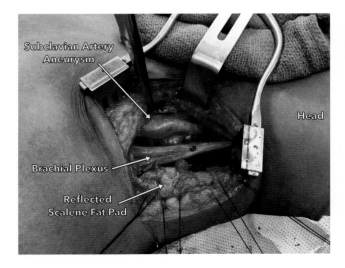

Figure 56.6 Subclavian artery aneurysm after scalenectomy and first rib removal.

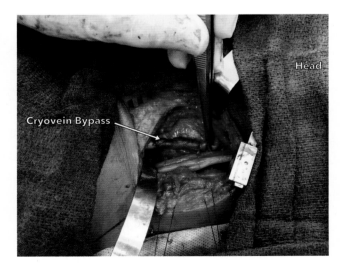

Figure 56.8 Arterial reconstruction with cryopreserved femoral vein graft.

described to perform SCA-axillary artery bypasses. The authors' conduit of choice has been cryopreserved femoral vein graft (**Figures 56.7** and **56.8**).

REFERENCES

1. Flinterman LE, Van Der Meer FJ, Rosendaal FR, et al. Current perspective of venous thrombosis in the upper extremity. *J Thromb Haemost.* 2008;**6**:1262–1266.

2. Azakie A, McElhinney DB, Thompson RW, et al. Surgical management of subclavian-vein effort thrombosis as a result of thoracic outlet compression. *J Vasc Surg.* 1998;**28**:777–786.

3. Sanders RJ, Hammond SL, Rao NM. Diagnosis of thoracic outlet syndrome. *J Vasc Surg.* 2007;**46**:601–604.

4. Tapson VF, Carroll BA, Davidson BL. The diagnostic approach to acute venous thromboembolism. Clinical practice guideline. American Thoracic Society. *Am J Respir Crit Care Med.* 1999;**160**:1043–1066.

5. Freischlag J. Venous thoracic outlet syndrome: transaxillary approach. *Oper Tech Gen Surg.* 2008;**10**:122–130.

6. Molina JE, Hunter DW, Dietz CA. Paget–Schroetter syndrome treated with thrombolytics and immediate surgery. *J Vasc Surg.* 2007;**45**:328–334.

7. Criado E, Berguer R, Greenfield L. The spectrum of arterial compression at the thoracic outlet. *J Vasc Surg.* 2010;**52**:406–411.

57

Neurogenic thoracic outlet syndrome

J. KARAM AND R. THOMPSON

CONTENTS

INTRODUCTION

The thoracic outlet region is comprised of three anatomic spaces: the scalene triangle; the costoclavicular space; and the pectoralis minor space. The neurovascular bundle, which consists of the subclavian artery (SCA), subclavian vein (SCV), and brachial plexus, courses through the scalene triangle to the costoclavicular space and then through the pectoralis minor space. Compression of the neurovascular bundle components anywhere along this trajectory can result in similar symptomatology because the vessels and nerves do not change substantially within the thoracic outlet region. Neurogenic thoracic outlet syndrome (NTOS) results from brachial plexus compression, which leads to a constellation of neurologic symptoms of the upper extremity. Variations in anatomy of the thoracic outlet region, as well as injuries and repetitive physical activities, can predispose a patient to the development of NTOS.

EPIDEMIOLOGY

There are approximately 2000–2500 first rib resection procedures performed annually in the USA; of these, NTOS accounts for >95% of all cases.[1] However, the lack of objective diagnostic criteria and inconsistent reporting standards for NTOS make it difficult to estimate the true incidence and prevalence. Also, the condition is likely underdiagnosed clinically in patients who seek medical attention and in symptomatic patients who fail to seek medical care.[2]

DIFFERENTIAL DIAGNOSIS

Because of the nonspecific and diffuse nature of symptoms, the differential diagnosis for NTOS can be broad and includes a variety of upper extremity neurologic and musculoskeletal conditions. Various cervical spine disorders can produce similar neurologic symptoms, including: arthritis; degenerative disc disease; post-traumatic strain; and spinal stenosis. Several impingement syndromes, such as acromioclavicular impingement, ulnar nerve (cubital tunnel) entrapment, and median nerve (carpal tunnel) compression syndrome, are also frequently on the differential diagnosis. Shoulder tendinitis, epicondylitis, and fibromyalgia should also be considered.

PHYSICAL EXAMINATION

Symptoms of NTOS include pain, dysesthesia, numbness, and weakness, that do not localize to a specific neuro-anatomic distribution. These neurologic symptoms are typically exacerbated by maneuvers that compromise the thoracic outlet, such as raising the arms overhead, or stretching the brachial plexus, such as dangling the arms. Various clinical tests are designed to elicit positional or effort-related sensory disturbances. With the Elevated Arm Stress Test (EAST; Roos Stress Test), patients are asked to adduct the shoulder to 90 degrees, flex the elbow to 90 degrees, and face the palms forward. With the arms in this position, the patient is asked to open and close the hands repeatedly for up to 3 minutes, or until the maneuver becomes intolerable. In addition, the Adson's maneuver is conducted by having the patient turn their head toward the affected side while extending the symptomatic arm and inhaling. Pulse changes and symptom exacerbation are then assessed. Although this test often does not specifically demonstrate nerve root compression, a positive Adson's sign suggests thoracic outlet compromise and can be associated with NTOS. Various other maneuvers, such as the Upper Limb Tension Test, also attempt to compromise the thoracic outlet and reproduce or exacerbate distal symptoms.

Tenderness to palpation over certain areas is also an important physical examination finding in the patient with NTOS. Palpation over the scalene triangle typically results in severe local discomfort, elicits pain that radiates down the axilla, or leads to the reproduction of distal sensory symptoms. Similarly, palpation over the pectoralis minor insertion can also lead to pain and symptom reproduction. Positive results on these physical examination tests and maneuvers serve to strongly support the diagnosis of NTOS in combination with a consistent clinical history.[3]

DIAGNOSTIC WORKUP

The diagnosis of NTOS is made clinically, with the assistance of specific clinical tests. Often, specific diagnostic testing for NTOS yields negative or equivocal results, thus diagnostic studies are frequently most useful for the exclusion of other conditions. Plain radiographs can aid in the diagnosis of NTOS if an osseous cervical rib is identified, but other imaging tests are typically uninformative.

Computed tomography or magnetic resonance imaging (MRI) studies are usually negative, because the factors causing brachial plexus compression are presumably beyond the resolution of such tests. Even if thoracic outlet anomalies are identified, correlation with the patient's symptoms cannot be definitively proven. However, exclusion of other conditions, such as degenerative disc disease or rotator cuff pathology, with these imaging modalities is important. Additionally, electromyography (EMG) and nerve conduction studies (NCS) are often performed when evaluating a patient with suspected NTOS and are also frequently negative in this condition. NTOS is not typically associated with permanent neurologic dysfunction; however, if EMG or NCS testing is positive in a patient with NTOS, the prognosis is poor even with adequate surgical decompression.[4]

PHYSICAL THERAPY

Before invasive intervention, trying physical therapy that is specifically directed toward the relief of NTOS symptoms is warranted. The approach to NTOS physical therapy is unique from therapy for other related conditions; thus, it should be conducted by a therapist with expertise in NTOS care. The Edgelow Neurovascular Entrapment Syndrome Treatment protocol has been tested extensively in patients with pain originating from the thoracic outlet. This approach focuses on correcting breathing and core motor control dysfunction and calming brachial plexus hyperesthesia. Adjunctive treatments, such as anti-inflammatory medications or muscle relaxants, can also provide benefit.[5]

DIAGNOSTIC BLOCKS

Test muscle blocks are frequently performed to help provide diagnostic information and guide NTOS therapy.[6] The pectoralis minor muscle block is performed by injecting local anesthetic into the pectoralis minor near the insertion site at the coracoid process. This is typically done by inserting a needle 2–3 cm below the clavicle, angled at 45 degrees, and pointed cephalad to prevent penetration into the pleural space. Aspiration during the procedure is important to ensure that the needle has not entered an axillary vessel. The response to the anesthetic injection is then assessed. Within a few minutes, the patient should start to have reduced symptoms at rest and improved tolerance during repeat physical examination.

Those patients who only receive a limited or partial response from pectoralis minor block, will also have an anterior scalene muscle (ASM) block performed. The procedure for an ASM block is performed similarly to the pectoralis minor block. With this procedure, the belly of the ASM can be targeted without guidance or with EMG and ultrasound, and local anesthetic is injected. Again, the patient is assessed for improvement in symptoms at rest or increased tolerance to physical examination maneuvers; a positive response with muscle block correlates with good outcomes for NTOS decompression surgery.

OPERATIVE TECHNIQUE

The authors focus their discussion on the supraclavicular approach for thoracic outlet decompression because it provides excellent exposure to the first rib, a cervical rib (if present), scalene muscles, and the brachial plexus. The authors also describe the adjunctive pectoralis minor tenotomy procedure via the deltopectoral approach.

Positioning

After the initiation of general anesthesia, the patient is positioned supine with the head of the bed elevated to 30 degrees. The neck is then extended and turned toward the opposite side from the surgical site. The upper extremity of the operative side is also prepped into the field, wrapped in a stockinet, and positioned across the abdomen. This enables movement of the extremity during the procedure, if necessary.

Exposure

The procedure begins with a transverse incision made 1–2 fingerbreadths above the clavicle within the supraclavicular fossa. On the medial side, the incision starts at the lateral border of the sternocleidomastoid muscle; laterally, the incision extends 6–8 cm, approaching the anterior edge of the trapezius muscle. The platysma muscle layer is then transected, exposing the supraclavicular scalene fat pad and the diagonally traversing omohyoid muscle, which is divided routinely. The scalene fat pad is then mobilized, starting at the lateral edge of the internal jugular vein, and is progressively dissected away from the surface of the ASM. As the fat pad is reflected, the ASM should be exposed, with the phrenic nerve crossing its surface. The surgeon should proceed with caution until the phrenic nerve is positively identified. Typically, the phrenic nerve can be easily distinguished, because it is the only peripheral nerve to run from lateral to medial as it courses distally. After the phrenic nerve is identified, the fat pad can be mobilized far enough laterally to expose the underlying brachial plexus roots; subsequently, it can be reflected on its pedicle and secured out of position with silk suture (**Figure 57.1**).

Scalenectomy

During dissection of the ASM, it is important to note the locations of the phrenic nerve, C5-C6 nerve roots, and the SCA, to avoid injury to these structures. In preparation for excision, the ASM should be mobilized circumferentially, down to the level of the attachment to the first rib. When the surgeon can pass a right-angle clamp under the ASM at its osseous attachment, the muscle can be divided at this location using curved Mayo scissors. It is preferable

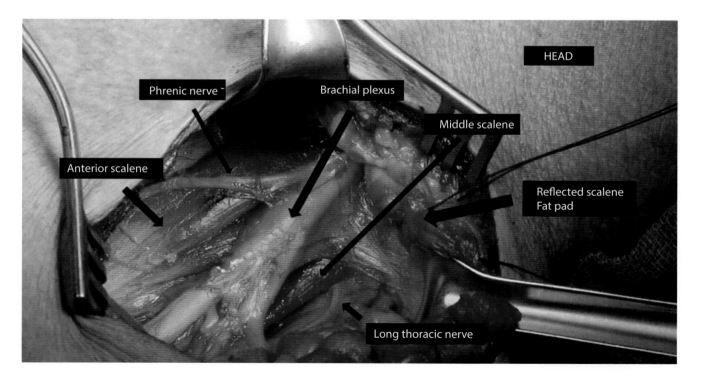

Figure 57.1 Operative image of the critical view of the essential structures in a standard supraclavicular thoracic outlet decompression.

to perform this step with scissors because cautery may induce thermal injury to adjacent structures. The muscle can then be lifted superiorly and detached from the underlying structures, typically using gentle finger dissection, to its origin at the C6 transverse process. Frequently, muscle fibers can interdigitate with roots of the brachial plexus; thus, care must be taken to avoid causing injury to these structures throughout the dissection. At its origin, the muscle can then be sharply divided while protecting adjacent nerve roots. Additionally, the scalenus minimus muscle, characterized by fibers that originate posteriorly to the C5-C6 nerve roots in the plane of the middle scalene muscle (MSM), may be apparent at this point. Because the scalenus minimus fibers pass between the brachial plexus nerve roots, it may be an additional source of neural compression and should also be excised.

With the ASM removed, the brachial plexus will be very apparent. It should be brought forward with gentle retraction to expose the MSM. Before dividing the MSM, the long thoracic nerve must be identified. This nerve exits the anterolateral border of the MSM and courses inferolaterally. The MSM insertion on the first rib is identified and dissected off the rib surface with electrocautery. Proximally, the MSM is sharply transected just distal to the course of the long thoracic nerve.

First rib resection

The posterior neck of the first rib is exposed with a periostial elevator. The lateral musculofascial attachments to the first rib are then released anteriorly from its posterior neck to the scalene tubercle. The pleural apex is bluntly dissected away from the inferior surface of the rib along its entire course. With the brachial plexus roots well protected, the neck of the first rib is sharply divided with a Stille bone cutter (Stille AB, Torshälla, Sweden). The cut edge of the posterior first rib is remodeled to a smooth surface with a Kerrison bone rongeur, protecting the C8 and T1 nerve roots from injury, to a level parallel with the transverse process; its edge is then sealed with bone wax (**Figure 57.2**).

The anterior portion of the first rib is then exposed underneath the clavicle and similarly divided just medial to the level of the scalene tubercle, with protection of the SCV, SCA, and brachial plexus nerve roots. The anterior edge of the rib is remodeled to a smooth surface and sealed with bone wax. After dividing additional intercostal muscle attachments, the first rib is removed from the operative field.

Cervical rib removal

When a cervical rib is present, the authors typically resect it after the middle scalenectomy is completed. It is exposed at its posterior origin and the neck of the rib is divided protecting the nerve roots origin (C8 and T1) from injury. The proximal end of the cervical rib is detached from its attachment of the first rib and removed as a specimen.

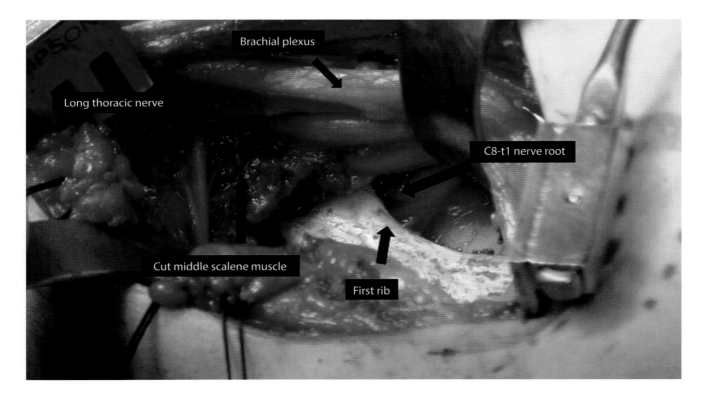

Figure 57.2 Operative image of the posterior aspect of the first rib with exposure of the C8- T1 nerve roots.

Brachial plexus neurolysis

Inspection of the brachial plexus nerve roots typically shows an extensive amount of dense postinflammatory scar tissue. This fibrous tissue is removed by performing a complete brachial neurolysis. During this step of the procedure, each of the nerve roots contributing to the brachial plexus is thoroughly identified and carefully protected from injury, including the C5-C8 spinal segments and T1.

To prevent or limit the development of perineural scar tissue that might contribute to recurrent NTOS, the authors use polylactide film wrapped around the brachial plexus, as a temporary physical barrier between the nerves and adjacent tissues. The advantage of this material is that it can be secured in place with sutures and may resist absorption for 2–3 months.

Pectoralis minor tenotomy

A small, vertical infraclavicular incision is made in the deltopectoral groove and carried through to the subcutaneous tissues. The pectoralis fascia is entered and the lateral edge of the pectoralis major is lifted and retracted medially. The space between the pectoralis muscles is developed bluntly; the pectoralis minor tendon is identified, encircled, then divided under direct vision close to the coracoid process with electrocautery for hemostasis. The edge of the muscle is oversewn with 2-0 silk suture. The clavipectoral fascia is also divided sharply just beneath the clavicle. This gives a palpable improvement in the subpectoral space, allowing relief if any neurovascular compression is found at this site.

Wound closure

The authors irrigate the wound with antibiotic solution, obtain hemostasis, and pay careful attention to any detectable lymphatic leak. The authors also check for any air leaks from the lung parenchyma. The opening in the pleural space is widened and the pleural cavity is suctioned. A closed-suction No. 19 Blake drain is brought through a lateral stab wound and placed extending into the pleural space. Two needle sheaths are placed percutaneously into the wound, through which continuous infusion catheters are passed and placed alongside the neurovascular bundle and the bed of the resected rib. The catheters are secured to the skin with nylon sutures; the drain is also secured. The authors connect the catheters to an elastomeric pump system for continuous infusion of local anesthetic (0.5% bupivacaine hydrochloride). The scalene fat pad is approximated over the brachial plexus and the wound is closed in layers.

POSTOPERATIVE CARE

The authors do not restrict arm movement postoperatively; physical therapy is initiated on the first postoperative day. The continuous bupivacaine hydrochloride perfusion catheter is removed on the third postoperative day. The closed-suction drain is removed in the clinic the day after discharge.

Pain control can be challenging in this patient population; care is taken to titrate narcotic medication. A strict bowel regimen is set in place.

Patients often complain of mild paresthesia in the C8-T1 distribution. An elevated hemidiaphragm can result from traction injury to the phrenic nerve.

It is imperative to establish a long-term follow-up plan for patients with NTOS. They require frequent medication alteration, evaluation for persistent or recurrent symptoms, and most importantly continued physical therapy.

CASE EXAMPLE

A 32-year-old woman (a hair stylist) presented with a 2-year history of left hand, arm, and neck pain. Her pain was exacerbated by arm elevation and overhead activities, severely restricting her ability to work. She also described numbness over the ulnar distribution of the arm with tingling and frequent bouts of tension headaches. She stated that her symptoms became apparent after a car accident, which caused a hyperextension strain to her neck with no cervical spine or skeletal injuries. Over the past 2 years, she had an extensive workup including cervical spine and shoulder MRIs that were read as normal, multiple epidural injections that gave minimal benefit, and intensive physical therapy. Her symptoms caused a significant decline in her ability to work. On exam, the patient had significant tenderness over the scalene triangle and pectoralis minor insertion with reproduction of symptoms in her affected arm. She had an EAST time of 40 seconds. Both ASM and pectoralis minor blocks produced temporary relief of her symptoms; she had minimal improvement in her symptoms with physical therapy. She was eventually scheduled for thoracic outlet decompression using a supraclavicular approach as well as pectoralis minor tenotomy. She recovered well from her surgery and progressed as expected with physical therapy.

REFERENCES

1. Hempel GK, Shutze WP, Anderson JF, et al. 770 consecutive supraclavicular first rib resections for thoracic outlet syndrome. *Ann Vasc Surg.* 1996;**10**:456–463.
2. Juvonen T, Satta J, Laitala P, et al. Anomalies at the thoracic outlet are frequent in the general population. *Am J Surg.* 1995;**170**:33–37.

3. Thompson RW, Petrinec D, Toursarkissian B. Surgical treatment of thoracic outlet compression syndromes. II. Supraclavicular exploration and vascular reconstruction. *Ann Vasc Surg.* 1997;**11**:442–451.

4. Freischlag J, Orion K. Understanding thoracic outlet syndrome. *Scientifica (Cairo).* 2014;**2014**:248163.

5. Watson LA, Pizzari T, Balster S. Thoracic outlet syndrome part 2: conservative management of thoracic outlet. *Man Ther.* 2010;**15**:305–314.

6. Sanders RJ, Hammond SL, Rao NM. Diagnosis of thoracic outlet syndrome. *J Vasc Surg.* 2007;**46**: 601–604.

58

Operative venous thrombectomy

ANTHONY J. COMEROTA AND RODRIGO RUIZ-GAMBOA

CONTENTS

INTRODUCTION

Although operative venous thrombectomy is infrequently required because of the increased safety and effectiveness of catheter-directed thrombolysis (CDT) for iliofemoral deep vein thrombosis (DVT), it remains a valuable treatment option in selected patients. Such patients include those with multiple traumas, those with active bleeding, those at high risk for bleeding into a critical site (intracranial), and pregnant patients refusing CDT.

The main reason to adopt a strategy of thrombus removal is the severe morbidity associated with post-thrombotic syndrome resulting from lower extremity DVT, especially iliofemoral DVT. Early removal of thrombus from the iliofemoral venous system improves long-term results and reduces venous pressures, often to normal levels.[1–4] Anticoagulation alone in the management of iliofemoral DVT has high morbidity, with up to 40% of patients complaining of venous claudication.[5]

The procedure is associated with relatively few complications. Eklof and Juhan reported their experience with 230 patients undergoing venous thrombectomy for iliofemoral DVT. They reported no pulmonary embolisms and only one mortality.[6] Based on multiple case series studies, they reported a long-term iliac vein patency of 80% in patients treated with venous thrombectomy for iliofemoral DVT (**Table 58.1**).

Table 58.1 Venous thrombectomy with arteriovenous fistula: long-term iliac vein patency

Study (authors)	Number	Follow-up (months)	Patent iliac vein (%)
Plate et al.[2]	31	6	76
Piquet[7]	57	39	80
Einarsson et al.[8]	58	10	61
Vollmar[9]	93	53	82
Juhan et al.[10]	150	102	84
Törngren and Swedenborg[11]	54	19	54
Rasmussen et al.[12]	24	20	88
Eklof and Kistner[13]	77	48	75
Neglén et al.[14]	34	24	88
Meissner and Huszcza[15]	27	12	89
Pillny et al.[16]	97	70	90
Hartung et al.[17]	29	63	86
Hölper et al.[18]	25	68	84
TOTAL	756	55 (mean)	80 (mean)

Note: Adapted with permission from Comerota AJ, Gale SS. Surgical venous thrombectomy for iliofemoral deep vein thrombosis. In: Greenhalgh RM, ed. *Towards Vascular and Endovascular Consensus*. London: BIBA Publishing; 2005.

PROCEDURAL AIMS

The aim of the procedure is to remove all thrombus, restore patency to the operated veins, and maintain unobstructed outflow from the iliofemoral venous segment into the vena cava. This is best achieved by opening thrombosed infrainguinal venous segments, correcting any underlying venous lesions or compression, and preventing rethrombosis by constructing an arteriovenous fistula (AVF) and providing adequate anticoagulation, often by the catheter-directed technique into the thrombectomized veins.

PREOPERATIVE CARE

The proximal and distal extent of the DVT should be clearly defined with venous duplex, computed tomography venography, magnetic resonance venography, or contralateral iliocavography.

The authors do not recommend routine use of vena cava filters, except in patients with nonocclusive thrombus in their vena cava. Options for protection from nonocclusive caval thrombus include permanent or retrievable filters or balloon occlusion of the proximal vena cava during thrombectomy. Heritable thrombophilia evaluations are no longer required because the risk for recurrence is governed by the extensive DVT, not the results of the thrombophilia test.[19]

TECHNIQUE OF CONTEMPORARY VENOUS THROMBECTOMY

General anesthesia is usually recommended for patients undergoing operative venous thrombectomy. A longitudinal inguinal incision under ultrasound (US) guidance exposes the common femoral vein (CFV), femoral vein, saphenofemoral junction, and profunda femoris vein (PFV) (**Figure 58.1a**). A longitudinal venotomy of the CFV is recommended to clearly visualize the origin of the saphenous and PFV branches. If an infrainguinal thrombus is present, the leg is elevated and compressed with a tightly wrapped rubber bandage, the foot is dorsiflexed, and the calf and thigh are squeezed. If the complete infrainguinal thrombus is removed, which is clinically evident when it occurs, balloon thrombectomy of the iliofemoral venous system is performed.

If the infrainguinal thrombus persists, one option for thrombus removal is to use an over-the-wire balloon thrombectomy catheter. First, a hydrophilic guidewire needs to be advanced antegrade through the valves and down to the tibial veins. If a guidewire cannot be passed through the infrainguinal valves, a cutdown is performed to expose the distal posterior tibial vein (PTV). Alternatively, this can also be done by cannulating the tibial vein under US guidance. A No. 3 Fogarty catheter is advanced from the distal PTV to and through the CFV venotomy. The silicone elastomer stem of an intravenous

catheter (12–14 G) is amputated from its hub and slid halfway onto the balloon catheter. Another balloon catheter (No. 4 Fogarty) is placed at the opposite end of the silicone elastomer sheath (**Figure 58.1a**). Pressure is applied to the two balloons by a single operating surgeon to ensure that the catheters remain secure inside the sheath. The No. 4 Fogarty balloon catheter is guided distally through the thrombosed venous valves and clotted veins (**Figure 58.1b**) to the level of the posterior tibial venotomy (**Figure 58.1c**). Thrombectomy is performed and repeated as necessary. Alternatively, if an over-the-wire balloon thrombectomy catheter is available, a guidewire can be passed proximally from the distal PTV and the infrainguinal thrombectomy is performed (**Figure 58.1d,e**).

After the infrainguinal balloon catheter thrombectomy, the infrainguinal venous system is flushed by placing a large red rubber catheter into the proximal PTV and vigorously flushing with a heparinized saline solution, using a bulb syringe to hydraulically express residual thrombus from the deep venous system (**Figure 58.1f**). An impressive amount of additional thrombus can be retrieved with this maneuver. Once the infrainguinal venous system is adequately cleared, a vascular clamp is applied below the femoral venotomy and the infrainguinal venous system is filled with dilute recombinant tissue plasminogen activator (rtPA) solution consisting of approximately 4–6 mg of rtPA in 200 mL of saline. The rtPA solution remains in the infrainguinal veins for the remainder of the procedure. This amount of local rtPA binds to fibrin-bound plasminogen in residual thrombus and promotes further clot dissolution; however, this dose does not cause a systemic lytic response because of the low-dose circulating rtPA and plasmin inhibitors. If the infrainguinal venous thrombectomy is not successful because of chronic disease, the femoral vein is ligated and divided below the PFV. PFV patency is ensured by direct thrombectomy, if necessary.

Iliofemoral venous thrombectomy is performed by passing a No. 8 or 10 venous thrombectomy balloon catheter partially into the iliac vein for several passes to remove the bulk of the thrombus before advancing the catheter into the vena cava. Proximal thrombectomy is routinely performed under fluoroscopic guidance with contrast material filling the balloon, especially if a vena caval filter is present, there is a clot in the vena cava, or resistance to catheter passage is encountered. During this part of the procedure, the anesthesiologist applies positive end-expiratory pressure to further reduce the risk of pulmonary embolization. If a clot is present in the vena cava, caval thrombectomy can be performed with a protective balloon catheter inflated above the thrombus as an alternative to vena caval filtration (**Figure 58.1g**).

After completion of the iliofemoral venous thrombectomy, intraoperative venography/fluoroscopy is performed to evaluate an underlying iliac vein stenosis (IVS) and assess the nature of the venous drainage into the vena cava. Intravascular US is gaining popularity and improves on single-view venography for detecting IVS. Any underlying IVS is corrected by balloon angioplasty and stenting.

If an iliac vein stent is used, a 14-mm-diameter or larger stent is recommended for the common iliac vein and a ≥12 mm one for the external iliac vein.

After the venotomy is primarily closed, an end-to-side AVF is constructed by anastomosing the amputated end of the proximal saphenous vein or a large proximal branch of the saphenous vein to the side of the superficial femoral artery (SFA). The anastomosis should be limited to 3.5–4.0 mm in diameter. An arterial punch (3.5 mm) is recommended for the SFA arteriotomy. The purpose of the AVF is to increase venous velocity but not venous pressure. CFV pressure is recorded before and after the AVF is opened. No increase in venous pressure should occur when the AVF is opened. If the pressure increases, this may be indicative of a residual stenosis or obstruction and the proximal iliac vein should be re-evaluated and treated accordingly. If the pressure remains elevated, the AVF is constricted to decrease flow and normalize pressure.

A piece of polytetrafluoroethylene or bovine pericardium is wrapped around the saphenous AVF and a large permanent monofilament suture (No. 0) is looped and clipped with approximately 2 cm left in the subcutaneous tissue (**Figure 58.1h**). This serves as a guide for future dissection if operative closure of the AVF becomes necessary. Since the

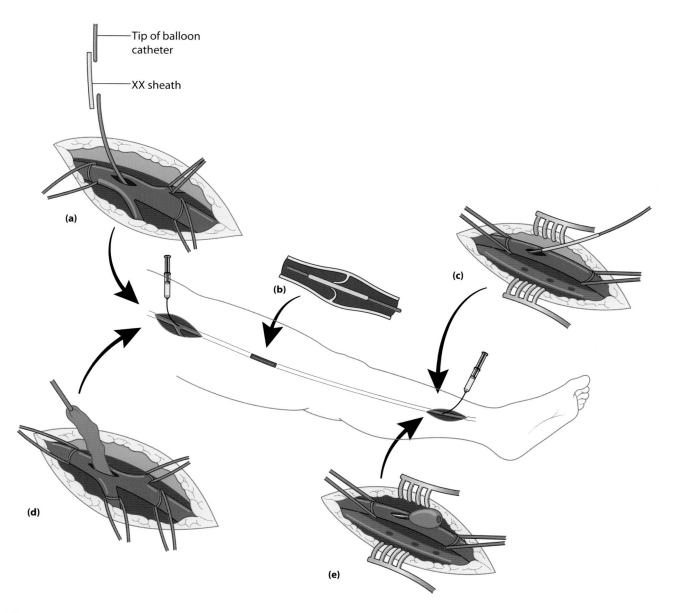

Figure 58.1 Surgical thrombectomy of iliofemoral venous thrombosis. (**a**) Longitudinal inguinal incision to expose the common femoral vein (CFV), femoral vein, saphenofemoral junction, and profunda femoris vein. (**b,c**) The balloon catheter is guided distally through the thrombosed venous valves and clotted veins using a silicone elastomer catheter attached to a small catheter passed from below. A thrombectomy is performed from the posterior tibial venotomy to the common femoral vein. (**d,e**) The passage of the balloon catheter is repeated as necessary.

(Continued)

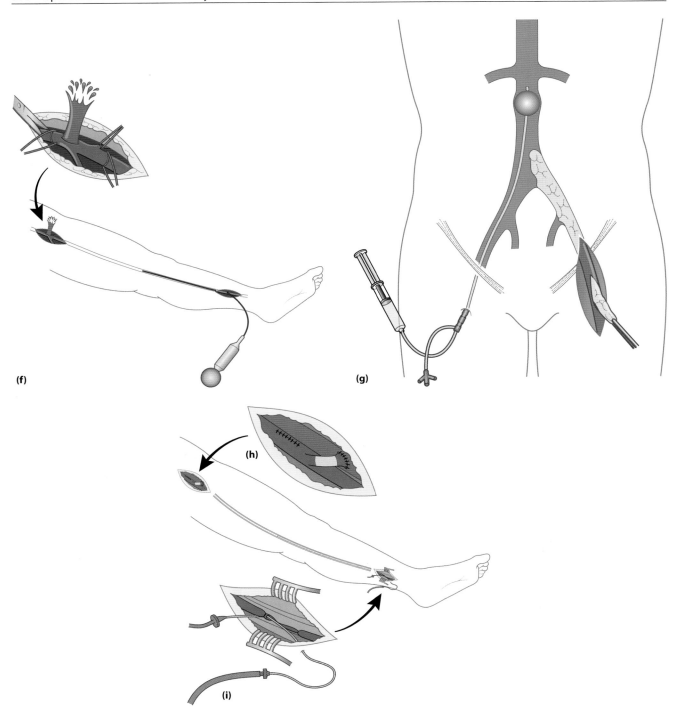

Figure 58.1 (Continued) Surgical thrombectomy of iliofemoral venous thrombosis. (**f**) After the infrainguinal balloon catheter thrombectomy, flushing of the infrainguinal venous system with a heparinized saline solution is performed by placing a large red rubber catheter into the proximal posterior tibial vein (PTV) and flushing vigorously with a bulb syringe. After flushing is complete, 250–300 mL of saline with 4–6 mg recombinant tissue plasminogen activator is infused into the deep venous system after the clamp is reapplied to the distal CFV. Proximal thrombectomy is then performed. (**g**) Iliocaval thrombectomy can be performed with a protective balloon catheter inflated above the caval thrombus, if it exists, as an alternative to vena cava filtration. A large venous thrombectomy catheter with an 8–10-Fr balloon is used to remove the clot from the iliofemoral venous segments. (**h**) Placement of a piece of polytetrafluoroethylene or bovine pericardium wrap around the saphenous arteriovenous fistula (AVF). A large, permanent monofilament suture is looped and clipped with approximately 2 cm left in the subcutaneous tissue. This serves to prevent dilation of the AVF and is also a guide for dissection, should surgical disconnection of the AVF become necessary. (**i**) Placement of a small infusion catheter (pediatric feeding tube) into the PTV via a separate stab incision in the skin. It is fixed in the proximal PTV for infusion of unfractionated heparin directly into the thrombectomized vein.

AVF is limited and cannot enlarge, the authors consider it permanent. Clinical experience has shown that approximately 15% of the iliofemoral segments rethrombose following elective closure of AVFs. These AVFs can also be closed with endovascular techniques, should the need arise.

A diligent search for transected lymphatics is performed with generous ligation and electrocoagulation. A closed-suction drain is generally placed in the wound to evacuate fluid that may accumulate postoperatively. The drain exits through a separate puncture site adjacent to the incision. The wound is closed with multilayered, running, absorbable suture to achieve both hemostatic and lymphostatic wound closure and ensure elimination of dead space.

If the PTV is exposed, the distal end of the vein is ligated. A small infusion catheter (pediatric feeding tube) is brought into the wound via a separate stab incision in the skin and inserted and fixed in the proximal PTV (**Figure 58.1i**). This catheter is used for postoperative anticoagulation with unfractionated heparin (UFH) and predischarge venography. If the PTV was accessed percutaneously, the catheter is left in place to serve the same purpose.

Anticoagulation via this catheter ensures maximum heparin concentration in the affected veins during their period of greatest thrombogenicity. A 2-0 monofilament suture is looped around the proximal PTV (and catheter) and both ends exit the skin adjacent to the wound. The ends of the suture are passed through the holes of a sterile button, which is secured snugly to the skin when the catheter is removed. Upward tension on the ends of the suture obliterates the proximal PTV at the time of catheter removal and eliminates the risk of bleeding; the suture is tied and secured above the skin by the button.

It is now the authors' preference to anticoagulate the patient postoperatively through a catheter in the thrombectomized deep venous system. If not placed during the surgical procedure, the catheter is placed in the femoral vein under US guidance. This results in the operated and stented veins receiving a much higher dose of heparin using a much lower systemic dose, thereby reducing the risk of rethrombosis while at the same time reducing the risk of wound hematoma.

Antibiotic ointment is applied to all wounds before the sterile dressing is applied. The patient's leg is wrapped snugly with sterile gauze and a multilayered dressing with elastic bandages from the base of the toes to the groin. The PTV catheter or other limb catheter, if present, exits between the layers of the bandage but is secured so that the patient can ambulate using an intravenous (IV) pole on wheels to support the infusion of UFH.

POSTOPERATIVE CARE

Therapeutic anticoagulation is continued with UFH through the leg catheter, attached to a pump on an IV pole with wheels so that the patient can ambulate. Before removal of the catheter, an ascending venogram is performed. Oral anticoagulation is started when the patient awakens and resumes oral intake. Heparin infusion and oral intake of heparin overlap for 4–5 days until the patient's international normalized ratio reaches 2–3. Heparin infusion is discontinued and oral anticoagulation is continued for an extended period, generally for ≥1 year. Use of direct-acting oral anticoagulants for long-term anticoagulation is becoming more popular; however, the authors prefer vitamin K antagonists for long-term anticoagulation for at least 6–12 months after the procedure.

Intermittent pneumatic compression garments are used on both legs postoperatively when the patient is not ambulating. Before discharge, the patient is fitted for 30–40 mmHg ankle gradient below-knee compression stockings and instructed to wear the stockings from

Table 58.2 Suggested guidelines for catheter-directed thrombolysis and venous thrombectomy for acute deep vein thrombosis

Guideline number	Description	Grade of recommendation[a]	Grade of evidence
1	In patients with symptomatic deep vein thrombosis (DVT) and large thrombus burden, particularly in iliofemoral DVT, a treatment strategy that includes thrombus removal is recommended.	1	B[b]
2	In patients with symptomatic iliofemoral DVT with symptoms <14 days duration, catheter-directed thrombolysis is suggested to reduce acute symptoms and post-thrombotic morbidity, if appropriate expertise and resources are available.	1	B
3	Pharmacomechanical thrombolysis, with thrombus fragmentation and aspiration, is suggested over catheter-directed thrombolysis alone in the treatment of iliofemoral DVT to shorten treatment time, if appropriate expertise and resources are available.	2	B
4	In patients with acute DVT, systemic thrombolysis is not recommended.	2	B
5	For patients with symptomatic iliofemoral DVT who are not candidates for catheter-directed thrombolysis, surgical thrombectomy is recommended.	1	B

[a] 1 = recommended, 2 = suggested.
[b] B: moderate-quality evidence.

waking in the morning until bedtime. Randomized trials have demonstrated at least a 50% reduction in post-thrombotic morbidity with the use of 30–40 mmHg ankle gradient compression stockings.[5,20,21]

When the patient is fully recovered and back to baseline activity, repeat venous duplex and venous function studies are performed to evaluate ultrasonic patency and vein valve function, which serve as a baseline for future studies.

GUIDELINES

Guideline recommendations are suggested in **Table 58.2**. All available evidence at the writing of this chapter was considered; therefore, the strength of these recommendations may differ from previously published guidelines. The authors are certain that the results of the ATTRACT trial (Acute venous Thrombosis: Thrombus Removal with Adjunctive Catheter-directed Thrombolysis) will have a major impact on future guidelines.

REFERENCES

1. Qvarfordt P, Eklöf B, Ohlin P. Intramuscular pressure in the lower leg in deep vein thrombosis and phlegmasia cerulae dolens. *Ann Surg.* 1983;**197**:450–453.
2. Plate G, Einarsson E, Ohlin P, et al. Thrombectomy with temporary arteriovenous fistula: the treatment of choice in acute iliofemoral venous thrombosis. *J Vasc Surg.* 1984;**1**:867–876.
3. Plate G, Akesson H, Einarsson E, et al. Long-term results of venous thrombectomy combined with a temporary arterio-venous fistula. *Eur J Vasc Surg.* 1990;**4**:483–489.
4. Plate G, Eklöf B, Norgren L, et al. Venous thrombectomy for iliofemoral vein thrombosis: 10-year results of a prospective randomised study. *Eur J Vasc Endovasc Surg.* 1997;**14**:367–374.
5. Delis KT, Bountouroglou D, Mansfield AO. Venous claudication in iliofemoral thrombosis: long-term effects on venous hemodynamics, clinical status, and quality of life. *Ann Surg.* 2004;**239**:118–126.
6. Eklof B, Juhan C. Revival of thrombectomy in the management of acute iliofemoral venous thrombosis. *Contemp Surg.* 1992;**40**:21–30.
7. Piquet P. Traitement chirurgical des thromboses iliocaves: exigences et resultats. [Chapter in French]. In: Kieffer E, ed. *Chirurgie de la Veine Cave Inferieure et de Ses Branches*; 1985. Paris: Expansion Scientifique Française. pp. 210–216.
8. Einarsson E, Albrechtsson U, Eklöf B. Thrombectomy and temporary AV-fistula in iliofemoral vein thrombosis. Technical considerations and early results. *Int Angiol.* 1986;**5**:65–72.
9. Vollmar JF. Robert May memorial lecture: advances in reconstructive venous surgery. *Int Angiol.* 1986;**5**:117–129.
10. Juhan C, Alimi Y, Di Mauro P, et al. Surgical venous thrombectomy. *Cardiovasc Surg.* 1999;**7**:586–590.
11. Törngren S, Swedenborg J. Thrombectomy and temporary arteriovenous fistula for ilio-femoral venous thrombosis. *Int Angiol.* 1988;**7**:14–18.
12. Rasmussen A, Mogensen K, Nissen FH, et al. Acute iliofemoral venous thrombosis. 26 cases treated with thrombectomy, temporary arteriovenous fistula and anticoagulants. [Article in Danish]. *Ugeskr Laeger.* 1990;**152**:2928–2930.
13. Eklof B, Kistner RL. Is there a role for thrombectomy in iliofemoral venous thrombosis? *Semin Vasc Surg.* 1996;**9**:34–45.
14. Neglén P, al-Hassan HK, Endrys J, et al. Iliofemoral venous thrombectomy followed by percutaneous closure of the temporary arteriovenous fistula. *Surgery.* 1991;**110**:493–499.
15. Meissner AJ, Huszcza S. Surgical strategy for management of deep venous thrombosis of the lower extremities. *World J Surg.* 1996;**20**:1149–1155.
16. Pillny M, Sandmann W, Luther B, et al. Deep venous thrombosis during pregnancy and after delivery: indications for and results of thrombectomy. *J Vasc Surg.* 2003;**37**:528–532.
17. Hartung O, Benmiloud F, Barthelemy P, et al. Late results of surgical venous thrombectomy with iliocaval stenting. *J Vasc Surg.* 2008;**47**:381–387.
18. Hölper P, Kotelis D, Attigan N, et al. Long-term results after surgical thrombectomy and simultaneous stenting for symptomatic iliofemoral venous thrombosis. *Eur J Vasc Endovasc Surg.* 2010;**39**:349–355.
19. Baglin T, Luddington R, Brown K, et al. Incidence of recurrent venous thromboembolism in relation to clinical and thrombophilic risk factors: prospective cohort study. *Lancet.* 2003;**362**:523–526.
20. Brandjes DP, Büller HR, Heijboer H, et al. Randomised trial of effect of compression stockings in patients with symptomatic proximal-vein thrombosis. *Lancet.* 1997;**349**:759–762.
21. Prandoni P, Lensing AW, Prins MH, et al. Below-knee elastic compression stockings to prevent the post-thrombotic syndrome: a randomized, controlled trial. *Ann Intern Med.* 2004;**141**:249–256.

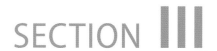

Endovascular and Open Venous Reconstructions

59

Endovascular/open central and peripheral venous reconstruction

SCOTT T. ROBINSON, TREVOR DOWNING, DAWN M. COLEMAN, DAVID M. WILLIAMS, AND THOMAS W. WAKEFIELD

CONTENTS

INTRODUCTION

Venous reconstruction techniques can be used to treat acute deep vein thrombosis (DVT) and chronic venous disorders (CVDs). Venous reconstruction may also be considered in other less common clinical scenarios, including venous disruption due to malignancy or trauma, and venous aneurysms. In contemporary vascular surgery practice, most of these conditions are treated with an endovascular approach. Open surgery is reserved for patients who have failed endovascular therapy and whose anatomy is favorable for surgical reconstruction.

The primary treatment for acute DVT remains systemic anticoagulation. However, treatment with anticoagulation alone relies on endogenous mechanisms of thrombolysis for clot resolution. This process can be slow in a setting of extensive iliofemoral DVT, which, over time, may result in post-thrombotic syndrome (PTS) and symptoms of CVDs. Recent advancement in catheter-based thrombolysis techniques has enabled effective and rapid removal of acute thrombus, which restores venous patency and preserves valvular competence. Thus, early intervention to decrease thrombus burden can potentially reduce the long-term morbidity of iliofemoral DVT.

CVDs encompass a spectrum of clinical manifestations that result from venous hypertension and valvular insufficiency. Symptoms associated with CVD include leg pain and heaviness, and often include skin changes that, in severe disease, may progress to ulceration. A standardized classification scheme, CEAP (clinical, etiologic, anatomic, pathophysiologic), was initially developed in 1995, and subsequently updated in 2004 to objectively categorize the variations in CVDs and potentially quantify the response to treatment.[1] The CEAP classification scheme is summarized in **Table 59.1**. Clinical severity scores range from C0 to C6, with C0 corresponding to no clinically identifiable venous disease and C6 corresponding to active venous ulceration. Etiology (E) is

Table 59.1 CEAP classification[a]

Clinical

C0: no visible or palpable signs of venous disease
C1: telangiectasies or reticular veins
C2: varicose veins
C3: edema
C4a: pigmentation or eczema
C4b: lipodermatosclerosis or atrophie blanche
C5: healed venous ulcer
C6: active venous ulcer
S: symptomatic (ache, pain, tightness, skin irritation, heaviness, muscle cramps)
A: asymptomatic

Etiologic

Ec: congenital
Ep: primary
Es: secondary
En: no venous cause identified

Anatomic

As: superficial veins
Ap: perforator veins
Ad: deep veins
An: no venous location identified

Pathophysiologic

Pr: reflux
Po: obstruction
Pr,o: reflux and obstruction
Pn: no venous pathophysiology identifiable

[a] Adapted from Eklöf B, Rutherford RB, Bergan JJ, et al. Revision of the CEAP classification for chronic venous disorders: consensus statement. *J Vasc Surg*. 2004;**40**:1248–1252. Copyright 2004, with permission from Elsevier.

classified as congenital, primary, secondary, or without cause. Congenital etiologies include diagnoses such as Klippel–Trénaunay syndrome, while a secondary etiology is most commonly PTS. The anatomic subgrouping (A) categorizes CVDs according to the pathway of the venous system that is affected (i.e., superficial, perforator, or deep veins). The final CEAP category groups CVDs according to a pathophysiologic cause (P), and includes reflux, obstruction, or both. An advanced CEAP classification scheme includes the addition of 18 named venous segments used to specify disease location.

The mainstay of therapy for CVDs is a good venous health program, which includes regular low-impact aerobic exercise, gradient compression with an elastic wrap or garment, and elevation of the affected extremity when not in use. Restoring patency to a chronic obstruction can potentially provide symptomatic relief in CVDs that have failed conservative management, potentially improving quality of life. Relief from venous obstruction is more commonly achieved through endovascular recanalization techniques, which include thrombolysis, recanalization, venoplasty, and venous stenting. Open surgical

reconstruction of venous occlusion is performed infrequently because of the increased perioperative morbidity in comparison to the ease and effectiveness of current endovascular therapies. Open surgical intervention should be limited to individuals with long-segment, chronic occlusion of the iliofemoral venous system who have failed endovascular management. Long-segment venous occlusion may be the result of external compression, as seen in May–Thurner syndrome, or from a mass effect caused by an adjacent tumor or aneurysm. Disruption of the iliofemoral venous system may also result from vascular trauma. The etiology of venous occlusion is relevant to operative decision-making, because the presence of malignancy may necessitate additional intervention or, in the case of metastatic disease, may preclude the patient from an operation entirely. Prior venous repair or ligation in a setting of vascular trauma may also render the occlusion less amenable to an endovascular strategy of repair, thus warranting surgical reconstruction. Numerous surgical venous reconstructions have been described, but with the advancement of endovascular technologies many are now of historical interest only. Two procedures that continue to have utility in the contemporary treatment of venous disease are: (1) saphenopopliteal bypass (SPB) for unilateral occlusion of the femoral vein; and (2) cross-femorofemoral venous bypass for unilateral external or common iliac vein (CIV) occlusion.

In recent years, the authors' practice has included the surgical management of peripheral venous aneurysms. Because of the rarity of this pathology, the natural course of venous aneurysms is not well defined. Although reported in multiple peripheral venous segments, aneurysms are most commonly located in the popliteal vein. Popliteal vein aneurysms (PVAs) are frequently asymptomatic, but can present as a painful, swollen mass behind the knee. The risk of venous aneurysm rupture is low; however, up to 50% of patients with PVAs present with pulmonary embolism (PE).[2] While no size criteria exist for PVAs, a venous segment is considered aneurysmal when it is 1.5 times the diameter of the native vessel. Because of the high morbidity associated with this pathology from the risk of PE, and the relatively low morbidity associated with repair, surgical treatment is typically recommended for any size of PVA. Several techniques for repair of venous aneurysms have been reported, but here we describe plication of a PVA.

ENDOVASCULAR TREATMENT

Indications for endovascular iliocaval recanalization are venous occlusion secondary to recurrent DVT, severe PTS, or significant limitations of daily activities. The foundation of endovascular venous recanalization centers on establishing wire access across the occlusion, balloon angioplasty, and stenting of the recanalized segments. In the authors' opinion, unassisted balloon angioplasty is not a durable treatment for chronic iliocaval thrombosis; therefore, stenting is usually required. The timing of recanalization is paramount to achieve a satisfactory result. If the patient has missed the customary 2–4-week window for thrombolysis of acute DVT, the authors often wait 3–4 months until the thrombus has contracted and partially organized because an organizing or early organized thrombus can be quite bulky, thereby limiting stent expansion.

Standard equipment for venous recanalization includes an angled tip catheter (e.g., vertebral tip) and straight, stiff hydrophilic guidewire (e.g., the GLIDEWIRE® Hydrophilic Coated Guidewire, Terumo Medical Corporation, Somerset, NJ, USA). Since these catheters and guidewires buckle on encountering resistance, the authors buttress them with ≥6-Fr sheaths. The sheath can then be methodically advanced over the catheter/wire combination to maintain the forward progress that has been made. For iliocaval reconstructions, the authors prefer to approach the obstruction from two sides; therefore, venous access routes most often include the right internal jugular vein (IJV) and both great saphenous veins (GSVs). In the authors' experience, GSV access affords ease of hemostasis relative to common femoral vein (CFV) access, especially in patients who require immediate full anticoagulation postprocedure. The GSV is superficial, easily compressible along the medial thigh, and accepts surprisingly large sheaths relative to its small vein size.

In the scenario where the obstruction is resistant to simple catheter and glidewire recanalization, sharp recanalization may be required with a transseptal needle, such as the BRK-1™ needle (St. Jude Medical, Inc., St. Paul, MN, USA). The operator can direct the needle toward a loop snare positioned on the other side of the obstruction. One can then ensnare the needle once it has passed the obstruction and exchange the inner 0.018-inch stylet for a 0.018-inch wire (preferably a 300-cm exchange length V-18™, Boston Scientific Corporation, Marlborough, MA, USA). This allows for through-and-through access. Alternatively, the operator can use a radiofrequency wire (Baylis Medical, Mississauga, ON, Canada) to pass the obstruction.

Recanalization should begin upstream and progress downstream (i.e., GSV to IJV) because this allows for intermittent contrast injections to guide the trajectory. Antegrade fluoroscopic venography usually fills extensive collaterals around the obstruction, but also often highlights the true lumen as a thin, straight channel (the so-called "string sign"). Retrograde injections do not similarly highlight the recanalization path. Progress is often slow and one must be willing to sacrifice 10–15 cm of forward progress if an apparent dead end is reached or extravasation is noted on contrast injection. In these scenarios, the catheter should be retracted by the operator and recannulation of the true channel attempted. The goal is that the wire either crosses the obstruction independently or sheaths become positioned in "dead space" adjacent to one another. Sharp recanalization/loop snare technique can then be used or side-by-side balloon angioplasty performed to unite the lumens.

Once the authors have crossed the obstruction, they confirm a safe track before large balloon dilation. One can accomplish this with contrast injections, CO_2 injections, or intravascular ultrasound (IVUS). The latter is particularly useful because it also provides anatomic relationships with nearby critical structures, for instance, the right renal or iliac arteries. After the operator deems the track safe, anticoagulation is initiated before sequential balloon dilation. The authors begin with the 8-mm balloon dilation of an iliocaval segment followed by contrast injection to exclude extravasation. If venography is unremarkable, they dilate the inferior vena cava (IVC) to 18 mm, the CIVs to 16 mm, and the external iliac veins (EIVs) and CFVs to 14 mm. The authors stent the IVC with an 18–20-mm self-expanding stent. Then, they estimate the CIV stent sizes, so that the square of the stent diameter is half the square of the stented IVC diameter (rounded up to the next size). If the estimated stent size is too small for the iliac veins, then the authors choose an appropriate stent size that allows for complete stent-wall apposition. In some cases, iliocaval thrombosis occurs with a filter-bearing IVC. If the authors cannot remove the filter, then they use a large self-expanding stent to sequester the filter outside of the functional IVC lumen.

Just as in the arterial system, long-term stent patency relies on adequate inflow and outflow. Venography of the femoral and deep femoral veins is performed to assess inflow before case completion. Typically, the authors avoid stenting below the saphenofemoral junction (SFJ) to preserve inflow from the GSV. However, occasionally, they stent into the femoral veins and angioplasty the stent interstices around the SFJ to augment flow. Rarely, an arteriovenous fistula (AVF) may also be required to provide the necessary inflow, or the combination of an open/endo phlebectomy and venoplasty.

OPEN SURGICAL TECHNIQUES

Saphenopopliteal bypass

Saphenopopliteal bypass (SPB) involves transplantation of the ipsilateral GSV to bypass femoral vein occlusions (**Figure 59.1**). The procedure was described in the 1970s by Husni[3] and by Frileux, Pillot-Bienayme and Gillot;[4] it can be used to treat unilateral occlusion of the femoral vein, especially if the profunda femoris vein (PFV) is an inadequate collateral channel or conduit. Preoperative venography and imaging with duplex ultrasound (US), including superficial vein mapping, is obtained. Usually, PFV flow compensates for femoral vein occlusion, but in the face of both femoral vein and PFV occlusion, SPB may be indicated. Appropriate candidates for the procedure must have preserved inflow and outflow, including a patent popliteal vein, GSV, SFJ, and patent proximal iliocaval venous outflow. In the event of ipsilateral iliac vein occlusion, SPB may be performed concomitantly with a cross-femorofemoral venous bypass to preserve outflow if the

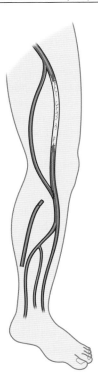

Figure 59.1 Saphenopopliteal bypass (illustration showing surgical incision, occluded vein segment, route of bypass). Note the distal GSV disconnected from the GSV used for the bypass).

iliac vein cannot be opened by an endovenous procedure. The decision to include a distal AVF to augment inflow is made intraoperatively by assessment of flow through the bypass.

At the authors' institution, patients undergo vein mapping in preoperative holding before proceeding to the operating room, at which time the GSV is identified and marked. The procedure is performed under general anesthesia (GA). The leg is prepped circumferentially including the ipsilateral groin. A medial longitudinal incision is made in the lower third of the thigh over the GSV. The GSV is mobilized and side branches are ligated with 3-0 silk ties. The popliteal fossa is then entered and the neurovascular bundle is identified. The popliteal vein is freed from the neurovascular bundle, and the patient is systemically anticoagulated with intravenous heparin until an activated clotting time (ACT) of 250 seconds is reached; this level of anticoagulation is maintained throughout the procedure. The desired anastomotic site on the popliteal vein is exposed, and the vein segment is isolated with silicone elastomer vessel loops. The GSV is transected with adequate length to perform the anastomosis. The GSV must be of sufficient length so that minimal tension is placed on the anastomosis when the knee is in full extension, but without such redundancy that the bypass graft kinks under knee flexion. A partially occluding vessel clamp is then applied to the popliteal vein. A longitudinal

venotomy is performed with a No. 11 blade and extended with Potts scissors. An end-to-side GSV-popliteal vein anastomosis is then completed with 6-0 polypropylene suture in an interrupted fashion to prevent purse stringing of the anastomosis. Before completing the anastomosis, the segment is back-bled and forward-bled to prevent embolization of air or debris. Care must be taken to preserve the orientation of the GSV so that it is not twisted or kinked.

Following completion of the anastomosis, inflow to the bypass may be assessed through a small side branch of the GSV. If an AVF is deemed necessary, an interposition graft or a direct anastomosis is performed between the popliteal artery and vein distal to the bypass anastomosis. Regarding the interposition graft, the area of the AVF is dissected so that the popliteal artery and vein can be adequately accessed. A 1–2-cm segment from a side branch or distal segment of the GSV is harvested. A side-biting clamp is applied to the popliteal artery distal to the saphenopopliteal anastomosis. An arteriotomy is created and then extended with an arterial punch. The arteriovenous anastomosis is then completed in an end-to-side manner with 6-0 polypropylene suture. A side-biting vascular clamp is then applied to the popliteal vein and a venotomy is created. An end-to-side anastomosis is performed with 6-0 polypropylene suture. Before completing the anastomosis, the AVF is back-bled and forward-bled to prevent embolism of debris. The AVF should be assessed for a thrill. Size and positioning of the interposition graft are crucial to achieve success with future embolization. The placement and angle of the interposition segment must allow for ease of endovascular access and the size must be appropriate for the deposition of coils; a 1–2-cm segment is generally ideal. Additionally, the authors obtain intraoperative duplex US to evaluate the anastomosis and bypass graft. A surgical BLAKE drain (Ethicon US, LLC, Somerville, NJ, USA) is placed before the incision is closed to prevent hematoma formation. After dressing the wound, a compression wrap is applied while the patient remains in the operating room.

Postoperatively, patients are started on low-molecular-weight heparin or oral anticoagulation. The authors encourage early ambulation, the use of elastic compression wraps or stockings and, while hospitalized, the use of intermittent pneumatic compression to encourage flow through the reconstruction. Patients with an AVF are seen in 8–12 weeks for venography and coil embolization of the AVF. This is done to avoid the complications associated with neointimal hyperplasia of the venous portion of the AVF, which could compromise long-term patency of the graft.

Palma procedure (cross-femorofemoral venous bypass)

Cross-femorofemoral venous bypass can be used to treat unilateral occlusions of the iliac veins if an endovenous

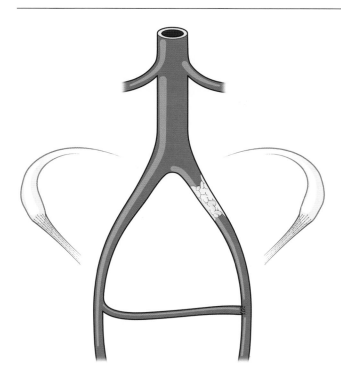

Figure 59.2 Palma procedure (illustration showing occluded left iliac vein segment and route of bypass).

approach fails or is not possible. The procedure was first described by Palma and Esperon in 1960;[5] it involves transposition of the contralateral GSV to the ipsilateral CFV (**Figure 59.2**). Preoperative venography and imaging with duplex US, including superficial vein mapping, is usually obtained. The decision to include a distal AVF to augment inflow is made intraoperatively by assessing the flow through the bypass.

Patients undergo vein mapping in preoperative holding before proceeding to the operating room, at which time the GSV is identified and marked. The procedure is performed under GA. The bilateral lower extremities are prepped circumferentially, as well as the abdomen. A vertical incision is made in the nonoccluded groin. The dissection is carried down to the SFJ. The GSV is then exposed through either a single medial thigh incision, or sequential small interrupted incisions down to the knee so that enough length is available to complete the bypass. Next, a vertical incision is then made in the affected groin, and the dissection is carried down to the deep vein system, exposing the CFV, PFV, and femoral vein. Great care should be taken in exposing the CFV because there are frequently large collaterals that have developed in response to the occlusion. It is best to preserve the existing collateral system as much as possible. A suprapubic subcutaneous tunnel is then created between the two groin incisions. Again, the presence of a unilateral iliac vein occlusion can result in extensive cross-pubic collateral veins. The suprapubic

tunnel should be made very carefully to prevent disruption of the collateral system. The contralateral GSV is then dissected free from surrounding tissues, and all side branches are ligated and divided with silk ties. The patient is then systemically heparinized to achieve an ACT of ≥250 seconds. The distal GSV is then ligated with a 0-0 silk tie, and the vein is mobilized toward the tunnel. Next, the contralateral GSV is then carefully passed through the tunnel to avoid any kinking or twisting. After the CFV is exposed and controlled, a longitudinal venotomy is created using a No. 11 blade and is extended to the appropriate length using Potts scissors. An end-to-side anastomosis is performed with the transposed GSV and CFV with 6-0 polypropylene suture in an interrupted fashion. Following completion of the anastomosis, flow in the bypass is assessed through a small side branch of the GSV. If there is concern for poor inflow, an AVF is created with a side branch or distal segment of the GSV interposition graft from the common femoral artery to the transposed GSV. The bilateral groin incisions are then closed in a layered fashion, with a surgical drain secured in each wound.

Postoperatively, patients are started on low-molecular-weight heparin or oral anticoagulation. Again, the authors encourage early ambulation, the use of elastic compression wraps or stockings and, while hospitalized, the use of intermittent pneumatic compression. Patients with an AVF are seen in 8–12 weeks postoperatively for venography and coil embolization of the AVF.

Popliteal vein aneurysm

Popliteal vein aneurysms (PVAs) are a rare entity that necessitate repair because of the associated high risk of PE. Several methods of repair have been described.[2] If there is redundant length of vein surrounding the aneurysm, resection with an end-to-end anastomosis of the proximal and distal segments of the vein can be performed. If additional length of vein is required for a tension-free anastomosis, resection with an interposition graft of the GSV or femoral vein can be performed. Alternatively, tangential aneurysmectomy and lateral venorrhaphy can be performed. Here, the authors describe a technique for PVA plication. In the presence of thrombus, the authors' technique is modified to include an open thrombectomy before plication. Preoperative diagnostic studies that are routinely obtained include duplex US and magnetic resonance venography (MRV) to evaluate congenital venous anomalies. A preoperative venogram is generally not indicated.

Patients undergo duplex US in preoperative holding before proceeding to the operating room, at which time the PVA is identified, marked, and assessed for thrombus. The patient is then transported to the operating room, where general anesthesia is induced and the patient is placed prone on the operating room table.

The leg is prepped from the foot to the thigh in a circumferential manner. A "lazy" S-shaped incision is made over the posterior knee overlying the popliteal space and preoperative site marking, with the superior extension of the incision medially, and the inferior extension of the incision laterally. The incision is carefully deepened with electrocautery through the subcutaneous tissue. During the dissection, the medial sural nerve should be identified and gently retracted and protected. Typically, the aneurysmal vein segment can be easily identified. The tibial nerve should be identified and gently dissected free from the artery and vein. Before beginning the repair, the authors use intraoperative duplex US to determine the native vessel diameter at the inflow and outflow of the aneurysm sac. This enables the authors to determine the specific luminal diameter required following plication. The popliteal vein is then encircled with silicone elastomer vessel loops at a nonaneurysmal segment both proximal to and distal from the dilation.

If preoperative duplex US does not identify thrombus within the aneurysm, a preoperative dose of 5000 IU/kg of subcutaneous heparin is given, but the authors do not typically administer systemic heparin. If there is no thrombus, the authors then perform an inward plication of the aneurysm with interrupted horizontal mattress sutures using polypropylene suture with felt pledgets. Care is taken to ensure that excess tissue becomes invaginated as the sutures are placed (**Figure 59.3a**). The authors use intraoperative US to guide the luminal size of the plicated vein to match the lumen of the vein proximal and distal to the aneurysm.

If thrombus is present on preoperative duplex US, then the patient is systemically anticoagulated until a target ACT of ≥250 seconds is obtained. Proximal and distal control is obtained. A longitudinal venotomy is created and extended to the appropriate length, and the thrombus is evacuated. The authors then plicate the aneurysm so that the aneurysmal tissue is everted, with an interrupted horizontal mattress technique using polypropylene suture with felt pledgets. Again, intraoperative US is used to guide the luminal size of the plicated vein to match the nonaneurysmal lumen. Excess aneurysmal tissue is then resected (**Figure 59.3b**).

Once plication is complete, the authors repeat the intraoperative duplex US to assess venous flow through the repair, ensure that the intraluminal diameter of the repair is like that of the native vessel, and evaluate any potential thrombus. The wound is then irrigated with antibiotic solution, and a layered closure is performed.

Postoperatively, the authors again encourage early ambulation and elastic compression. Before discharge, the authors obtain a duplex US DVT scan. If thrombus is present at this time, the authors will consider a 3-month course of anticoagulation. Otherwise, they do not routinely place patients on an extended course of anticoagulation if they have not opened the vein, since intimal integrity is preserved and there is no nidus for thrombus formation.

RESULTS AND MAJOR COMPLICATIONS

Endovascular venous reconstruction

Endovascular iliocaval recanalization is an effective method of improving venous outflow with low associated morbidity. Currently, there are no randomized trials comparing iliocaval stenting to best medical therapy; however, several studies have demonstrated the efficacy of the procedure in restoring venous patency. In a large case series of 982 patients, Neglén and collaborators demonstrated primary and secondary patency rates at 72 months of 67 and 93%, respectively.[6] Importantly, significant clinical improvement was noted through quality of life scores. The authors employ these techniques routinely at their institution; in their experience, endovascular iliocaval recanalization is an important element of clinical care for the treatment of CVD.[7]

Technical difficulties involving guidewire-resistant obstructions can be overcome with patient, anatomically precise sharp recanalization. Short segments of extravascular passage in the region of chronic thrombosis have not been a significant problem. Although the authors have not encountered major iliac vein or IVC tears, this complication can be addressed using a self-expanding stent graft. The type of stent graft would be dependent

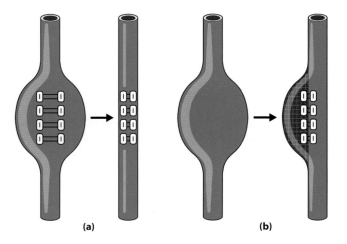

(a) (b)

Figure 59.3 **(a)** Popliteal vein aneurysm plication. Note the pledgeted sutures. **(b)** Popliteal vein aneurysm excision of redundant vein tissue (dark with cross-checks) with closure. Note the pledgeted sutures.

on vessel size. A GORE® VIABAHN® Endoprosthesis (W. L. Gore & Associates, Flagstaff, AZ, USA) can be used for vessels up to 11 mm; if larger sizes are needed, aortic endograft cuffs or limb extenders must be used. Unintended guidewire perforations and false passages readily thrombose so long as the operator has not initiated anticoagulation before crossing the obstruction and validating the pathway. Furthermore, the regions of extravascular passage are often compressed by the self-expanding stent in the final channel and the low-pressure venous system affords opportunity for thrombosis. Regions of concern during sharp recanalization are around the iliac artery bifurcation and near the renal artery. Techniques to avoid arterial injury include using IVUS to provide spatial anatomy or placing arterial catheters to perform intermittent arteriograms to avoid transgressing these structures. Double-J ureteral stents are occasionally placed to similarly avoid ureteral injury while recanalizing at the pelvic brim.

Saphenopopliteal bypass

In a recent series of 17 patients at the authors' institution by Coleman and collaborators, primary patency was preserved in 53% of patients following SPB, with primary assisted patency and secondary patency of 69 and 75%, respectively.[8] Most importantly, symptoms of venous claudication resolved in 83% of patients, indicating that a clinical benefit is seen with this procedure. In the same series, morbidity was relatively benign. Complications from the procedure included surgical site infection, hematoma (potentially requiring reoperation), and early graft occlusion.

Palma procedure

In a series of 25 patients at the Mayo Clinic, Garg and collaborators reported a 5-year primary patency of 70% and a secondary patency of 78% in patients who underwent a Palma procedure using a vein as the conduit.[9] These results suggest that the Palma procedure is an effective method of relieving unilateral iliac vein obstruction. Complications from the procedure include surgical site infection, hematoma, and early graft occlusion.

Popliteal vein aneurysm repair

At present, the data pertaining to PVA repair is sparse. However, a recent review of the literature consisting of 25 patients indicated that the procedure is effective at preventing recurrent PE, with no reports in the literature of PE after repair.[2] This same review noted a complication rate of 20%, which included transient peroneal

nerve palsy, hematoma, wound infection, and postoperative thrombosis of the repaired segment.

CASE EXAMPLES

Case example 1

A 22-year-old, previously healthy woman presented with back pain and bilateral leg fatigue of 6 days' duration that worsened until 2 days before admission when she developed severe leg swelling. This prompted a visit to the emergency department where US demonstrated bilateral DVT up to the iliac veins. An MRA/MRV demonstrated absence of contrast in the infrahepatic IVC, bilateral CIVs, and EIVs with a large network of paracaval collaterals suggestive of chronic IVC thrombosis or IVC atresia. She underwent immediate venography with thrombolysis, suction thrombectomy, and balloon angioplasty from above-knee popliteal veins into the EIVs. The patient returned 6 months later to undergo IVC and bilateral iliofemoral vein recanalization, balloon angioplasty, and stenting. In the interim, anticoagulation was maximized with D-dimer and high-sensitivity C-reactive protein values decreasing from 3.49 (high) to 0.17 (normal) and 20.0 (high) to 1.8 (normal), respectively. Inferior venocavogram at the time of recanalization showed occlusion of the suprarenal IVC and innumerable small collateral channels extending caudally, which was consistent with chronic occlusion (**Figure 59.4**). Bilateral iliofemoral venography showed diminutive right iliac veins and occlusion of the left iliac veins (**Figures 59.5 and 59.6**). The authors noted numerous retroperitoneal, lumbar, and deep pelvic collateral channels coursing toward the expected location of the infrarenal IVC confirming chronic iliocaval occlusion. The authors deployed three 18-mm WALLSTENT™ endoprostheses (Boston Scientific Corporation) in the IVC, two kissing 12-mm WALLSTENT™ endoprostheses in the CIVs (**Figure 59.7**), and multiple bilateral, overlapping 14-mm WALLSTENT™ endoprostheses in the EIVs and rostral CFVs (**Figure 59.8**). The authors discharged the patient on 1 mg/kg low-molecular-weight heparin twice daily, and 75 mg clopidogrel and 81 mg aspirin daily. Surveillance venogram 6 months later showed patent IVC and bilateral iliofemoral stents with minimal in-stent stenosis.

Case example 2

A 47-year-old man presented with right leg pain and swelling 1 year after a gunshot wound to his thigh. At the time of the injury, he underwent primary repair of the right superficial femoral artery (SFA) at the bifurcation with the profunda femoris artery, and ligation of the femoral vein. Preoperative venography revealed

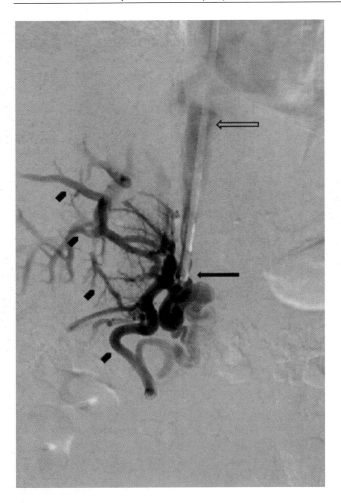

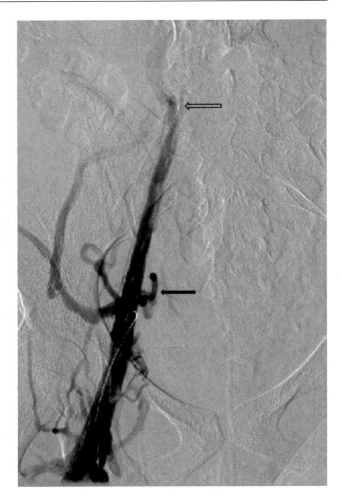

Figure 59.4 Inferior venocavogram through a 9-Fr, 30-cm sheath from right internal jugular vein access of a 22-year-old woman (case example 1). The tip of the sheath is embedded in the occluded suprarenal inferior vena cava (IVC) (solid arrow). Contrast fills a relatively normal-appearing intrahepatic IVC (open arrow), but no contrast is noted to reflux into the infra-renal IVC. A large network of retroperitoneal and accessory hepatic caudate vein collaterals (arrowheads) are highlighted around the distal sheath.

Figure 59.5 Antegrade right common femoral digital subtraction venogram through a 6-Fr, 30-cm great saphenous vein sheath (later upsized to 10 Fr) (case example 1). Contrast fills the diminutive right external iliac (EIV) and common iliac (CIV) veins. Deep pelvic collaterals arise from around the cau-dal EIV (incidentally marked with a Rosen wire (Cook Medical Inc., Bloomington, IN, USA); solid arrow) and the rostral CIV appears occluded near the top of the image (open arrow).

a 4-cm occlusion of the femoral vein with a large collateral network providing flow from the femoral vein to CFV. The GSV and proximal CFV were patent (**Figure 59.9**). The initial operative plan was to perform an interposition bypass of the occlusion with the contralateral GSV. However, the groin dissection was extremely difficult because of scar tissue from his prior trauma and surgery. Because of the proximal ligation of the femoral vein, an adequate proximal target could not be identified. However, during the dissection, the GSV was exposed and appeared to be in good condition. Therefore, the decision was made to perform a SPB. The incision was extended to above the knee, and the distal femoral vein/proximal popliteal vein were exposed in Hunter's canal. The GSV was mobilized and

an end-to-side anastomosis was performed between the GSV and popliteal vein. The patient recovered well and patency of his bypass was confirmed with duplex US at follow-up after 3 months.

Case example 3

A 28-year-old woman presented with a chronically occluded right CIV stent. The patient had multiple attempts at recanalization and thrombolysis, but ultimately reoccluded her stents despite remaining on therapeutic anti-coagulation. Genetic testing revealed a prothrombin G20210A mutation, which likely contributed to her hyper-coagulable state. She experienced heaviness and swelling

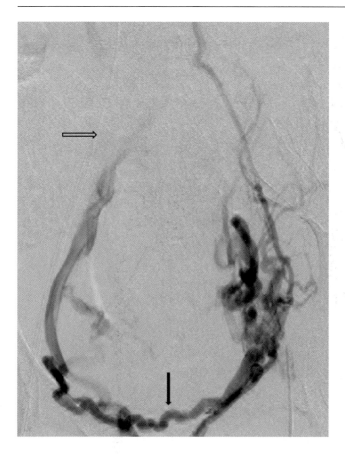

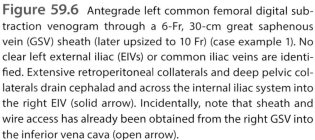

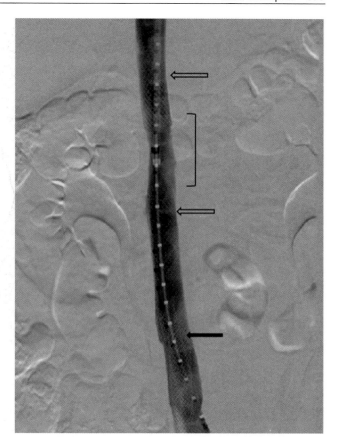

Figure 59.6 Antegrade left common femoral digital subtraction venogram through a 6-Fr, 30-cm great saphenous vein (GSV) sheath (later upsized to 10 Fr) (case example 1). No clear left external iliac (EIVs) or common iliac veins are identified. Extensive retroperitoneal collaterals and deep pelvic collaterals drain cephalad and across the internal iliac system into the right EIV (solid arrow). Incidentally, note that sheath and wire access has already been obtained from the right GSV into the inferior vena cava (open arrow).

Figure 59.7 Inferior venocavogram at procedure completion demonstrating widely patent 18-mm WALLSTENT™ endoprostheses (Boston Scientific Corporation, Marlborough, MA, USA) within the suprarenal and infrarenal inferior vena cava (IVC; open arrows) as well as kissing 12-mm WALLSTENT™ endoprostheses within the common iliac veins (solid arrow). A short, approximately 5-cm, segment of the IVC at the renal veins was intentionally not stented to preserve renal vein inflow (bracket).

of the right leg because of her thrombus burden, and elected to undergo a cross-femorofemoral venous bypass for symptom relief. During her initial procedure, the left GSV was used as a conduit and tunneled to the right groin where an end-to-side anastomosis was performed with the right CFV. An AVF was then created with an additional short segment of GSV as an interposition graft between the SFA and the bypass graft (**Figure 59.10**). Following this procedure, she recovered well, and returned 6 weeks later for interval embolization of the AVF. However, venography at that time revealed that the bypass graft was adequately dilated to the level of the AVF, but was occluded between the AVF and the anastomosis with the right CFV. The decision was made to revise the bypass, so the patient was taken to the operating room and the right groin was reexplored. The sclerosed segment of bypass graft was ligated, and the segment of AVF was then used for inflow as a new venous conduit by transposition to the prior

anastomosis site on the CFV (**Figure 59.11**). The revised bypass has remained open for 3 years. The repair remained patent and stable through the patient's first pregnancy and delivery of her first child. Her venous claudication has significantly improved and she is fully functional.

Case example 4

A 54-year-old woman with a history of varicose veins of the right leg presented to vascular surgery clinic for treatment for spider veins on the medial aspect of her right knee. Her symptoms included aching and throbbing behind her right knee with prolonged standing and mild swelling of her ankle; she had no prior history of venous thromboembolism. Preoperative US demonstrated a right PVA with maximum diameter of 2.65 cm without the presence of thrombus (**Figure 59.12a,b**). Additional imaging with

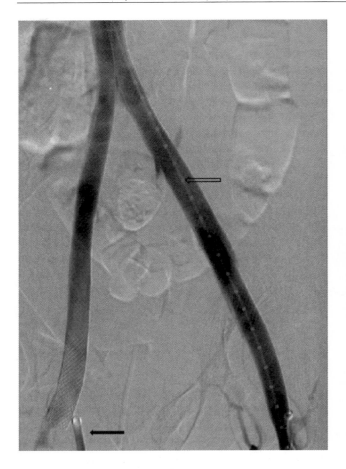

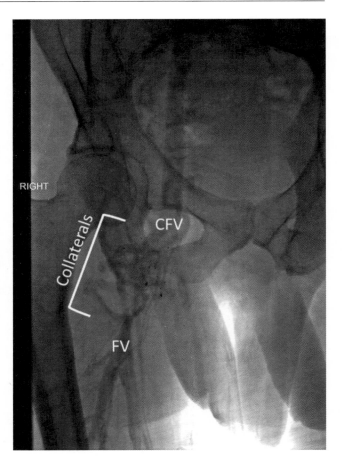

Figure 59.8 Bilateral iliofemoral digital subtraction venography from right 10-Fr great saphenous vein sheath (solid arrow) and left 5-Fr marking Omni™ Flush catheter (AngioDynamics, Latham, NY, USA) inserted from the right internal jugular vein (open arrow) (case example 1). Overlapping 14-mm WALLSTENT™ endoprostheses (Boston Scientific Corporation, Marlborough, MA, USA) extend from the bilateral common femoral veins to the common iliac veins (CIVs) and transition into kissing 12-mm CIV stents. Contrast opacifies widely patent, reconstructed iliofemoral veins with robust outflow into the inferior vena cava. No extravasation of contrast is noted along the stented segments.

Figure 59.9 Preoperative venogram of a 47-year-old man (case example 2) showing occlusion of the right femoral vein and large collateral network. CFV: common femoral vein; FV: femoral vein.

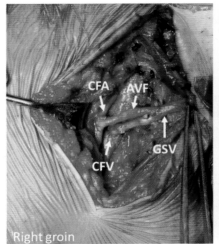

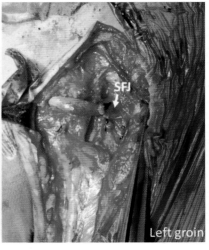

Figure 59.10 Completion of Palma procedure with arteriovenous fistula in a 28-year-old woman (case example 3). AVF: arteriovenous fistula; CFA: common femoral artery; CFV: common femoral vein; GSV: greater saphenous vein; SFJ: saphenofemoral junction.

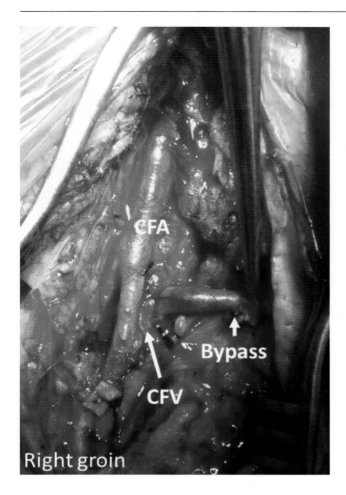

Figure 59.11 Revision of the Palma procedure with take-down of arteriovenous fistula (AVF) and use of the AVF vein segment as interposition between the common femoral vein and the patent portion of the bypass (case example 3). Note the interval removal of the AVF. CFA: common femoral artery; CFV: common femoral vein.

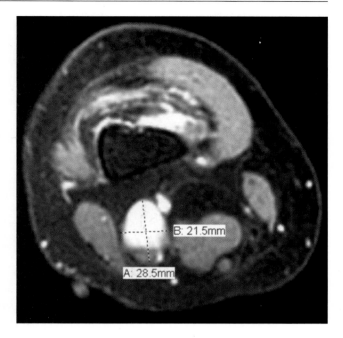

Figure 59.13 Magnetic resonance venography of popliteal vein aneurysm (case example 4). The image shown is an axial T1 fast spoiled gradient-echo FS postcontrast magnetic resonance imaging.

MRV confirmed the presence of the PVA (**Figure 59.13**) and the patient agreed to proceed with surgical repair. No thrombus was present within the aneurysm on preoperative US, thus the PVA was inwardly plicated to achieve a diameter equal to the native vessel (**Figure 59.14a,b**). On the second postoperative day, a diagnostic vascular US was obtained. This showed that the repaired popliteal vein segment was patent and the patient was discharged home. The repaired vein segment remained patent and the patient was without DVT or PE after 5 months of follow-up.

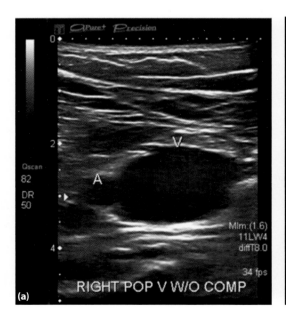

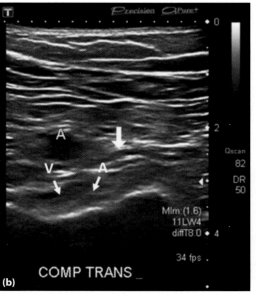

Figure 59.12 Preoperative duplex ultrasound of popliteal vein aneurysm (a) with and (b) without compression in a 54-year-old woman (case example 4). A: artery; V: vein.

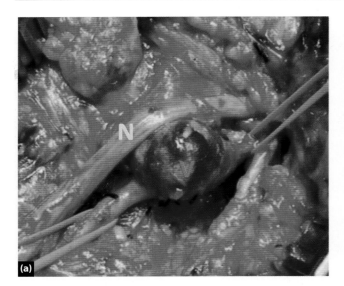 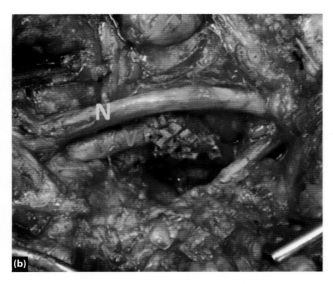

Figure 59.14 Intraoperative images of popliteal vein aneurysm **(a)** before and **(b)** after plication of the aneurysm (case example 4). N: tibial nerve; V: popliteal vein.

REFERENCES

1. Eklöf B, Rutherford RB, Bergan JJ, et al. Revision of the CEAP classification for chronic venous disorders: consensus statement. *J Vasc Surg.* 2004;**40**: 1248–1252.

2. Sessa C, Nicolini P, Perrin M, et al. Management of symptomatic and asymptomatic popliteal venous aneurysms: a retrospective analysis of 25 patients and review of the literature. *J Vasc Surg.* 2000;**32**: 902–912.

3. Husni EA. In situ saphenopopliteal bypass graft for incompetence of the femoral and popliteal veins. *Surg Gynecol Obstet.* 1970;**130**:279–284.

4. Frileux C, Pillot-Bienayme P, Gillot C. Bypass of segmental obliterations of ilio-femoral venous axis by transposition of saphenous vein. *J Cardiovasc Surg (Torino).* 1972;**13**:409–414.

5. Palma EC, Esperon R. Vein transplants and grafts in the surgical treatment of the postphlebitic syndrome. *J Cardiovasc Surg (Torino).* 1960;**1**:94–107.

6. Neglén P, Hollis KC, Olivier J, et al. Stenting of the venous outflow in chronic venous disease: long-term stent-related outcome, clinical, and hemodynamic result. *J Vasc Surg.* 2007;**46**:979–990.

7. Williams DM. Iliocaval reconstruction in chronic deep vein thrombosis. *Tech Vasc Interv Radiol.* 2014;**17**:109–113.

8. Coleman DM, Rectenwald JE, Vandy FC, et al. Contemporary results after sapheno-popliteal bypass for chronic femoral vein occlusion. *J Vasc Surg Venous Lymphat Disord.* 2013;**1**:45–51.

9. Garg N, Gloviczki P, Karimi KM, et al. Factors affecting outcome of open and hybrid reconstructions for nonmalignant obstruction of iliofemoral veins and inferior vena cava. *J Vasc Surg.* 2011;**53**:383–393.

Index

Note: page numbers in *italics* refer to figures and tables.